SPORTS INJURIES OF THE SHOULDER

Conservative Management

SPORTS INJURIES OF THE SHOULDER

Conservative Management

Edited by

Thomas A. Souza, D.C., C.C.S.P.

Chairman, Department of Diagnosis
Clinical Professor, Department of Clinics
Palmer College of Chiropractic-West
San Jose, California
Lecturer, Department of Continuing Education
Sports Diplomate Program
Western States Chiropractic College
Portland, Oregon
Diplomate, American Academy of Pain Management
Modesto, California

Churchill Livingstone

New York, Edinburgh, London, Madrid, Melbourne, Tokyo

Library of Congress Cataloging-in-Publication Data

Sports injuries of the shoulder : conservative management / edited by
  Thomas A. Souza.
        p. cm.
    Includes bibliographical references and index.
    ISBN 0-443-08844-6
    1. Shoulder—Wounds and injuries. 2. Sports—Accidents and
injuries. 3. Shoulder—Mechanical properties.   I. Souza, Thomas A.
    [DNLM: 1. Athletic Injuries—diagnosis.   2. Athletic Injuries—
therapy. 3. Shoulder—anatomy and histology. 4. Shoulder—injuries.
WE 810 S764 1993]
RD557.5.S76 1993
617.5 ' 72044—dc20
DNLM/DLC
for Library of Congress   93-24468
                                                                CIP

Distributed in the United Kingdom by Churchill Livingstone, Robert Stevenson House, 1–3 Baxter's Place, Leith Walk, Edinburgh EH1 3AF, and by associated companies, branches, and representatives throughout the world.

The procedures and protocols described in this book are intended as generic suggested approaches without prior knowledge of the specific training of a given practitioner or the multidimensional needs of an individual patient. It is recommended that hands-on training be pursued prior to the application of these techniques. In particular, application of adjustive techniques is not recommended without hands-on training. The author is not responsible for misapplication of a specific approach.

The Publishers have made every effort to trace the copyright holders for borrowed material. If they have inadvertently overlooked any, they will be pleased to make the necessary arrangements at the first opportunity.

Copy Editor: *Lorene K. Johnson*
Production Supervisor: *Patricia McFadden*
Cover Design: *Regina Dahir*

Printed in the United States of America

First published in 1994   7 6 5 4 3 2 1

To Jim and Doris Souza, my parents,
for their unconditional love and support.

And to my wife, Francie,
and sons, Aaron and Wesley
for their patience and love, without whom
this text would not be possible.

Contributors

Christopher A. Arrigo, M.S., P.T., A.T.C.
Physical Therapist, HEALTHSOUTH Sports Medicine and Rehabilitation Center, Birmingham, Alabama

Joan Davis, D.C., D.A.C.B.R.
Associate Instructor, Department of Clinics, Palmer College of Chiropractic-West, San Jose, California; Consultant, San Francisco Magnetic Resonance Center, San Francisco, California; Diplomate, American Chiropractic Board of Radiology, Elizabeth, New Jersey

Edward Feinberg, D.C., C.C.S.P.
Associate Professor, Department of Clinical Practice, Palmer College of Chiropractic-West, San Jose, California; Post Graduate Faculty, Sports Chiropractic Certification Program, Western States Chiropractic College, Portland, Oregon; Post Graduate Faculty, Cervical Spine Trauma, Palmer College of Chiropractic-West, San Jose, California; Certified Chiropractic Sports Practitioner, American Chiropractic Association Sports Council, Colorado Springs, Colorado; Private Practice, Saint Claire Chiropractic, Santa Clara, California

Joseph H. Introcaso, M.D., D.M.D.
Assistant Professor, Division of Neuroradiology, Department of Radiology, Northwestern University Medical School, Chicago, Illinois; Attending Staff, Division of Neuroradiology, Department of Radiology, Northwestern Memorial Hospital, Chicago, Illinois

Warren D. King, M.D.
Physician, Division of Sports Medicine, Palo Alto Medical Clinic, Palo Alto, California; Team Physician, San Jose Sharks, San Jose, California; Team Physician, San Francisco Giants, San Francisco, California; Assistant Director, Center for Sports Health, Sequoia Hospital, Palo Alto, California; Director, Pacific Coast Rugby Football Association, San Francisco, California

Christian H. Neumann, M.D., D.M.D.
Associate Clinical Professor, Department of Radiology, University of California, San Francisco, School of Medicine, San Francisco, California; Director of MRI Services, Department of Radiology, Desert Hospital, Palm Springs, California

Steve A. Petersen, M.D.
Assistant Professor, Department of Orthopaedic Surgery, Wayne State University School of Medicine, Detroit, Michigan; Chief of Adult Reconstruction and Shoulder Surgery,

Department of Orthopaedic Surgery, Hutzel Hospital, Detroit, Michigan; Chief of Adult Reconstruction and Shoulder Surgery, Department of Orthopaedic Surgery, Veterans Administration Medical Center, Allen Park, Michigan

Thomas A. Souza, D.C., C.C.S.P
Chairman, Department of Diagnosis, and Clinical Professor, Department of Clinics, Palmer College of Chiropractic-West, San Jose, California; Lecturer, Department of Continuing Education, Sports Diplomate Program, Western States Chiropractic College, Portland, Oregon; Diplomate, American Academy of Pain Management, Modesto, California

Howard R. Unger, Jr., M.D.
Staff, Abdominal Imaging Service, Department of Radiology, Wilford Hall USAF Medical Center, Lackland, Texas

Kevin E. Wilk, P.T.
National Director of Research and Clinical Education, HEALTHSOUTH Rehabilitation Corporation, Birmingham, Alabama; Associate Clinical Director, HEALTHSOUTH Sports Medicine and Rehabilitation Center, Birmingham, Alabama; Director of Rehabilitative Research, American Sports Medicine Institute, Birmingham, Alabama

Foreword

In my sixteen years since graduation from chiropractic school, I have needed to restudy and continually educate myself in the understanding and management of the problems of the shoulder. The development of Sports Medicine/Chiropractic has seen phenomenal growth and sophistication in scope and general interest. The practitioner who relies on conservative management of the shoulder has always been aware of the need for in-depth resources. With *Sports Injuries of the Shoulder: Conservative Management*, both the educator and practitioner now have a text that will assist them in every facet of conservative management.

This text has several unique chapters that devote extensive discussion to the following areas: shoulder biomechanics of several major sports, weight training for prevention and rehabilitation, examination as it relates to anatomy and biomechanics, relationship to the cervical spine and other related structures, and mobilization, adjustive, and PNF techniques. Several distinguished contributors also provide authoritative information on subjects such as MRI, sonography, and isokinetic exercise. Extensive illustrations provide a valuable aid to the exercises discussed in the text.

The authors have made every effort to provide the practitioner with a comprehensive text that not only includes hundreds of references but also gives an understanding for diagnosing and providing treatment protocols for the shoulder. This text will also provide any practitioner attempting to master the complexities of the shoulder with valuable and interesting information for the nineties and beyond. I look forward to using this text in my teaching and as a guide in the management of my patients.

Jan M. Corwin, D.C., C.C.S.P.
1988 U.S. Olympic Team Medical Staff

Preface

Whereas the 1980s was the decade of the knee, the 1990s is the decade of the shoulder. Although much of the basic understanding of the shoulder's structures and functions has remained unchanged since the original observations of Codman in the 1930s, a change in attitude toward surgical treatment and prevention of sports-related shoulder injuries has emerged. Some of the major changes in thinking have occurred with regard to the role of surgery. Surgery was often used as a means of "exploring the possibilities" with little more than guess-work with regard to elimination of suspected pathology.

With the increased athletic demand for post-surgical function, a new appreciation for the biomechanics of the shoulder complex has developed, particularly with regard to the general concept of stability and the requisite, balanced muscular demands to maintain this stability. Through electromyographic studies, selective cutting experiments, and careful radiographic evaluation of joint mechanics, new concepts of function have evolved.

Other stabilizing factors have also been recognized including negative pressure in the joint. The stabilizing role of the scapula has become evident providing a "moving platform" on which the humerus can function. The looseness of the shoulder has also proved to be a significant and common thread with many shoulder injuries. A nontraumatic form of "functional" instability may lead to impingement and its concomitant entities such as tendinitis and bursitis.

With a new specialty focus for chiropractors and other healthcare professionals on sports-related injuries, it becomes necessary to explore in more detail the function of the shoulder when challenged to extremes. This text, *Sports Injuries of the Shoulder: Conservative Management* is an attempt at synthesizing current information into a practical approach in the evaluation, conservative treatment, and prevention of sports-related injuries. The topics presented are not only written for the sports-related practitioner but for all those whose patients are amenable to conservative care. Where appropriate, surgical management is recommended.

This text represents a growing trend toward cooperation among all healthcare practitioners to better serve their patients. It is hoped that the knowledge gained will also help facilitate communication among all who treat the athletic patient.

Thomas A. Souza, D.C., C.C.S.P.

Acknowledgments

In an attempt to express my gratitude to some of the many people who were instrumental in the development and completion of this text, I would like to thank the following:

John Boykin for his mentorship; Gigi Chu and Thelma Adams for their many hours of devoted help; models Thomas Milus, D.C., Pamela Rients, D.C., Mehdi Moossavi, D.C., Mark Hayden, Gary Lang, A.T.C., and David Rivera; Robert Cook, D.C. and Maggie Craw, D.C. for photography; Frank Mainzer, M.D. and Victor Prieto, M.D. for radiographs; Supreme Courts of Sunnyvale, California and Richard Gardner, D.C., for the use of their weight training facilities; and all those who have assisted in time and support for this endeavor. Thank you.

Contents

1

Anatomy

THOMAS A. SOUZA

In simple terms the shoulder is often thought of as a ball and socket joint, the glenohumeral articulation. Functionally, however, the shoulder is a complex composed of three anatomic and one functional joint. The anatomic joints are (1) the glenohumeral, (2) the acromioclavicular, and (3) the sternoclavicular. The functional scapulothoracic joint describes the movement of the scapula on the thorax without synovial articulation. Without this functional joint, shoulder movement would be limited to 90 degrees or less of abduction.[1] Pushing and throwing motions would be extremely limited without the component of scapular retraction, protraction, and elevation. Additional functional considerations are the subacromial space, thoracic outlet, and the first sternocostal and costovertebral joints (Fig. 1-1). Each of these areas may cause mechanical or neurologic ramifications if dysfunctionally involved.

Nonpathologic function of the glenohumeral joint is dependent on proper functioning of the other articulations. In addition, it is essential to understand that many of the current models of function have been developed with either the shoulder acting alone or in combination with upper extremity movement. Realistically, descriptions of function assuming only an upright position may be inadequate. A prone or supine body position, or a forward flexed, rotated, or laterally bent trunk, may alter forces and resultant muscle demands in ways not described in the simple biomechanical constructs currently proposed.

OSSEOUS STRUCTURES

Viewed from above, the scapula grasps the upper limb by the humeral head (Fig. 1-2). Fixed and suspended by the axial skeleton via clavicular articulations and muscular attachments, the scapula performs its important function of providing a stable base on which the humerus may perform. The direct articulation of the humerus with the posterior mobile scapula, therefore, allows for a large range of movement that is dependent on proper positioning between them.

Clavicle

The clavicle, derived from the Greek word meaning key or bolt, acts as a stabilizing strut in the shoulder complex. The clavicle is not found in animals that use the forelimbs for support. In animals that, like humans, need to climb, grasp, hold, and elevate, it appears to serve a function of keeping the arm free of the body wall while allowing transmission of the supporting force of the trapezius to the scapula through the coracoclavicular ligaments.

The medial third of the clavicle is convex whereas the distal two-thirds is concave. This configuration has been described as an **S** or italic letter *F* shape, which conforms to the general contour of the chest wall and functionally causes a coupled rotation element with elevation of the arm. Opposite movement occurs between the acromial and sternal ends with shoulder elevation: elevation of the distal end causes depression of the proximal end.

The clavicle is the first long bone of the body to ossify, occurring during the fifth intrauterine week. It is, however, the last long bone to develop and close an epiphysis. About 80 percent of growth in the clavicle occurs medially.[2] Medial end epiphysis fusion may occur as late as age 25 years in men[3]. One study indicated that full fusion may occur as late as 31 years of age.[4] It is possible that assumed sternoclavicular dislocations may in fact represent fractures through the physeal plate.[5]

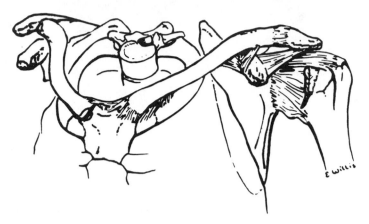

Fig. 1-1. Bones and joints of the shoulder complex. (From Dempster,[84] with permission.)

Articulation of the medial end of the clavicle is with the manubrium and first rib. This is a rather incongruent articulation, with only 50 percent of the medial end truly articulating.[6] The remaining 50 percent lies superior to the sternocostal articulation, allowing for a great degree of mobility but sacrificing stability, which must be provided by strong ligamentous structures.

The distal articulation with the acromion, like the proximal articulation, is synovial. It serves mainly as a mechanical connection with the scapula (i.e., movement of the scapula is partially transferred to the clavicle). Ligaments connecting the distal third of the clavicle with the coracoid process of the scapula provide stabilization of the acromioclavicular joint. In addition,

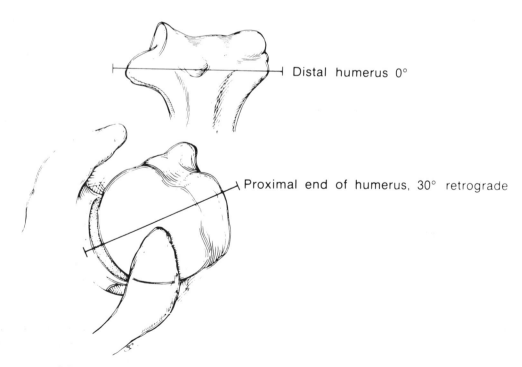

Distal humerus 0°

Proximal end of humerus, 30° retrograde

Fig. 1-2. Scapulohumeral orientation demonstrating 30 degree retroversion. (From Perry,[52] with permission.)

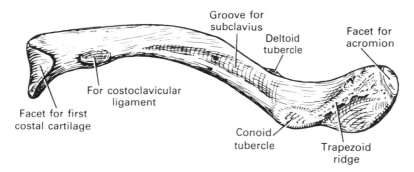

Fig. 1-3. The undersurface of the left clavicle. (From McKinn[85] with permission.)

the coracoclavicular ligaments impose a coupling that transforms the somewhat independent clavicle and acromion units into a single moving unit within certain ranges of shoulder elevation.

The clavicle, by acting as a functional strut, serves as a site for muscular attachment connecting the head, sternum, rib cage, scapula, and humerus. Insertions include the upper trapezius, which attaches at the posterior superior distal end, and the subclavius, which attaches to the inferior surface of the middle clavicle (Fig. 1-3). Origins include the deltoid on the lateral third, the pectoralis major from the medial two-thirds, the sternocleidomastoid from the middle third, and some fibers from the sternohyoid.

Scapula

The scapula has a triangular body with three superior extensions: the glenoid, the acromion, and the coracoid. The glenoid serves as a structural attachment to the upper limb, the acromion to the trunk, and the coracoid for ligamentous and muscular anchoring. A line of demarcation on the superior/posterior surface (the scapular spine) separates the scapula into two separate compartments muscularly.

The scapula is angled somewhere between 30 and 45 degrees anterior to the coronal plane in relationship to the spine.[7] The distance between the scapula and clavicle is functionally variable (Fig. 1-4). At rest it is approximately 60 degrees; retraction increases this to 70 degrees while protraction decreases this distance to 50 degrees.[1]

The anterior surface of the scapula serves mainly as an attachment for the serratus anterior and subscapularis (Fig. 1-5). It does not truly articulate with the thorax; however, it does act as a functional joint. As a joint it is still susceptible to processes such as osteoarthritic spur formation or irritation from the underlying ribs. This scapulothoracic joint is protected by bursae that preexist or develop in response to stress. They may be the source of irritation and pain.

The scapula functions to maintain a moving support platform for the humeral head allowing greater overall range of motion. This positioning also allows for proper functional length of the muscles that act to stabilize the shoulder. An additional role is suggested by Rowe and Sakellarides.[8] They feel that the scapula acts as a a shock absorber when there are direct blows to the arm, in particular to the extended arm.

The glenoid is a pear-shaped concave expansion of the superior apex of the scapula. The narrow end is superior with the broader section inferior. The glenoid has one-half of the contour and one-third the surface area of the humeral head with which it articulates.[9] This arrangement allows for mobility with little stability.

The glenoid serves as the point of attachment for the glenoid labrum, the capsule, the triceps, and the long head of the biceps muscle. In pathologic states these structures may be torn from their attachments with avulsion or serve as sites for ectopic bone formation.

New concepts regarding the direction of "facing" for the glenoid are now surfacing. Basmajian and Bazant[10] believed that the angulation of the glenoid slightly superior aided in the static stability of the glenohumeral joint. Recent studies, however, indicate a slightly downward angulation (as much as 5 degrees),[11] which

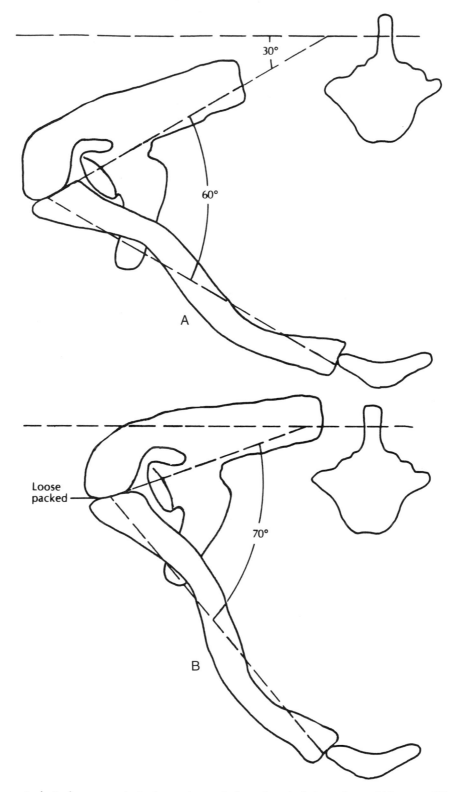

Fig. 1-4. Acromioclavicular, sternoclavicular, and scapulothoracic articulations shown **(A)** at rest, **(B)** in retraction, and (*Figure continues.*)

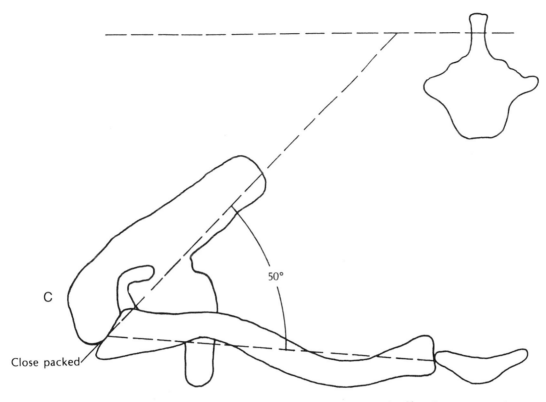

Fig. 1-4. (*Continued*). **(C)** in protraction. (From Hertling and Kessler,[86] with permission.)

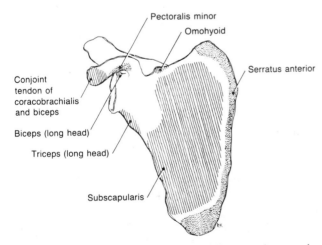

Fig. 1-5. Anterior view of the scapula showing the muscle origins of the anterior surface (*striped pattern*) and the muscle insertions (*dotted pattern*). Ligaments and their origins and insertions are not illustrated. (From Jobe[87] with permission.)

would imply a nonosseous support system. However, the majority of authors still feel that there is enough superior angulation to act as a major element in support of the dependent arm.

The version or angulation of the glenoid in relation to the coronal plane demonstrates a slight degree of retroversion. This has been documented to be between 2 and 7 degrees by computed tomography (CT).[12,13] In patients with posterior instability this value is in the range of −9 to −10 degrees as demonstrated by CT.[14] Similar relationships have been suggested by Das et al.[15] with anterior instability in relation to anteversion of the glenoid but these have not been documented at present.

The acromion is actually the lateral extension of the scapular spine. The angle of inclination of the acromion may be significant in determining predisposition to certain rotator cuff pathology.[16,17] Classified as types 1 to 3, the type 1 slope is essentially nonexistent (hori-

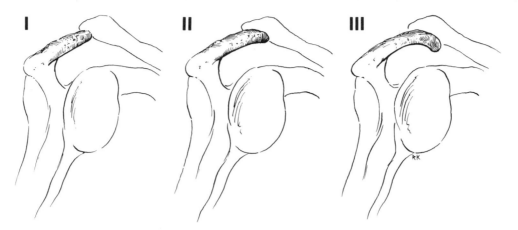

Fig. 1-6. The three types of acromion morphology defined by Bigliani and Morrison. Type I, with its flat surface, provided the least compromise of the supraspinatus outlet, whereas type III's sudden discontinuity or hook was associated with the highest rate of rotator cuff pathology in a series of cadaver dissections. (From Jobe,[87] with permission.)

zontal). Types 2 and 3 becomes progressively more sloped. A type 3 slope is associated with a "hooked" acromion, which has been linked to impingement (Fig. 1-6).

The coracoid is an anchoring point for the scapula providing insertions for the coracohumeral and cora-

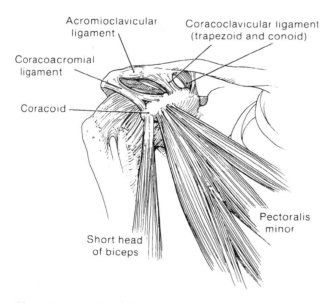

Fig. 1-7. Anatomy of the coracoid and associated muscular and ligamentous attachments. (From Tullos and Bennett[89] with permission.)

coacromial ligaments, the insertion of the pectoralis minor, and the origin of the coracobrachialis (Fig. 1-7). This arrangement establishes ligamentous and muscular connections between the rib cage and scapula, and the scapula and humerus. In addition to its static insertional function, some authors[18] feel that at 90 degrees of abduction and beyond, the coracoid may provide some protection to anterior dislocation of the shoulder.

There is a secondary ossification center of the coracoid that may be mistaken as an avulsion fracture in individuals in their midteens. It has a shell-like configuration radiographically.[19]

Humerus

The proximal humerus is composed of a neck and a bulbous humeral head (Fig. 1-8). The neck of the humerus is sometimes described as having an anatomic and surgical neck. The distinction is used because of the tendency for fractures to occur more frequently at the surgical neck. Humeral head landmarks include the greater and lesser tubercles, which serve as sites of attachment for muscles that contribute fine control of the shoulder. In between these tubercles lies the bicipital groove. Anomalies of the groove may contribute to certain shoulder disorders. Hitchcock[20] noted that the medial wall that is formed by the lesser tubercle is variable in height and may be associated

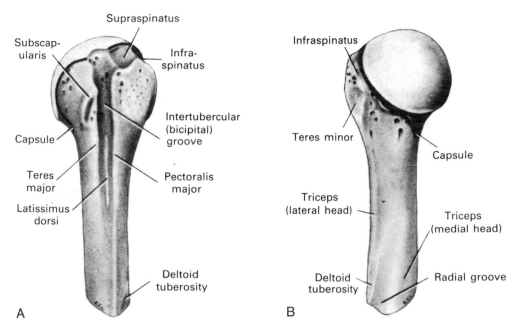

Fig. 1-8. (A) Anterior and **(B)** posterior view of proximal humerus. (From McKinn[85] with permission.)

with a supratubercular ridge (Fig. 1-9). Seventy percent of individuals have a height between 60 and 90 degrees in relationship to the floor of the groove. DePalma[6] believes that in the remainder of the population instability and/or irritation of the bicipital tendon may occur if a coexistent supratubercular ridge is found. This

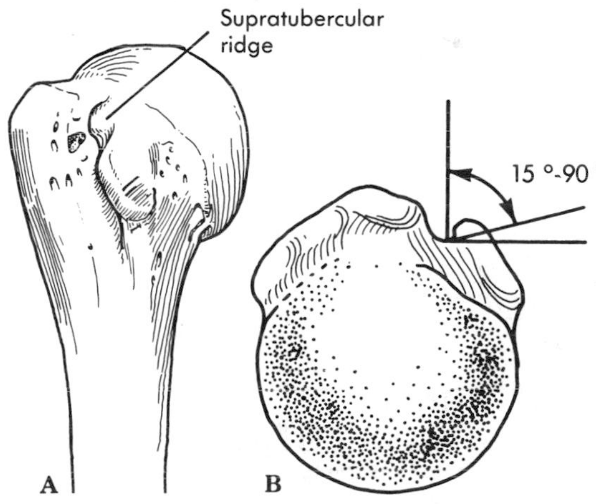

Fig. 1-9. (A) Bicipital groove with supratubercular ridge. **(B)** Angle of inclination, of medial wall. (From Hurley,[88] with permission.)

ridge is an osseous extension of the superior portion of the lesser tubercle.

Stability of the biceps tendon in the intertubercular groove would logically be ascribed to the transverse ligament. This ligament runs perpendicular over the biceps tendon. However, it appears that the coracohumeral ligament is the primary restraint to biceps tendon dislocation.[21] Dislocation of the long head of the biceps has been implicated as a cause of tendinitis; however, dislocation is a rare occurrence.[22] Impingement is more likely the cause of tendinitis, possibly due to the shape of the intertubercular groove or status of the transverse ligament.

The size of the humeral head may be an important factor in the stability of the shoulder. Saha[23] described three sizes based on the relationship between the humeral head and the glenoid. They are classified by the humeral head either being equal to, greater than, or lesser than the glenoid. Humeral heads greater than the glenoid were found to be more unstable.[24]

The humeral head is slightly retroverted when compared to the humeral epicondyles (Fig. 1-2), measuring between 30 and 40 degrees depending on the author reviewed.[1] Abnormalities in humeral head version have not been found to relate to instability patterns as have glenoid version abnormalities. The angle relationship between the shaft and head of the humerus is between 130 and 150 degrees.[1]

The proximal humeral epiphysis fuses in the late teens for females, whereas males reach fusion approximately 1 year later. Approximately 80 percent of the growth of the humerus is attributed to the proximal epiphysis.[6] The proximal epiphysis may be the site of a pathology referred to as "Little League" shoulder wherein disruption of the epiphysis is due to repetitive torque trauma in the young pitcher.

STERNOCLAVICULAR JOINT

The sternoclavicular joint (Fig. 1-10) is supplemented by a fibrocartilaginous disc that serves to increase the congruency between the clavicle and its articulation with the manubrium and first rib. Additionally it divides the joint in two with the superior portion of the disc attaching to the clavicle and the inferior portion to the first rib. As with many synovial articulations there is support from a capsule, ligaments, and musculature. The primary restraint is from the capsule, sternoclavicular, interclavicular, and costoclavicular ligaments.

The costoclavicular ligaments are divided into anterior and posterior bundles that have an angulation similar to the intercostal musculature crossing in opposite directions. They limit passive elevation of the clavicle and limit to some degree protraction and retraction.[25] At the lateral crossing of these bundles on the clavicle there is a bursa.

The interclavicular ligament joins the two sternoclavicular joints with attachment also to the sternum. It is a variable structure either absent or not palpable in 22 percent of individuals.[19] It is not of primary concern with injury.

The anterior and posterior sternoclavicular ligaments provide the majority of support for the sternoclavicular joints. These are also referred to as the capsular ligaments. The stronger of the two, the posterior element, prevents depression of the lateral clavicle.[19] Additional muscular support is provided minimally by the sternohyoid, sternothyroid, and sternocleidomastoid muscles.

The tendency of the sternoclavicular joint is to dislocate in a superior, anterior, and medial direction. This is a rare occurrence. Posterior dislocation is a rare but life-threatening event due to the proximity of the great vessels, lungs, and trachea.[3] Although instability is usually a consequence of trauma, as with the glenohumeral joint, some degree of inherent individual "looseness" may be present.[26]

Scapular movement is dependent on movement at both the sternoclavicular and acromioclavicular joints. Initially, during the first 30 to 90 degrees of shoulder elevation, 30 to 50 degrees of elevation occurs at the sternoclavicular joint between the clavicle and disc. Clavicular rotation slightly before and above this range occurs between the disc and sternum allowing for full elevation of the arm. Total rotation about the long axis is between 44 and 50 degrees. Fusion limits abduction of the arm to 90 degrees.[3]

The nerve to the subclavius supplies the sternocla-

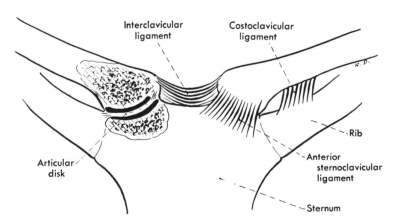

Fig. 1-10. Anatomy of the sternoclavicular joint. (From Hollinshead and Jenkins,[57] with permission.)

vicular joints with some additional contribution from the supraclavicular nerve.

A normal sternoclavicular joint will not show changes of degeneration until around the seventh decade.[27]

ACROMIOCLAVICULAR JOINT

The acromioclavicular joint (Fig. 1-11) also contains a fibrocartilaginous disc to help remediate the problem of inherent incongruency between the acromion and clavicle. The joint is surrounded by a capsule and supported by an array of ligaments. The acromioclavicular ligament connects the two bones by wrapping around in a circular manner reinforcing the capsule. The main stabilizing function seems to be prevention of posterior rotation and translation.[28]

The coracoclavicular ligaments, although not directly inserted into the joint, peripherally provide sta-

bility to vertical translation. There are two ligaments in this complex: the medioposterior conoid and the lateroanterior trapezoid. In addition to stability, tension on the coracoclavicular ligaments during arm elevation causes indirectly a rotary component to the scapula via the acromioclavicular joint.

Although the acromioclavicular and coracoclavicular ligaments will resist abnormal motion, their primary function is to guide motion between the clavicle and scapula. The conoid ligament is crucial to the rotation of the clavicle with shoulder elevation.[28]

The acromioclavicular joint serves as a stabilizing point for the shoulder in addition to allowing translation of forces from the clavicle to the scapula and vice versa. The need for this articulation becomes more apparent with heavy overhead lifting maneuvers.[1]

The acromioclavicular joint has been determined by DePalma[6] to have varying morphologic presentations. These are usually divided into three types (Fig. 1-12). Type I is essentially a vertical articulation with progres-

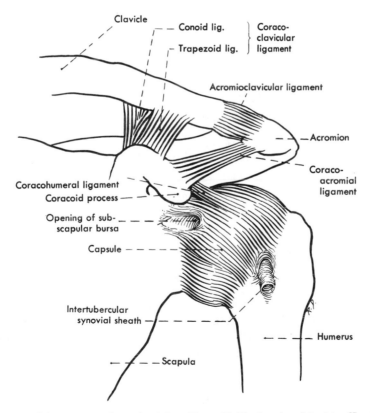

Fig. 1-11. Anatomy of the acromioclavicular joint. (From Hollinshead and Jenkins,[57] with permission.)

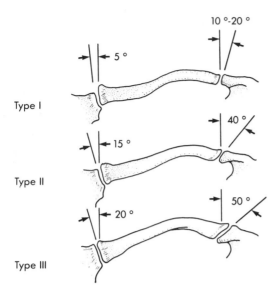

Fig. 1-12. Variations in the sternoclavicular and acromioclavicular articulations. (From Hurley,[88] with permission.)

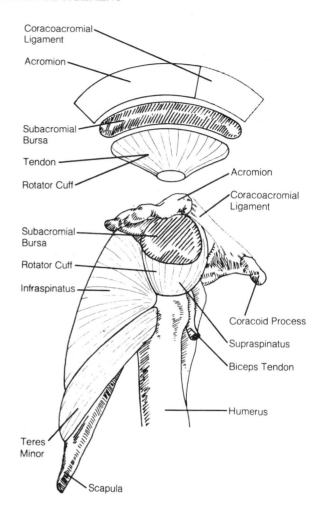

Fig. 1-13. The coracoacromial arch. (From Brunet et al.,[90] with permission.)

sion to a more oblique presentation in type III. The clinical significance of this variation is the observation by DePalma that degenerative acromioclavicular joints were more often type I. He attributes this finding to an inherent increase in shear forces coupled with the observation that type I joints were generally smaller, thereby increasing the local contact force. In general, degeneration of the disc and articular cartilage occurs at a much earlier age than for the sternoclavicular joint. DePalma noted changes in individuals in their twenties with significant degeneration visible in individuals in their forties.[27]

CORACOACROMIAL ARCH

The coracoacromial arch (Fig. 1-13) is formed by the coracoacromial ligament. Connections are from the coracoid process to an insertion that fans out over and under the acromion. Although the coracoacromial ligament might anatomically be considered part of the acromioclavicular joint, it seems to contribute little if any support to the joint. It acts as a superior roof of protection for the humerus and may prevent excessive superior migration but may inadvertently act as a

source of irritation. The coracoacromial ligament crowns what is sometimes considered an accessory joint, creating a functional space that is occupied by the tendons of the rotator cuff, biceps, and the subdeltoid bursa. The spaciousness of the subacromial space varies markedly with an average of 9 to 10 mm. Values in males vary from 6.6 to 13.8 mm, and in females from 7.1 to 11.9 mm.[29] Positions or pathologies that limit this available space may impose irritation of the occupying structures. The most common example is elevation of the arm without concomitant external rotation.

GLENOHUMERAL JOINT

Capsule

The glenohumeral capsule is strong yet loose guaranteeing maximum strength with optimum mobility. The strength is inherent because of the orientation of fibers coupled with thickenings. These thickenings are referred to as separate glenohumeral ligaments anteriorly, the posterior capsule, and the distinct coracohumeral ligaments. This static stability is supplemented by the extrinsic tightening effect of the insertions of the rotator cuff musculature into the capsule.

The capsule is twisted in orientation so that abduction of the arm increases tension on the anterior capsule, which in turn imposes an external rotation to the humerus. This aids in clearing the humeral head from the coracoacromial arch. Other end-range tightening effects cause the humeral head to translate in the direction opposite tension. For example, when the arm is raised to 90 degrees abduction and externally rotated, the tension in the anterior capsule causes a posterior translation of a few millimeters.[30]

There is considerable variability in the presence and substantiality of the shoulder ligaments. Their ability to restrain or protect movement patterns is dependent on their abundance in size and thickness coupled with the availability of other ligamentous and muscular support. Recent studies are challenging views held in the past regarding function based on purely anatomic observations. Positional demands require an interplay between sections of an individual ligament and among other ligaments. A summary of the findings of Terry et al.[31] is presented in Table 1-1.

Coracohumeral Ligament

The coracohumeral ligament (Fig. 1-14) traverses horizontally from the lateral aspect of the coracoid to the greater tuberosity just lateral to the bicipital groove. In so doing it covers the superior glenohumeral ligament anterosuperiorly. The coracohumeral ligament blends with the capsule prior to its insertion. It is believed to be phylogenically the past insertion for the pectoralis minor. In fact, in approximately 15 percent of the population the tendon crosses to the humeral head in addition to the coracoid process.[32] The coracohumeral ligament is located in the interval between the subscapularis and supraspinatus and may represent more of a "folding" of the capsule.

The function of the coracohumeral ligament is subject to debate. Basmajian and Bazant[10] believed that it was a major protector of inferior stability in conjunction with the superior glenohumeral ligament. Several investigators have recently concluded, however, that the coracohumeral ligament is simply a thin capsular fold in most individuals and represents no significant stabilization to inferior translation.[33,34] It was also observed that when more substantial in presentation it did provide some inferior stability function.

Although its function as a humeral head stabilizer is debatable, most authors agree that the coracohumeral ligament serves as a major restraint to subluxation and dislocation of the long head of the biceps tendon. In concert with edges of the supraspinatus and subscapularis muscle, it acts to prevent mainly medial translation of the biceps tendon.[35-37]

Glenohumeral Ligaments

Glenohumeral ligaments (Fig. 1-15) are thickenings of the anterior capsule and are divided into superior, middle, and inferior bands. Positional changes call into play different fibers. In the resting position tension is placed mainly on the superior and middle glenohumeral ligaments. As abduction progresses there is a gradual switch in tension to the inferior glenohumeral ligament. Most authors feel that this is the major restraint to anterior dislocation.[31,34]

It has been observed by dissection that there is variability in the size of individual ligaments. The authors[31,34] suggested that this may be due to a hypertrophy caused by chronic selective stresses or simply congenital variation. If due to a reactive hypertrophy, there are clinical applications in regards to potential protection capabilities.

Superior Glenohumeral Ligament

Beneath the coracohumeral ligament lies the superior glenohumeral ligament. Attachments are on the anterior labrum forward of the biceps tendon and on the superior aspect of the lesser tuberosity close to the bicipital groove. There are three common variations of glenoid origin ranging from close approximation to

Table 1-1. Passive Shoulder Restraints[a]

Ligament	Movement Restricted	Coupled Movement
Coracohumeral	Flexion and extension	Internal rotation—posterior capsule External rotation—anterior glenohumeral
Anterior glenohumeral	Extension, abduction, and external rotation (or a combination)	External/internal rotation—superior Flexion/external rotation—middle Abduction/extension/external rotation—inferior
Posterior capsule	Flexion, abduction, internal rotation	Internal rotation—superior and middle Abduction or abduction/internal rotation—inferior

[a] The main passive restraints are the glenohumeral ligaments, the posterior capsule, and the coracohumeral ligament. The glenohumeral ligaments are further divided into superior, middle, and inferior components.
(Data from Terry et al.[31])

either the biceps or middle glenohumeral attachment to total separation.[18] Its presence is more consistent than the coracohumeral ligament, ranging between 90 and 97 percent.[38,39] However, a substantial ligament was present only 50 percent of the time according to Warner et al.[34] Variations include presentations that are gradations of mild to moderate thickening of the joint capsule. When not substantially present, negative intra-articular pressure is important for stabilization of the abducted shoulder.[30] It is suspected that a deficiency of the rotator interval may in fact represent a deficient superior glenohumeral ligament, increasing the possibility of anterior or inferior instability.[40]

The superior glenohumeral ligament serves as the primary restraint to inferior translation with the arm at the side.[40] Although it has not been found to contribute to anterior posterior stability in the adducted or 90 degree abducted arm, Warren et al.[41] have demonstrated that posterior dislocation was not possible with the arm in the typical flexed, adducted, and internally rotated position, unless the superior glenohumeral ligament was sectioned.

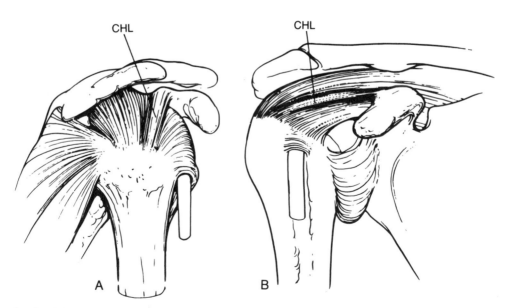

Fig. 1-14. The **(A)** lateral view and **(B)** anterior view of the coracohumeral ligament *(CHL)*. The CHL is a strong band originating from the base of the lateral border of the coracoid process, just below the coracoacromial ligament, and merging with the capsule laterally to insert on the greater tuberosity. This ligament may have importance as a suspensory structure for the adducted arm. (From O'Brien et al.,[18] with permission.)

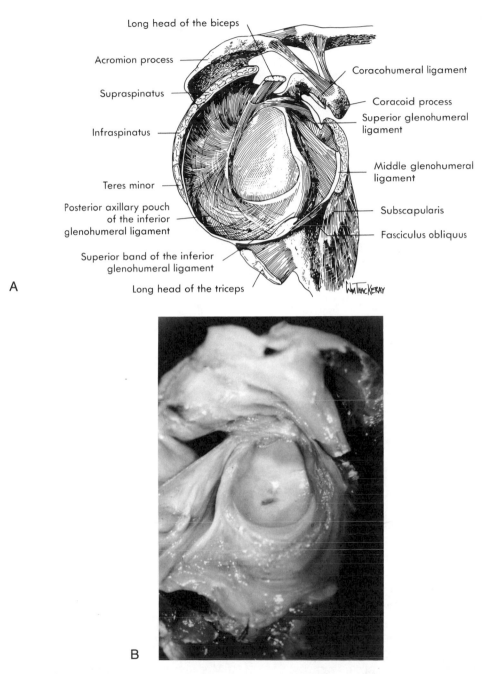

A

Long head of the biceps

Acromion process

Supraspinatus

Infraspinatus

Teres minor

Posterior axillary pouch
of the inferior
glenohumeral ligament

Superior band of the inferior
glenohumeral ligament

Long head of the triceps

Coracohumeral ligament

Coracoid process

Superior glenohumeral
ligament

Middle glenohumeral
ligament

Subscapularis

Fasciculus obliquus

B

Fig. 1-15. **(A)** Schematic drawing of right glenohumeral capsuloligamentous complex. Note superior, middle, and inferior glenohumeral ligaments. The superior ligament is variable in its presence. **(B)** Cadaveric specimen of left glenohumeral capsuloligamentous complex. Compare with schematic drawing. (From Skybar et al.,[91] with permission.)

Middle Glenohumeral Ligament

The middle glenohumeral ligament functionally plays more of an intermediary role, serving a secondary role in stability. This is probably due to the extreme variability of presentation with observations of total absence in 27 percent of individuals by O'Brien et al.[39] and absence or poor definition in 30 percent of individuals examined by DePalma et al.[38] When substantial the middle glenohumeral ligament may be as thick as the biceps tendon. In general, this ligament arises below the superior glenohumeral ligament and attaches medial to the lesser tuberosity. However, there are several common variations.

Secondary stabilization roles of the middle glenohumeral ligament include resistance to inferior translation with the arm adducted and externally rotated, and resistance to anterior translation with the arm abducted 45 degrees.

In their investigations O'Connell et al.[42] showed that the middle glenohumeral ligament plays a significant role in preventing anterior translation at 90 degrees abduction. They found that the inferior glenohumeral ligament was the major restraint, but that the middle glenohumeral ligament developed substantial tension. Primary stabilization with this ligament by default may occur with damage to the anterior band of the inferior glenohumeral ligament.[43]

Inferior Glenohumeral Ligament Complex

The primary restraint with abduction of the arm is the inferior glenohumeral ligament (Fig. 1-16). With the advent of arthroscopy, it was determined that the inferior glenohumeral ligament was a complex composed of three distinct structures: an anterior band, posterior band, and axillary pouch.[39] These structures act reciprocally forming a "hammocklike" structure. The reciprocity occurs because of an accommodation in shape such that when the abducted arm is externally rotated the anterior band fans out to support anteriorly as the posterior band becomes cordlike supporting the humeral head inferiorly. The opposite occurs with abduction and internal rotation.

The inferior glenohumeral ligament arises from either the glenoid neck or labrum in varying locations. Using a clock face analogy, O'Brien et al.[39] found the anterior band originating from a 2 to 4 o'clock position

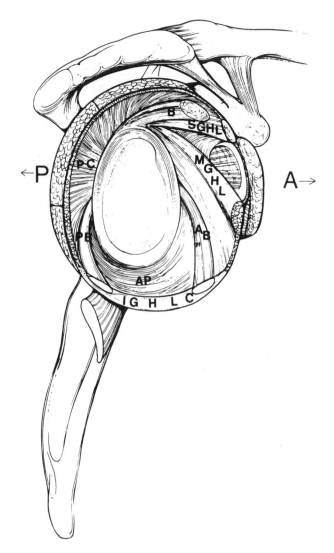

Fig. 1-16. Anatomic depiction of the glenohumeral ligaments and inferior glenohumeral ligament complex *(IGHLC)*. *P,* posterior; *A,* anterior; *SGHL,* superior glenohumeral ligament. (From O'Brien et al.,[18] with permission.)

and the posterior band from 7 to 9 o'clock. Insertion has two common presentations. A collarlike attachment to the anatomic neck is common. Another pattern is a **V** shape with the anterior and posterior bands attaching to or close to the articular surface and the axillary pouch attaching as the apex further away from the articular surface. The humeral attachment is in between the insertions of the triceps and the subscapularis muscles. The inferior glenohumeral ligament is thicker than either the anterior or posterior capsule in most individuals.

The anterior stabilizing function of the inferior glenohumeral ligament is primarily with increasing abduction. The past belief of preventing inferior translation in the relaxed "arm by the side" position was overemphasized. Warner et al.[34] demonstrated that the inferior glenohumeral ligament did not contribute to inferior stability. Unpublished data by Bowen, in 1991, indicate a secondary ability but confirm lack of a primary role.

The reciprocal function of the anterior and posterior bands of the inferior glenohumeral ligament (Fig. 1-17) is very important. With abduction at 45 and 90 degrees, Warner[34] demonstrated that the combination of both the anterior and posterior bands prevented inferior translation. When internal rotation was introduced, the anterior band slipped under the humeral head preventing inferior translation. With external rotation, the posterior band slipped under the humeral head preventing inferior translation.

Schwartz et al.[43] have demonstrated additional roles for the inferior glenohumeral ligament regarding anterior to posterior stability. They found that (1) the anterior band was the major stabilizer with 30 degrees horizontal extension and also neutral extension, and (2) the posterior band was the major stabilizer at 30 degrees horizontal flexion.

Posterior Capsule

The posterior capsule is the thinnest capsular structure. It attaches to the 9 to 12 o'clock area. The area is posterior to the biceps and superior to the inferior glenohumeral ligament. The ability of the posterior capsule to prevent posterior dislocation is limited.[41] In fact, intact anterior structures are probably as important to posterior stability. Interestingly, Oversen and Nielsen[44,45] observed through sectioning various aspects of the capsule and posterior cuff musculature that anterior subluxation was possible when lesions were present in either the posterior capsule or cuff.

The assumed responsibility of ligaments and capsule by logical static observation is often incorrect. The superior glenohumeral ligament is far more important than the inferior glenohumeral ligament with regard to inferior instability in the relaxed arm position; the anterior capsule is more important to posterior insta-

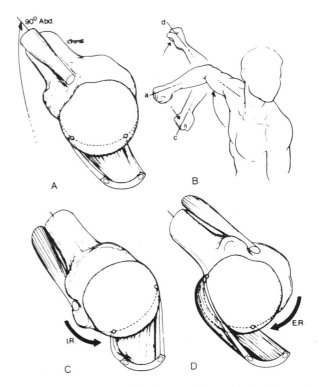

Fig. 1-17. The inferior glenohumeral complex is tightened during abduction **(a)**. During abduction and internal or external rotation different parts of the band are tightened **(b)**. With internal rotation the posterior band fans out to support the head and the anterior band becomes cordlike or relaxed, depending on the degree of horizontal flexion or extension **(c)**. Upon abduction and external rotation, the anterior band fans out to support the head and the posterior band becomes cordlike or relaxed, depending on the degree of horizontal flexion or extension **(d)**. (From O'Brien et al.,[18] with permission.)

bility than casually assumed; and the posterior capsule contributes to anterior stability.

Coupled movement is more representative of functional positions. These movements selectively strain divisions of the capsule. For example, the anterior glenohumeral ligaments, in general, restrict extension, abduction, and external rotation. Coupled movement such as extension with internal rotation places more stress on the superior band, whereas abduction with external rotation places more stress on the inferior band.[41]

Synovial Recesses

Recesses may form at the insertion points of the anterior capsule. These are referred to as synovial recesses (Fig. 1-18) and act as entryways for the synovial sheath of the biceps and the subscapular bursa. The recess is formed by a more medial attachment onto the scapular neck. The more medial the insertion the larger the recess. DePalma[6] and others[18] have classified these as types. The most common is that above the middle glenohumeral joint. The clinical significance of these recesses is that they are in effect defects in the continuity of the capsule. Theoretically, these may serve as a potential cause of instability.

Glenoid Labrum

The glenoid labrum (Fig. 1-19) is a structure, in many ways, analogous to the meniscus in the knee. Structurally it serves to deepen the glenoid receptacle. This stabilizing role is further augmented by capsular and tendinous marriage. The labrum is composed of these

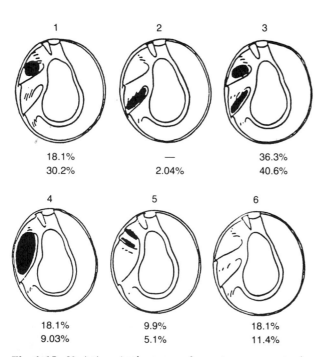

1	2	3
18.1%	—	36.3%
30.2%	2.04%	40.6%
4	5	6
18.1%	9.9%	18.1%
9.03%	5.1%	11.4%

Fig. 1-18. Variations in the types of anterior recesses in the capsule. The original percentages of DePalma are listed *(top lines)* along with percentages from more recent anatomic studies *(bottom lines)*. (From O'Brien et al.,[18] with permission.)

interdigitations from the capsule, the nearby hyaline cartilage, synovium, and periosteum. It is essentially devoid of fibrocartilage consisting of dense fibrous tissue with some elastic fibers. The role of the labrum in stabilizing the glenohumeral joint is still debated; however, it appears that the patency of the glenohumeral ligament attachments to the glenoid and labrum are essential to stability.[3]

MUSCLES

Muscles of the shoulder complex may be divided on a functional or anatomic basis. The functional division is further divided into those muscles operating on the scapula and those on the glenohumeral joint. Further classification is based on generalized function: whether the muscles are stabilizers and positioners, accelerators (creating motion), or decelerators of active or passive movement. Specific functional considerations of movement would include whether the muscle is primarily a flexor, extensor, rotator, etc. acting eccentrically or concentrically.

The muscles may be divided into superficial (which mainly elevate the shoulder), deep (which primarily stabilize the shoulder), and peripheral muscles (which assist with strength movement). This division allows much overlap yet reflects the general function of muscles in relation to the joint they affect. In other words, the larger peripheral muscles function primarily to provide strength with gross movement due to their long lever arm and size. The smaller deeper muscles provide stability (rotator cuff).

Scapular Guidance Musculature

The scapula serves as the origin for muscles that act on the humerus. In addition, it serves as the insertion point for muscles that govern its own movement, thereby indirectly affecting humeral movement. Primarily these muscles act on their insertions on the medial and superior borders and the scapular spine. They are stabilized at either the spine or the rib cage. The more superior the insertion the more upward lift of the scapula as a whole. The lower the insertion on the medial border the more likely the scapula will elevate at its glenoid end. The trapezius inserts all along

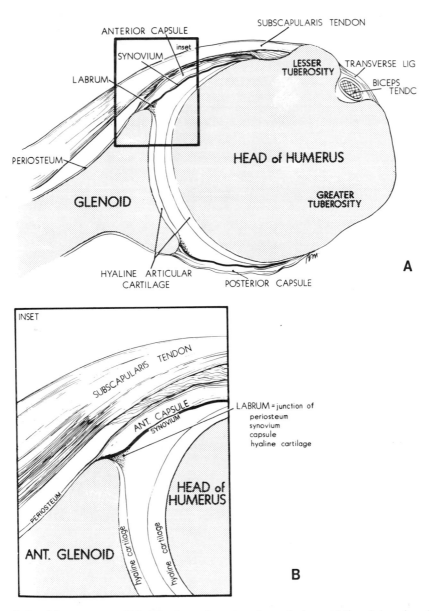

Fig. 1-19. Normal shoulder anatomy. **(A)** A horizontal section through the middle of the glenohumeral joint demonstrating normal anatomic relationships. Note the close relation of the subscapularis tendon to the anterior capsule. **(B)** A close-up view in the area of the labrum. The labrum is essentially devoid of fibrocartilage and is composed of tissues from the nearby hyaline cartilage, capsule, synovium, and periosteum. (From Rockwood and Green,[3] with permission.)

the medial border, thereby assuming different functions based on the fibers incorporated.

The primary muscles include the levator scapulae, all the divisions of the trapezius, the rhomboids, and the serratus anterior. This posterior musculature anchoring at the spine includes the entire cervical, thoracic, and lumbar segments.

The levator scapulae and upper trapezius are the upper group that help elevate the medial border of the scapula causing mainly dropping of the glenoid border. The middle trapezius and rhomboid fiber alignment, in a neutral arm position, act to protract (adduct) the scapula. These muscles often act eccentrically to decelerate a forward moving arm and shoulder in sports.

Although not often included as shoulder muscles, spinal muscles are, in fact, necessary for positioning of the humerus in many throwing activities. To maintain a relative position of 90 degrees abduction, varying degrees of lateral trunk bending are incorporated. It has been demonstrated that when throwing heavier objects, the arm becomes more vertical.[46] This positioning is necessary for stability of the glenohumeral joint and is accomplished by contralateral spinal extensor contraction including the erector spinae and the quadratus lumborum.

Trapezius

The trapezius (Fig. 1-20) is a broad muscle divided into three sections. It is rather superficial lying above the rhomboids, levator scapulae, and serratus anterior. Fiber attachments on the spine are from the nuchal line down the spinouses of the cervical and thoracic regions inclusive. This includes the supraspinous ligaments. Variations include a lower border somewhere between T8 and L2, and an upper origin at the external occipital protuberance.[47]

The insertions are reversed triangles connected at their bases. The upper fibers attach to the lateral clavicle. The middle attach to the acromion. The lower fibers travel upward and laterally to insert on the base of the scapular spine.

The primary and secondary actions of the trapezius include: (1) primarily acting as a positioner (with the serratus anterior) of the glenoid through elevation of the lateral border of the scapulae (mainly upper and lower fibers), (2) retraction of the scapulae (mainly

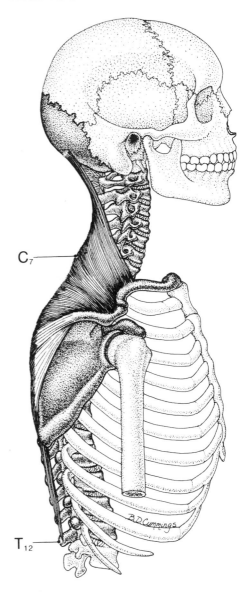

Fig. 1-20. Side view of right trapezius. (From Travell and Simons,[92] with permission.)

middle fibers), and (3) relief of strain on the sternoclavicular ligament. During elevation there is a selective use of mainly the upper fibers.[48] However, to some degree there is an upper to lower recruitment of trapezius fibers. This is less evident during pure flexion when retraction of the scapula is counterproductive. With loss of trapezius function, the shoulder can only be abducted 90 degrees.[49,50] However, forward flexion is less restricted. It is important to note that with grade

II and III acromioclavicular separations, the attaching fibers of the trapezius and deltoid are often torn.

Motor innervation is from the spinal accessory nerve (cranial nerve XI) with sensory supply from C2 to C4. Arterial supply appears to be twofold: from the transverse cervical artery (mainly upper fibers of trapezius) and the dorsal scapular artery (mainly lower fibers).[51]

Levator Scapulae

The levator scapulae (Fig. 1-21) originate off of the posterior tubercles of the transverse processes of the first four cervical vertebrae. Running obliquely inferiorward they insert on the superior medial border of the scapula with some fibers inserting further down the medial border. Their primary action is to lift the superior border of the scapula.[52] Acting together with the scapula fixed, the right and left levator scapulae act as checkreins to forward flexion of the neck. Interestingly, the levator scapulae have a larger mass than the upper trapezius compared by cross-section.[44] The innervation is from C3 and C4 and occasionally from the dorsal scapular nerve. Blood supply is mainly via the dorsal scapular artery.

The levator scapulae are often involved when fatigue postures (slumped or stooped) are maintained, producing a local tender mass at the superior medial border attachment. This may become a chronic focus referred to as the levator scapulae syndrome, scapulocostal syndrome, or superior scapula syndrome. It is often confused with disorders of the glenohumeral joint.[53]

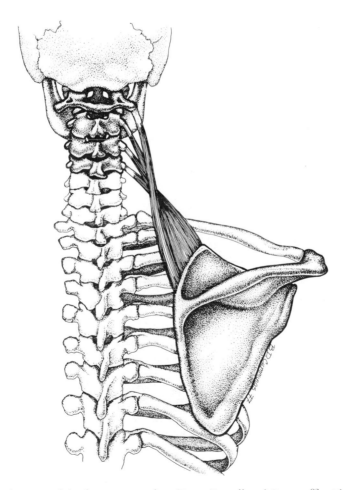

Fig. 1-21. Attachments of the levator scapulae. (From Travell and Simons,[92] with permission.)

Serratus Anterior

The serratus anterior (Fig. 1-22) has, in the past, been inaccurately assessed regarding its function at the shoulder. Activated with all shoulder movements, the serratus operates at a higher percentage more often than any other shoulder muscle.[44,54] Recent evidence suggests that it is an integral component for the successful completion of the scapulohumeral movement couple, protracting the scapula and providing a stable base for the humeral head.[55] Innervation is from the long thoracic nerve (C5 to C7). Stretch of the long thoracic may occur over the second rib when the head is tilted laterally while depressing the shoulder.[56] Blood supply to the serratus is from the lateral thoracic artery and/or the thoracodorsal artery.[57]

The serratus anterior has a broad anterior origin from the first eight to nine ribs. Usually it is divided into three divisions. The first arises from the first two ribs as a single slip. The second has three slips from ribs 2 to 4. The third originates from ribs 5 to 9 as separate slips. Traveling with the ribs posteriorly, the upper fibers insert on the costal scapular surface medially. The lower fibers, which are believed to be the most important for scapular movement, insert on the inferior-medial border of the costal surface of the scapula.

Rhomboid Major and Minor

The rhomboid minor lies superior to the major originating from the seventh cervical and first thoracic vertebrae (Fig. 1-23). The rhomboid major originates off of the second through fifth thoracic vertebrae and their

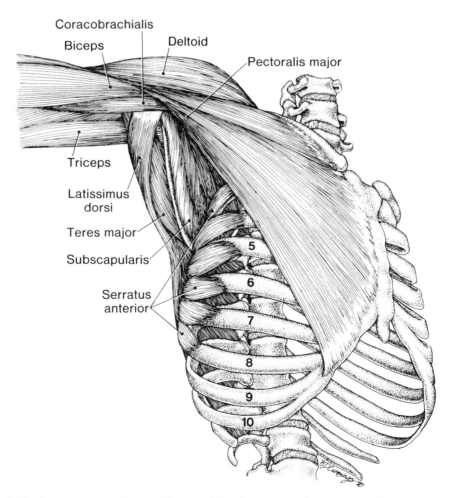

Fig. 1-22. Anterior musculature of the shoulder. (From Travell and Simons,[92] with permission.)

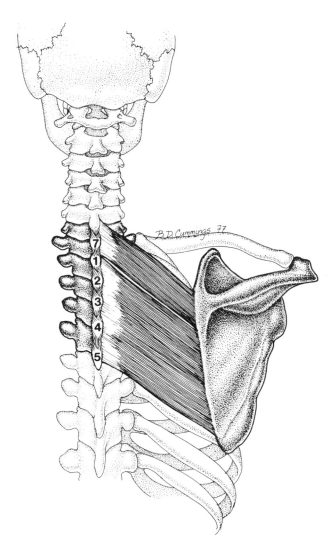

Fig. 1-23. Rhomboid major and minor attachments. (From Travell and Simons,[92] with permission.)

respective supraspinous ligaments. Both insert on the medial border of the scapula. Innervation is from the dorsal scapular nerve (C5). The dorsal scapular nerve either originates with the nerve to the subclavius or the C5 branch of the long thoracic nerve. Arterial supply is from the dorsal scapular artery.

Essentially the rhomboids serve a similar function to the middle trapezius fibers causing retraction of the scapula. This also translates into a stabilizing function for the medial border of the scapula. This action is eccentrically demanding during the follow-through phases of throwing activities. In addition, because of

their oblique orientation, they may perform some degree of scapular elevation function.

Pectoralis Minor

The pectoralis minor (Fig. 1-24) originates off of the second through fifth ribs and inserts on the medial base of the coracoid. As mentioned previously, there are variations of attachment sites in 15 percent of the population. Often this represents a shadowing of the coracohumeral ligament. The medial pectoral nerve (C6 to T1) innervates the pectoralis minor with vascular supply from the pectoral branch of the thoracoacromial artery or the lateral thoracic artery.

The pectoralis minor is a contingency muscle, that is, there must be prior positioning of the scapula before the muscle is called into action. If the scapula is retracted and laterally depressed the pectoralis functions as a protractor. If the scapula is rotated upward, the pectoralis minor will rotate the scapula down.

Glenohumeral Guidance Musculature

Muscles that directly influence glenohumeral motion originate off of either the scapula/clavicle, the rib cage, or the thoracic/lumbar spine. As mentioned previously, the larger peripheral muscles are used for strength and gross movement, whereas the smaller muscles are stabilizers. Insertions medial to the greater tuberosity (with the exception of the anterior deltoid) will usually result in an adduction/internal rotation action. Those inserting on or lateral to the greater tuberosity are external rotators.

The primarily axial skeleton muscles that influence humeral motion are large broad muscles. The anterior component is the pectoralis group and the posterior component is the latissimus dorsi. Both insert close to each other on either side of the intertubercular groove having similar actions of adduction/internal rotation. These muscles are primary accelerators in throwing sports and swimming. The pectorals may help the subscapularis in decelerating the horizontally extended/externally rotated shoulder as in the cocking phase of most throwing sports.[58,59]

Latissimus Dorsi

The latissimus dorsi (Fig. 1-25) has an extensive attachment off of the thoracolumbar fascia including the thoracic and lumbar spinous processes, and the iliac crest

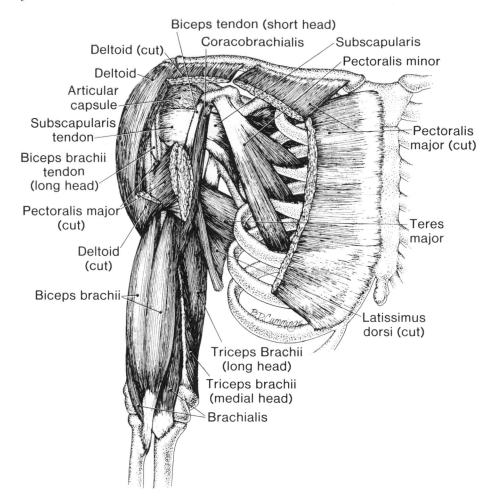

Fig. 1-24. Pectoralis minor and other deep muscles of the shoulder. (From Travell and Simons,[92] with permission.)

and sacrum; there is a direct connection between the spine/pelvis and the shoulder. Spiraling up under the axilla it inserts into the humerus medial to the intertubercular groove. Originating posteriorly and inserting anteriorly, the latissimus also aids in extension in addition to the shared role of adduction/internal rotation with the pectorals. Innervation is from the thoracodorsal nerve (C6 to C8).

In sports participation, the latissimus dorsi serves several functions:

1. Pulls the raised arm down forcefully; used mainly in throwing and hitting sports.
2. Supports the trunk via strong adduction; for example the "iron cross" on the still rings and the support position on parallel bars.
3. Raises the body when the arms are fixed.

The pectoralis major assists in these functions.

Pectoralis Major

The pectorals originate off of the medial clavicle, manubrium, sternum, and costal cartilage of the first six ribs. Usually the upper fibers are described as the clavicular division; the lower are called the sternal division. The clavicular fibers run downward whereas the sternal division has fibers that run straight laterally and others that ascend up and under the clavicular division.

They insert in a conjoined tendon at the inferior lesser tubercle, just lateral to the intertubercular groove. The insertion is distinct in that the upper fibers off of the chest insert lower on the humerus whereas the lower chest fibers insert above the clavicular fibers. This twisted insertion normalizes the length of all the fibers and results in slightly different functions based on fiber origin. Innervation is from the medial and lateral pectoral nerves (C5 to T1).

The pectoralis major (Fig. 1-26) assists the latissimus dorsi in the above-mentioned functions of forceful downward movement of the raised arm and trunk support. Additionally, the pectorals assist in raising and rotating the trunk in positions where the arms are fixed

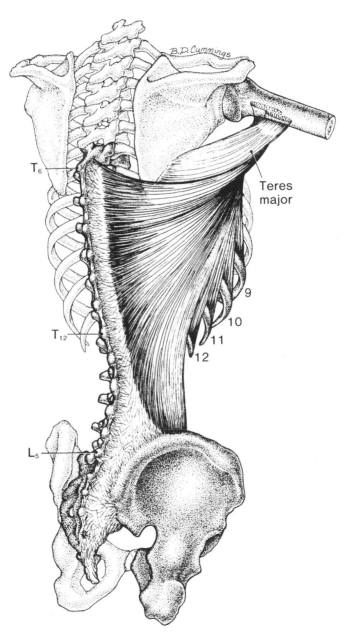

Fig. 1-25. The latissimus dorsi muscle attachments. (From Travell and Simons,[92] with permission.)

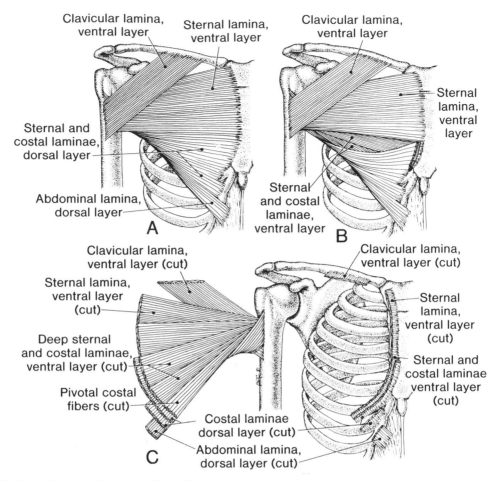

Fig. 1-26. Semischematic drawings of the fiber arrangement in the pectoralis major muscle. **(A)** Usual ventral view. **(B)** Ventral view with the superficial dorsal-layer fibers retracted to show the deep lamina of the ventral layer when it attaches to the humerus. **(C)** Muscle reflected laterally to show the dorsal aspect of the seldom seen "playing card" arrangement of the deep lamina of the ventral layer. The dorsal layer swings around the other fibers to attach on the humerus dorsal to them. (From Travell and Simons,[92] with permission, as adapted from Ashley GT: The manner of insertion of the pectoralis major muscle in man. Anat Rec 113:301, 1952.)

such as in pole vaulting. All the muscle fibers function with forceful downward movement of the raised arm. There is some isolation in function due to fiber orientation:

1. Horizontal adduction is accomplished mainly by the straight fibers of the sternocostal section (e.g., discus throwing).
2. Forward movement of the extended arm is due mainly to contraction of the clavicular portion (e.g., bowling).

3. Internal rotation is due mainly to the clavicular and straight portions of the sternal section (e.g., throwing and swimming).
4. Adduction is due mainly to contraction of the sternal section, both horizontal and ascending fibers (e.g., support phases of gymnastics).

Deltoid

Originating off of the lateral clavicle, scapular spine, and acromion, the deltoid converges into a small insertion point of the humerus, the deltoid tubercle (Figs.

1-22 and 1-24). There is a complex arrangement of the middle division that allows greater force production within a shorter distance of movement. It is bipenniform with oblique fiber orientation. Interconnecting tendons arise from the deltoid tubercle and travel superiorly. The anterior and posterior divisions consist of fusiform long fiber bundles that travel more directly to the insertion point. Innervation is from C5 and C6 through the axillary nerve. Paralysis of the axillary nerve will result in a decrease of strength with elevation, although full elevation may be accomplished by other muscles and body position.[60] Arterial supply is mainly from the posterior humeral circumflex with some anastomosis with the deltoid branch of the thoracoacromial artery.

The deltoid is primarily the "elevator" muscle. Some or all of its three divisions are involved in every mode of elevation: flexion, abduction, and extension. The middle third is the prime facilitator of abduction in the scapular plane (30 to 40 degrees anterior to the coronal plane) with some assistance from the anterior deltoid. Above 90 degrees, the posterior deltoid is called into action. Coronal plan elevation is also primarily the middle third; however, there is more contribution of the posterior and less of the anterior deltoid. Forward flexion is mainly the anterior deltoid with assistance from the middle deltoid. Movements such as horizontal adduction and abduction differ significantly in the contribution of the deltoid. Horizontal adduction involves only a 12 percent contribution by the deltoid, whereas horizontal abduction involves 60 percent contribution.[44]

Rotator Cuff

The rotator cuff originates from anterior, posterior, and lateral surfaces of the scapula. Its insertions grasp the humeral head in a manner similar to the grip of a hand on a baseball. Although all act as stabilizers of humeral head movement, each muscle accomplishes this task through different actions. The supraspinatus is primarily involved with abduction. The infraspinatus and teres minor are primarily external rotators, and the subscapularis is primarily an internal rotator. In addition to dynamically maintaining stability, the tendons of these muscles may act as mechanical blockage to excessive movement, such as the subscapularis, which aids in anterior stability up to 90 degrees abduction.[40]

Supraspinatus

The supraspinatus muscle belly occupies the supraspinous fossa created by the scapular spine on the posterior surface of the scapula (Fig. 1-27). Its tendon passes laterally under the acromioclavicular arch to insert on the greater tubercle of the humerus. Through this passage, the tendon is susceptible to impingement on overhead movements if:

1. The glenoid fails to rotate upward during elevation
2. The humerus does not externally rotate
3. The subacromial space is narrowed by other processes

The supraspinatus couples with the deltoid in achieving abduction. Nerve and blood supply is from the suprascapular nerve (C5 and C6) and vessels.

Infraspinatus

Arising from the posterior surface of the scapula below the scapular spine, the infraspinatus tendon passes laterally to insert on the posterior aspect of the greater tubercle (Fig. 1-27). The posterior location of the muscle and its tendon assures mainly an external rotation aspect of its function. It is stronger than the teres minor, yet both function in external rotation/horizontal extension components of sports such as the cocking phase of the throwing mechanism.[57,58] Both act as decelerators of the acceleration and follow-through phases of throwing. Nerve and blood supply is also from the suprascapular nerve (C5 and C6) and vessels that travel through the suprascapular notch, a potential site of entrapment.

Teres Minor

The teres minor (Fig. 1-27) arises from the lateral border of the scapula above the origin of the teres major. Its tendon passes under the long head of the triceps to insert in very much a conjoined tendon with the infraspinatus. Due to the close proximity of their insertions, the infraspinatus and teres minor are often functionally grouped together. Their primary function in movement is external rotation. They also are primary stabilizers of the humeral head in the glenoid fossa. Clinically it is difficult to separate them on the basis of strength testing. The infraspinatus/teres minor also serve to decelerate the rapidly forward moving/internally rotating arm as mentioned previously.

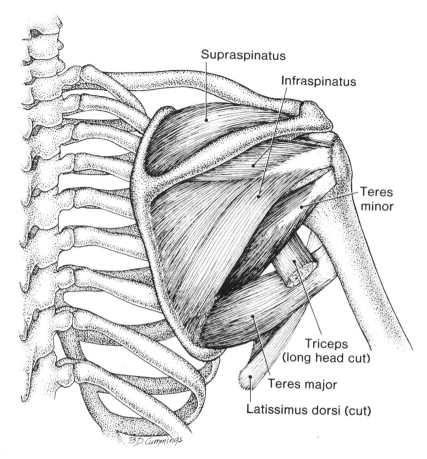

Fig. 1-27. Posterior rotator cuff and teres major. (From Travell and Simons,[92] with permission.)

The lower border of the teres minor serves as the "roof" for two vascular spaces: the triangular and quadrilateral. Nerve supply from the axillary nerve (C5 and C6) is shared with the deltoid.

Subscapularis

The subscapularis (Fig. 1-24) is plastered against the anterior surface of the scapula. Its tendon passes laterally to insert on the lesser tubercle close to the insertions of other internal rotators such as the pectoralis major, latissimus, and teres major. Its tendon does not cross under the acromioclavicular arch so is less affected in impingement syndromes. Nerve supply is from two sources, the upper and lower subscapular nerves (C5 and C6). Blood supply is essentially from the subscapular artery.

Functions of the subscapularis include

1. Passive stabilization to anterior translation of the humerus. This is due to an unusually dense collagen makeup[40,61]
2. Internal rotation of the humerus
3. Stabilization of the humeral head through the depressor effects of the lower fibers

The function of the subscapularis in sports may vary depending on the degree of training. It has been demonstrated that the subscapularis is primarily used as an internal rotator in professional pitchers whereas in amateurs it plays more of a stabilizer function, decreasing its contribution in assisting acceleration.[62] Recently it has been suggested by Belle and Hawkins[63] that the subscapularis may play an even more important role through eccentric contraction. While testing electromyographically external rotation in neutral and with abduction, the subscapularis demonstrated substantially more activity than the agonist (infraspinatus).

Teres Major

The teres major (Fig. 1-27) attaches below the teres minor on the lateral aspect of the scapula. Its tendon passes anterior to insert medial to the latissimus dorsi on the humerus. Its function has not been studied as thoroughly as other shoulder muscles but appears to aid in internal rotation, adduction, and extension of the shoulder. It therefore resembles the latissimus dorsi and assists in pulling the raised arm down and forward such as in freestyle swimming or cross-country skiing. In addition, it assists the latissimus dorsi in strong adduction/supportive movement as in the front support swing on the horizontal bars. The "iron cross" is an example of a supportive position that incorporates the latissimus dorsi, lower portion of the pectoralis major, and the teres major. The teres major has been shown to become active only against strong resistance.[64] It is postulated that it functions mainly to draw the lower portion of the scapula toward the humerus, a kind of "scapular elevator."[65] Nerve supply is from the subscapular nerve (C5 and C6).

Biceps

Although not considered primarily a shoulder muscle, the biceps (Fig. 1-24) does have attachments about the shoulder and has been demonstrated, in pathologic states at least, to serve a function of stability.[66] There are two heads, the long and short. The long head arises from the supraglenoid rim in intimate connection with the glenoid labrum. The tendon passes with a synovial lining over the superior aspect of the humerus into the biceps groove. The proximal tendon is intra-articular yet extrasynovial. The tendon then passes down the anterior aspect of the arm, crossing the elbow to insert on the radius. The short head comes off of the coracoid process and joins the long head at 7.5 cm above the elbow inserting in a conjoined tendon. Nerve supply is from the musculocutaneous nerve (C5 and C6).

Functioning mainly as an elbow supinator and flexor, the biceps does serve to assist in shoulder flexion along with the anterior deltoid and coracobrachialis. Its function as a stabilizer of the humeral head is apparent with pathology of the shoulder, in particular instability.[67] This is in part due to a compressive force

produced at higher ranges of elevation. The tendon of the long head of the biceps was also found to be enlarged when pathology such as rotator cuff tear or instability was present. Burkhead[68] believes that the bibiceps plays at least some role as a humeral head depressor at higher degrees of elevation.

Another feature of the tendon of the long head of the biceps that may be clinically important is its stability in the bicipital groove. Developmental or acquired anomalies may account for attrition or instability, as mentioned previously. In the past it was believed that the stability of the tendon was maintained by the transverse ligament. It is now generally agreed that the stability is more a function of the coracohumeral ligament and the supraspinatus and subscapularis insertions.[69]

Coracobrachialis

Similar in location to the short head of the biceps, the coracobrachialis (Fig. 1-24) originates off of the coracoid process. Unlike the short head of the biceps it inserts onto the anteromedial aspect of the humerus. Its function is similar to the short head in that it aids in flexion with more importance in adduction. Nerve supply is from the musculocutaneous nerve (C5 and C6).

Triceps

Again not primarily a shoulder muscle, the triceps (see Figs. 1-24 and 1-27) may influence shoulder movement if pathology exists at the insertion into the inferior glenoid rim. As the name implies there are three heads. The long head originates off of the inferior rim of the glenoid posteriorly, and the middle and lateral heads originate off of the posterior humerus itself, extending posteriorly to the olecranon. Innervation is from the radial nerve via C7 and C8.

VASCULAR SUPPLY

The vascular supply of the shoulder (Fig. 1-28) is dependent on an inconsistent array of blood vessels. Often redundancy is built into the supply with two or three arteries or branches serving the same muscle.

Inconsistencies are found with the thoracoacromial, suprahumeral, and subscapular arteries, three of the arteries that potentially supply the rotator cuff. The ef-

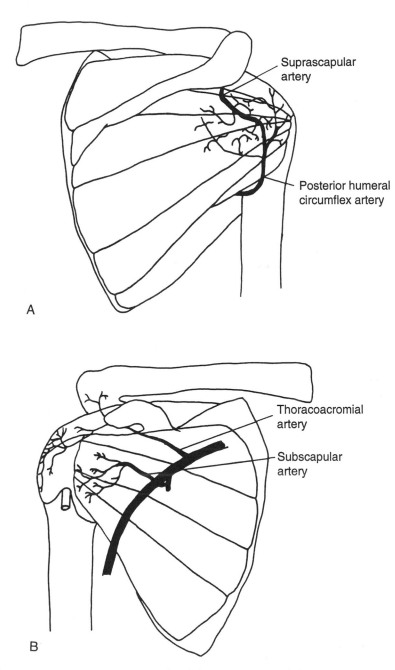

Fig. 1-28. Vascular supply of the rotator cuff muscles: **(A)** posterior view; **(B)** anterior view, showing the thoracoacromial and subscapular arteries. (*Figure continues.*)

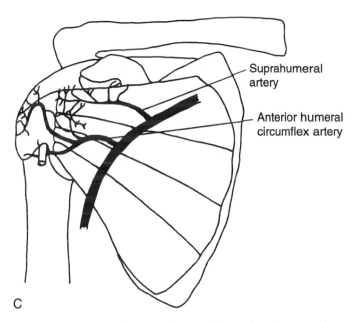

Suprahumeral
artery

Anterior humeral
circumflex artery

C

Fig. 1-28. (*Continued*). **(C)** Anterior view, showing the suprahumeral and anterior humeral circumflex arteries. (From Hertling and Kessler,[86] with permission.)

fect is on the supraspinatus muscle, which is primarily fed by the thoracoacromial arteries, and on the subscapularis muscle, which is supplied by the anterior humeral circumflex and the thoracoacromial arteries. The infraspinatus and teres minor are supplied by the posterior humeral circumflex and the suprascapular arteries, both of which are usually present.

The supraspinatus seems especially vulnerable in regards to its vascular supply. In addition to the inconsistencies of supply, the tendon may be directly compressed or impinged in the subacromial arch. The blood supply entry into the tendon varies from the norm. Normally tendons receive their supply from small vessels entering at a right angle to the tendon.[70,71] Stretch has little effect on this arrangement. However, the supraspinatus contains blood vessels that travel parallel to the fibers (longitudinal). Therefore, any stretch on the tendon may stretch the vascular supply thereby reducing patency.

One final concern is the critical zone that seems to be present slightly proximal to the supraspinatus insertion point. This area seems to be relatively avascu-

lar when compressed or stretched with various positions.[72] Stretching occurs over the humeral head with the relaxed arm-by-the-side position. It seems also to be the area most often caught in impingement with abduction and internal rotation. The combination may lead to degenerative changes.

NEURAL SUPPLY

Neural supply to the shoulder for motor and sensory control is primarily from the brachial plexus originating in the cervical region. Sympathetic supply originates primarily in the thoracic region mainly T2 to T6 and as far down as T8.[73] Entry into the arm is via the brachial plexus from the cervical ganglia.

Brachial Plexus

Motor and sensory supply to the glenohumeral joint and muscles is primarily from the C5 and C6 levels (Fig. 1-29). Innervation of the major muscle surround-

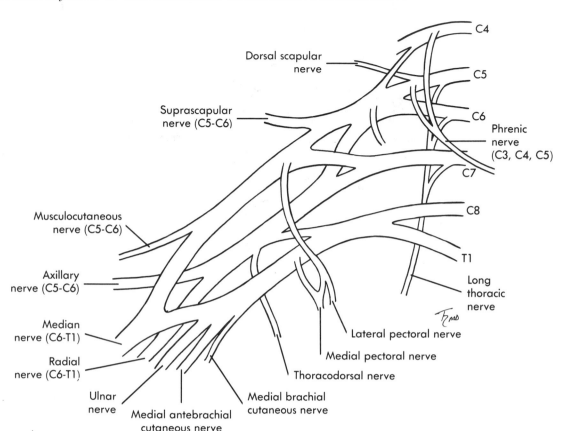

Fig. 1-29. Diagram of the brachial plexus. (From Hershman,[94] with permission.)

ing the shoulder is often paired. The supraspinatus and infraspinatus are supplied by the suprascapular nerve, the teres minor and deltoid by the axillary nerve, and the teres major and subscapularis by the subscapular nerve.

The construction of this neural network is such that many levels may contribute to a single peripheral nerve. In addition, the nerves pass through an array of potential entrapment sites, fixed points of stretch, or compression sites. Starting at the intervertebral foramina, the nerves that comprise the brachial plexus must run between the anterior and middle scalenes, the clavicle and first rib, and the pectoralis minor. In addition, the suprascapular nerve may become stretched across or compressed at the suprascapular notch at the medial third of the spine of the scapula, an injury associated with throwing and heavy lifting. It is important to remember that all spinal nerves contain sensory (both afferent and efferent), motor, and sympathetic

elements. Any element or combination may be affected. Structures related on a spinal segmental basis may refer pain to other structures within this related group, such as scleratogenous and myotogenous pain.

Table 1-2 and 1-3 summarize innervation of the muscles governing shoulder movement. Figures 1-30 and 1-31 illustrate the capsular innervation of the shoulder. The following is a description of some of the major peripheral nerves about the shoulder.

Suprascapular Nerve

The suprascapular nerve originates off of the upper trunk of the brachial plexus at Erb's point. It is formed from nerve roots C5 and C6, and occasionally there is a contribution from C4. The nerve courses behind the upper trapezius. Upon reaching the superior border of the scapula, the nerve passes through the scapular notch. The notch is covered by the transverse scapular

Table 1-2. Muscles Controlling Scapular Motion, Nerve Supply, and Innervation

Scapular Motion	Muscle	Nerve Supply	Segment Level
Lateral rotation of inferior angle	Trapezius (upper and lower fibers)[a]	Accessory	Cranial XI; C3,4
	Serratus anterior[b]	Long thoracic	C5,6 (7)
	Levator scapulae[a]	Dorsal scapula	C3,4 (5) (roots)
Elevation	Trapezius (upper fibers)	Accessory	Cranial XI; C3,4
	Levator scapulae	Dorsal scapula	C3,4, (5) (roots)
	Rhomboid major	Dorsal scapula	(C4) C5 (roots)
	Rhomboid minor	Dorsal scapula	(C4) C5 (roots)
Depression	Serratus anterior	Long thoracic	C5,6 (7)
	Pectoralis major[c]	Lateral pectoral	C5,6 (lateral cord)
	Pectoralis minor	Medial pectoral	C8, T1 (medial cord)
	Latissimus dorsi	Thoracodorsal	C6,7,8 (posterior cord)
	Trapezius lower fibers	Accessory	Cranial XI; C3,4
Protraction	Serratus anterior	Long thoracic	C5,6 (7)
	Pectorallis minor	Medial pectoral	C8,T1
	Latissimus dorsal	Thoracodorsal	C6,7,8
Retraction	Trapezius	Accessory	Cranial XI; (C3,4)
	Rhomboid major	Dorsal scapula	(C4) C5
	Rhomboid minor	Dorsal scapula	(C4) C5
Medial (downward) rotation	Rhomboid major	Dorsal scapula	(C4) C5
	Rhomboid minor	Dorsal scapula	(C4) C5
	Levator scapulae	Dorsal scapula	C3,4 (C5)

[a] Acting as force couples.
[b] Mainly lower four digitations.
[c] Acting through the clavicle.
( ) = Subsidiary segments.
(From Reid,[93] with permission.)

ligament. In addition to motor supply to the supraspinatus, sensory branches supply the posterior capsule and acromioclavicular joint. Passing laterally, the nerve then passes around the base of the spine of the scapula to pass through the spinoglenoid notch. The infraspinatus is supplied after passage through this notch. About 50 percent of the normal population have a spinoglenoid ligament, an aponeurotic band that separates the supraspinatus and infraspinatus.[74,75] There are no cutaneous branches.

The literature reports varied etiologies of suprascapular nerve irritation in sports. Many are idiopathic[76]; however, some are due to traction injuries in throwing,[77] direct trauma from fracture or dislocation,[78] and possible transient problems due to compression or tractioning during supine weightlifting. Specific sports include throwing sports, backpacking, weightlifting, and volleyball.

Axillary Nerve

The axillary nerve, formed from the fifth and sixth spinal nerve roots, arises from the posterior cord at the level of the coracoid process. Comparatively it has a very short route. Passing under the coracoid process and continuing anteriorly, it supplies the subscapularis. Near the inferior border of the subscapularis it joins the posterior humeral circumflex artery passing posterior through an open area referred to as the quadrilateral space. This space is bounded by the teres major and minor, the long head of the triceps, and the shaft of the humerus. Branches to the inferior medial joint capsule occur during this route. Dividing into anterior and posterior branches, the teres minor, deltoids, and the skin overlying the deltoid are supplied.

Injury prior to entering the quadrilateral space is primarily due to stretch. The shorter the distance from the brachial plexus the more effect stretch has on the nerve. The three most common causes are (1) dislocation,[79,80] (2) fracture of the proximal humerus, and (3) a direct blow to the shoulder.[81] Another possible cause is blunt trauma to the axilla resulting in hematoma and adhesions that compress the axillary nerve.[82] The most common sports in which axillary nerve injury occurs are football, wrestling, gymnastics, mountain climbing, and rugby.[83]

Table 1-3. Glenohumeral Muscle Action and Innervation

Motion	Muscle	Nerve Supply	Segmental Intervention
Abduction	Deltoid[a]	Axillary	C5,6 (posterior cord)
	Supraspinatus[a]	Suprascapular	C5,6 (trunk)
	Infraspinatus[b]	Suprascapular	C5,6 (trunk)
	Subscapularis[b]	Subscapular	C5,6 (posterior cord)
	Teres minor[b]	Axillary	C5,6 (posterior cord)
	Biceps (long head)	Musculocutaneous	C5,6 (7) (lateral cord)
Adduction	Pectoralis major[a]	Lateral pectoral	C5,6 (lateral)
	Latissimus dorsi[a]	Thoracodorsal	C6,7,8 (posterior cord)
	Teres major	Subscapular	C5,6 (posterior cord)
	Subscapularis	Subscapular	C5,6 (posterior cord)
Flexion	Deltoid (anterior fibers)[a]	Axillary	C5,6
	Pectoralis major (clavicular lateral pectoral fibers)	Lateral pectoral	C5,6
	Coracorbrachialis	Musculocutaneous	C5,6 (7)
	Biceps (against significant resistance)	Musculocutaneous	C5,6 (7)
Extension	Deltoid (posterior fibers)[a]	Axillary	C5,6
	Latissimus dorsi[a]	Thoracodorsal	C6,7,8
	Teres major	Subscapular	C5,6
	Teres minor	Axillary	C5,6
	Triceps (long head)	Radial	(C5) C6,7,8 (T1) posterior cord
Horizontal adduction	Pectoralis major[a]	Lateral pectoral	C5,6
	Deltoid (anterior fibers)[a]	Axillary	C5,6
Horizontal abduction	Deltoid (posterior fibers)[a]	Axillary	C5,6
	Teres major[b]	Subscapular	C5,6
	Teres minor[b]	Axillary	C5,6
	Infraspinatus[b]	Suprascapular	C5,6
Medial (internal) rotation	Pectoralis major[a]	Lateral pectoral	C5,6
	Latissimus dorsi	Thoracodorsal	C6,7,8
	Deltoid (anterior fibers)	Axillary	C5,6
	Teres major	Subscapular	C5,6
	Subscapularis (when arm is adducted)	Subscapular	C5,6
Lateral (external) rotation	Infraspinatus[a]	Suprascapular	C5,6
	Teres minor	Axillary	C5,6
	Deltoid (posterior fibers)	Axillary	C5,6

Actions are described in the plane of the body.
[a] Prime movers.
[b] Control and centralize position of the head of the humerus in the glenoid.
(From Reid,[93] with permission.)

Long Thoracic Nerve

The long thoracic nerve is purely motor supplying the very important serratus anterior. It arises from the ventral rami of C5, C6, and C7 and is sometimes referred to as the external respiratory nerve of Bell. Due to its long, relatively superficial course, it is susceptible to injury either through direct trauma or stretch. Injury has been reported in almost all sports, including weightlifting, archery, rowing, gymnastics, tennis, squash, soccer, shooting, discus throwing, football, ballet, bowling, basketball, and wrestling. With weightlifting, pull-overs may be the culprit due to the stretch effect with elevation of the arms combined with spinal extension.

Musculocutaneous Nerve

The origin of the musculocutaneous nerve is from the C5 and C6 levels with occasional contribution from C7. It arises from the lateral cord of the brachial plexus at about the level of the pectoralis minor. Coursing through the coracobrachialis (which it innervates) it enters the arm to supply the biceps and brachialis.

At about 2 to 5 cm above the cubital crease, the musculocutaneous nerve divides, giving off a sensory branch that is divided into anterior and posterior fibers.

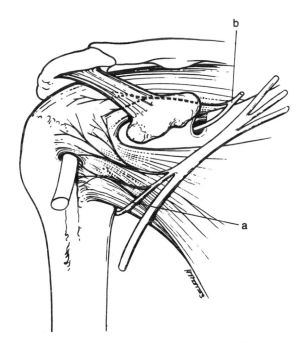

Fig. 1-30. Anterior innervation of the shoulder. The **(a)** axillary and **(b)** suprascapular nerves innervate the capsule and glenohumeral joint with occasional musculocutaneous contribution. (From O'Brien et al.,[18] with permission.)

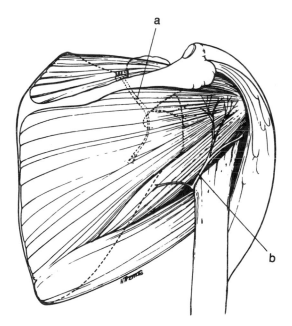

Fig. 1-31. Posterior innervation of the shoulder. The primary nerves are the **(a)** suprascapular and **(b)** the axillary. (From O'Brien et al.,[18] with permission.)

REFERENCES

1. Inman VT, Saunders JBDeCM: Observations on the function of the clavicle. Calif Med 65:158, 1946
2. Ogden JA, Conologue GS, Bronson ML: Radiology of post-natal skeletal development: the clavicle. Skeletal Radiol 4:196, 1979
3. Rockwood CA Jr, Thomas SC, Matsen FA: Subluxations and dislocations about the glenohumeral joint. p. 722. In Rockwood CA Jr, Green DP, Bucholz RW (eds): Rockwood and Green's Fractures in Adults. 3rd. Ed. JB Lippincott, Philadelphia, 1991
4. Webb PAO, Suchey JMM: Epiphyseal union of the anterior iliac crest and medial clavicle in a modern multiracial sample of American males and females. Am J Phys Anthropol 68:457, 1985
5. Rockwood CA: Disorders of the sternoclavicular joint. p. 477. In Rockwood CA, Matsen FA (eds): The Shoulder. Vol. 1. WB Saunders, Philadelphia, 1990
6. DePalma AF: Surgery of the Shoulder. JB Lippincott, Philadelphia, 1983
7. Bechtol C: Biomechanics of the shoulder. Clin Orthop 146:37, 1980
8. Rowe CR, Sakellarides HT: Factors related to recurrences of anterior dislocations of the shoulder. Clin Orthop 20: 41, 1961
9. Kent BE: Functional anatomy of the shoulder complex. Phys Ther 51:867, 1971
10. Basmajian JV, Bazant FJ: Factors preventing downward dislocation of the adducted shoulder joint. J Bone Joint Surg 41A:1182, 1959
11. Walker PS: Human Joints and Their Artificial Replacement. Charles C Thomas, Springfield, IL, 1977
12. Cyprien JM, Vasey HM, Burdet A, Bonuin JC: Humeral retroversion and glenohumeral relationship in the normal shoulder and in recurrent shoulder dislocation (scapulometry). Clin Orthop 175:8, 1983
13. Laumann U, Kramps HA: Computer tomography on recurrent shoulder dislocation. In Bateman JE (ed): Surgery of the Shoulder. CV Mosby, St. Louis, 1984
14. Brewer B, Wubben R, Carrera G: Excessive retroversion of the glenoid cavity. J Bone Joint Surg 68A:724, 1986
15. Das SP, Saha AK, Roy GS: Observations on the tilt of the glenoid cavity of the scapula. J Anat Soc India 15:144, 1966
16. Morrison DS, Bigliani LU: The clinical significance of variations in acromial morphology. Presented to the Society of American Shoulder and Elbow Surgeons Third Open Meeting, San Francisco, CA, 1987
17. Neer CS, Poppen NK: Supraspinatus outlet. Presented to the Society of American Shoulder and Elbow Surgeons Third Open Meeting, San Francisco, CA, 1987

18. O'Brien SJ, Arnoczky SP, Warren RF, Rozbruch SR: Developmental anatomy of the shoulder and anatomy of the glenohumeral joint. p. 16. In Rockwood CA, Matsen FA (eds): The Shoulder. Vol. 1. WB Saunders, Philadelphia, 1990

19. Rockwood C, Wilkins K, King R: Fractures in Adults. JB Lippincott, Philadelphia, 1984

20. Hitchcock HH: Painful shoulder: observation on role of tendon of long head of biceps brachii in its causation. J Bone Joint Surg 30A:263, 1948

21. Petersson CJ: Spontaneous medial dislocation of the long head of the biceps brachii: an anatomic study of prevalence and pathomechanics. Clin Orthop 211:224, 1986

22. Neer CS: Impingement lesions. Clin Orthop 173:70, 1983

23. Saha AK: Dynamic stability of the glenohumeral joint. Acta Orthop Scand 42:491, 1971

24. Sarrafian SK: Gross and functional anatomy of the shoulder. Clin Orthop 173:11, 1983

25. Bearn JG: Direct observations on the function of the capsule of the sternoclavicular joint in clavicular support. J Anat 101:159, 1967

26. Cyriax EF: A second brief note on "floating clavicle". Anat Rec 52:97, 1932

27. DePalma AF: Degenerative Changes in the Sternoclavicular and Acromioclavicular Joints in Various Decades. Charles C. Thomas, Springfield, IL, 1957

28. Fukuda K, Graig EV, An K, Cofield RH et al: Biomechanical study of the ligamentous system of the acromioclavicular joint. J Bone Joint Surg 68A:434, 1986

29. Petersson CJ, Redlund-Johnell I: The subacromial space in normal shoulder radiographs. Acta Orthop Scand 55:57, 1984

30. Harryman DT, Sidles JA, Clark JM et al: Translation of the humeral head on the glenoid with passive glenohumeral motion. J Bone Joint Surg 72A:1334, 1990

31. Terry GC, Hammon D, France P, Norwood LA: The stabilizing function of passive shoulder restraints. Am J Sports Med 19:26, 1991

32. Williams PL, Warwick R, Dyson M, Bannister LH (eds): Gray's Anatomy. 36th ed. WB Saunders, Philadelphia, 1980

33. Cooper D, Warner JD, Deng X et al: Anatomy and function of the coracohumeral ligament. Presented at the Annual Meeting of the Society of American Shoulder and Elbow Surgeons, New Orleans, LA, 1990

34. Warner JP, Deng X, Warren RF et al: Static capsuloligamentous restraints to superior-inferior translation of the glenohumeral joint. Presented at the Annual Meeting of the Orthopaedic Research Society, Anaheim, CA, 1991

35. Paavolainen P, Bjorkenheim JM, Slatis P, Paukku P: Operative treatment of severe proximal humeral fractures. Acta Orthop Scand 54:374, 1983

36. Meyer AW: Spolia anatomica: absence of the tendon of the long head of the biceps. J Anat 48:133, 1914

37. Meyer AW: Spontaneous dislocation of the long head of the biceps brachii. Arch Surg 13:109, 1926

38. DePalma AF, Gallery G, Bennett GA: Variational anatomy and degenerative lesions of the shoulder bone. Instruction Course, Am Acad Orthop Surg 16:255, 1949

39. O'Brien SJ, Neves MC, Armoczky SP et al: The anatomy and histology of the inferior glenohumeral complex of the shoulder. Am J Sports Med 18:449, 1990

40. Bowen MK, Warren RF: Ligamentous control of shoulder stability. Clin Sports Med 10:757, 1991

41. Warren RF, Komblatt IB, Marchand R: Static factors affecting posterior shoulder stability. Orthop Trans 8:89, 1984

42. O'Connell PW, Nuber JW, Milekis RA, Lautenschlager E: The contribution of the glenohumeral ligaments to anterior stability of the shoulder joint. Am J Sports Med 18:579, 1990

43. Schwartz RE, O'Brien SJ, Warren RF et al: Capsular restraints to anterior-posterior motion of the abducted shoulder: a biomechanical study. Orthop Trans 12:727, 1988

44. Oversen JM, Nielsen S: Anterior and posterior instability. Acta Orthop Scan 57:324, 1986

45. Oversen J, Nielsen S: Posterior instability of the shoulder: a cadaver study. Acta Orthop Scand 57:436, 1986

46. Atwater AE: Biomechanics of overarm throwing movements and of throwing injuries. Exer Sports Sci Rev 7:43, 1979

47. Beaton LE, Anson BJ: Variations of the origin of the m. tarpezius. Anat Resc 83:41, 1942

48. Inman VT, Saunders JB de CM, Abbott LC: Observations on the function of the shoulder joint. J Bone Joint Surg 26:1, 1944

49. Horan FT, Bonafede RP: Bilateral absence of the trapezius and sternal head of the pectoralis major muscles: a case report. J Bone Joint Surg 59A:133, 1977

50. Dewar FP, Harris RI: Restoration of function of the shoulder following paralysis of the trapezius by fascial sling fixation and transplantation of the levator scapulae. Ann Surg 132:111, 1950

51. Salmon J, Dor J: Les arteres des muscles des membres et da tronc. Paris Masson et Cie (Librairie de L'academie de medecine), 1933

52. Perry J: Biomechanics of the shoulder. p. 3. In Rowe C (ed): The Shoulder. Churchill Livingstone, New York, 1988

53. Estwanik JJ: Levator scapulae syndrome. Phys Sports Med 17:57, 1989

54. Scheving LE, Pauly JE: An electromyographic study of some muscles acting on the upper extremity in man. Anat Rec 135:239, 1959

55. Nuber GW, Jobe FW, Perry J et al: Fine wire electromyography analysis of muscles of the shoulder during swimming. Am J Sports Med 14:7, 1988

56. Horwitz MT, Tocantins LM: Isolated paralysis of the serratus anterior (magnus) muscle. J Bone Joint Surg 20A:720, 1938

57. Hollinshead WH, Jenkins DB: Functional Anatomy of the Limbs and Back. 5th Ed. WB Saunders, Philadelphia, 1981

58. Jobe FW, Tibone JE, Moynes DR et al: An EMG analysis of the shoulder in pitching and throwing: a preliminary report. Am J Sports Med 11:3, 1983

59. Jobe FW, Moynes DR, Tibone JE et al: An EMG analysis of the shoulder in pitching: a second report. Am J Sports Med 12:218, 1984

60. Colachis CS, Jr, Strohm BR, Brecher VL: Effects of axillary nerve block on muscle force in the upper extremity. Arch Phys Med Rehabil 50:645, 1969

61. Turkel SJ, Pamio MW, Marshall JL, Girgis FG: Stabilizing mechanisms preventing anterior dislocation of the glenohumeral joint. J Bone Joint Surg 63A:1208, 1981

62. Gowan ID, Jobe FW, Tibone JE et al: A comparative electromyographic analysis of the shoulder during pitching: professional versus amateur pitchers. Am J Sports Med 15:586, 1987

63. Belle RM, Hawkins RJ: Dynamic electromyographic analysis of the shoulder muscles during rotational and scapular strengthening exercises. In Post M, Morrey BF, Hawkins RS (eds): Surgery of the Shoulder. CV Mosby, St. Louis, 1990

64. Broome HL, Basmajian JV: The function of the teres major muscle: an electromyographic study. Anat Rec 170:309, 1971

65. Jobe CM: Gross anatomy of the shoulder. p. 34. In Rockwood CA, Matsen FA (eds): The Shoulder. Vol. 1. WB Saunders, Philadelphia, 1990

66. Glousman R, Jobe FW, Tibone JE et al: Dynamic electromyographic analysis of the throwing shoulder with glenohumeral instability. J Bone Joint Surg 70A:220, 1988

67. Glousman R, Jobe F, Tibone J et al: Dynamic EMG analysis of the throwing shoulder with glenohumeral instability. J Bone Joint Surg 70A:220, 1988

68. Burkhead WZ: The biceps tendon. p. 791. In Rockwood CA, Matsen FA (eds): The Shoulder. Vol. 2. WB Saunders, Philadelphia, 1990

69. Paavolainen P, Slatis P, Alto K: Surgical pathology in chronic shoulder pain. p. 313. In Bateman JE, Welsh RP (eds): Surgery of the Shoulder. BC Decker, Philadelphia, 1984

70. Watterson PA, Taylor GI, Crock JG: The venous territories of muscles: anatomical study and clinical implications. Br J Plast Surg 41:569, 1988

71. Taylor GI, Palmer JH: The vascular territories (an-

giosomes) of the body: experimental study and clinical implications. Br J Plast Surg 40:113, 1987

72. Rathbun JB, Macnab I: The microvascular pattern of the rotator cuff. J bone Joint Surg 52B:540, 1970

73. Keele CA, Neil E (eds): Samson Wright's Applied Physiology. 12th Ed. Oxford University Press, London, 1971

74. Ferretti A, Cerullo G, Russo G: Suprascapular neuropathy in volleyball players. J Bone Joint Surg 69A:260, 1987

75. Mestdagh H, Drizenko A, Ghesten P: Anatomical basis of suprascapular nerve syndrome. Anat Clin 3:67, 1981

76. Drez D: Suprascapular neuropathy in the differential diagnosis of rotator cuff injuries. Am J Sports Med 4:43, 1976

77. Bryan WJ, Wild JJ: Isolated infraspinatus atrophy: a common cause of posterior shoulder pain and weakness in throwing athletes? Am J Sports Med 14:113, 1976

78. Zoltan JD: Injury to the suprascapular nerve associated with anterior dislocation of the shoulder: case report and review of the literature. J Trauma 19:203, 1979

79. Blom S, Dahlback LO: Nerve injuries in dislocations of the shoulder joint and fractures of the neck of the humerus. Acta Chir Scand 136:461, 1970

80. Pasila M, Jarona H, Kiviluto O et al: Early complications of primary shoulder dislocations. Acta Orthop Scand 40: 260, 1978

81. Berry H, Bril V: Axillary nerve trauma following blunt trauma to the shoulder: a clinical and electrophysiological review. J Neurol Neurosurg Psychiatry 45:1027, 1982

82. Leffer RD, Seddon H: Infraclavicular brachial plexus injuries. J Bone Joint Surg 47B:9, 1965

83. Bateman JE: Nerve injuries about the shoulder in sports. J Bone Joint Surg 49A:785, 1967

84. Dempster WT: Mechanisms of shoulder movement. Arch Phys Med Rehabil 1:49, 1965

85. McKinn RMH: Last's Anatomy: Regional and Applied. 8th Ed. Churchill Livingstone, Edinburgh, 1990

86. Hertling D, Kessler RM: Management of Common Musculoskeletal Disorders: Physical Therapy Principles and Methods. Harper & Row, Philadelphia, 1990

87. Jobe CM: Gross anatomy of the shoulder. p. 44. In Rockwood CA, Matsen FA (eds): The Shoulder. Vol. 1. WB Saunders, Philadelphia, 1990

88. Hurley JA: Anatomy of the shoulder. p. 27. In Nicholas JA, Hershman EB (eds): The Upper Extremity in Sports Medicine. CV Mosby, St. Louis, 1990

89. Tullos HS, Bennett JB: The shoulder in sports. p. 111. In Scott WN, Nisonson B, Nicholas JA (eds): Principles of Sports Medicine. Williams & Wilkins, Baltimore, 1984

90. Brunet ME, Haddad RJ, Porche EB: Rotator cuff impingement syndrome in sports. Phys Sports Med 10:87, 1982

91. Skybar MJ, Warren AF, Altchek DW: Instability of the shoulder. p. 181. In Nicholas JA, Hershman EB (eds): The

Upper Extremity in Sports Medicine. CV Mosby, St. Louis, 1990

92. Travell JG, Simons DG: Myofascial Pain and Dysfunction: The Trigger Point Manual. Williams & Wilkins, Baltimore, 1983

93. Reid D: Sports Injury Assessment and Rehabilitation. Churchill Livingstone, New York, 1992

94. Hershman EB: Brachial plexus injuries. Clin Sports Med 9:313, 1990

2

General Biomechanics

THOMAS A. SOUZA

When discussing the biomechanics of any single part of the body it becomes clear that all models can, at best, determine a limited, and more importantly, isolated concept of function. Descriptions usually include bone movement in relationship to another bone, joint movements (accessory), and muscle function related to a single joint.

In reality the body functions as a whole unit. Seemingly distant and unrelated dysfunction may be the cause or effect of dysfunction in the part being analyzed. Therefore, on an isolated basis, models of joint function appear clearer than actual function in vivo. An example of this isolationalist approach assumes that a muscle will function a particular way based on its location, size, length, etc. However, when analyzed in a functional group electromyographically, it becomes apparent that other factors come into play in the determination of body preference with muscle recruitment.[1] An example is the observation that the subscapularis, an internal rotator, contracts vigorously during attempts at external rotation (stabilizing).[2]

A currently unattainable goal would include the study of all muscular function during a given movement (no matter how isolated it may appear) to determine all the components of normal function. Video analysis is an early attempt at indirectly determining body positions through a given movement. However, it does not necessarily indicate which specific muscles are needed and the hierarchy of their recruitment.

LEVERAGE AND MECHANICAL ADVANTAGE

In order to create motion in the shoulder (as in other joints) a force is applied at the humerus to overcome a resistance that is equal to the weight of the arm plus any load added. The perpendicular distance from the line of action of force to the fulcrum is referred to as the moment arm or lever arm. Within a lever system there are two opposing forces: the effort force and the resistance. Each, as an applied force, forms a lever arm. A moment of force or torque is equal to the product of the length of this lever times the force applied (moment = force × distance). Therefore a change in either force or distance (length of lever arm) requires a change in the other component to maintain an equilibrium.

A lever system includes three components: (1) fulcrum or axis of rotation, (2) a resistance force, and (3) an effort force to overcome the resistance load. This interaction takes place through a rigid (or somewhat rigid) lever arm (bone). The lever arm created by a resistance load is referred to as the resistance arm. The lever arm created by the effort load is referred to as the force arm.[3]

The mechanical efficiency of a system is based on a ratio between these two lever arms. In other words, to be mechanically efficient in sustaining or moving a resistance the load arm should be equal to or longer than the resistance arm (Fig. 2-1). Yet there are factors other than strength that constitute efficiency. Most joints in the body are class 3 levers, meaning that the point of force application is between the fulcrum and the resistance load (Fig. 2-2). This is not very efficient for strength purposes yet provides a lever that increases linear velocity. The linear velocity of an object at the end of a lever is equal to the product of the lever's length and angular velocity. This becomes obvious when swinging a tennis racket or throwing a ball. The trade-off is that more force is needed due to the increase in the resistance load and/or length of the lever arm.

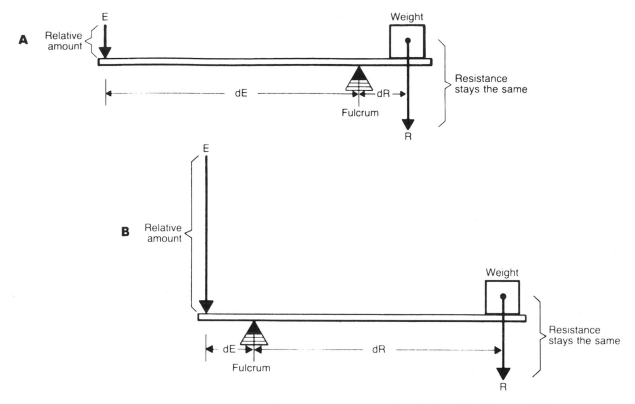

Fig. 2-1. Moment of force and mechanical advantage *(MA)* demonstrated with effort *(E)*, effort arm *(dE)*, resistance *(R)*, and resistance arm *(dR)*. **(A)** *MA* > 1; **(B)** *MA* < 1. (From Leveau,[62] with permission.)

Several factors affect the length of lever arms, including (1) the position of the arm: global position (e.g., flexed, extended, rotated), whether the elbow is flexed or extended, the position of the body (e.g., lateral flexion of the trunk); (2) the insertion point of muscles into the level arm (bone); and (3) the point and magnitude of resistance force application (e.g., tennis racket, shot put, baseball, dumbbells)

CENTER OF GRAVITY

Gravity acts on the arm at a point where weight on either side of this point is essentially equal. This is the center of gravity. The center of gravity location for the extended arm is 43 percent distal to the shoulder joint[4] and remains unchanged as the arm is raised. The reason it is not in the center of the segment is because the proximal portion of each segment generally contains more musculature.

The center of gravity is a fixed point when the arm is in a position other than vertical. However, the distance of the line perpendicular to the line of force to the fulcrum increases (as does the resistance) as the arm is raised to 90 degrees. It then decreases beyond this point.

With the arm outstretched (the elbow extended) one may view the demand torque as equal to the sum of the torques produced at several segments: the humerus, forearm, and wrist (Fig. 2-3). In this way, any change in the position of the arm (in particular elbow flexion) will alter the relationship of each center of gravity to the axis point (shoulder joint). This changes the functional lever arm with a concomitant increase or decrease in demand torque. For example, when the shoulder is at 90 degrees abduction, elbow flexion of 90 degrees moves the center of gravity of the forearm and wrist forward to the level of the elbow. This effectively decreases the total demand torque of the arm 22 percent.[4] Elbow flexion introduces an internal

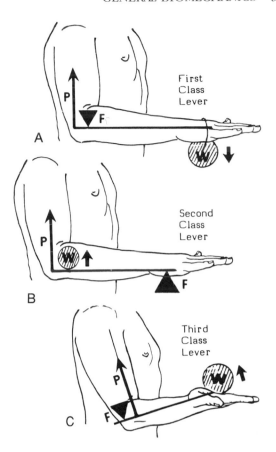

Fig. 2-2. Mechanical arrangement of bones as levers and muscles as sources of power. *P,* power; *W,* weight; *F,* fulcrum; *arrow,* direction of movement. **(A)** The arm is used as a first-class lever in pressing weight downward, with the triceps serving as the power source. **(B)** The arm is used as a second-class lever in elevating the body as in doing push-ups, with the triceps serving as the source of negative power. **(C)** The arm is used as a third-class lever in lifting a weight vertically, with the biceps serving as the source of power. (From Schafer,[63] with permission.)

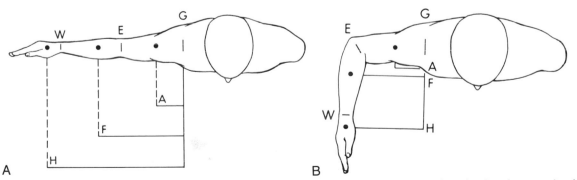

Fig. 2-3. Shoulder torque variations with arm alignment. **(A)** Elbow extended. Lever length of each more distal segment is progressively increased. *G,* glenohumeral joint axis; *E,* elbow; *W,* wrist; *dot,* mass center of that bony segment; *A,* upper arm mass center lever length; *F,* forearm mass center level length; *H,* hand mass center level length. **(B)** Elbow flexed 90 degrees. Upper arm level length is unchanged. The forearm and hand masses center levers are now equal to the length of the humerus. Forearm and hand masses also are anterior to the shoulder joint axis. (From Perry,[5] with permission.)

torque due to its anterior position in relation to the humeral axis. This demonstrates that any change of position for the benefit of mechanical efficiency shifts demands to other supportive structures.[5]

This simple system is not what occurs in the body. There are many forces acting on a body segment including several effort forces and occasionally more than one resistance force. Further, the forces are not always acting perpendicular to the lever arm. Muscle insertions are often not centered and so introduce a rotational torque. At the fulcrum (in this case the shoulder joint) there is also a joint reaction force. This is equal to the sum of component forces acting on the levers.

JOINT REACTION FORCE

When the arm is abducted 90 degrees and externally rotated the joint reaction force is equal to the compressive force, the anterior shear, and inferior shear forces created by the contraction of the muscles resisting gravity. The resultant of these forces is directed 12 degrees anteriorly requiring restraint by the anterior capsule and muscles (primarily the subscapularis) (Fig. 2-4 to 2-6). With extension of the arm added to this position even more anterior shear is added with an increase in the demand of anterior restraint.[6]

The tensile strength of the anterior capsular structures is estimated to be less than 20 kg.[6] Unfortunately the anterior shear force may reach between and 40 to 60 kg with contraction of shoulder musculature.[7]

MUSCULAR EFFECTS

The effectiveness of the shoulder musculature on positioning the arm, moving a hand-held load, and accelerating a load is dependent on the mechanical efficiency of its inherent design. Muscularly several factors enter into this equation:

1. Muscle type
2. Fiber orientation

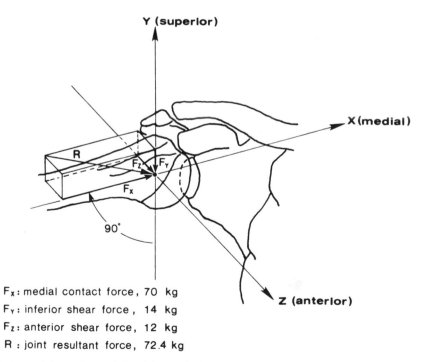

F_X: medial contact force, 70 kg
F_Y: inferior shear force, 14 kg
F_Z: anterior shear force, 12 kg
R : joint resultant force, 72.4 kg

Fig. 2-4. Equilibrium of the unloaded shoulder with the arm at 90 degrees abduction and 90 degrees external rotation. Note that there are inferior and anterior shearing forces. The anterior shear force is the key factor contributing to the anterior dislocation of the shoulder. (From Morey and Chao,[7] with permission.)

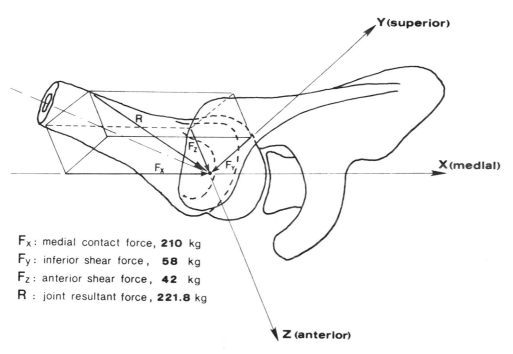

F_X: medial contact force, **210** kg
F_Y: inferior shear force, **58** kg
F_Z: anterior shear force, **42** kg
R : joint resultant force, **221.8** kg

Fig. 2-5. With the shoulder abducted 90 degrees, externally rotated 90 degrees, and extended 30 degrees, and with the intrinsic muscles maximally contracting, significant anterior shear force is produced, which may exceed the tensile strength of the capsule structure. This is believed to be the most frequent cause of anterior dislocation. (From Morey and Chao,[7] with permission.)

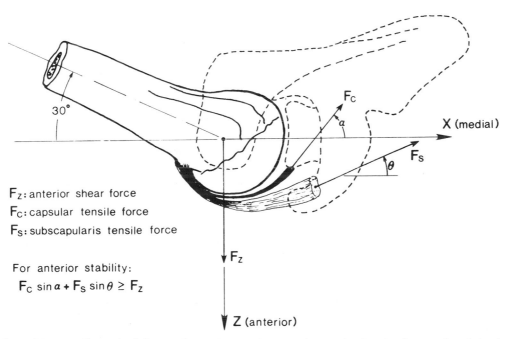

F_z: anterior shear force
F_c: capsular tensile force
F_s: subscapularis tensile force

For anterior stability:
$$F_C \sin \alpha + F_S \sin \theta \geq F_Z$$

Fig. 2-6. With externally applied forces, the static anterior capsular mechanism is disrupted and the humeral head dislocates. In order to prevent such a lesion, the vertical component of F_c (capsular force) and F_s (subscapularis tension) must be greater than or equal to the anterior shear force, F_z. (From Morey and Chao,[7] with permission.)

41

3. Muscle size
4. Length of the fibers
5. Type of contraction
6. Speed (with concentric)
7. Lever length (a function of position) and type

If a muscle is primarily made up of type I slow twitch (ST) fibers it will have a tendency to maintain long sustained contractions (posture) with relatively slow fatigue and a high oxidative capacity.[8] Part of smaller motor units, ST fibers are innervated by highly active motor neurons that fire at low frequencies. The conduction time is relatively slow. Type II or fast twitch (FT) fibers are the opposite. They are designed for fast contraction innervated by motor neurons that are more "purpose demand" activated, firing at high frequencies with short conduction time. Their fatigue rate is much quicker. Usually they are part of larger motor units indicating a more precise function result.

Further design criteria include the orientation of muscle fibers. Longitudinal fibers allow for maximum

shortening resulting in greater speed. Oblique fiber orientation is a design for strength (Fig. 2-7). This oblique angulation allows a greater number of muscle cells to be included in a given space. The amount of maximum force generated by a muscle is, in fact, determined by the number of motor cells contained. A measure of a muscle's physiologic cross-section is used for this determination.[9] With longitudinal fibers an anatomic transverse section is all that is needed and is relatively accurate. The difficulty arises in evaluating pennate muscle fibers that angle toward a central insertion point. A very detailed dissection must be done to count several bundles in order to estimate indirectly the perpendicular areas of all the fibers. Other approaches include computed tomography (CT) with the use of transverse sections.[10] From a clinical point of view it becomes obvious that larger muscles such as the pectorals and the latissimus are able to generate more force than smaller muscles such as the rotator cuff. The difficulty arises in trying to determine differences between muscles that are apparently closer in

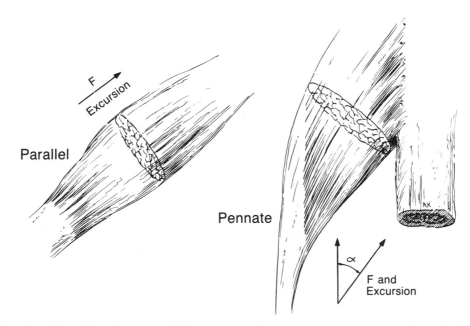

Fig. 2-7. Muscles whose fibers have a parallel arrangement have maximum excursion and speed of contractility, as both force and excursion are parallel to the long axis of the muscle. In a pennate arrangement, multiple numbers of fibers with shorter length can be stacked to obtain a greater cross-sectional area. Not all of this strength is in the desired direction, nor is excursion. The effective force and excursion are projections of these vectors on the described directions, the magnitudes of which are products of the cosine of the angle times the excursion or force magnitude. (From Jobe,[64] with permission.)

GENERAL BIOMECHANICS 43

size or making the assumption that larger muscles functionally participate more to a movement than a smaller agonist. For example, the serratus anterior and trapezius are of equal size, but their participation is far from equal.[11]

The type of contraction required for a muscle may affect its force capabilities. With isotonic contractions there is a distinct favorability for the eccentric phase (contraction with lengthening). This is due to two major factors: the advantage of passive tension and the lack of effect by speed of contraction. Passive tension can increase the efficiency of a muscle from 13 to 20 percent.[12] Concentric (shortening while contracting) contractions are decreased as much as 50 percent with speeds of 214 degrees/s.[13] Another asset of eccentric contraction is most evident during the end of cocking and beginning of acceleration, while throwing a ball, when a plyometric event occurs. The eccentrically contracting anterior musculature aids the following concentric contraction through prestretch and usage of elastic energy.

The position of a muscle relative to a joint can affect the fiber length and the lever length. There is a point referred to as the resting length, which represents the best connection or bonding between actin and myosin.[5] This is apparently at 90 percent of its maximum length.[14,15] Either an increase or a decrease in this length may result in a decrease in available force. Arm elevation is an example of how joint position may change the insertion point of pull from below to above

the center of rotation. Interestingly, this point in relation to muscle length and distance from the fulcrum would continue to change in the shoulder except for the scapula, which maintains a relatively constant position between the muscle and the glenohumeral joint throughout this range.

When a muscle contracts it creates a force at both its sites of attachment and at the joint across which it works. When this force is directed parallel to the joint it causes a shear stress. If, however, it is more perpendicular to the plane of the joint (glenoid) it creates a compressive force.[16,17] Shear forces have a tendency to create instability and degeneration. If the shear force is not neutralized by either the compressive forces of the inherent muscles or other muscles, strain will occur to both dynamic and static stabilizing structures. In general, compressive forces provide both stability and aid in diffusion of nutrients for the articular cartilage of the joint.

The major muscles involved in this equilibrium for the shoulder are the deltoid and rotator cuff.[13] Because of their relative oblique orientation to the shoulder, each has a component of shear and compressive force with contraction. This relationship changes with arm position, changing the relative pull of the muscle resulting in either an increase or decrease in either component.

The rotator cuff group, in general, pulls mainly horizontal and downward with a strong ratio of compression over shear. The deltoid's angle of pull initially

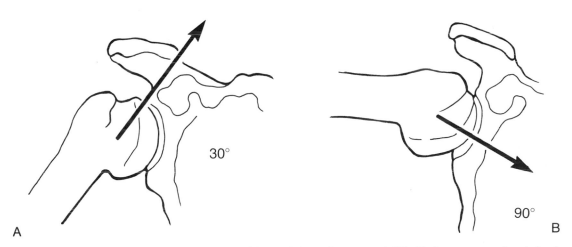

Fig. 2-8. Direction of the joint forces with shoulder in **(A)** 30 degrees and **(B)** 90 degrees scapular abduction. (From Perry,[5] with permission.)

is quite vertical and results in a shear dominance. As elevation progresses above 60 degrees, compression becomes dominant. Combined muscle function establishes stability with a maximum at 90 degrees (Fig. 2-8). Maximum shear is at 60 degrees.[5] It is interesting to note that the position of maximum stability is unfortunately a position most associated with impingement.[18]

This scenario is a simple description of elevation without either a component of flexion or extension in the horizontal plane included. However, many positions such as those found in throwing require horizontal extension. In the late phase of cocking, the position of external rotation, abduction, and horizontal extension may change the angulation of the external rotators (infraspinatus/teres minor) to increase the anterior shear force assisting in a tendency toward anterior dislocation or subluxation. This tendency must be neutralized by the effect of anterior capsular structures and the subscapularis muscle/tendon.

OSTEOKINEMATICS

In the past, movement of a body part was described in reference to the long axis of the moving bone. Terms such as angular movement (decrease or increase in the angle between bones), circumduction, rotation, and sliding were used. These descriptions are not very helpful in illustrating realistic movement between bones and at the joint. MacConaill and Basmajian[19] introduced a new concept of description that allows a separation in analysis between movement that is bone on bone and movement at the joint.

Movement between bones is more easily defined through a reference point, a mechanical axis of movement. This axis is a line drawn through the moving bone, through the center of movement on the opposing surface and perpendicular to that surface. Rotation about this axis is referred to as *spin*. All other movement is regarded as *swing*. Swing is further subdivided into (1) pure or cardinal swing, and (2) impure or

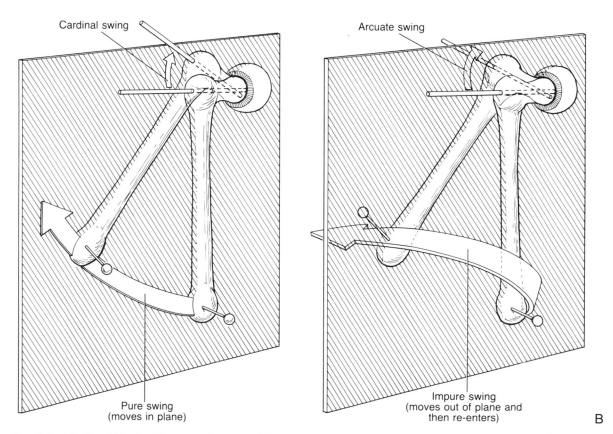

Fig. 2-9. MacConaill's classification of swing: **(A)** pure swing; **(B)** arcuate swing. (From Barak et al.,[65] with permission.)

arcuate swing. Pure swing occurs when movement does not involve any concurrent spin (rotation). A line drawn between the starting and final positions equals the shortest distance between these points. Impure swing includes simultaneous spin (rotation) with another movement. An arc of movement usually occurs with movement from one to point another; therefore, the distance between two points of movement is greater than with pure swing (Fig. 2-9).

Using these principles of description, rotation of the humerus with the arm at the side finds the mechanical axis of the joint not perpendicular to the long axis of the humerus. Therefore, even though rotation is occurring it is not spin but swing. For spin to occur the shoulder would have to be abducted 90 degrees so that the mechanical axis coincides with the long axis of the humerus. Then internal and external rotation would represent spin.

An impure swing occurs where both swing and rotation occur simultaneously. This type of rotation is referred to as conjunct rotation. Pure swing is possible if the angulation anteriorly is neutralized by abduction in the plane of the scapula. This has been designated as between 30 and 40 degrees anterior to the coronal plane.[20] In this position no relative rotation occurs. It is interesting that this is often the position that is strongest in function. Patients with shoulder pain often seek this position for accomplishing elevation.[5]

Clinically, conjunct rotation is important because as it occurs a twisting of the capsule results. In the resting position (arm at the side) the capsule is oriented lateral and inferior with a medial twist. As abduction progresses to 90 degrees (other than in the scapular plane), the twisting increases. This twisting will result in a "locking" of the joint unless an opposite conjunct rotation occurs. In order for the humerus to attain full elevation, external rotation must occur untwisting the joint capsule.

ARTHROKINEMATICS

MacConaill and Basamajian[19] have also described patterns of accessory movement (movement that is involuntary, occurring between joint surfaces). These movements include spin, glide (slide), and roll. Spin, similar to osteokinematic spin, involves movement around a stationary mechanical axis. When one point on a surface comes into contact with new points on another

surface, slide or glide occurs. Roll occurs when new points on one joint surface come into contact with new points on another joint surface. Roll would tend to occur in joints that are not congruent, often with a convex surface moving on a concave surface like the shoulder. However, this theoretic construct does not hold true for the shoulder. Radiographic evidence suggests that very little roll occurs with shoulder movement.[21] Some roll occurs at the beginning of movement as a stabilizing attempt. However, movement beyond this point is primarily glide because the center of contact with the glenoid remains relatively stationary. These principles, then, may be more applicable to passive movement than to active movement of the shoulder.

In reality movement in most joints is a combination of rolling and gliding. Often the initiation of movement involves rolling (e.g., the knee) followed by gliding.[22] Muscular dysfunction, instability, or bony pathology may result in an increase or decrease of the rolling or gliding component. This is inherently dangerous to the joint. As rolling progresses it places a stretch demand on the capsular/ligamentous restraint of the joint leading to further damage such as dislocation or fracture. An excess of the sliding component may result in capsular or ligamentous sprains or strains of muscles used to accommodate for capsular/ligamentous laxity.

There is a relationship between joint surfaces that may have clinical impact for anyone involved with manual therapy. This is the convex/concave rule that states that when a convex surface moves on a stationary concave surface, gliding occurs in the opposite direction of bone movement.[19] Applicability in the shoulder relative to hypomobility occurs when trying to increase range of motion while passively moving the humerus (Fig. 2-10). A caudal glide should be imposed as the humerus is lifted into abduction. The opposite is true for concave surfaces moving on a stationary convex surface where the glide is in the same direction of bone movement. It is important to realize that these are not voluntary functional movements of the humerus but acquired passively to help aid in normal function.

Another important concept regarding normal biomechanics and the biomechanics of injury is the close-packed/open-packed position.[19] Each joint has a position where it is maximally congruent. Partially this is due to the bony fit of the joint. In addition, a soft tissue component is added by movement. This movement

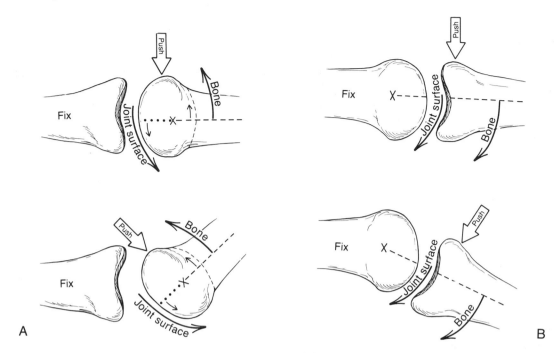

Fig. 2-10. **(A)** Convex surface moving on concave surface. **(B)** Concave surface moving on convex surface with a combination of roll, spin, and glide occurring in both simultaneously. (From Barak et al.,[65] with permission.).

involves an impure swing with conjunct rotation. This movement tightens the capsule and ligaments of the joint causing compression of the joint surfaces and adding to the inherent stability (or inflexibility). The close-packed position for the shoulder is abduction with external rotation.

In addition to stability it has been postulated that alternating in and out of a close-packed position may, in fact, be necessary for proper nutrition and lubrication of the articular cartilage. This pumping effect may aid in the diffusion of nutrients and fluid, "squeezing" out synovial fluid.[19] In other words a certain amount of joint compression force is necessary for a healthy joint as long as it alternates with noncompressive intervals and does not include significant shear force. Most common joint movements involve alternation between close-packed and loose-packed positions. Immobilized joints lack this normal process and may develop articular cartilage changes as a result.[23,24]

A loose-packed position is an incongruent position that allows a certain amount of joint play. The ligaments and capsule are essentially untensed. This is the functional position where movement is allowed to occur.

In these positions an examiner may test for any restrictions in accessory movements that are necessary for nonpathologic motion to occur. Arthrokinetic movements of roll and glide are assessed using the convex/concave rule. If, for example, the joint has lost some accessory movement, the joint will theoretically reach the close-packed position earlier than normal, causing undue compression and restriction of further movement. Further, the loose-packed position is the maximum position for accommodation of intra-articular swelling. Therefore, each joint will assume a loose-packed position when pressure buildup occurs inside the joint.

If the close-packed position is maintained at the time of an injury, dislocation or fracture is likely. Loose-packed injury positions usually result in sprains of the capsule and ligaments.

STATIC STABILITY

Primary passive restraint in the shoulder is provided by the glenohumeral ligaments, the posterior capsule, and the coracohumeral ligaments.[25] Tension on the capsule is created, statically and dynamically, by position due to the blended insertions of the rotator cuff musculature with the capsule. The various components of this system share responsibility with transference of tension not only to specific aspects of the capsule but to specific divisions of each section.[25]

In vitro studies have produced interesting results; however, it must be remembered that dynamic muscular contribution was not one of the analyzed components.[25,26] It is true, though, that these strain gauge measurements correlate well with electromyographic evidence.[27] The coracohumeral ligament restricts and protects flexion and extension of the shoulder, mainly because of its coronal orientation. When coupled with rotation, tension is partially transferred to the capsule. Internal rotation stresses mainly the middle and inferior sections of the posterior capsule while external rotation stresses primarily the middle and inferior sections of the anterior glenohumeral ligament. Comparatively, while the strain is shared in these coupled movements, flexion with internal rotation only mildly reduces the tension in the anterior coracohumeral ligament from 67 to 53 percent while flexion with external rotation reduces this tension considerably from 67 to 18 percent.[25]

The anterior glenohumeral ligament has been divided into three divisions: superior, middle, and inferior. As a whole unit the anterior glenohumeral ligament tenses with external rotation, extension, and abduction or a combination of any of these positions. The superior section supports the arm in the resting neutral position with decreasing contribution as the arm is elevated. The superior section is also tightened with the coupled movement of extension and internal rotation. The middle glenohumeral ligament provides support with the superior section in the resting position. Its contribution continues through about 45 degrees of elevation with a decreasing contribution past 90 degrees.[26] The coupled movement pattern that creates the most tension is flexion with external rotation. The inferior glenohumeral ligament is without tension in the resting position. However, past 90 degrees it is the main stabilizer. The greatest tension is developed in the inferior glenohumeral ligament with the coupled movement of extension, abduction, and external rotation (the cocking position for throwing). This position creates a shared responsibility with the anterior coracohumeral ligament. Figures 2-11 to 2-17 illustrate

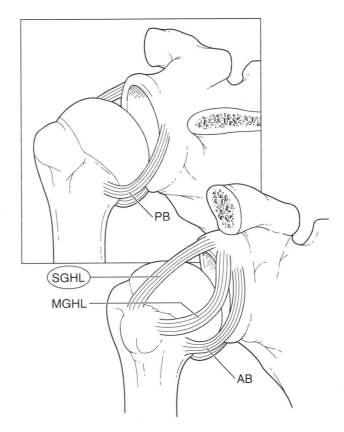

Fig. 2-11. Diagram of the functional anatomy of an adducted shoulder in neutral rotation. The superior glenohumeral ligament *(SGHL)* is the primary restraint to inferior translation. The anterior and posterior bands of the inferior glenohumeral ligament *(AIGHL* and *PIGHL)* play a lesser role. *PB,* posterior band; *AB,* anterior band; *MGHL,* middle glenohumeral ligament. (Adapted from Bowen and Warren,[66] with permission.)

the reciprocal actions of the inferior glenohumeral ligament with varying degrees of abduction coupled with internal and external rotation.

The posterior capsule is tightened with flexion, abduction, and internal rotation or a combination of these movements. Similar to the anterior capsule the posterior is divided into three divisions: superior, middle, and inferior. The superior and middle segments are tightened with internal rotation. The inferior section is tightened with abduction or a combination of abduction and internal rotation.[25]

Another aspect of capsular tightening has recently been discovered. Harryman et al.[28] have demonstrated

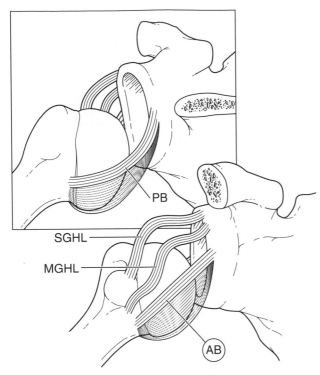

Fig. 2-12. Capsular tension at 45 degrees abduction; neutral rotation. (Adapted from Bowen and Warren,[66] with permission.)

that end-range tightening produces humeral head movement opposite to the section of the capsule that tightens. This movement is a matter of millimeters, however, and is considered functionally significant. For example, flexion produced anterior movement due to tightening of the posterior capsule. Operative tightening of the posterior capsule increased significantly the anterior and superior movement of the humeral head. Extension caused posterior movement due to tightening of the anterior capsule. These are important clinical considerations for the manipulative therapist, chiropractor, and surgeon.

Other contributions to static stability are less effective. They include (1) bony articulation (e.g., glenoid version, anteversion/retroversion), (2) glenoid labrum, and (3) negative pressure within the joint.

Bony Articulation

The glenohumeral joint is inherently unstable. With only a 25 to 30 percent glenoid contact with the humeral head, little stability is evident.[20] Some have sug-

gested a relationship to instability based on a variable humeral contact referred to as the glenohumeral index. This is calculated by dividing the maximum diameter of the glenoid by the maximum diameter of the humeral head. Saha has calculated this to be an average ratio of 0.75 in the sagittal plane and 0.6 in the transverse plane.[30] Others have found similar values.[31] Currently there appears to be no solid clinical or research evidence to suggest a major role by this factor, due partially to the minimal contribution in the average individual and the lack of noticeable extremes of this ratio.

Glenoid Labrum

The glenoid labrum functions to add stability to the glenohumeral joint. This is accomplished through deepening the socket and serving as an attachment site for the glenohumeral ligaments. The labrum is analagous to the knee meniscus in both type of injury and function. Like the meniscus, loss of labral integrity may

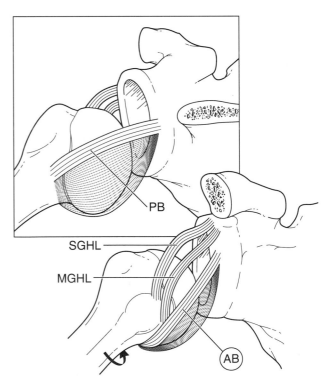

Fig. 2-13. Capsular tension at 45 degrees abduction; internal rotation. (Adapted from Bowen and Warren,[66] with permission.)

lead to instability and degenerative changes.[32,33] It will be interesting to see whether research indicates an important proprioceptive role for the labrum as it has for the meniscus and cruciates in the knee.[34]

The labrum has a varied presentation with individual shoulders. It may be quite thick or simply vestigial. Due to observations that the labrum flattens with certain movements (in particular external rotation) it is assumed that the labrum is in fact only an extension of the capsule (a source of added attachment).[35] However, Howell et al.[36] found a substantial structure with an average size of 9.0 mm superior to inferior and estimated anterior to posterior depth to be approximately 2.5 mm.[36] Currently it is not possible to determine the degree of contribution of this structure.

It appears that there are generally two mechanisms of injury common to the labrum. The first mechanism involves repetitive activity either in throwing activities such as pitching, tennis serves (in particular the deceleration phase), swimming, or weight training (bench

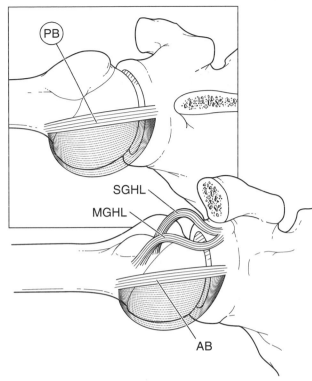

Fig. 2-15. Capsular tension at 90 degrees abduction; neutral rotation. (Adapted from Bowen and Warren,[66] with permission.)

and overhead presses).[37,38] The second mechanism involves direct trauma, which usually involves a fall on an outstretched arm or with the lead shoulder of a batter or golfer grounding the bat or club, respectively. Interestingly, there is disagreement as to whether the traumatic injury is due to entrapment between the humeral head and glenoid rim or due to a violent biceps contraction resulting in avulsion injury.

Damage associated with overhead sports appears to affect the upper labrum. The attachment of the long head of the biceps to the anterosuperior labrum is proposed as the site and etiology of injury. In an attempt to decelerate the rapidly extending elbow during the deceleration phase of throwing a strong eccentric contraction of the biceps may pull on the labral attachment. Andrews and Angelo[37] demonstrated that electrical stimulation of the biceps lifted the superior labrum off of the glenoid in some patients viewed arthroscopically. These tears are not usually associated with instability[39] and represent what Pappas et al.[40] refer to as "functional instability." Therefore, laxity

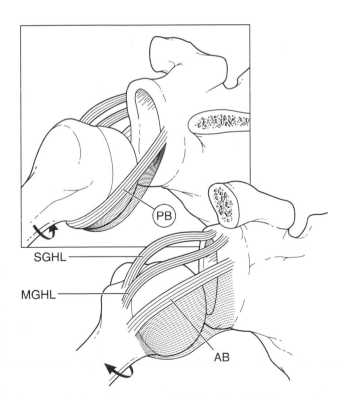

Fig. 2-14. Capsular tension at 45 degrees abduction; external rotation. (Adapted from Bowen and Warren,[66] with permission.)

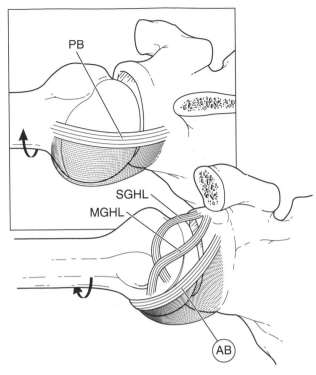

Fig. 2-16. Capsular tension at 90 degrees abduction; internal rotation. (Adapted from Bowen and Warren,[66] with permission.)

In addition, loss of labral integrity may remove a mechanical buttress to anterior translation similar to loss of anterior stability with lesions of the medial meniscus. This factor plays an important role in surgical decision making. If the labrum is resected, symptoms may initially be relieved, but with the creation of an unstable shoulder likely to become symptomatic in the future.

Negative Pressure

A negative pressure is apparently maintained in the glenohumeral joint. The degree of contribution has not been determined; however, given the lack of bony constraint coupled with minimal muscle activity in the resting position, it seems tenable that it may be significant. This was demonstrated by Kumar and Balasubramaniam.[42] If this negative pressure is interrupted by an arthrotomy or puncture, inferior subluxation of the humeral head occurs. The negative pressure effect may

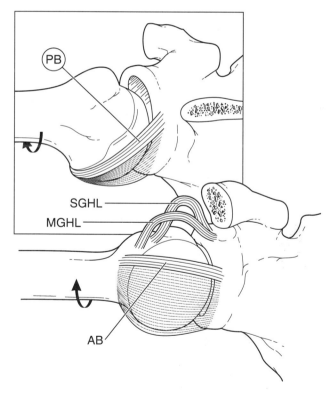

Fig. 2-17. Capsular tension at 90 degrees abduction; external rotation. (Adapted from Bowen and Warren,[66] with permission.)

may not be evident or reported by the athlete; however, signs of mechanical interference with normal motion are usually present. Glenoid labrum tears may then be present without instability, found mainly superiorly. Traumatic instability due to dislocation/subluxation usually involves damage to the labrum inferiorly.

Another mechanism for upper quadrant labrum tears is referred to as a superior labrum anterior and posterior (SLAP) lesion, with tearing extending anterior to posterior. It is proposed that an entrapment or compression occurs when an athlete falls on an outstretched arm as might occur with a player diving to catch a ball. This is in contrast to the avulsion type injury described by Andrews and Angelo.[37]

Damage to the inferior labrum is more associated with dislocation/subluxation. These tears or detachments in association with the glenohumeral ligament are often referred to as a Bankart lesion.[41] Functionally, this represents a loss of firm attachment for the anteroinferior glenohumeral ligament, which serves as the major restraint to anterior and inferior instability.

also explain the audible "pop" heard with shoulder adjustments.[43]

DYNAMIC STABILITY

In general, the rotator cuff musculature is responsible for the dynamic stability of the glenohumeral joint. There is a haziness in the use of dynamic because the simple presence of a muscle/tendon will statically provide stability in certain positions. Dynamically, though, muscles contribute to stability through contraction causing a compression force of the humeral head into the glenoid and contraction causing a tightening of the capsular insertions of the rotator cuff (the musculotendinous glenoid).

Stability is provided indirectly by the "nonrotator cuff" (scapular musculature). Through the combined effort of mainly the serratus anterior and upper trapezius an adaptive repositioning of the scapula occurs providing a stable base for humeral movement. This positioning also guarantees the proper lever length for the rotator cuff musculature.

SHOULDER MOVEMENT

Descriptions of shoulder movement vary consistently. Often this variation is due to an attempt to clarify some other description overlap. Normal movement patterns such as flexion/extension, internal/external rotation, and abduction/adduction are relatively standard in use. The one exception is the use of medial and lateral rotation as a substitute for internal and external rotation, respectively. The more common complication involves descriptions of horizontal movement of the shoulder. Horizontal movement anteriorly is referred to as either horizontal flexion or horizontal adduction (occasionally called anteversion). Movement posteriorly in the horizontal plane is referred to as either horizontal extension or horizontal abduction (occasionally called retroversion). If the subject is prone this same movement is called elevation in the horizontal plane.

The difficulty arises when trying also to describe scapular movement. Movement anterior and lateral is referred to as either abduction or protraction. Movement posterior and medial is referred to as either adduction or retraction.

The term *elevation* is commonly used as an umbrella term that includes either flexion, abduction, or a combination. As mentioned previously it is also used to describe movement into horizontal extension when the subject is lying prone.

A new descriptive term, *scaption,* has been introduced by Townsend et al.[1] The observation that abduction in the coronal plane is not in alignment with the orientation of the scapula (glenoid) has led many to specify elevation or abduction in the scapular plane as a description separate from abduction. This lengthy description has become cumbersome and led to the use of the term scaption, which combines the terms scapula with flexion (or elevation). Functionally, this position is significant and commonly recommended as the testing position of muscles rather than the straight coronal movement of abduction.[44]

Codman's Paradox

A source of confusion and discussion was observed by Codman[29] regarding rotational movement of the humerus. He noticed that when a movement other than rotation was performed by the humerus, an apparent rotation of the humerus still occurred when comparing the starting and ending positions (Figs. 2-18 and 2-19). For example, using the medial epicondyle as a reference point, if the arm is flexed 90 degrees and then horizontally extended into a 90 degree abducted position the medial epicondyle is pointing perpendicular to the coronal plane. When the arm is then lowered from this position to the resting position next to the side, the medial epicondyle indicates external rotation of the humerus has occurred even though the coupled sequential movements of flexion and horizontal abduction were the only movements involved.

The rotational aspect is, in part, due to the oblique orientation of the humerus with the glenoid. Movement must be in reference to the scapular plane; therefore, with any pure movement into flexion, abduction, etc. there is inherently a rotational component relative to the coronal plane.

Morrey and An[45] offer the explanation that rotation is sequence dependent and not additive. In other words, rotation about the x axis and then the y axis results in a different end position than rotation about

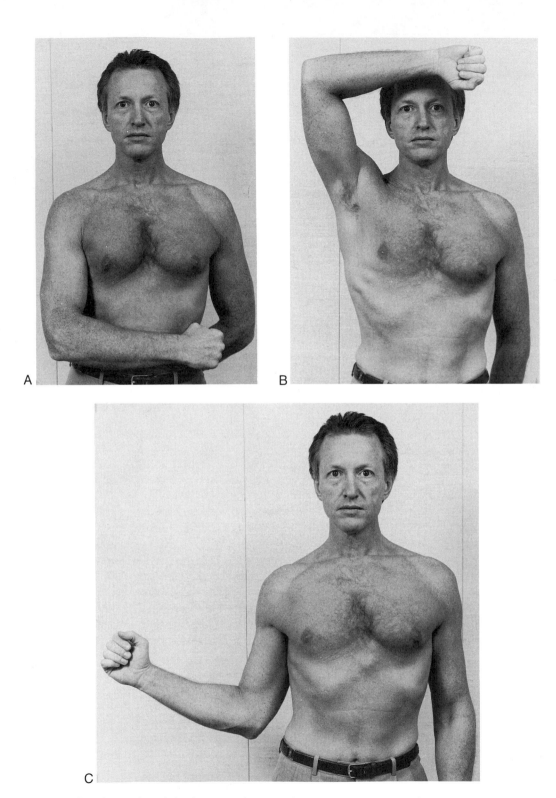

Fig. 2-18. Codman's paradox. **(A)** The patient's arm is by the side with internal rotation across the body. **(B)** The patient flexes the arm fully. **(C)** The patient lowers the arm to the side. Even though beginning in internal rotation, without any subsequent attempt at rotational movement, the final position finds the arm in external rotation.

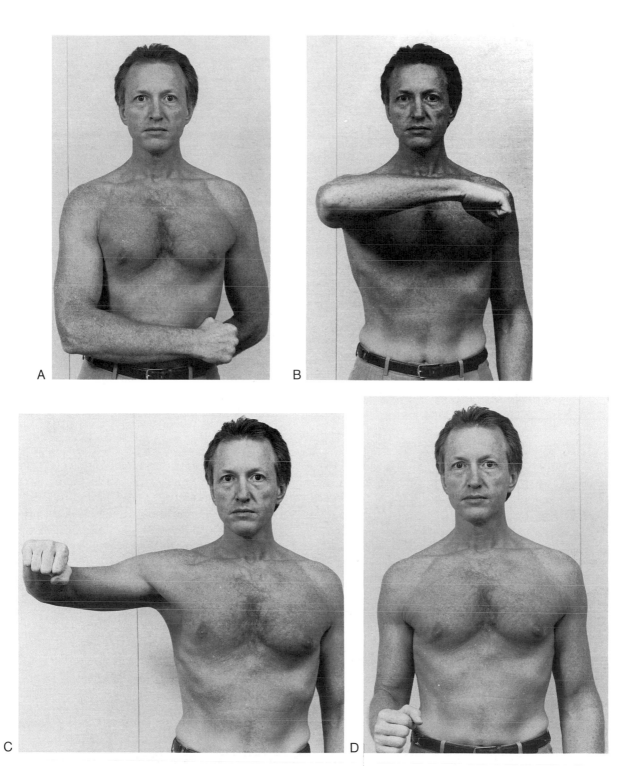

Fig. 2-19. Codman's paradox. **(A)** The patient begins again with the arm at the side in internal rotation. **(B)** The patient lifts (flexes) the arm to 90 degrees. **(C)** The patient then horizontally extends the arm. **(D)** The arm is lowered to the side. Although the initial position is with the arm in internal rotation, the final position finds the arm in neutral rotation without any attempt at rotation during the sequence of movement.

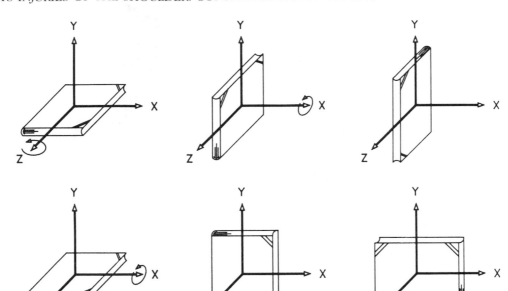

Fig. 2-20. Finite orientation is dependent on the sequence of serial rotations around the orthogonal axes. (From Morrey and An,[67] with permission.)

the x axis and then the z axis. Figure 2-20 demonstrates that even though rotation about the z and x axes occurs, the end position is different contingent upon which rotation occurs first.

Resting Position

Contrary to previous assumptions, the shoulder is not supported by its bony architecture.[5] The support in the resting position is essentially soft tissue and specifically capsular and ligamentous. Electromyographic analysis demonstrates no significant muscular activity with the unchallenged arm at rest.[46] If chronically loaded, ligamentous tension will eventually lead to ischemia, pain, and stretching. Relief occurs when intermittent muscle activity (usually involving movement) interrupts this tension.

When challenged by either a weight or tug, shoulder musculature responds preferentially.[30] The supraspinatus accompanied by weak posterior deltoid activity has been demonstrated electromyographically. Interestingly, no activity in the triceps, biceps, or middle deltoid was reported. Perry[5] suggests this isolated supraspinatus activity is directly tied to fiber orientation

giving the supraspinatus the greatest advantage. The deltoid has a similar angulation; however, isolated activity would result in more shear force and less compressive force. There should theoretically be either an increase of the supraspinatus and posterior deltoid activity or a recruitment of other musculature when inferior instability or a second/third degree sprain of the acromioclavicular joint is present. It would also be interesting to measure activity when there is a strong grip of the ipsilateral hand. The most common example is squeezing a tennis ball as an initial toning exercise for shoulder rehabilitation.

Walking on a treadmill demonstrates a continued role for the supraspinatus for stability. In addition, muscle recruitment becomes necessary for primary deceleration of forward and backward arm swing. The middle and posterior deltoid decelerates forward arm swing while the latissimus dorsi and teres major assist.

Shoulder Elevation

Shoulder elevation will first be considered because it represents the prototype movement of the shoulder in particular with sports. Elevation illustrates several salient features with regards to most shoulder movement:

1. Need for concomitant scapular movement for stabilization (Fig. 2-21).
2. Need for force-couple functioning of shoulder musculature.
3. Multiaxis and plane-of-motion components of many shoulder movements.
4. Interdependence of the sternoclavicular, acromioclavicular, scapulothoracic, and glenohumeral joints for full nonpathologic function of the shoulder.

The primary ingredients of elevation are humeral and scapular movement (Fig. 2-22). The relationship between the two has been approximated at 2:1 in favor of glenohumeral movement.[30] There is a variability of reported ratios from 2.5:1 to 1.25:1.[13] Doddy et al.[47] found the ratio to be 7:1 during the first 30 degrees. This indicates that there is little scapular movement initially. They felt the ratio was close to 1:1 from 90 to 150 degrees. Variations on this observation have oc-

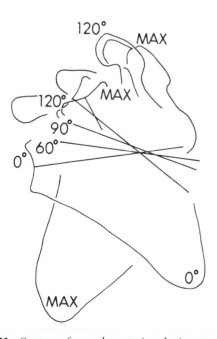

Fig. 2-21. Centers of scapular rotation during arm elevation tend to cluster about two points. Base of scapular spine (0 to 90 degrees). Base of coracoid process (120 degrees to max). (From Perry,[5] with permission.)

curred. The ratio during the first 30 degrees according to Jobe et al.[48] is 4:1 but is 5:4 during the remainder of abduction. It is important to consider relative absence of participation of the scapula in the terminal phases of elevation (initiation and conclusion). In other words, during the majority of elevation the ratio is closer together. Averaged throughout the full range of elevation the scapular component appears to be 2 degrees for every 3 degrees of humeral movement. If resistance to arm elevation is added the scapular component begins earlier.[36]

The center of the humeral head is the instant center of motion. It remains relatively stable. The variability is within 5 mm when measured on consecutive elevation films taken at 30 degree intervals.[20] This implies a true ball and socket arrangement. Similar to the abnormality of excursion found in patients with shoulder pathology, the instant center of motion may also be displaced.[20]

Howell et al.[36] have demonstrated posterior gliding occurring with horizontal extension coupled with external rotation. This is a common position used in throwing sports. When measured radiographically it was found that there is a 4 mm posterior glide of the humeral head in normal subjects. Interestingly, lack of this obligate translation occurred in some patients with instability. Harryman et al.[28] have demonstrated the same movement of the humeral head with flexion, extension, abduction, and adduction. Movement was always in the opposite direction of capsular tightening. Therefore, extension caused posterior movement and flexion caused anterior movement. This movement could not be eliminated by muscular control. However, an increase in the movement occurred with tightening of the capsule. For example, tightening of the posterior capsule increased anterior translation.

The instant center of the scapula begins at the inferior border. Through the first 30 degrees of abduction and the first 60 degrees of flexion there is some mild variability as the scapula centers itself for further elevation of the shoulder. From 60 degrees to 120 degrees the instant center is close to the base of the spine of the scapula. Further elevation shifts the center to the base of the glenoid.[4]

The progressive shifting of the instant center location is directly related to movement patterns of specific joints of the shoulder complex. Also coupling and uncoupling of these joints during elevation (abduction

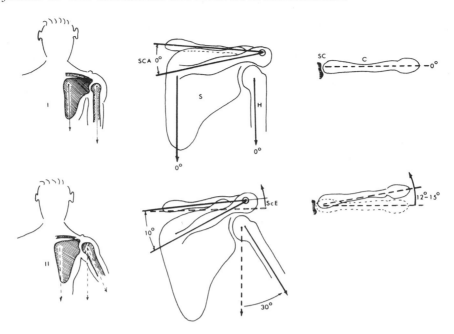

Fig. 2-22. Accessory movement of the scapulohumeral rhythm other than the glenohumeral movement. Movement of the arm through all phases of abduction involves all joints of the shoulder girdle in a synchronous manner.

Phase I: The resting arm: 0 degrees scapular rotation *(S);* 0 degrees spinoclavicular angle *(SCA);* 0 degrees movement at the sternoclavicular joint *(SC);* no elevation of the outer end of the clavicle *(C);* no abduction of the humerus *(H).*

Phase II: Humerus abducted 3 degrees: the outer end of the clavicle is elevated 12 to 15 degrees with no rotation of the clavicle; elevation occurs at the sternoclavicular joint; some movement occurs at the acromioclavicular joint as seen by an increase of 10 degrees of the *SCA* formed by the clavicle and the scapular spine. *(Figure continues.)*

or flexion) allows alternating periods of stability with little movement for long phases and flexibility with greater amounts of movement possible for short phases. For example, initial scapular elevation occurs at the sternoclavicular joint during the first 120 degrees. Beyond this point movement of the acromioclavicular joint and clavicular rotation of approximately 40 degrees allows further scapular motion.[49]

Dvir and Berme[50] describe four phases of elevation. Phase 1 is the setting phase and as explained above represents scapular stabilization. Then as the conoid ligament becomes taut there is a uniting of the previously independent units of the clavicle and scapula. This claviscapular linkage then rotates around an imaginary axis that extends from the sternoclavicular joint through a point at the medial spine of the scapula during phase 2.

Phase 2 ends with tightening of the costoclavicular ligament. At this point the clavicle begins to rotate and the scapula follows. During phase 3 the scapula rotates

about an axis extending through the acromioclavicular joint. This provides a stable yet moving platform for the humeral head. When the trapezoid ligament becomes taut, phase 4 begins as the claviscapular linkage is reestablished until further movement is structurally limited.

Static Stability

In the resting position with the arm at the side there is tension in the superior and middle glenohumeral ligaments, which act as the primary restraint. As the arm is elevated tension is released from the superior and gradually develops in the middle and inferior glenohumeral ligaments. At 90 degrees abduction and beyond the primary restraint is from the anterosuperior band of the inferior glenohumeral ligament.[26] Scapular plane elevation creates the least amount of tension.[51] Coronal plane elevation introduces a com-

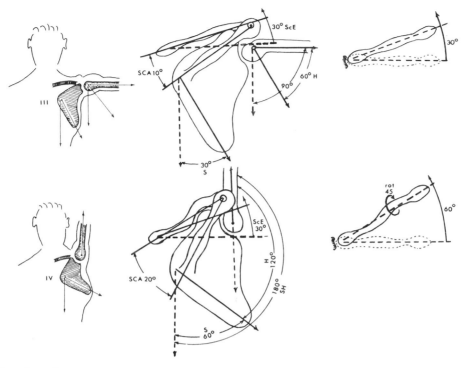

Fig. 2-22. *(continued).*

Phase III: Humerus *(H)* abducted to 90 degrees (60 degrees glenohumeral, 30 degrees scapular): the clavicle is elevated to its final position, 30 degrees; no rotation of clavicle has occurred (all movement is at the sternoclavicular joint); no change in the *SCA.*

Phase IV: Full overhead elevation (SH = 180 degrees; *H* = 120 degrees; *S* = 60 degrees): outer end of the clavicle has not elevated further (at the sternoclavicular joint), but the *SCA* has increased (to 20 degrees). Because of the clavicle's rotation and its "cranklike" form, the clavicle elevates an additional 30 degrees. The humerus through this phase has rotated, but this has not influenced the above degrees of movement. (From Calliett,[68] with permission.)

ponent of external rotation requiring tension in the anterior glenohumeral ligament.

With the arm at the side internal rotation is limited by soft tissue and bony restriction of the thorax; however, some tension is placed on the posterior capsule. External rotation adds considerable tension to the anterior capsule. Capsular restraint is introduced as axial rotation is performed in increasing degrees of elevation.

Muscular Participation (Fig. 2-23)

Elevation (Abduction and Scaption [Fig. 2-24])

For years it was assumed that the initiation of elevation was via the supraspinatus, which acted alone to bring the humerus to a position of mechanical advantage for the deltoid. This belief was primarily due to Codman's observation that patients with large rotator cuff tears could not initiate abduction yet could hold the arm when passively raised above 70 to 90 degrees (principle of Codman's Test).[20] Like many clinical observations, there are several contradictory electromyographic and theoretical considerations.[52] The supraspinatus, because of size and position, could accomplish elevation to 30 degrees but with a 98 percent effort. A 200 percent effort would be needed for elevation to the horizon. Muscles cannot function at this intensity without adequate rest.[53] Elevation to 30 degrees could only occur once, followed by a long refractory period; hardly an efficient system. The deltoid, because of size and leverage, can alone elevate the arm to the horizontal with only a 55 percent effort.[49]

Working together the anterior and middle deltoid plus the supraspinatus can function each with an inten-

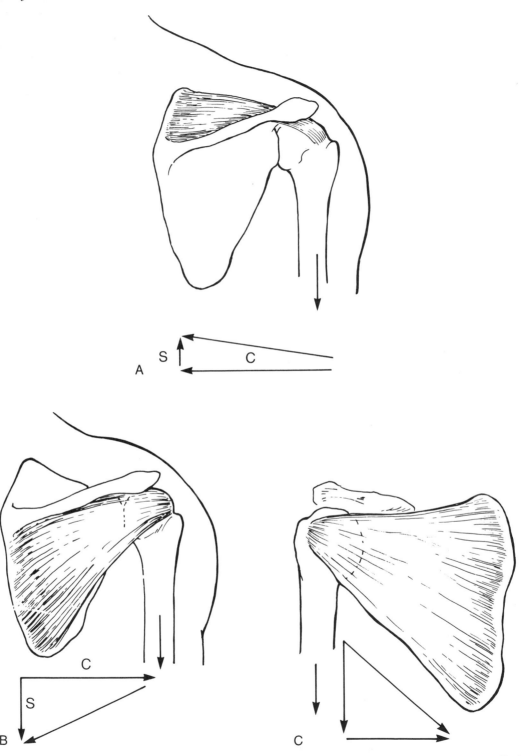

Fig. 2-23. (A) Supraspinatus joint forces, compression dominant. Depressor muscles of the rotator cuff, shear force is strong and downward: **(B)** Infraspinatus. **(C)** Subscapularis. (From Perry,[5] with permission.)

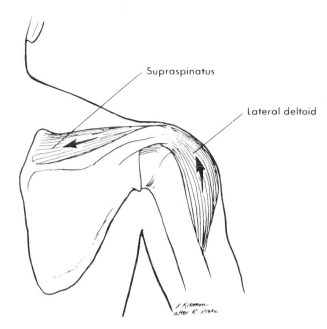

Fig. 2-24. Abductors of the shoulder and arm. (From Bogumill,[69] with permission.)

sity of only 35 percent (Fig. 2-25). This would allow some endurance capacity not allowed by independent action.

Another function of this combination is a force-couple that protects against humeral migration superiorly by an unopposed deltoid contraction. Due to the angle of pull, the deltoid creates more of a shear force with the arm at the side. Balancing with a compressive force is the supraspinatus, which has a more horizontal arrangement pulling the humeral head into the glenoid. Assistance by other rotator cuff muscles seems to be minimal yet consistent (Fig. 2-26).

The function of the deltoid is dependent on plane of motion and degree of elevation. Scapular plane elevation involves mainly the middle and anterior deltoid.[54] Coronal plane elevation, because of its relative horizontal extension component, calls into play more of the posterior deltoid. An isolated movement of forward elevation (flexion) is primarily due to the anterior deltoid while extension involves more the posterior deltoid.

During the first 30 degrees of elevation in the scapular plane, the middle deltoid has the main advantage. By 60 degrees the anterior and middle share an equal advantage. Above 90 degrees the anterior deltoid be-

comes dominant. The functional length of the deltoid is determined by the relationship between the scapula (glenoid) and the humerus. If the scapula does not rotate, the functional length decreases to a point where further function is limited.[55] Via rotation the scapula allows the deltoid to continue to function above 90 degrees efficiently.

A significant detour from normal deltoid function seems to occur as an inhibitory reaction to supraspinatus tendinitis. One electromyographic study indicated that in shoulders with supraspinatus tendinitis at approximately 45 degrees of abduction, the middle deltoid decreased its activity significantly.[56] The added strain to the supraspinatus (already compromised) may lead to a cycle of unrelenting injury.

Of course, elevation of the shoulder involves more than muscular contraction at the glenohumeral joint. Requisite for full elevation is movement of the scapula, positioning itself under the humeral head to maintain proper lever length and functional length of the previously mentioned muscles. The primary muscles involved in movement of the scapula are the upper trapezius (which elevates the lateral scapula), the lower trapezius (which pulls downward on the medial border of the scapula), and the serratus anterior (which pulls the scapula forward on the chest wall) (Figs. 2-27 and 2-28). This movement occurs primarily between 60 and 120 degrees of abduction.[57] The scapula is rotating around an axis centered at the root of the spine of the scapula. Beyond this point the predominant action is from the lower trapezius coupled with the serratus anterior and the contralateral erector spinae (Fig. 2-29). This coupling allows further elevation of the arm through rotation of the scapula and sidebending of the trunk. Any interference with the ability of the scapula to translate across the thorax will affect the ability of the humeral head to elevate fully. This may be due to weakness of the scapular musculature or any number of restrictive elements about the shoulder or spine.

Normal elevation is assumed to be 180 degrees; however, fewer than 4 percent of men and 28 percent of women can achieve this range.[57,58] Limitations may involve the last few degrees of elevation. Numerous factors account for this including a kyphotic thoracic spine, scoliosis, and muscle contracture. Weakness due to instability may limit full elevation as does the painful compression of an involved acromioclavicular joint or subacromial impingement.

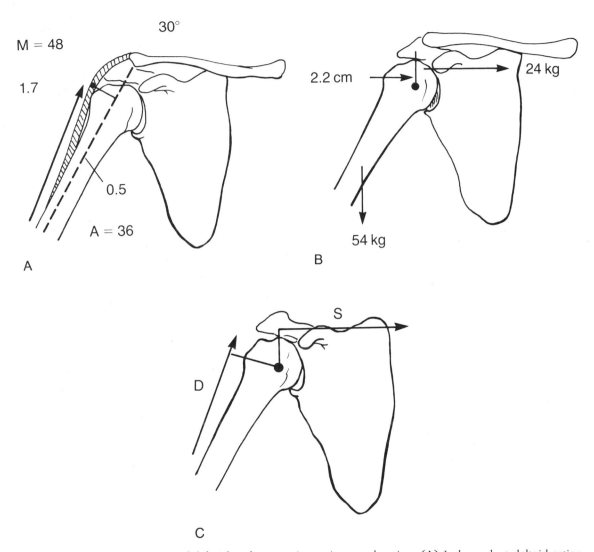

Fig. 2-25. Relative effectiveness of deltoid and supraspinatus in arm elevation. **(A)** Independent deltoid action at 30 degrees equals 54 percent of maximum capability. **(B)** Independent supraspinatus capability equals 98 percent of available torque. 2.2 cm = lever length; 24 kg = muscle force; 54 kg = demand torque by arm weight. Shoulder position = 30 degrees abduction. **(C)** Combined deltoid *(D)* and supraspinatus *(S)* action reduces effort to 35 percent for each muscle. Arrows indicate direction of dominant muscle force. (From Perry,[53] with permission.)

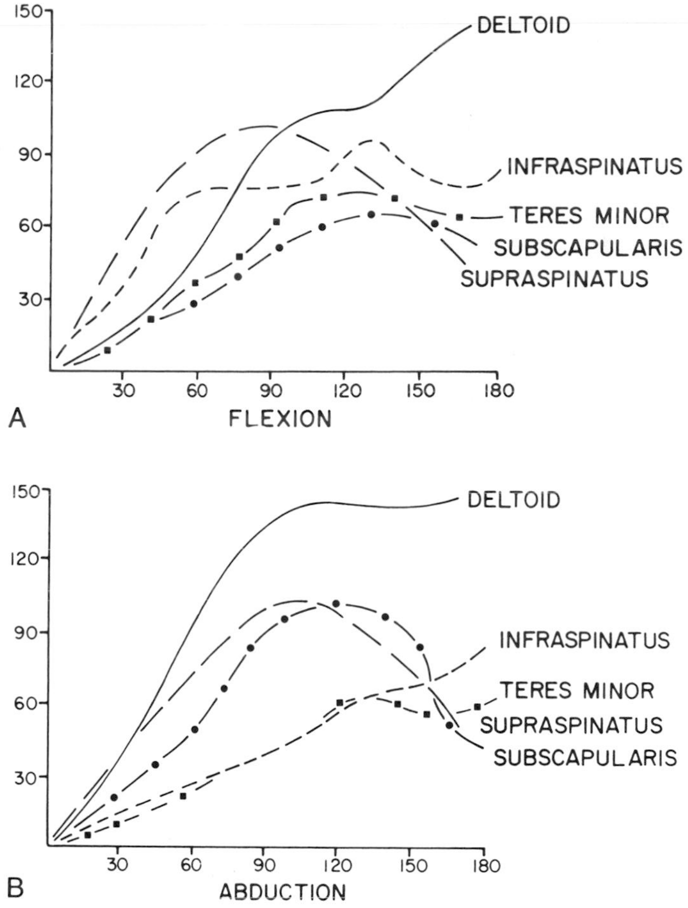

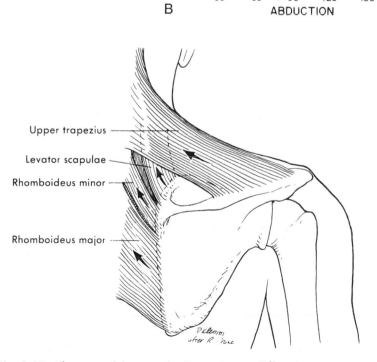

Fig. 2-26. Relative intensity of deltoid and rotator cuff muscle action during arm elevation (dynamic electromyographic values) for **(A)** flexion and **(B)** abduction. Vertical scale, microvolts of electromyography; horizontal scale, degrees of arm elevation. (From Perry,[53] with permission.)

Fig. 2-27. Elevators of the scapula. (From Bogumill,[69] with permission.)

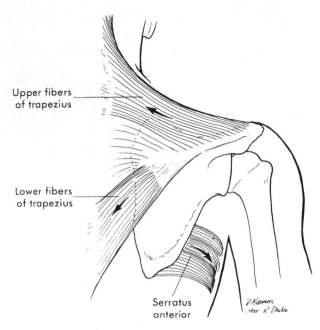

Upper fibers
of trapezius

Lower fibers
of trapezius

Serratus
anterior

Fig. 2-28. Upward rotators of the scapula. (From Bogumill,[69] with permission.)

Flexion

Flexion (Fig. 2-30) is quite similar to abduction in regards to scapular movement; however, the setting phase may last longer, through the first 60 degrees.[57] Further, initiation of flexion is primarily directed by the anterior deltoid. Additional assistance is given by the coracobrachialis, the clavicular section of the pectoralis major, and the biceps. From 60 to 120 degrees there is similar action in the scapular musculature as was found in abduction, including upper trapezius and serratus anterior activity for rotation of the scapula. Again recruitment of the lower trapezius, serratus anterior, and the contralateral erector spinae are needed to flex beyond 120 degrees. As with abduction there is a gradual, consistent recruitment of the rotator cuff musculature. However, with flexion there appears to be less involvement of the teres minor/infraspinatus group.

Passive restraint is provided primarily by the inferior glenohumeral ligament and the posterior capsule.[25]

Extension

Extension of the arm (Fig. 2-30) is a rather limited movement as compared to flexion (approximately 60 degrees).[59] The musculature involved includes the posterior deltoid, latissimus dorsi, teres major, and the triceps. Pure extension occurs infrequently in sports. Bowling introduces more of a passive extension. Underhand pitching or throwing is similar with less resistance. The recovery phase in freestyle and butterfly swimming strokes are more common examples. It must be noted that in this scenario the arm has the added resistance of water and gravity.

Extension is limited by the restraint of the coracohumeral ligament and to a lesser degree some portions of the anterior glenohumeral ligament.[26]

Adduction

Adduction (Fig. 2-31) is an extremely powerful movement that is used primarily for stabilization of the shoulder with the trunk. An example is the iron cross on the still rings or support maneuvers on the parallel bars or pommel horse.[60]

Scapula fixating muscles include the rhomboids, the trapezius, and the serratus anterior. The pectoralis major and latissimus dorsi are strong agonists for adduction. In fact, literally every shoulder muscle is involved in this movement.

Internal/External Rotation

Internal rotation (Fig. 2-32) is inherently a stronger movement than external rotation due to the participation of more and larger musculature. The pectoralis major, latissimus dorsi, subscapularis, anterior deltoid, and teres major assist in this movement. A relatively common pattern in sports, internal rotation is found in martial arts (in particular judo and wrestling), swimming (in particular during the pull-through phase of most strokes), and fencing. Relatively more range of internal rotation as compared to external rotation is found with abduction of the arm to 90 degrees (except in pitchers).[61]

External rotation (Fig. 2-33) is a weaker movement determined by only a few muscles: the teres minor, infraspinatus, and posterior deltoid. Again, it is common to martial arts, swimming (in particular the breast stroke), and fencing. Of the total 180 degrees found in the neutral position, external rotation accounts for 108 degrees or 60 percent.[57] This decrease as the arm is elevated primarily because of restrictions in the joint capsule.

In general, internal rotation is limited by the poste-

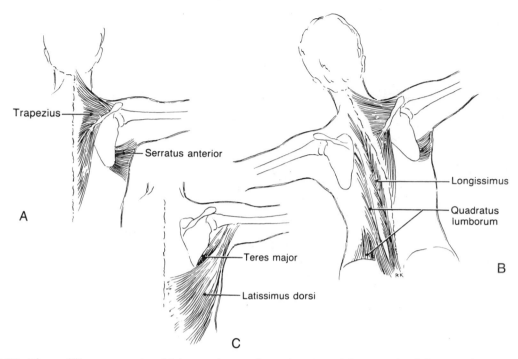

Fig. 2-29. Three different ways in which muscles produce elevation of the scapula. **(A)** Pure elevation of the scapula in the scapular plane, as might be performed in a throwing motion. **(B)** In throwing a heavier object, to allow the glenoid to bear extra weight more elevation of the scapula is necessary. Because the muscles of the shoulder are already operating at optimum points of their length-tension curve, further elevation must be obtained by using the contralateral flexion of the spine. **(C)** An upward moment on the upper limb, as in the iron cross maneuver, must be resisted by a greater force in the latissimus dorsi. The resultant caudad-directed joint reaction vector must meet the bone of the glenoid. This scapular elevation is produced by the teres major. (From Jobe,[64] with permission.)

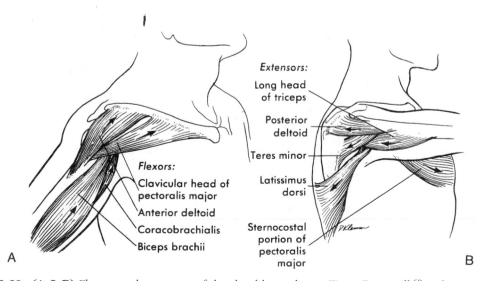

Fig. 2-30. (A & B) Flexors and extensors of the shoulder and arm. (From Bogumill,[69] with permission.)

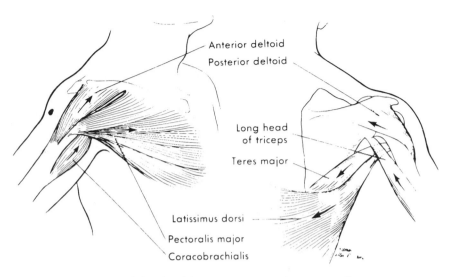

Fig. 2-31. Adductors of the shoulder and arm. (From Bogumill,[69] with permission.)

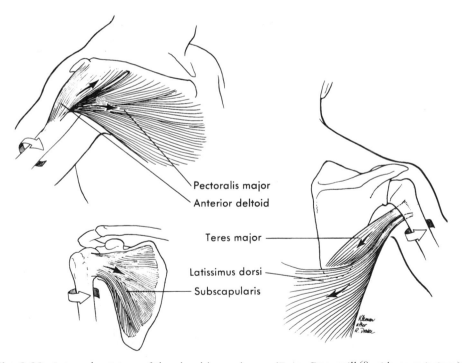

Fig. 2-32. Internal rotators of the shoulder and arm. (From Bogumill,[69] with permission.)

rior capsule whereas external rotation is limited by and anterior glenohumeral ligament.[25]

Horizontal Flexion/Extension

An extremely ubiquitous pattern of movement found in sports is horizontal flexion/extension. Most throwing sports, swimming, and racquet sports utilize the approximately 180 degrees of movement provided by this plane of motion. Horizontal flexion is the predominant component equal to 135 degrees or 76 percent of the total movement.[5] In addition to a greater range, the musculature participation is comprised of the strongest shoulder movers, the pectoralis major assisted by the anterior deltoid. Horizontal flexion is necessary for the follow-through movement of throwing and the forehand movement of racquet sports.

Horizontal extension is a component of the windup in discus throwing and certain maneuvers in gymnastics. The primary muscles are the posterior musculature of the shoulder and back. This includes the teres minor, infraspinatus, and posterior deltoid for the shoulder; and the middle trapezius and rhomboids for the scapula.

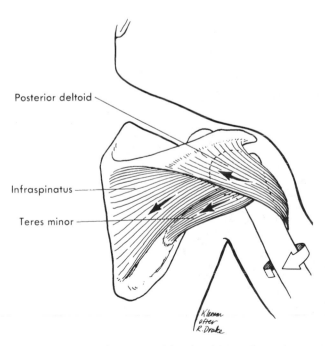

Fig. 2-33. External rotators of the shoulder and arm. (From Bogumill,[69] with permission.)

Horizontal extension coupled with external rotation is a movement pattern common to most throwing sports during the cocking phase. The primary muscles are again the infraspinatus, teres minor, and posterior deltoid for the shoulder; and the middle trapezius and rhomboids for the scapula. This position is responsible for considerable stretch-tension in the anterior musculature and capsule. Due to the position of the deltoid in relation to the axis of rotation, the more extension involved, the more of a fulcrum is created that forces the humeral head anterior. Surprisingly, the external rotators such as the infraspinatus and teres minor can reduce this tendency by decreasing the effect of the posterior deltoid.[53] Protection is also accomplished by the passive stretching of the anterior musculature, in particular the subscapularis.

The position of horizontal extension with external rotation was studied by Howell et al.[36] who found posterior translation in the normal control group. Anterior translation occurred only in those individuals with a previous history of recurrent dislocation or subluxation. In addition, it became clear that positional reduction, not muscular correction, of the normal posterior translation was the only alleviating factor. In other words, contraction of the anterior musculature was unable to reduce the humeral head to its normal center. The suspicion is that the posterior translation is due to tension in the capsule or perhaps may be related to articular congruence. It must be remembered that this study was performed supine, which adds a gravity component to the tendency toward posterior translation.

The inferior portion of the glenohumeral ligament is the main restraint to horizontal adduction (in particular coupled with external rotation). The inferior portion of the posterior capsule, likes its anterior neighbor, restricts horizontal adduction when combined with external rotation, and the superior and middle components with internal rotation.[25]

Scapular Positioning

Retraction

Sometimes referred to as scapular adduction, retraction of the scapula (Fig. 2-34) is a necessary component of extension movements of the humerus. The most common example is with the arm at 90 degrees abduction. The medial musculature, specifically the middle

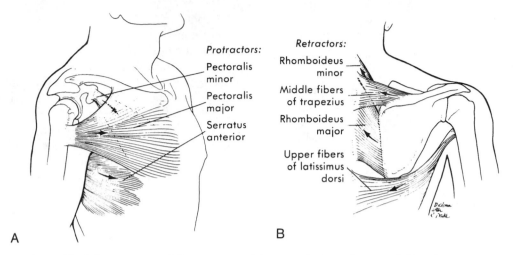

Fig. 2-34. (A) Protractors; **(B)** retractors of the scapula. (From Bogumill,[69] with permission.)

trapezius and rhomboids, are activated to pull the medial border of the scapula toward the spine. Retraction is necessary for movement patterns in rowing, the recovery phase of swimming, and the cocking phase of throwing.

Protraction

Protraction (see Fig. 2-34) is often referred to as scapular adduction. This movement is an extremely important component of forward arm movements such as

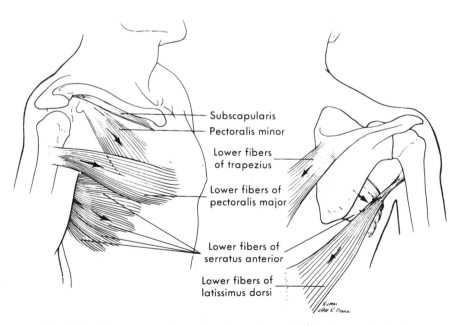

Fig. 2-35. Depressors of scapula. (From Bogumill,[69] with permission.)

the acceleration phase of throwing sports, punching in boxing and martial arts, and lunge movements in fencing. The serratus anterior is the primary muscle involved. Failure to move the scapula forward reduces the amount of speed and range of motion possible due to articular blockage. Any forward movement of the humerus must be accompanied by protraction of the scapula (glenoid) to provide a stable base for movement.

Scapular Depression

The scapula depresses (Fig. 2-35) when the trunk is lifted such as rising from a chair. In regards to sports, many positions in gymnastics require a support of the trunk by the arms. Examples include the iron rings and pommel horse and various floor positions. The main muscles that initiate the movement are the inferior digitations of the serratus anterior and the lower trapezius muscles. Additional stabilization is provided by the pectoralis major and latissimus dorsi acting at the glenohumeral joint.

REFERENCES

1. Townsend H, Jobe FW, Pink M, Perry J: Electromyographic analysis of the glenohumeral muscles during a baseball rehabilitation program. Am J Sport Med 19:264, 1991
2. Belle RM, Hawkins RJ: Dynamic electromyographic analysis of the shoulder muscles during rotational and scapular strengthening exercises. p. 32. In Post M, Morrey BF, Hawkins RS (eds): Surgery of the Shoulder. CV Mosby, St. Louis, 1990
3. Barham JN: Mechanical Kinesiology. CV Mosby, St. Louis, 1978
4. Demster W: Space requirements of the seated operator. WADC A Technical Report. p. 55. Offices of Technical Services, U.S. Department of Commerce, Washington, D.C., 1955
5. Perry J: Biomechanics of the shoulder. p. 1. In Rowe CR (ed): The Shoulder, Churchill Livingstone, New York, 1988
6. Reeves B: Experiments on the tensile strength of the anterior capsular structures of the shoulder region. J Bone Joint Surg 50:B856, 1968
7. Morey BF, Chao EY: Recurrent anterior dislocation of the shoulder. p. 39. In Dumbleton J, Black J (eds): Clinical Biomechanics. Churchill Livingstone, New York, 1981
8. Bergstrom J: Muscle electrolytes in man. Scan J Clin Lab Invest 68(suppl): 1962
9. Ikai M, Fukunaga T: Calculation of muscle strength per unit of cross-sectional area of human muscle. A Angew Physiol Einschl Argeitphysiol 26:26, 1968
10. Haggmark T, Jansson E, Svane B: Cross-sectional area of the thigh muscle in man measured by computed tomography. Scand J Clin Lab Invest 38:355, 1978
11. Weber EF: Ueber die langenderhaltnisse der fleischfasen dur muskeln im allgemeinen. Berlin Verh K Sach Ges Wissensch math-Phys 63, 1951
12. Schmidt GL: Biomechanical analysis of knee flexion and extension. J Biomechan 6:79, 1973
13. Perry J: Anatomy and biomechanics of the shoulder in throwing, swimming, gymnastics, and tennis. Clin Sports Med 2:247, 1983
14. Tabury JC, Tabary C, Tardieu C et al: Physiological and structural changes in the cat's soleus muscle due to immobilization at different lengths by plaster casts. J Physiol 224:231, 1972
15. Tardieu C, Huet E, Bret MD et al: Muscle hypoextensibility in children with cerebral palsy: 1. clinical and experimental observations. Arch Phys Med Rehabil 63:97, 1982
16. Inman VT, Saunders JR, Abbott LC: Observations on the function of the shoulder joint. J Bone Joint Surg 26:1, 1944
17. Poppen NK, Walker PS: Forces at the glenohumeral joint in abduction. Clin Orthop 136:165, 1978
18. Hawkins RJ, Kennedy JC: Impingement syndrome in athletics. Am J Sports Med 8:151, 1980
19. MacConaill MA, Basmajian JV: Muscles and movements: a basis for human kinesiology. Williams & Wilkins, Baltimore, 1969
20. Poppen NK, Walker PS: Normal and abnormal motion of the shoulder. J Bone Joint Surg 58A:195, 1976
21. Walker PS: Human Joints and Their Artificial Replacement. Charles C Thomas, Springfield, IL, 1977
22. Smidt DL: Biomechanical analysis of knee flexion and extension. J Biomechan 6:79, 1973
23. Ely LW, Mensor MC: Studies on the immobilization of the normal joints. Surg Gynecol Obstet 57:212, 1963
24. Dowson D: Modes of lubrication in human joints. In: Lubrication and Wear in Living and Artificial Joints. Vol. 181. Institute of Mechanical Engineers, London, 1967
25. Terry GC, Mannon D, France P, Norwood LA: The stabilizing function of passive shoulder restraints. Am J Sports Med 19:26, 1991
26. O'Connell PW, Nuber GW, Mileski RA, Lautenschlager E: The contribution of the glenohumeral ligaments to

anterior stability of the shoulder joint. Am J Sports Med 18:579, 1990

27. Jobe FW, Tibone JE, Perry J et al: An EMG analysis of the shoulder in throwing and pitching: a preliminary report. Am J Sports Med 11:3, 1983

28. Harryman DT, Sidles JA, Clark JM et al: Translation of the humeral head on the glenoid with passive glenohumeral motion. J Bone Joint Surg 72A:1334, 1990

29. Codman EA: The Shoulder. Thomas Todd, Boston, 1934

30. Saha AK: Dynamic stability of the glenohumeral joint. Acta Orthop Scand 42:491, 1971

31. Maki S, Gruen T: Antropometric study of the glenohumeral joint. Paper presented at the 22nd annual Orthopedic Research Society meeting, New Orleans, LA, January 28–30, 1973

32. Levy IM, Torzilli PA, Warren RF: The effect of medial meniscetomy on the anterio/posterior motion of the knee. J Bone Joint Surg 64A:883, 1982

33. Andrews JR, Kupferman SP, Dillman CJ: Labral tears in throwing and racquet sports. Clin Sports Med 10:901, 1991

34. Cerulli G, Ceccarini A, Alberti PF et al: Mechanoreceptors of some anatomical structures of the human knee. p. 50. In Muller W, Hackenbruch W (eds): Surgery and Arthroscopy of the Knee. Springer-Verlag, Berlin, 1988

35. Moseley JB Jr., Overgaard B: The anterior capsular mechanism in recurrent dislocation of the shoulder. J Bone Joint Surg 44B:913, 1962

36. Howell SM, Galiant BJ, Renzi AJ, Marone PJ: Normal and abnormal mechanics of the glenohumeral joint in the horizontal plane. J Bone Joint Surg 70A:227, 1988

37. Andrews JR, Angelo BL: Shoulder arthroscopy for the throwing athlete. Tech Orthop 3:75, 1988

38. McMaster WC: Anterior glenoid labrum damage: a painful lesion in swimmers. Am J Sports Med 14:383, 1986

39. Ellman H: Shoulder arthroscopy: current indications and techniques. Orthopaedics 11:45, 1988

40. Pappas AM, Goss TP, Kleinmen PK: Symptomatic shoulder instability due to lesions of the glenoid labrum. Am J Sports Med 11:279, 1983

41. Bankart ASB: The pathology and treatment of recurrent dislocation of the shoulder. Br J Surg 26:23, 1938

42. Kumar VP, Balasubramaniam P: The role of atmospheric pressure in stabilizing the shoulder: an experimental study. J Bone Joint Surg 67B:719, 1985

43. Unsworth A, Dowson D, Wright V: Cracking joints: a bioengineering study of cavitation in the metacarpalphalangeal joint. Ann Rheum Dis 30:348, 1971

44. Greenfield BH, Donatelli R, Wooden MJ, Wilkes J: Isokinetic evaluation of shoulder rotational strength between the plane of scapula and the frontal plane. Am J Sports Med 18:124, 1990

45. Morrey BF, An K-N: Biomechanics of the shoulder. p. 208. In Rockwood CA, Matsen FA (eds): The Shoulder. Vol. 1. WB Saunders, Philadelphia, 1990

46. Basmajian JV, Bazant FJ: Factors preventing downward dislocation of the adducted shoulder joint. J Bone Joint Surg 41A:1142, 1959

47. Doddy SG, Waterland JC, Freedman L: Scapulohumeral goniometer. Arch Phys Med Rehabil 51:711, 1970

48. Jobe FW, Moynes DR, Brewster CE: Rehabilitation of shoulder joint instabilities. Orthop Clin North Am 18:473, 1987

49. Freedman L, Munro RH: Abduction of the arm in the scapular plane: scapular and glenohumeral movements. J Bone Joint Surg 18A:1503, 1966

50. Dvir Z, Berme N: The shoulder complex in elevation of the arm: a mechanism approach. J Biomechan 11:219, 1978

51. Johnston TB: The movements of the shoulder joint. Br J Surg 25:252, 1937

52. Howell SM, Imobersteg AM, Seger DH, Marone PJ: Clarification of the role of the supraspinatus muscle in shoulder function. J Bone Joint Surg 68A:398, 1986

53. Perry J: Muscle control of the shoulder. p. 17. In Rowe CR (ed): The Shoulder. Churchill Livingstone, New York, 1988

54. Nuber CW, Bowman ID, Perry JP et al: EMG analysis of classical shoulder motion. Trans Orthop Res Soc 11, 1986

55. Lucas DB: Biomechanics of the shoulder joint. Arch Surg 107:425, 1973

56. Michaud M, Arsenault AB, Gravel D et al: Muscular compensatory mechanism in the presence of tendinitis of the supraspinatus. Am J Phys Med 66:109, 1987

57. Doody SG, Freedman L, Waterland JC: Shoulder movements during abduction in the scapular plane. Arch Phys Med Rehabil 51:595, 1970

58. Freedman L, Munro R: Abduction of the arm in the scapular plane: scapular and glenohumeral movements. J Bone Joint Surg 48A:1503, 1966

59. Matsen FA III: Biomechanics of the shoulder. In Frankel VH, Nordin M (eds): Basic Biomechanics of the Skeletal System. Lea & Febiger, Philadelphia, 1980

60. Weineck J: Functional Anatomy in Sports. CV Mosby, St. Louis, 1990

61. Boone DC, Azen SP: Normal range of motion of joints in male subjects. J Bone Joint Surg 61A:756, 1979

62. Leveau BF: Basic biomechanics in sports and orthopaedic therapy. p. 76. In Gould JA, Davies GJ (eds); Orthopaedic and Sports Physical Therapy. CV Mosby, St. Louis, 1990

63. Schafer RC: Clinical Biomechanics. 2nd Ed. Williams & Wilkins, Baltimore, 1987

64. Jobe CM: Gross anatomy of the shoulder. p. 49. In Rock-

wood CA, Matsen FA (eds): The Shoulder. Vol. 1. WB Saunders, Philadelphia, 1990

65. Barak T, Rosen ER, Sofer R: Mobility: passive orthopaedic manual therapy. p. 201. In Gould JA, Davies GJ (eds): Orthopaedic and Sports Physical Therapy. CV Mosby, St. Louis, 1990

66. Bowen MK, Warren RF: Ligamentous control of shoulder stability based on selective cutting. Clin Sports Med 10: 757, 1991

67. Morrey PF, An K-N: Biomechanics of the shoulder. p. 215. In Rockwood CA, Matsen FA (eds): The Shoulder, Vol. 1. WB Saunders, Philadelphia, 1990

68. Calliett R: Shoulder Pain. 2nd Ed. FA Davis, Philadelphia, 1983

69. Bogumill GP: Functional anatomy of the shoulder and elbow. p. 193. In AAOS: Symposium on Upper Extremity Injuries in Athletes. CV Mosby, St. Louis, 1986

3

The Shoulder in Throwing Sports

THOMAS A. SOUZA

The common denominator for many sports is the requirement to throw. Although there are obvious differences among many of these activities there is a surprising similarity in the gross movement used.[1] The pitching motion in baseball is the prototype movement that will be discussed. Inherent in the throwing action is the need for contribution of the entire body from the foot to the shoulder. This concept of kinesiological linkage is paramount in understanding proper form and function. Although focusing on the shoulder's participation in the throwing act, it must be understood that with proper technique, only about one-half of the force is generated by the shoulder.[2,3] The contribution of specific shoulder musculature to the propulsion of the ball may be affected by abnormal conditions endemic to the shoulder such as impingement or instability or by distant problems such as lack of trunk flexibility, low back pain, or foot problems.[4,5]

The description of the stages of throwing is complicated by the lack of consistency in terminology and division of phases. Table 3-1 illustrates examples of varied divisions.[6–10] Depending on the source of explanation and the need for detail, throwing is divided among three major phases with further subdivisions into early and late phases. To add to the confusion, authors will use the same term to describe different events due to an overlap definition. For example, the standard use of the term cocking (specifically early cocking) is included in Kulund's use of the term windup[11] and substituted by Michaud with the term acceleration I.[9] The deceleration phase described by some authors as included in the initial component of the follow-through phase by others is described as a separate phase.[10] In addition, there is difficulty in describing the movements used given the complexity of shoulder motion and the inherent coupling effect with any form of shoulder movement.

PITCHING

The phases of throwing (Fig. 3-1) are divided based on the position of the ball and the thrower's body position. Four major phases are used[6]:

Wind-up—a preparatory phase used for balance and "coiling" involving mainly a flexed body posture. Both hands hold the ball.

Cocking—the "stored energy" phase, which is divided into an early and late phase. The early phase begins with release of the ball into the throwing hand. Foot contact with the contralateral foot initiates the late component.

Acceleration—begins with the arm at maximum external rotation and ends with ball release. This is the "explosive" phase.

Follow-through—essentially the "energy dissipation" phase where the arm and body move together. The point of maximum internal rotation of the arm divides this phase into early and late phases (or deceleration and follow-through by some authors).[10]

Windup

The windup is a highly individualized phase occasionally modified as in pitching from the "stretch" in baseball[12] (used to discourage base running). This phase

Table 3-1. Variations in the Description of Pitching Phases

Author	Division of the Throwing Act
Tullos and King,[34] McLeod[10]	Windup, cocking, acceleration, deceleration, follow-through
Perry and Glousman[42]	Windup, cocking (early and late phases), acceleration (early and late phases), follow-through
Michaud[9]	Windup, acceleration I, acceleration II, follow-through
Blackburn[13]	Windup, cocking, acceleration, ball release, deceleration, follow-through

allows the athlete to establish a rhythm and balance. Additionally, the body is in a position that, in a sense, allows a "running start" from a static posture. In other words, at the end of windup the trunk and lower body are rotationally as far away from the release position as possible. Hence, more force can be generated resulting in an increase in speed or distance.

Depending on individual style, the windup usually lasts between 0.5 and 1 second.[13] The contralateral leg is raised significantly in preparation for foot plant thus raising the center of gravity. This is crucial to the creation of potential energy. The trunk is rotated to the pitching arm side. The contribution of shoulder musculature is minimal. The majority of muscular activity is occurring in the lower extremity and trunk. Windup ends with a switch in the center of gravity over the pivot foot.

The leg lift is variable dependent on the style, flexibility, and fatigue of the pitcher. If lifted too high, it may throw the pitcher off balance; too low a lift may increase the need for upper extremity forces due to the decrease in lower extremity participation.[12]

Cocking

Cocking prepares the arm for acceleration by placing it in an extreme position of stretch. This prestretch is essential in generating a more forceful contraction during acceleration.[5] This position will allow the arm to travel the greatest amount of distance, which translates into the most amount of force that can be applied to the ball prior to its release.

Cocking begins with transfer of the ball to the throwing hand while weight is maintained over the ipsilateral leg. The late phase of cocking begins with foot plant and ends with the shoulder reaching maximum external rotation. Interestingly, the shoulder does move forward from horizontal extension to neutral while the humerus continues to maximally externally rotate during the end stage of cocking.[14]

The scapula is retracted maximally during cocking through the assistance of the middle trapezius and rhomboids. The shoulder is in a position of extreme horizontal extension (abduction); about 30 degrees. External rotation is approximately 120 to 160 degrees; abduction at 90 degrees.[10] In the early phases of cocking, the deltoid is of prime importance for abduction. Later the rotator cuff musculature is called into play for stabilization and external rotation of the arm.[6] The elbow is flexed to about 90 degrees while the wrists and metacarpals are extended.

The cocking position of abduction, horizontal exten-

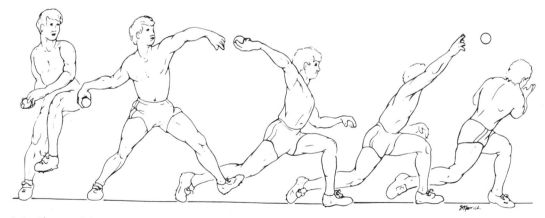

Fig. 3-1. Phases of the pitch, from left to right: windup, early cocking, late cocking, acceleration, follow-through. (From Perry and Glousman,[89] with permission.)

sion, and external rotation places maximum tension on the anterior inferior glenohumeral ligament. Some tension is also generated in the anterior coracohumeral ligament and the anterior superior glenohumeral ligament.[15] This may result in posterior translation of the humeral head.[16]

A review of lower body participation from windup through cocking is essential in understanding the throwing act. Beginning with the windup, the leg is flexed to about 90 degrees, tucked into the body facing 90 degrees to the plate. In the late phase of cocking, the left foot (in a right-handed pitcher) is planted facing the plate leaving the trunk and pelvis behind in relative external rotation. The foot plant essentially establishes the beginning of pelvic and trunk rotation.

As we will see a transfer of momentum to the upper body and extremity will occur throughout the throwing act, analogous to a whipping action, where the most distal segment the hand (holding the ball) is propelled forward by a coordinated sequence of movement initiated in the lower body.[17]

At foot plant, the arm is nearing an extreme stretch position. This places stress on anterior stabilization, both dynamic and static. The internal rotators such as the pectoralis major, subscapularis, and latissimus are attempting to decelerate the arm eccentrically. The anterior capsule, in particular the inferior band,[18] is under maximal tension. The amount of external rotation possible is determined by these structures. In other words, tightness of any of these structures will limit the amount of rotation decreasing the distance the arm travels resulting in a less efficient throw.

The late stage of cocking involves trunk rotation to the opposite side (left side with a right-handed pitcher). Accompanying trunk rotation is a movement of the scapula forward (abducted or protracted) to provide a firm support for the humerus, which moves from horizontal extension to neutral. The serratus anterior and rotator cuff musculature are very important for this coordinated movement.

Acceleration

Acceleration begins when forward shoulder movement is complete providing a stable support for the whipping of the elbow and arm. The trunk moves forward over the contralateral support leg. Movement at the shoulder is primarily internal rotation. The elbow

moves from a flexed position of 90 degrees to 20 to 30 degrees of extension. The ball is accelerated from 0 to 80 miles per hour and sometimes higher. All of these movements occur in a very short period of time (80 milliseconds).[10]

Arm movement begins from a maximal externally rotated position. Suddenly, there is a switch from an eccentric contraction to a concentric contraction of the internal rotator musculature.[6] This is essentially an example of a plyometric action where movement stored in the eccentric phase is then released in the concentric phase. There is a massive call for internal rotation of the shoulder. For this to occur there must be stabilization of the scapula and of the humeral head in the glenoid so that internal rotation takes place around a fixed point. The rhomboids and middle trapezius are contracting eccentrically while the serratus anterior and upper trapezius are contracting concentrically to keep the shoulder positioned with stability. Halfway through acceleration the humerus is decelerated by the supraspinatus, teres minor, and infraspinatus. This effectively transfers the momentum to the forearm.

There is a visual illusion with some forms of pitching that the shoulder is abducted to various degrees depending on the style of pitching. Yet much of this appearance is produced by lateral bending of the trunk. Examples are when a pitcher is said to throw overhead, side-arm, or three-quarter. When examined these discrepancies were explained by body position with the arm being essentially in the same position of 90 degrees abduction.[17]

A review of preceding events demonstrates that acceleration is developed by a series of components. The rotation of the trunk and lower extremity with concomitant backward movement of the arm sets up the plyometric movement to follow. Later as the lower body motion is substantially decreased, the upper body is whipped forward over this stable base. Finally this movement is assisted by the push-off of the right leg and foot. In essence this is exactly what happens throughout the throwing act. There is a sequence of whipping initiated in the lower extremity moving up to the trunk, the shoulder, the elbow, and wrist. Each of these components is carried forward by the somewhat sudden slowing of the previous link.

Coiling of the joint capsule is an important factor in the development of potential energy. During the cocking phase there is a twisting of the capsule, developing tension that is released during acceleration.[6] It has been estimated that the capsule may have the same stretch qualities as the subscapularis tendon, which would result in approximately a 13 percent increase in length. Perry[1] estimates that this "coiled spring" effect can develop torsional strains exceeding 17,000 kg/cm.

The acceleration phase causes an increase in posterior capsular tension by 75 percent while the anterior inferior glenohumeral ligament relaxes.[15] This combination of events may render the anterior-superior labrum at risk of damage. This has been confirmed as a possible acceleration injury mechanism.[19]

Forward movement of the scapula is also an important contributor to efficient acceleration. An adaptive repositioning of the glenoid must occur for the rotating and forward moving humerus. This is dependent specifically on proper functioning of the serratus anterior. Gowitzke and Milner[20] represent a surfacing consensus that the serratus anterior has been underestimated regarding its function during throwing.

Muscularly, the demand is primarily on the internal rotators of the shoulder: the pectoralis major, teres major, latissimus, and subscapularis. They are contracting concentrically to accelerate the arm while the posterior musculature that stabilizes the scapula and shoulder contract eccentrically. These muscles include the rhomboids, middle and upper trapezius, and the infraspinatus/teres minor. The triceps concentrically extends while the biceps and brachialis eccentrically decelerate the elbow and forearm.

The wrist is pronated to some degree with most pitches with ball release. This radioulnar pronation begins about 10 milliseconds prior to ball release due to contraction of the pronator teres. Apparently the exception to the rule is the curveball where pronation occurs after ball release. There is an extreme valgus force applied to the elbow during acceleration. The fastball creates the most valgus force to the elbow followed by the slider and the curveball.[21]

Acceleration ends with ball release. This is a variable event and difficult to evaluate even with high-speed cameras. The average time for ball release is between 6 and 10 milliseconds.[10]

Follow-through

With follow-through the shoulder continues into horizontal flexion and internal rotation. Jobe et al.[22] calcu-

late that with a 90-mile-per-hour pitch only 88.2 joules of energy are imparted to the ball while 212 joules are left to be dissipated by the body. In an attempt to dissipate the massive forces generated in acceleration, the torso rotates forward. This rotation allows the shoulder to decrease the relative speed of movement with the body and transfer energy away from the arm. If the arm was allowed to continue forward without this coordinated movement is would literally be pulled out of socket. In fact, during follow-through there is as much as a 2.5 cm gapping of the glenohumeral joint.[12] The deceleration forces equal twice that of acceleration. However, injury is no more likely to occur given that deceleration forces are applied over a longer period of time.[10] Capsular tension is increased particularly in the middle and inferior posterior capsules and the anterior superior glenohumeral ligament.[15]

As follow-through ends the pitcher comes off of the ipsilateral foot to continue rotation on the planted contralateral foot. Often two or three steps are taken to further dissipate the excess energy.

Muscularly the majority of activity is in the posterior musculature acting to decelerate the forward moving arm straining the infraspinatus/teres minor, middle trapezius and rhomboids, and the serratus anterior. There is stretching and traction of the posterior capsular structures.[10]

Summary Analysis

Atwater[17] compares the throwing act to a whipping motion generated in the larger more powerful lower body segments transferred to increasingly smaller segments via relative slowing of the preceding proximal segment. Jobe et al.[22] draw the analogy between a spinning skater and a thrower; both follow the law of conservation of rotational energy. The formula $\frac{1}{2} IW^2$ represents rotational energy where W is the rate of rotation, and I the moment of inertia. Inertia is dependent on the mass of the object rotating and its distance from the axis of rotation. The spinning skater can only take advantage of the latter component by bringing the arms in tightly thereby reducing the distance to the axis of rotation and increasing the speed of rotation.

The thrower indirectly takes advantage of this law more from the perspective of decreasing the rotating body mass. Although the weight of the pitcher remains the same, the rotating body component decreases relatively in mass throughout throwing to the point of ball release. For example, in the late phase of cocking when the upper body is moving relative to the stationary lower body, the angular movement of inertia is virtually halved. Again when the torso slows relative to the upper extremity, the mass of the moving segment is dramatically decreased, enormously increasing acceleration (rotation). During follow-through it is necessary to reverse the process and transfer kinetic energy to a slower moving segment. This occurs by muscles decelerating the smaller segments. As they catch up with the slower lower half of the body energy is dissipated through the larger muscle groups.

Muscular Contributions

Muscular activity about the shoulder (Fig. 3-2) can be grossly divided into two major groupings.[23] The first group positions that arm for acceleration by placing it in maximum external rotation, horizontal extension, and 90 degrees abduction. This includes the deltoid, trapezius, supraspinatus, infraspinatus, teres minor, and biceps brachii. The majority of activity occurs in the early and particularly the late phase of cocking. The second group accelerates the ball. It consists of the large pectoralis major and latissimus dorsi, the subscapularis, the serratus anterior, and the triceps brachii. Their activity continues into the follow-through phase. The anterior musculature in addition to decelerating the posterior movement of the humerus is maximally prestretched to accentuate the forceful concentric contraction that begins the acceleration phase. Other reciprocal activity is evident between the triceps and biceps particularly during acceleration.

As previously noted there is minimal muscular activity during windup. During the early phase of cocking when the arm is being positioned into abduction, the deltoid and supraspinatus are the prime initiators. In the late phase of cocking the supraspinatus activity increases while the deltoid decreases. The infraspinatus and teres minor also show activity increasing through the cocking phase. These three rotator cuff muscles demonstrate mild inhibition through the acceleration phase (allowing forward movement of the shoulder while providing stabilization). Follow-through then demands an increase in activity of these muscles for deceleration and stabilization.[6]

The subscapularis joins its rotator cuff partners during the cocking phase contracting eccentrically. During acceleration there is a maximum concentric contraction to provide a major component of the internal rotation demand for the humerus assisted by the latissimus dorsi.

The clavicular head of the pectoralis major and the serratus anterior demonstrate the greatest activity just prior to maximum external rotation. This activity continues throughout the acceleration phase with diminishing activity during the follow-through.[6]

The upper trapezius maintains minimal activity throughout cocking and acceleration. Activity increases during follow-through to help decelerate the forward moving scapula.

Biceps activity is controversial, but most studies indicate a major role at the elbow and not at the shoulder.[6] This is evidenced by an increase in activity during the late phase of cocking when elbow flexion is a requirement and not during acceleration or follow-through

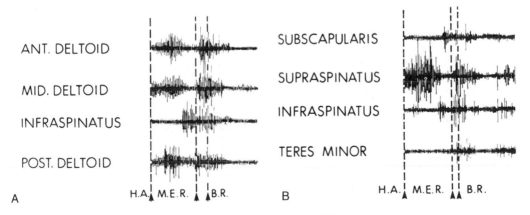

Fig. 3-2. Muscle action during a typical baseball pitch. **(A)** Deltoid; **(B)** rotator cuff. Phases of pitching: *HA*, hands apart; *MER*, maximum external rotation; *BR*, ball release. (From Perry,[30] with permission.)

when a stabilization role for the shoulder would be represented by an increase in activity.

Spinal Contributions

As mentioned earlier, the contributions of the shoulder account for only about half of the force generated in throwing.[3] Much of the remainder of the power is produced through massive rotation of the body. Beginning at the leg, rotation next occurs at the pelvis and spine. During windup the spine is slightly extended or in neutral. However, at the end of windup the spine is flexed. At foot plant in the late phase of cocking the pelvis rotates toward the planted foot with the spine extended and rotated. During the first phase of acceleration the spine is in maximum extension. Due to the explosive contraction of antagonists switching from external to internal rotation during acceleration the vertebral column is maximally loaded in addition to the joints of the shoulder complex.[24] Similar to the shoulder prestretch/contraction sequence with cocking and acceleration, the trunk flexors are prestretched followed by contraction to accelerate the trunk into flexion through follow-through. The spinal extensors then contract eccentrically to decelerate the forward flexing trunk.

Depending on the type of throwing style (overhead, three-quarter, or side-arm) there is lateral bending of the spine. Bending is away from the throwing arm side with an overhead throw and toward the same side with a three-quarter or side-arm throw.[17]

The cervical spine movement is primarily based on the thrower's attempt to visualize the target. For this reason, as the trunk rotates toward the throwing arm side, the cervical spine must be rotated to the opposite side. During the late phase of cocking and early phase of acceleration the cervical spine is also laterally flexed away from the throwing arm side. Limitation of any of the above movements due to stiffness, pain, or spinal segmental dysfunction will theoretically limit the effectiveness of the throw.

Differences Between Amateurs and Professionals

The activity of throwing may visually appear to be similar when observing the professional and amateur; however, the gross mechanism used and the selective call for muscle activity differs considerably.[23] The muscular activity of the amateur is in many ways similar to that of a professional with instability.[25] The uninjured professional selectively uses the larger muscles for acceleration and incorporates the trunk and lower body in a more efficient manner than the amateur. Fine control becomes more reflex in the professional.

Most divergence of muscle patterns appears in the late phase of cocking. However, the biceps appears to demonstrate marked activity throughout the entire cycle in the amateur, especially in the late phase of cocking and the follow-through. This may represent an attempt at stabilization.[23]

Posterior rotator cuff activity was kept to a minimum in the professional during acceleration whereas the subscapularis was one of the primary muscles used. The infraspinatus, teres minor, and supraspinatus were all incorporated by the amateur during acceleration. The professional seems to reflexly inhibit these muscles to incorporate selectively the subscapularis and latissimus dorsi during acceleration.[23]

The differences between the amateur and the professional are certainly in large part due to training. Atwater[17] observes that another major difference lies in the perceived gross intention of the throwing act. With untrained females she noted that their throwing actually was more analogous to a hard "push" of the ball rather than the "flinging" seen in the professional. This uncoordinated movement is due to the inability to generate momentum in one body part and pass it on to the next sequential neighbor without losing it. In error the body and arm move together throughout the movement.

Adaptations to Throwing

There are some inevitable adaptations in a professional thrower.[7] These are reactions to stresses applied over time. Soft tissue changes include hypertrophy of the upper extremity (in particular the forearm flexors) and

Table 3-2. Adaptive Changes Due to Pitching

Soft Tissue
    Increase in external rotation (total range of motion remains normal)
    Hypertrophy of the internal rotators
    Stretching of the anterior capsule
Osseous
    Hypertrophy of the dominant side humerus
    Possible bony outgrowth at the triceps insertion at the posterior inferior capsule

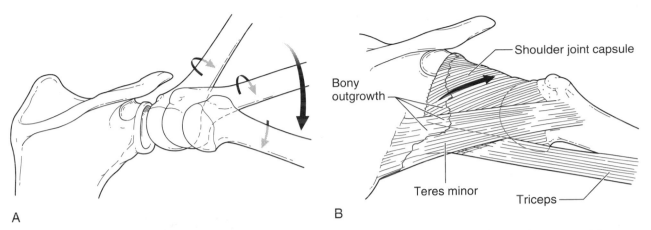

Fig. 3-3. (**A & B**) During follow-through of a throw, the humeral head leaves the glenoid (exaggerated for emphasis). The humerus pulls on the capsule, triceps, and teres minor, causing a bony outgrowth. (Adapted from Kulund,[11] with permission.)

stretching of anterior capsular structures on the throwing arm side due to the excessive amount of external rotation used (Table 3-2). These changes may lead to a visual drooping of the dominant shoulder also often seen with tennis players. Eventually repetitive external rotation stress may lead to a pathologic condition of anterior instability.

The excessive amount of external rotation required during cocking leads to an interesting imbalance. Even though there is an adaptation of increased external rotation and a proportionate decrease in internal rotation, the total range of rotation is normal compared to the nondominant side.[7] One would expect that this increase in external rotation would be accompanied by a hypertrophy of the external rotators, yet the opposite is true. The internal rotators hypertrophy often with a concomitant weakness in the horizontal abductors and external rotators.[26]

There are two significant bony adaptations to the professional throwing shoulder. The first is the expected cortical hypertrophy of the humerus of the throwing arm.[7] This change is necessary to handle the enormous torsional strains applied to the humerus especially during acceleration.

The second adaptive change is not a desirable one. Stresses applied to the posterior capsule, teres minor, and triceps during the deceleration of follow-through may cause ossification at the posteroinferior glenoid (Fig. 3-3). This change is referred to as a Bennett's lesion. It may avulse bone and interfere with normal pitching mechanics and also become a source of pain.[27]

Pathomechanics

Specific Pathology Due to Position

Positional stresses (Table 3-3) usually fall into three categories: (1) overstretching, (2) overcontraction (repetitive contraction over time), and (3) compression.

Table 3-3. Phase Related Injuries with Throwing

Phase	Possible Injury	Cause
Cocking	Anterior capsular fibrosis	Excessive external rotation
	Tearing of the capsule or glenoid labrum	Inadequate stabilization
	Impingement of rotator cuff	Positional plus lack of sufficient stabilization
Acceleration	Strains of the pectorals, laterals, subscapularis, and triceps	Powerful contraction from a stretched position
	Spiral fracture of humerus or epiphyseal damage in the young pitcher	Extreme torsional stress from external to internal rotation
Follow-through	Irritation of the suprascapular nerve, the middle trapezius, and rhomboid	Excessive scapulothoracic movement compensating for a decrease in glenohumeral movement
	Tendinitis or strain of the infraspinatus/teres minor	Deceleration overstress
	Bennett's lesion—avulsion or ectopic bone on posterior/inferior capsule	Excessive pull of triceps tendon and/or posterior capsule

Knowledge of the positional requirements of each phase of pitching enables one to predict the most likely consequences. Injury to muscle can be further broken down into either a concentric or eccentric injury based on the requirements of a particular phase of pitching. The location of pain may be a helpful indicator as to the cause of the underlying pathology (Figs. 3-4 and 3-5).

The windup, at least as defined by most authors, is essentially a passive upper body position. Therefore, the demands are low with a low risk of injury. During the cocking phase the demand is increased with several common problems occurring. These include eccentric muscle injury to the anterior musculature, instability with potential stretch injury to the anterior capsule, and compressive/impingement injury to the posterior glenoid area.

As the anterior musculature is repeatedly maximally stretched prior to contraction there is the likelihood of anterior symptomatology due to insertional tendinitis of the anterior deltoid, pectoralis major, latissimus dorsi, and long head of the biceps as noted by Albright et al.[28] Barnes and Tullos[29] found that out of 29 baseball players with anterior shoulder pain, 3 had insertional tendinitis of the pectoralis major and 2 had tendinitis of the latissimus dorsi (including a rupture). Subluxation of the long head of the biceps may occur.[11] The possibility of tendinitis and other inflammatory reactions is increased by the mechanical error of "opening up too soon" where the body rotates forward too early.

The later phase of cocking requires an excessive amount of external rotation and horizontal extension. This demands a flexible anterior capsule and musculature. There is often a fine line between required flexibility and instability. The posterior deltoid has a line of action distant from behind the glenohumeral joint center. Therefore contraction imposes an anterior force on the humeral head that increases as the humerus horizontally extends. Protection from this occurrence is twofold. First, the obvious protection is from the subscapularis, which acts both statically as a mechanical constraint to forward movement and dynamically through contraction. Second, assistance from the infraspinatus and teres minor appears to reduce the participation of the posterior deltoid because of their action as external rotators.[30]

Chronic stretching will lead to fibrosis of the capsule and in some cases lead to anterior instability. As the capsule is being stretched in this position, the glenoid

labrum is being abutted. This will often lead to fibrosis or tearing. If instability is present, this process may also involve the posterior capsule and labrum.

Poppen and Walker[31] demonstrated that in the normal shoulder (after initial abduction) the humeral head remained relatively centered throughout most

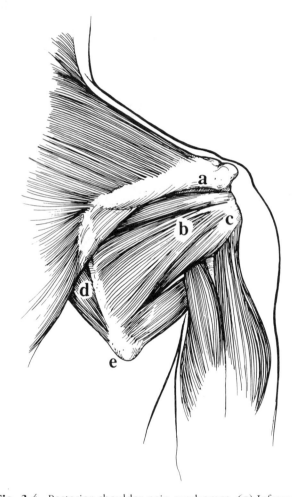

Fig. 3-4. Posterior shoulder pain syndromes. *(a)* Infraspinatus traction tendonitis. Pain under the posterior acromial arch is not likely due to traction tendinitis on the posterior rotator cuff tendons. *(b)* Infraspinatus fibrosis and internal rotation contractures. Repeated infraspinatus microtears may occur during follow-through, leading to muscle fibrosis. A secondary internal rotation contracture will develop. *(c)* Posterior capsule sprain. Follow-through stretches the posterior capsule, leading to joint line tenderness and pain on instability testing. *(d)* Rhomboid strain. Any of the periscapular muscles may be strained from the forces of follow-through. *(e)* Periscapular bursitis. Deep burning pain beneath the scapula may be due to a scapulothoracic bursa. (From Bryan,[90] with permission.)

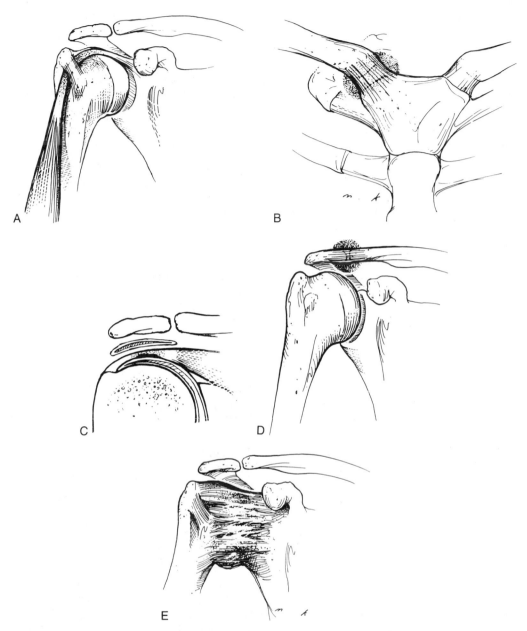

Fig. 3-5. Anterior shoulder pain syndromes. **(A)** Long head biceps tendonitis: uncommon in throwers but often confused with anterior instability syndromes. **(B)** Sternoclavicular sprain: hard swings with a bat or a vigorous weightlifting program may loosen the ligaments connecting the clavicle to the sternum. **(C)** Rotator cuff dysfunction syndromes: traction tendonitis secondary to the repititive stress of cocking-acceleration and anterior instability leads to subacromial pain. When symptoms are severe and performance is significantly impaired, consider the presence of a partial rotator cuff tear. Burning "at rest" pain may also indicate an inflammed bursa. **(D)** Acromioclavicular dysfunction. Three different situations are encountered: gross instability from old separation, popping or snapping from a torn acromioclavicular cartilage, distal clavicle osteolysis—pain over joint with x-rays demonstrating cysts in distal clavicle secondary to slight instability and/or chronic acromioclavicular cartilage tear. **(E)** Anterior capsule ligament/capsule sprain: repititive stretching in the cocking phase may stretch the anterior restraining structures leading to joint line pain; fraying of the labrum may occur but is of little clinical significance. (From Bryan,[90] with permission.)

movement. However, Howell et al.[32] tested the shoulder in the horizontal plane and found that in normal shoulders the humeral head rested approximately 4 mm posterior to the center of the glenoid. Positional changes such as flexion or rotation out of the cocked position caused anterior translation. Yet isometric contraction of anterior musculature such as the pectoralis major or anterior deltoid had no effect in recentering the humeral head. Given that the position of cocking normally allows posterior translation and that forceful contraction coupled with positional movement out of cocking causes anterior translation, it could theoretically be suggested that the articular cartilage (and the labrum) are subjected to enormous shear forces.

These exaggerated movements occur at 90 degrees of abduction with external rotation. It is possible therefore to cause irritation of the rotator cuff or biceps tendon. Impingement is more likely to occur if an underlying abnormality such as instability or a preexisting tendinitis or bursitis is present.

The acceleration phase demands rapid internal rotation from the anterior musculature. Rotary torque produced by the throwing arm is estimated by Gainor et al.[33] to be 14,000 inch-lb. Angular velocity of internal rotation was measured by Pappas et al.[8] to be 9,198 degree/s at the shoulder. The elbow extension velocity was 6,933 degrees/s.[8]

This torsional strain may lead to fractures of the proximal humerus. Tullos and King[34] feel that the spontaneous "ball-throwing" fracture of the humerus is likely due to stress (stress fracture). In the young pitcher with unclosed growth plates, epiphyseal damage is possible.[35] On rare occasions, there are total ruptures of the anterior muscles such as the pectoralis or subscapularis.[36] Most injuries involve first and second degree strains.

Repetitive resistance to the torsional strains of acceleration may also lead to synovitis of the sternoclavicular and acromioclavicular joints. Over time fibrosis and capsular thickening may develop. Calcification and possible early degeneration may occur.[37]

During follow-through (which includes deceleration as described by some authors) the demand is placed on the eccentrically contracting external rotators. Therefore, the majority of injury could be described as traction injury. Tendinitis of the infraspinatus and teres minor are possible. As mentioned earlier, there is a traction on the posterior capsular attachments of the triceps where ossification and possible avulsion may occur. Ossification at this point, the posteroinferior rim of the glenoid, is referred to as a Bennett's lesion.[38] This lesion is reflective of the tremendous amount of distraction applied to the humerus. The humerus may leave the glenoid by as much as 2.5 cm.[11] Additionally it is suspected that a Bennett's lesion is also due to posterior subluxation of the humeral head and/or posterior "cuffitis" slightly distal to the scapular attachment of the teres minor.

Due to the repeated trauma to the posterior capsule during cocking and follow-through it is possible for insidious posterior instability to develop. This development is seen in other athletes using repetitive overhead movements.[37]

Richardson[37] believes that the majority of posterior shoulder pain in throwers is due to a combination of capsulitis and tendinitis. Noting also that although the Bennett's lesion is more associated with the follow-through phase, irritation and pain are often found in the cocking phase.

With both normal follow-through movement and in particular when glenohumeral movement is restricted, there is a concomitant increase in scapulothoracic movement. Scapular traction injury is not uncommon. Neural tractioning involves the suprascapular nerve, while soft tissue involvement includes the rhomboids, middle trapezius, and levator scapulae.

The suprascapular nerve supplies the infraspinatus and supraspinatus. Irritation through stretch and compression occurs at a point where it passes through the suprascapular notch in the spine of the scapula. When affected, the ability of proper rotator cuff fraction is jeopardized.[39]

Medial scapular border pain is often associated with the follow-through phase of throwing and is usually the result of tendinitis of the rhomboids, middle trapezius, or levator scapulae. Excessive movement can initiate the development of adventitial bursae on the anterior surface of the scapula or irritate the bursa found at the inferior or superomedial pole of the scapula.[37]

Specific Types of Pitches

Pitches may be divided into different types based on arm delivery such as overhand, three-quarter arm, side-arm, and underhand. Although appearing at different levels of arm position, Atwater[17] discovered that the position is relative to side-bending rather than abduction of the shoulder. Using the face of a clock and viewing the pitcher from behind, a 12 o'clock pitch would represent a true overhand pitch. Pitching at 1 or 2 o'clock positions would represent a three-quarter overhand throw. Pitched from a 3 o'clock position, the throw would represent a true side-arm pitch. All represent positions of 90 degrees abduction, but changes in trunk flexion combined with flexion/extension of the elbow result in these apparent differences.

Overhand

Overhand pitches are also referred to as overhead and overarm. Overhand pitchers apparently generate more speed.[40,41] The increase in speed is probably due to the long moment arm. The axis of motion and moment arm are represented in Figure 3-6. The pitch appears overhead, and therefore pitched with full shoulder abduction. However, the angle is directed by lateral

bending of the trunk toward the left (in a right-handed pitcher).

Advantages to the overhand throw, in addition to speed, include a higher plane of flight, and possibly less occurrence of shoulder symptoms.[28] The one significant disadvantage is that the long moment arm is more difficult to control. Balance is one of the factors. The more side-leaning the more difficult the balance.

Three-quarter

The three-quarter pitch is produced with a neutral trunk and vertical forearm. It is called the 90 degree flexion throw by Collins.[40] The axis of rotation and moment arm are represented in Figure 3-7. The speed of the three-quarter pitch is not as fast due to the shorter lever arm. Short arming the ball and generally more valgus stress to the elbow may result in a higher injury rate with this pitch.

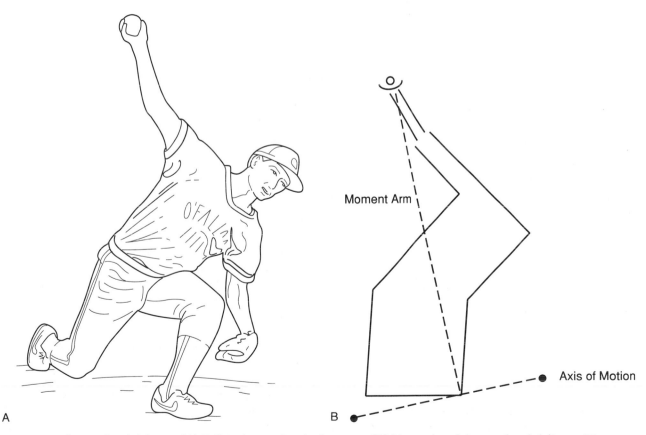

Moment Arm

Axis of Motion

A

B

Fig. 3-6. Overhand delivery. **(A)** Ball in the overhand release arc; **(B)** kinematics of the overhand delivery. (Fig. **A** adapted from Braatz and Gogia[24]; Fig. **B** from Braatz and Gogia,[24] with permission.)

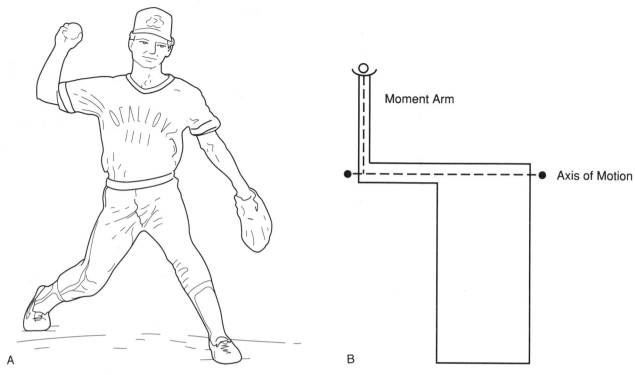

Fig. 3-7. Three-quarter arm delivery. **(A)** Three-quarter arm acceleration; **(B)** kinematics of the three-quarter arm delivery. (Fig. **A** adapted from Braatz and Gogia[24]; Fig. **B** from Braatz and Gogia,[24] with permission.)

Side-arm

The side-arm delivery is performed with an erect trunk and extended elbow. This position places more stress on the clavicular section of the pectoralis major and the anterior deltoid. The axis of motion and moment arm are represented in Figure 3-8. Due to the long moment arm, Collins[40] rates this as the second fastest pitch position.

Disadvantages to the side-arm delivery is that elbow injury is more likely due to the extension that occurs early in acceleration.[28] Also muscular protection of the anterior shoulder may be less. Finally, due to the flat plane of release, breaking pitches and changing speed on pitches is more difficult.

Underhand

The underhand pitch is the opposite of the overhand throw with relationship to side bending. With the underhand throw the right-handed pitcher bends the trunk toward the right. The axis of motion and moment arm are represented in Figure 3-9. Difficult to master, the underhand pitch has the advantage of confusing the batter due to the low trajectory.

Pitches can also be divided by the finger and thumb placement on the ball, which results in different speed and trajectory types. Different types of pitches require different muscular contribution both for the acceleration and the deceleration phases. All pitches involve some degree of pronation of the forearm.[21] The fastball requires the most amount of pronation. The brachioradialis and the pronator teres are the main muscles used with the fastball. The curveball uses more supinator and wrist extensor activity. Obviously this type of pitch effects less the shoulder and more the elbow, forearm, and wrist.

Interestingly, it would appear that the fastball would require the most deceleration; however, the rate of elbow extension is the prime determinant of deceleration needed. The curveball requires the most amount of deceleration force even though it is a slower pitch than the fastball. This is due to the rate of elbow extension being faster than for a slider or fastball.

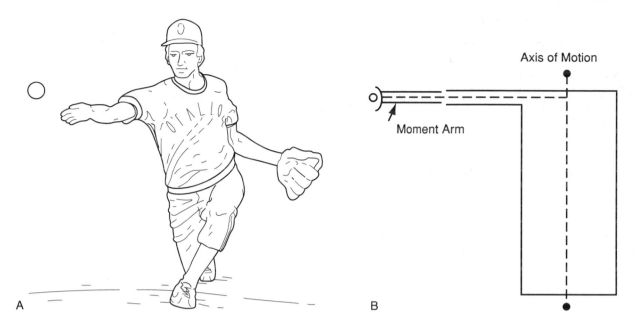

Fig. 3-8. Side-arm delivery. **(A)** Early follow-through from the side-arm motion; **(B)** kinematics of the side-arm delivery. (Fig. **A** adapted from Braatz and Gogia[24]; Fig. **B** from Braatz and Gogia[24] with permission.)

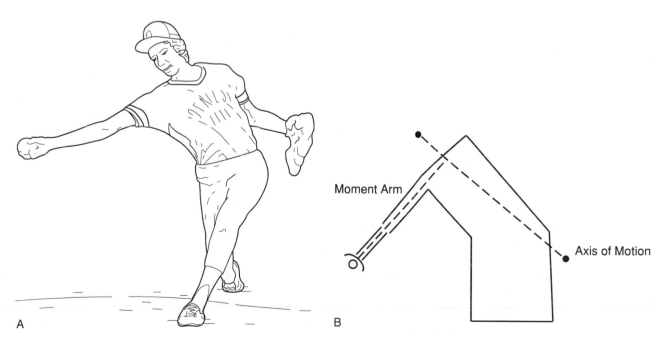

Fig. 3-9. Underhand delivery. **(A)** Release point during an underhand pitch; **(B)** kinematics of the underhand delivery. (Fig. **A** adapted from Braatz and Gogia[24]; Fig. **B** from Braatz and Gogia,[24] with permission.)

Impingement

Impingement occurs less often as a result of pitching due to the use of 90 degrees of shoulder abduction coupled with external rotation. As mentioned earlier, any deviation that visually appears to occur such as elevation or lowering of the arm is in fact due to body leaning. Although impingement is not commonly found with pitching, a pitcher with impingement or tendinitis of the supraspinatus may reflexly inhibit the supraspinatus.[42] This will increase the need for deltoid action during abduction especially during the late phase of cocking, risking upward movement of the humerus and further exacerbating the prior tendinitis or impingement. This will also decrease the available stability of the shoulder during late cocking.

A preliminary study by Michaud et al.[43] contradicts the observation of unopposed deltoid action with impingement. They found that the middle deltoid was inhibited with patients demonstrating supraspinatus tendinitis. Electromyographic activity significantly decreased at 45 degrees of abduction.

There is also a decrease in activity of the internal rotators such as the pectoralis major, the subscapularis, and latissimus dorsi. Decreased activity of the serratus anterior is also present. This lack of stabilization will eventually result in stretching of the anterior capsular structures possibly leading to instability. The lack of maximum internal rotation muscularly results in a slower and less efficient throw.[43]

Instability

Functional instability in a pitcher is not an unusual event. Due to the extreme stretching of soft tissue structures about the shoulder during cocking and follow-through, laxity is often a result. Instability may also occur at ball release when there may be a strong contraction of the biceps (Fig. 3-10). The bicipital attachment to the upper glenoid and labrum may be detached leading to a labral tear with associated instability.[44]

When pitchers with documented instability have been evaluated there have been some interesting findings.[25] There is a mild increase of activity in the supraspinatus during late cocking and acceleration. The biceps also mildly increases activity during acceleration. The proposed explanation is that this muscular activity

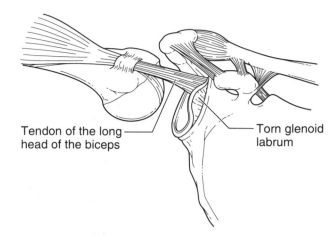

Fig. 3-10. After a baseball pitcher releases the ball, his biceps muscle contracts strongly. This contraction may result in the long head of the biceps pulling the upper part of the glenoid barium from the glenoid. (Adapted from Kulund,[11] with permission.)

Tendon of the long head of the biceps

Torn glenoid labrum

is an attempt at stabilization. This may lead to overload stress to these muscles.

Decreased activity was found again in the internal rotator group and the serratus anterior. This apparent reflex inhibition denies the needed stabilization during the cocking phase in an attempt to decrease the forces during the acceleration phase. Lack of scapular protraction may reduce subacromial space leading to or aggravating impingement of tendons or the subacromial bursa. Unfortunately, this creates a vicious cycle.

Adding to the complexity of the problem, there appeared to be a slight reflex inhibition of the infraspinatus that, depending on your point of view, may protect or aggravate anterior instability.[25]

Scapulothoracic Movement

A potential factor with inefficient throwing is the interruption of normal scapulothoracic movement. There are a number of possible causes, but, one final outcome: lack of stabilization for the humeral head with consequential soft tissue strain and possible impingement. If the scapula is not allowed to position itself under the humeral head for support, then muscular and capsular strain will result. Blockage of movement is seen with the following situations:

1. Tendinitis of the medial scapular musculature
2. Rib pain and/or subluxation
3. Adventitial scapular bursae or adhesions
4. Subscapular bursitis
5. The "snapping scapula" syndrome

Most of the above problems limit scapula movement through a combination of mechanical restriction and painful inhibition of muscular action. The snapping scapula syndrome is usually due to either a large osteochondroma or dysfunctional musculature. Clinically this may be evident by a large thud when the arm is raised. Rowe[45] feels that muscular tension is also a common cause. Tightening of the scapulothoracic muscles while elevating the arm causes the scapula to grind against the rib cage. He advises patients to "leave the shoulder muscles out of it" and concentrate on moving the hand only. Patients who are given strengthening exercises may inadvertently irritate their problem.

A common location for scapulothoracic bursitis is at the inferomedial angle of the scapula. Due to the repetitive stresses at the scapulothoracic area, inflammation and fibrosis may result. Pain is most often felt during early and late cocking and acceleration.[6] With follow-through, the pain is relieved. Many pitchers attempted to relieve the irritation and pain by pitching side-arm or leaving out the wind-up. Unfortunately, this does not effectively relieve the pain and at the same time interferes with delivery. Conservative care is recommended. Surgery is rarely indicated.

A relatively common abnormality of scapulothoracic movement is excessive movement (lack of stabilization against the thorax). This dysfunction of the serratus anterior is an important factor in many shoulder problems.[5,6]

Congenital Contributions

A suspected factor in the development of what pitchers refer to as a glass arm is a variation in the shape of the intertubercular groove.[46] These variations usually fit into two patterns. One involves the development of a ridge (Meyer's ridge). This may predispose the individual to pressure and direct irritation of the biceps tendon. Evidence of frequency in the general population was noted by Hitchcock and Bechtol[47] to be 67 percent. Another factor is the depth and angle of the groove

itself. These variations may lead to lack of stability and allow chronic dislocations of the biceps tendon. Added to this potential is the fact that internal rotation of the humerus reduces the stability. This position is needed during acceleration. Although dislocation is possible, it is believed that the vast majority of biceps problems are due to impingement and not to the rare dislocation.[48]

Proper Technique and Common Biomechanical Errors

An interesting observational summary and training method is the 90 degree rule advocated by McFarland.[49] The 90 degree position may exist with the leg, shoulder, elbow, or trunk. There are several positions that may be used as marker points.

1. In the "gathered" position of the windup, the stride leg knee should be bent at least 90 degrees (Fig. 3-11). This is crucial for balance and coordination.
2. On planting the stride leg, the knee should be bent at least 90 degrees (Fig. 3-12). This is important for shock absorption and transfer of momentum.
3. The angle between the body and shoulder should be 90 degrees during the early phase of acceleration (Fig. 3-13). This avoids opening up too soon.
4. During early cocking, the lead arm should never be more than 90 degrees abducted (Fig. 3-14). This

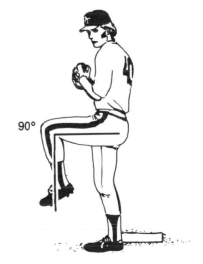

Fig. 3-11. 90 degrees: the gathered position. (From McFarland,[49] with permission.)

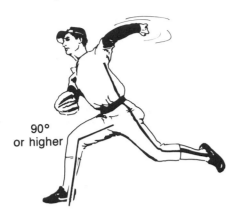

Fig. 3-12. 90 degrees: planting stride leg. (From McFarland,[49] with permission.)

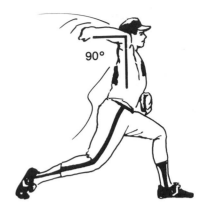

Fig. 3-15. 90 degrees: elbow with body, end of cocking. (From McFarland,[49] with permission.)

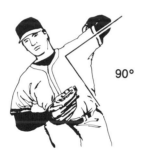

Fig. 3-13. 90 degrees; body and shoulder early acceleration. (From McFarland,[49] with permission.)

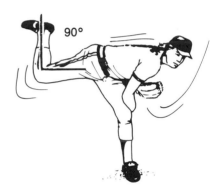

Fig. 3-16. 90 degrees: back leg and hip during follow-through. (From McFarland,[49] with permission.)

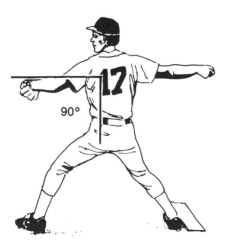

Fig. 3-14. 90 degrees: leg arm abduction, early cocking. (From McFarland,[49] with permission.)

position emphasizes another concept by McFarland called the "T position." With this concept the pitcher is taught to rotate the trunk as a unit keeping the arms essentially horizontal.

5. At the end of cocking and early acceleration, the elbow should form at least a 90 degree angle with the body when viewed from the side (Fig. 3-15). This will generate more torque production to delivery of the ball.

6. During follow-through, the back leg knee and hip should be at 90 degrees (Fig. 3-16). This allows absorption of the deceleration forces and maintains balance.

Advice from professional pitchers such as Tom Seaver[12] illustrates common mistakes made by amateurs in an attempt to simulate the strength and speed of a professional (Table 3-4). Examples include (1) rushing, (2) overthrowing, (3) crossing the arm over the body, and (4) pitching with a stiff lead leg.

Rushing is one of the best examples of a young or inexperienced pitcher's attempt at speed. The coordination between the upper and lower halves of the body is sacrificed. The lower body's contribution is neutralized resulting in an overlag of the arm. This decreases the efficiency of the throw and adds unneeded stress to the throwing arm.

Overthrowing is again an attempt at an increase in speed at the sacrifice of coordination. The excessive forces are applied to the throwing arm predisposing the athlete to injury.

As mentioned previously, it is extremely important to understand the contribution of the lower body in the production of the throwing act. A simple demonstration involves having the pitcher sit and throw. It becomes obvious that the distance thrown is easily cut in half and the speed of the ball is greatly diminished.

On follow-through it is extremely important to allow the momentum generated to be dissipated through trunk rotation. If the arm flings across the chest with no accompanying rotation of the trunk or body, all the deceleration forces are applied to the shoulder.

Planting the leg with excessive external rotation causes the athlete to open up too soon. The elbow has a tendency to drop, adding strain to both the elbow and the shoulder. The stress to the elbow is a valgus force. Planting the leg with too much internal rotation causes excessive arm crossover. This is referred to as staying closed too long. The planted left foot points more toward third base with a right-handed pitcher. Essentially, the body's momentum is decreased trans-ferring much of the stress to the arm. This crossover causes excessive stretching of the posterior structures with concomitant compression of anterior structures.

If the pitcher plants with a hyperextended leg landing on the heel a sudden deceleration of the body occurs. Often this is seen with pitchers trying to throw a fastball. Again the responsibility of achieving the speed is taken away from the body and given to the arm. As a result, shoulder injury is more likely to occur.

Little Leaguer's Shoulder

Little Leaguer's shoulder was first described in 1965 and consists of slippage or erosion of the epiphyseal plate of the humerus of the throwing arm.[50] Radiographic manifestations may include widening of the epiphyseal line, rarefaction on the metaphyseal side of the growth plate, and in rare occasions include a triangular metaphyseal avulsion as is seen in type II Salter fractures. Damage to the epiphyseal plate is caused by the extreme repetitive rotatory torque forces generated during the acceleration phase and distractive forces during follow-through. Although designated as a pitcher's ailment, catchers who must throw with less windup are also prone.

There have been rules set up to limit the amount of non-relief pitching in Little League. Unfortunately, this only applies to one team. Often a good pitcher is used by more than one team so that the rule is in effect nullified. In other words, each team may apply the rule, but if the pitcher is on more than one team, the effects are accumulative.

Another possible concern with young throwers with shoulder pain is the possibility of a fracture through a thin-walled unicameral bone cyst. Essentially a radiographic diagnosis, the helpful distinguishing factor is the presentation of a swollen tender shoulder.

OTHER THROWING EVENTS

It is far beyond the scope of this text to discuss all throwing events in the detail that would do them justice. As a result, some isolated examples are used to help demonstrate similarities and possible individual differences. Further reading is suggested for more in-depth consideration.

In the following discussion of other throwing sports

Table 3-4. Biomechanical Errors Leading to Injury

Error	Results
Rushing	Lack of synchronization between upper and lower body leading to an arm that lags too far behind
Overthrowing	Tendency to use the arm for propulsion decreasing the contribution of the lower body; overuse injury of arm
Throwing across the body	Lack of synchronization between the legs decreasing the effectiveness of the lower body; overuse injury to the shoulder
Lack of front leg flexibility	Leads to "bullwhipping" of throwing arm

it is important to realize that thorough electromyographic literature is not as prevalent as for pitching (with the exception of tennis). Most biomechanical evaluations are written in terms of physics and engineering, often concentrating on the apparatus used and the environment of the event rather than the muscular contributions. Therefore, these discussions offer little to the coach or physician seeking usable information in training and rehabilitation. As a result evidence for suggested coaching techniques or rehabilitation programs are almost purely theoretical and observational. The practical transference of the biomechanical discussions is difficult if not impossible. Therefore, until electromyographic evaluation coupled with cinematographic analysis is available, logic, coupled with observation, are the most one can utilize for these endeavors.

Javelin Throwing

The modern day javelin weighs less than 2 lb with a fixed length. This was a relatively late development in the 1950s. Prior to the development of the modern aerodynamic javelin, the design remained much the same as in the first ancient Olympic Games. The shaft was at least 260 cm and weighed at least 800 g.[51]

As with pitching or throwing a baseball, the speed and distance of the javelin are the result of combined forces generated from the entire body acting to transfer momentum sequentially to the arm/hand/javelin (Fig. 3-17). The obvious differences include the need for balance of a longer projectile and the assistance of a running phase prior to release. A braking force at release allows the transfer of horizontal movement to the arm and javelin. Biomechanical analysis of javelin

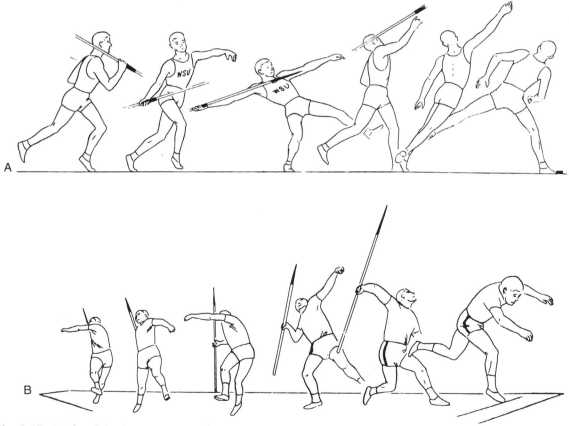

Fig. 3-17. Javelin. **(A)** The Finnish style utilizes the low cross-stepping approach, which allows progressive and steady acceleration. **(B)** The American approach utilizes a high cross-step style and a throw in which the shoulders are perpendicular to the direction of throw; this can lead to shoulder impingement and elbow medial capsular injury. (From Schneider et al.,[91] with permission.)

throwers in the 1976 Olympics in Montreal revealed some interesting differences between the more efficient European throwers and the less efficient U.S. throwers.[52,53]

Although running at high speed would at first glance seem to guarantee a faster, therefore lengthier throw, it appears to be only half of the equation. By evaluating the efficient throwers it became evident that the rotational torque developed by the body was the important missing ingredient in the U.S. throwers. The U.S. throwers attempted to reach maximum speed in the run before release. This necessitated keeping the pelvis forward and keeping the sagittal plane of the body perpendicular to the throw. They also incorporated an overhead toss.

The European throwers twisted the trunk so that the shoulders were 90 degrees and the hips 45 degrees rotated out of the plane of the throw. This angulation decreased the efficiency of the running speed prior to release; however, the rotational torque generated by this position added the needed force to produce longer throws. Further, as in other throwing sports, the successful throwers demonstrated a smooth transition of forces from the lower to upper body and from acceleration through deceleration. An adapted style of rapid cross-steps is used, turning the feet slightly toward the release arm side, which further increases efficiency. About 10 to 12 strides are used prior to release.

The most common injuries to the shoulder include impingement syndrome with an overhead throw and supraspinatus/teres minor strain with a side-arm throw. Sudden use of the biceps or any sporadic muscular attempt about the shoulder may lead to a glenoid labrum tear. Due to the angled release of the javelin coupled with the forces produced, the acromioclavicular joint is commonly sprained.

Discus

The discus is one of the most ancient sports events (Fig. 3-18). Via Homer's epic poetry it appears the discus may have occurred as early as 1300 BC In 708 BC the discus throw was part of the pentathlon. Originally, the discus was much heavier and was launched from a pedestal. Momentum was generated by a repetitive rotational rocking motion.

In 1910 a 2.5 m throwing circle was introduced that allowed a one and one-half turn pattern. A one and three-quarters turn was introduced in the 1930s with a hop. These advances plus the use of a 2 kg discus resulted in dramatic increases in distance.

Often a rubber discus is used to minimize hazards of off-throws. In addition, the high school discus is limited to 3 lb, 9 oz to decrease loads on the adolescent musculoskeletal system. A strapped discus is often used in practice to develop coordination and balance.

By lowering the knees and trunk, the hips travel a wider arc generating more momentum. The center of gravity should be kept ahead of the feet. The feet are kept close to the body counteracting the centrifugal force generated. Momentum is produced through a smooth transference of lower body energy to the upper body and discus. This is accomplished by two or three preliminary swings followed by rotation and/or a jump. The discus is released with a snap of the wrist.

Common injury patterns include allowing the arms to lag behind the lower body creating anterior shoulder stretch forces. This may lead to capsular sprain or subluxation. Additionally, the power snap at the wrist may lead to sprain or de Quervain's syndrome. Holding the discus more horizontal will place extra stress on the pectoralis major. This also allows the athlete to turn more quickly in the turns. Finally, the discus thrower's upper body is held rather rigid straining the lumbar, thoracic, and lumbar spine.

Shot Put

Like many of the Olympic throwing events, the shot put is an ancient event recorded as early as 632 B.C. in Ireland and Scotland. Then a 14 lb stone was tossed. The current 16 lb shot put used in college, Amateur Athletic Union (AAU), and Olympic events was first introduced in 1876. In 1904, the restrictions of the 7 ft circle were introduced. The lead-centered shot put is made of iron, bronze, or brass. Limitations on weight for younger participants are 12 lb for high school age and 8 lb for grade school.

The style of throwing has changed (Fig. 3-19) evolving from a straight style to a low set rotational style along a straight line introduced in the 1950s. In the 1970s the switch to the more efficient "discus-like" style was introduced by the Russians. With this ap-

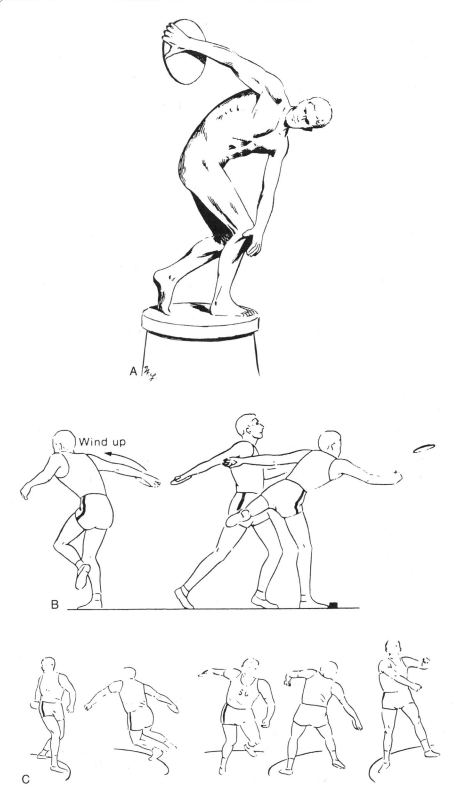

Wind up

A

B

C

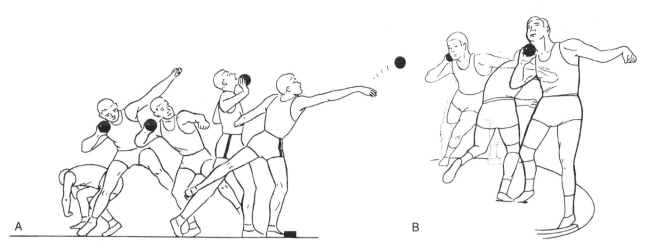

Fig. 3-19. Shot put. **(A)** Originally the shot was pushed forward, utilizing a hop and pivot to store and effectively dissipate energy; to this a starting crouch was added to gradually raise the center of gravity much as a sprinter uses the blocks. **(B)** A whirling discus style has recently been introduced in competition that may eventually prove to be more effective. (From Schneider et al.,[91] with permission.)

proach there is a total of 540 degrees of rotation. To take advantage of the centrifugal force generated, the weight is kept behind the center of gravity.

In general, shot putting is more analogous to an explosive push rather than a throw. The optimal release angle is considered to be about 41 degrees. Eventually, the shot putter launches the shot from the fingertips. However, early in the season the athlete uses the hand for propulsion. To prevent injury a rubberized or indoor shot is used during training. This somewhat diminishes the tremendous torque forces produced.

The shot put was studied comparing the throwing of the more successful Eastern European throwers and the less efficient U.S. throwers.[54,55] Some important differences became apparent. One of the most important was that the successful throwers gradually developed acceleration throughout the throw imparting maximum velocity at the release. U.S. throwers had a tendency to accelerate too quickly at the beginning of the throw.

Dessureault[56] has noted important differences be-

tween poor and world-class throwers. The better throwers extended their bodies more outside the rear of the circle before beginning the initial movement across the circle. Also the right knee was flexed. The better performers had more horizontal as compared to vertical velocity. Many of the better throwers left the ground at release. After the glide, the majority of better throwers were in contact with the ground for a shorter period of time.

There are two methods of delivery, the "straight-line" (glide) and rotational style (spin). The glide style is divided into several phases. The initial phase accelerates the body and shot together ending with the rear foot leaving the ground. The second or glide phase is a period of time when the athlete leaves the ground briefly (airborne) ending with rear-foot contact. The third phase beginning with rear-foot contact ends with front-foot contact. The fourth phase is the push-off ending with release of the shot put.

Difficulties arise in three areas. First, the less efficient thrower will accelerate too quickly, decelerate, and then accelerate at push-off. Secondly, a decrease

Fig. 3-18. Discus. **(A)** Originally the discus was thrown from a pedestal. **(B)** Additional momentum was gained with the institution of a throwing circle, which allowed a pivot rotation energy amplification process. **(C)** A linear rotation pattern shown above has since developed that further amplifies momentum. (From Schneider et al.,[91] with permission.)

in the lower body component may be caused by raising the center of gravity throughout the throw. This causes the athlete to "open-up" too soon and lose the full contribution of the body. More successful throwers maintain the same center of gravity throughout the throw. Thirdly, less efficient throwers remain in the air longer than necessary during the gliding phase. The more time spent in the air, the less time there is to push-off. Therefore, by decreasing the gliding phase (airborne) more force can be imparted prior to release.

Injury patterns in shot putting are, like many sports, errors of technique. Sprains and strains of the paraspinals, gluteals, external or transverse obliques, hip capsule, and other joints occur as a result of the tremendous torque forces generated. Injury to the anterior cruciate of the knee may occur when the athlete plants under the toe bar. This practice is an attempt at stopping momentum, preventing a foul, and gaining balance. However, the momentum generated continues through internal rotation of the planted leg. The fingers are involved due to the weight of the shot and pushing-off too early. The strain is at the extensor wad (lateral epicondylitis) in the elbow. In the fingers the volar plate, collateral ligaments, and lumbricals may be injured.

Hammer-Throw

Like the shot put, the hammer-throw (Fig. 3-20) originated in Ireland, although slightly later at about 500 B.C. Evolution to more modern day techniques began in the 1860s when, in American collegiate sports, a 16 lb shot on an oak handle was used. The restriction of a 7 ft throwing circle was introduced about 15 to 20 years later. In addition, two circular turns were intro-

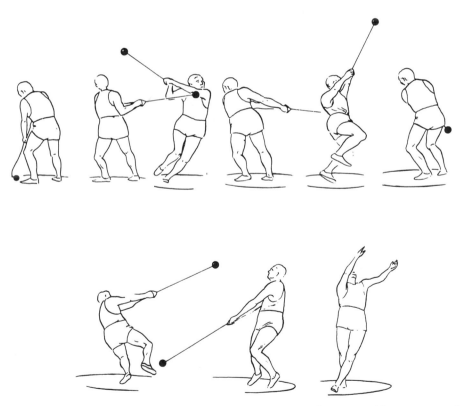

Fig. 3-20. Hammer-throw. This event is all technique in that the center of gravity and leverage must be perfectly balanced in order to generate momentum and energy. Using abdominal and back muscles to lock the upper body in position over the lower body, energy is stored and amplified by reciprocating crossed-extensor reflex during rotation. (From Schneider et al.,[91] with permission.)

duced. The three-turn technique began in the 1950s. The Europeans were able to generate four turns by the mid-1960s.

Although not a common sport event, this Olympic event was also studied by Ariel[57] in relation to the 1976 Games in Montreal. Again several distinct differences were evident. The shorter throws by the U.S. team were due to the inability to develop an increase in speed throughout the turns. Also the more efficient throwers used a double support, two-footed phase. This allows for more time to impart force via the legs. The U.S. group was also airborne longer producing the opposite effect. Center of gravity was also a key element in effective delivery. The lower the center of gravity the more horizontal thrust could be developed across the throwing circle. Finally, a continuous movement of the center of gravity toward the direction of throw was crucial. The best release angle is estimated at between 42 and 44 degrees.

The hammer-throw is accomplished by the athlete sitting back against the centrifugal force generated by the hammer. This sitting back position helps relax the shoulder and increase the traveling radius. A pull inward will decrease the radius and also prevent pelvic rotation. According to Doherty,[58] there is a 6 ft gain in distance for every inch added to the radius. The shoulders and hips are locked as the athletes expend a majority of their energy balancing on the balls of the feet and toes.

The demands on the shoulder are rather unique in this sport. The stabilizing functions of the shoulder are challenged maximally. Distraction forces are enormous and must be resisted. The demand on the posterior deltoid and triceps are likely high, but no electromyographic data have been presented to support this observation.

The natural stresses of the hammer-throw are on the hip due to the sitting back component of delivery. Strains of the back, abdominal muscles, and iliotibial band, and sprains of the hip capsule and public symphyses are not uncommon.

Injury is usually due to several technique errors. Allowing the hammer to get ahead of the athlete may cause subluxation of the posterior shoulder. Any disruption of the smooth progressive rhythm of the throw will lead to a jerk that may strain the shoulder, neck, hip, and back. An attempt to increase height of the throw by a sudden backward lean may damage the rhomboids, levator scapula, or rotator cuff. Lateral collateral ligament sprain of the knee may occur if the athlete attempts terminal elevation instead of gradually developing elevation throughout the delivery. Pulling on the hammer causing flexion of the elbows may lead to medial or lateral epicondylitis.

Tennis

There is an obvious similarity between throwing and racquet sports. The difference is that the racquet extends the length of the lever arm, which results in a mechanical advantage in force delivery. However, an increase in the length of the lever arm functionally equals more stress to the shoulder, elbow, and wrist due to increased weight. Therefore, the body must accelerate and decelerate an addition to itself. Another difference between throwing and racquet sports is the continuous demand not found with pitching. Added to this aerobic demand is a tremendous proprioceptive demand that is constantly changing requiring coordinated total body function. Add to this the different demands of various possible strokes. The focus of the following discussion will be on tennis; however, the principles can be transferred to other racquet sports. It must be pointed out that racquetball and similar "fast" court games do not allow the same body contribution found in tennis, thereby placing more demands on the distal upper extremity, in particular the elbow and wrist.

Strokes

In simple terms there are three major strokes: the serve (and the overhead smash), the backhand groundstroke, and the forehand groundstroke. The major difference between the serve and the groundstroke is the abducted positional requirement. Each stroke is further subdivided into stages, but in general, the two phases of activity are (1) preparation for ball contact, and (2) contact and acceleration of the ball. Like throwing, much of the preparation is through body positioning with the shoulder "along for the ride."

Serve

The serve is divided into four stages (Fig. 3-21 and Table 3-5):[14]

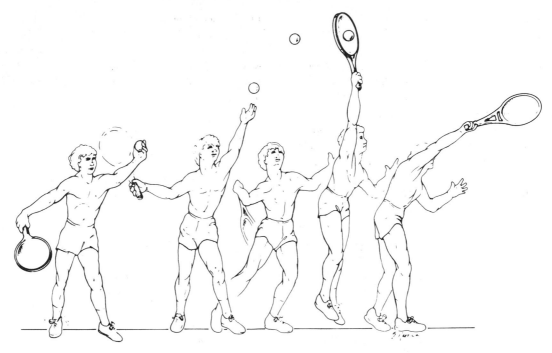

Fig. 3-21. Phases of the tennis serve, from left to right: wind-up, early cocking, late cocking, acceleration, follow-through. (From Perry and Glousman,[89] with permission.)

Windup—preparatory phase; largely a passive event for the shoulder. It starts with the initiation of the serve to ball release from the opposite hand.
Cocking—starts with ball release and ends when the shoulders are essentially level in a neutral position.
Acceleration—begins with internal (medial) rotation of the arm and ends with ball contact.
Follow-through—begins with ball contact and ends with completion of the serve.

Windup. The windup is an excellent example of the body positioning the shoulder without the need for much intrinsic shoulder musculature activity. By lateral trunk flexion coupled with rotation of the trunk and lower extremity, the shoulder is positioned into horizontal extension, abduction, and slight external rotation. The weight of the racquet also assists in passively extending the shoulder.

Cocking. Shoulder activity increases in this stage, yet abduction is still assisted by trunk positioning of rota-

tion and lateral flexion. As a result, middle deltoid activity is rather minimal.[59] Stabilization demands increase as evidenced by an increase to moderate activity of the supraspinatus and infraspinatus. The serratus activity is quite high in this stage indicating the need for scapular stabilization. Coupled with abduction and external rotation of the shoulder is elbow flexion requiring moderate activity of the biceps brachii.

The reciprocal phasing activity referred to by Perry[1] is called into play as the subscapularis increases in activity to decelerate the external rotation of the shoulder. This eccentric activity helps develop a subsequent plyometric activity of the subscapularis in the next phase.

During the late stages of this phase, forward momentum is begun in the legs and progresses through the hips and the trunk.

Acceleration. The momentum developed in the late stages of cocking by the lower extremity and trunk is assisted by strong activity in the subscapularis, pectoralis major, and latissimus dorsi in an effort to adduct

Table 3-5. Stages of Various Types of Tennis Strokes

Stroke	Stages
Serve	*Windup*—start of the service motion to ball release. Shoulder is abducted, extended, and externally rotated. Trunk laterally bends and rotates. Lower extremity rotation. *Cocking*—ball release until point of maximum shoulder external rotation. Muscular action similar to windup with addition of scapular rotation. *Acceleration*—internal rotation of the shoulder until ball impact. Shoulder internal rotation and adduction with simultaneous trunk flexion and elbow extension. *Follow-through*—ball impact to completion of serve. Muscularly there is a continuance of above decelerating functions.
Forehand groundstroke	*Racquet preparation*—begins with shoulder turn; ends with weight transfer to the front foot. Abduction and external rotation of the shoulder with trunk and lower extremity rotation. *Acceleration*—begins with weight transfer to front foot followed by forward racquet movement, ending with ball contact. Internal rotation and adduction of the shoulder is accompanied by elbow extension and scapular protraction. *Follow-through*—ball impact to completion of stroke. Muscular events similar to acceleration but at a lower level of activity.
Backhand groundstroke	*Racquet preparation*—begins with shoulder turn and initiation of weight transfer from back to front foot. Internal rotation and adduction of the shoulder accompanied by trunk and lower extremity rotation. *Acceleration*—begins with weight transfer to the front foot and forward movement of the racquet prior to ball impact. There is external rotation and abduction at the shoulder while the scapula is retracted and the elbow extended. *Follow-through*—begins with ball impact and ends when the stroke is complete. The forces generated in acceleration are diminished and decelerated by the posterior shoulder and scapular musculature.

and internally rotate the shoulder.[59] Even though this is the shortest of all phases, the muscle activity is the most powerful.

Although not requiring external rotation or even deceleration of internal rotation, the infraspinatus activity is rather high indicating more of a stabilization func-tion. This is also evident by the moderate activity of the supraspinatus and the high activity of the serratus anterior.[59] Other muscles found to have a relatively high output include the lower trapezius and internal/external abdominal obliques.[60]

As in throwing, there is an increase in biceps activity toward the end of acceleration to decelerate the rapidly extending elbow.

Follow-through. In the early stage of follow-through there is a continuance of the internal rotation muscle activity. This decreases while external rotator muscle activity increases in an attempt to slow down the forward flung arm and racquet. Stabilization is required with a consistent level of activity of the supraspinatus and serratus anterior.

Groundstrokes

The forehand and backhand groundstrokes (Table 3-5) are divided into three phases that are relatively self-explanatory: racquet preparation, acceleration, and follow-through.

Forehand (Fig. 3-22). As in the serve, racquet preparation (analogous to the windup with a serve) is a period of minimal shoulder activity. Arm and racquet position are primarily directed by trunk and lower extremity rotation.

Acceleration requires forceful contraction of the internal rotators, particularly the pectoralis major and subscapularis. Stabilization is provided mainly by the serratus anterior. Supraspinatus and infraspinatus activity is rather minimal. Biceps activity is increased during acceleration to decelerate the rapidly extending elbow. Follow-through calls into play the infraspinatus/teres minor to decelerate the forward moving arm and racquet.

Backhand. The backhand (Fig. 3-23) represents the reverse requirements of the forehand. Acceleration requires forceful external rotation and abduction calling into play marked activity of the infraspinatus, supraspinatus, and middle deltoid. Internal rotator activity is minimal with no substantial increases during follow-through. This suggests that deceleration is more of a body controlled event or the result of soft tissue restraint.

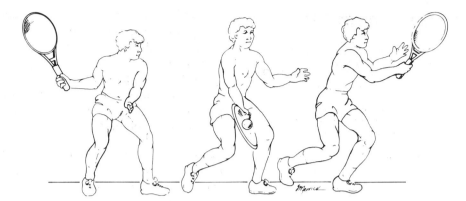

Fig. 3-22. Phases of the tennis forehand, from left to right: preparation, acceleration, follow-through. (From Perry and Glousman,[89] with permission.)

Generalized Muscle Requirements for Tennis Strokes

All strokes require full body participation with a reliance on efficient trunk and lower body rotation for proper positioning of the shoulder (Table 3-6). With this contribution the shoulder is for the most part passively positioned. The elbow is usually decelerated by moderate to marked activity of the biceps brachii muscle. If internal rotation and adduction are components of the acceleration phase, external rotator activity is required to decelerate the advancing arm and racquet. Another common requirement with most strokes is the stabilization provided by the serratus anterior positioning the glenoid under the humerus to provide a fixed point for rotation, whether external or internal.

Similar to findings comparing professional and amateur pitchers, the serve in tennis shows more selective recruitment with the professional. Miyashita et al.[61,62] confirmed in a small sample study that there were short silent periods of muscular activity before the sudden bursts for selected muscles. Further, they found that the electromyographic patterns of most muscles were somewhat similar when comparing the professional pitcher and tennis server with the exception of the trapezius, deltoid, and biceps.

Performance Factors Influencing Injury

Factors that contribute to injury involve the following:

1. Extrinsic factors including racquet size and con-

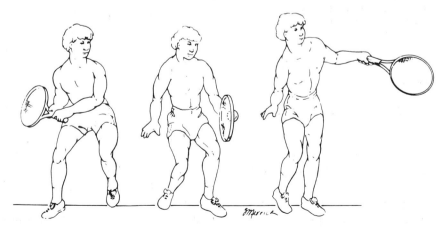

Fig. 3-23. Phases of the tennis backhand, from left to right: preparation, acceleration, follow-through. (From Perry and Glousman,[89] with permission.)

Table 3-6. Muscular Activity Related to Stroke Phases

Peak Muscles Activity	Stroke Relationship
Subscapularis, pectoralis major, and serratus anterior	Serve and forehand
Middle deltoid, supraspinatus, and infraspinatus	Backhand (during acceleration and follow-through)
Biceps brachii	Serve (cocking and follow-through); forehand and backhand (acceleration and follow-through)

struction (including grip size), string tension, and playing surface.
2. Proper conditioning and form.

Racquet and Grip Size

Theoretically, for the "all-around" player, a midsize racquet is the best compromise for force production and restriction of overload stresses. It has a 20 percent larger head translating into a larger "sweet spot."

Suggestions fall under two general guidelines when determining the proper tension for a racquet:

1. For control, string the racquet at the upper end of the manufacturer's tension range. For power, string slightly below the lower end tension suggested by the manufacturer.
2. Stiff racquets generally require higher tension than a flexible racquet.

It is specifically recommended that the strings be nylon and be strung between 62 and 67 lb. The strings will not last as long at a high load due to increased tension. The grip is usually an open throat construction that should decrease twisting on hits that are off-center.

Oversize racquets are often recommended for the novice due to the even larger "sweet spot," which gives a psychological boost making up for deficiencies in timing. These racquets should be strung between 72 and 80 lb with nylon.

The length of the racquet has been shown to be correlated with the size of the player and resulting efficiency. The smaller player generally does better with a smaller racquet.[63,64]

Grips should be leather assuring a firm contact. They should be long enough for a two-handed grip. Replacement should be every 6 months on average to avoid

the smoothness that may occur with usage resulting in a tendency to slip and turn.

The size of the grip is important; however, agreement as to which is better in decreasing forces at the elbow and shoulder has not been reached.[65] Some authors recommend an adjustment to a larger grip if the patient develops symptoms[66]; others recommend a smaller grip.[67] One study failed to distinguish either advantage. Nirschl[68] in 1973 developed a method that seems practical. He suggested measuring along the radial side of the ring finger from the tip to the palmar crease to determine proper grip handle size (Fig. 3-24).

Racquet construction has evolved dramatically over the last two decades with numerous choices being available to the consumer. There is insufficient biomechanical data upon which to base a decision. Theoretically, graphite offers the advantage of light weight with known vibration-dampening characteristics. In gen-

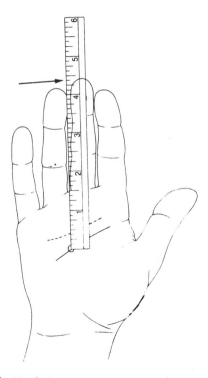

Fig. 3-24. Hand size measurement to determine proper grip handle size. Measurement of the ring finger along the radial border from the proximal palmar crease to the ring finger tip is a good technique for determining proper grip handle size. (From Nirschl,[83] with permission.)

eral, the more expensive the racquet the more graphite used in construction.

Playing Surface

A wet surface will increase the chance of injury from a stability standpoint. In addition, the ball becomes heavier when it is wet increasing the stress load to the upper extremity. It is also believed that clay courts may have some disadvantages because they are generally considered to be faster.

Form and Conditioning

In general, efficient stroke mechanics is similar to the mechanics in throwing sports. The efficiency is dependent on the summation of forces from the foot to the racquet, continuity of those forces and timing of the force transference and application. If the force generated in a particular body link is not transferred to the next sequential component it is diminished. The timing of this transference is crucial to optimum usage, such that if a body part does not decelerate quickly passing on the force generated, it is lost. If this occurs throughout the process, the end result is markedly diminished. Moving "into a shot" (stepping toward the direction of the shot) takes advantage of angular momentum maximizing transference of ground reaction forces to the ball.

Groppel[69] and Nirschl[68] summarize some of the common improper mechanics that occur in tennis:

1. Timing the body to the ball instead of the stroke
2. Exhibiting a "tray" effect when serving
3. Use of a one-handed backstroke leading with the elbow
4. Use of wrist motion at just prior to ball contact to make up for a poorly executed stroke
5. Doing too much, too soon, too fast

Serving

Serving has been compared to pitching a baseball, but there is a fundamental difference. A baseball pitcher throws down from the mound. A tennis player serves the ball up and over the net. This type of motion is more analogous to other throwing acts such as an outfielder throwing toward home plate. If the server did hit straight ahead, instead of up, the center of the racquet would have to be 10 ft in the air, even with a hard hit.[70]

When the ball is tossed it should be positioned in front of and to the right of the body (with a right-handed player). Training texts suggest that the ball be in front of the right shoulder and be at a height slightly higher than the racquet when extended. Theoretically, Beerman and Sher[71] demonstrated that a player has eight times the time to hit the ball when thrown at the level of the "sweet spot" of the racquet than when it is thrown 1.2 m above this point. In fact, this height would give the player less time due to the fact that the ball would be traveling at approximately 5 m/s. Plagenhoef[72] demonstrated that most world-ranked players make ball contact just after it begins to drop.

A comparison between two serve techniques, foot-up (FU) and foot-back (FB), was performed by Elliot and Wood[73] using cinematography and dynamometry. Vertical ground reaction forces were larger for the FU group providing a better up-and-out trajectory compared to the FB group. Larger horizontal trajectory forces were created with the FB technique that may provide an assistance in quickly approaching the net following the serve.

It has been assumed that the summation process seen in other throwing activities starting in the lower extremity was also true of the tennis serve. Elliot et al.[74] and others[75] demonstrated that this is a correct assumption. In addition, the lower limb contribution indirectly acted to increase the range of racquet movement. This occurs when the vertical lift from the lower extremity accelerated the shoulder leaving the racquet and forearm essentially "behind," with the racquet traveling down the back of the server.

Forehand and Backhand

The summation process for hitting the ball has also been found to occur in the forehand and backhand.[76,77] There is an interesting finding regarding final velocity. The peak angular velocity decreases at impact apparently meeting the demands of accuracy. Van Gheluwe,[76] and Ariel and Braden[77] have demonstrated with world class tennis players that the peak angular velocity of the racquet slowed averaging around 350 to 500 degrees/s reduction at impact.

Hobart[78] and Holcomb[79] determined that forward rotation of the pelvis on the front leg was the main

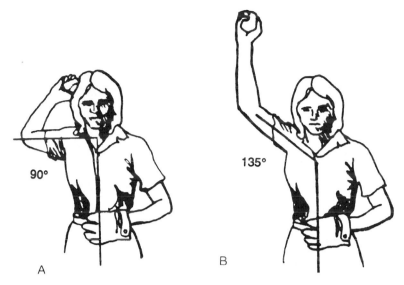

Fig. 3-25. Elevated technique to protect shoulder and medial elbow. **(A)** The 90 degree angle position is most damaging because the shoulder shear forces are greatest in this position. In addition, forces on the medial elbow are great. Therefore, this position increases the chances of injury to both the shoulder and medial elbow. **(B)** High arm elevations are more protective to the shoulder tendon cuff (shoulder scapular elevation releases the tight coracoacromial canal and diminishes rotator cuff shear forces). Higher elevations also diminish medial elbow force load. (From Nirschl,[83] with permission.)

contributor to forward movement of the racquet for both the forehand and backhand. Advanced players always demonstrated an increase in distance that the racquet traveled forward as compared with less trained individuals. Comparisons also indicated that electromyographic activity decreased with advanced players with concomitant increase in racquet velocity and overall stroke efficiency.[80]

Choosing between a one-handed and two-handed backhand is probably one of individual preference. The one exception would be when the player is injured, in which case the reduction of forces with the two-handed stroke is preferred. The need for coordination is probably also decreased to some degree due to controlling only two body segments as compared with five when using the single-hand stroke.[81] Apparently, accuracy is not an issue even when beginners were tested.[82]

Other Factors Influencing Injury

When injured, in particular with impingement or tennis elbow, a player should follow the above recommendations for racquet and grip size, construction, string tension, and playing surface. In addition,

Nirschl[83] recommends the use of a higher elevation serve position to avoid impingement. At 90 degrees there is increased compression at the subacromial space (Fig. 3-25), and the elbow is bent at an angle that increases valgus forces. At around 135 degrees of elevation, subacromial impingement is less and the elbow angle has increased decreasing the amount of valgus loading.

Counterforce bracing has been recommended for both the elbow and shoulder to reduce the tension on the extensor wad and biceps, respectively. The effect is thought to be one of displaced insertional tension, taking the tension off the injured area.

Golf

Although not technically a throwing sport, some aspects of golf are analogous to tennis and seem appropriate for discussion in the context of this chapter. Golf is a sport that is often regarded as nonstressful, requiring little conditioning and specific muscle training. However, given that there is a large number of older athletes participating, a closer look at the mechanics and muscular function is justified.

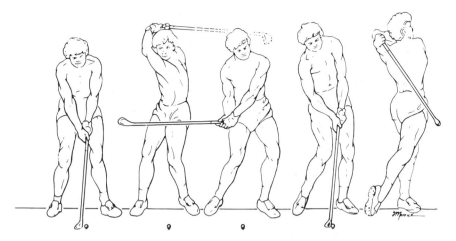

Fig. 3-26. Phases of the golf swing, from left to right: takeaway, forward swing, early acceleration, late acceleration, follow-through. (From Perry and Glousman,[89] with permission.)

Traditionally, the golf swing is divided into three or four stages[84] (Fig. 3-26):

Takeaway—This represents the movement pattern from addressing the ball to the end of the backswing (Fig. 3-27).

Forward swing—This phase begins with the end of the backswing and ends when the club reaches horizontal.

Acceleration—This movement begins at the horizontal position until ball contact (Fig. 3-28). (Forward swing and acceleration are often combined into a stage called impact.)

Follow-through—This is the final phase of movement beginning at ball contact through the end of the swing. Pink et al.[85] divide this phase into an early and late component. Early follow-through is from ball contact to horizontal club; late follow-through is from horizontal club to the completion of the movement (Fig. 3-29).

There are some significant differences between golfing and other similar sports. The overhead activity is minimal, usually never higher than 90 degrees with little opportunity for the end-range pathologies seen in baseball or swimming. There is much less internal

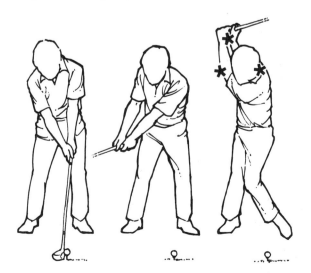

Fig. 3-27. Takeaway. (From McCarroll,[92] with permission.)

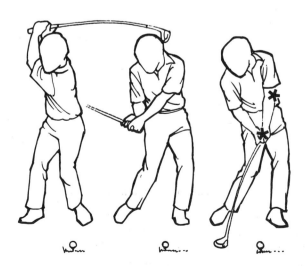

Fig. 3-28. Impact. (From McCarroll,[92] with permission.)

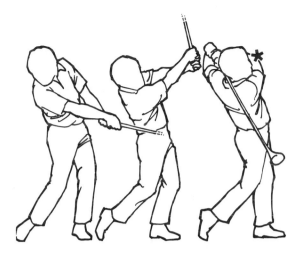

Fig. 3-29. Follow-through. (From McCarroll,[92] with permission.)

rotation requirements in the acceleration and follow-through phases of golf compared to baseball pitching and tennis. The bilateral participation is surprisingly equal in commitment to the production of the swing.

Similarities between golf and other related sports include the need for lower body contribution to the development of power through the swing. The lower body and pelvis rotate "ahead" of the upper body during acceleration then decelerate as the momentum is imparted to the arms and club. The right arm (of a right-handed golfer) acts in a similar manner to the drive arm of a forehand in tennis, the left as a backhand. However, the relationship of body position to force delivery is out of phase compared to tennis.

Electromyographic evaluation of the professional golfer has been performed by several authors.[42,84,86,87] The evidence is rather consistent and points to some important considerations in the development of training and preventive programs for golfers. To date, studies on amateur golfers have not been performed. It might seem logical to transfer the findings found on a comparison study of amateur and professional pitchers, which indicated the ability of professionals to fine-tune their muscle activity.[23] This indicated that less stability function of the cuff musculature was needed. These same differences may be evident in the amateur, and if so, may indicate more of a propensity to injury.

Muscular Participation

Muscular participation by phase for a right-handed golfer is as follows:

Takeaway

Right arm—Activity is generally minimal with some firing of the infraspinatus and supraspinatus. The subscapularis and posterior deltoid are also fired but with even less activity.

Left arm—The major muscle appears to be the subscapularis. Other participating muscles of almost equal contribution are the infraspinatus, supraspinatus, latissimus dorsi, and pectoralis major. A small contribution of the anterior deltoid was also noted.

Forward Swing

Right arm—The major muscles include the subscapularis, latissimus dorsi, and pectoralis major all acting as internal rotators. The contribution of the infraspinatus and supraspinatus decreases while there is a small increase in the firing of the anterior deltoid.

Left arm—Activity of the rotator cuff, pectoralis major, and anterior deltoid remain about the same. There is a sharp increase in latissimus dorsi activity and a small increase in the posterior deltoid activity.

Acceleration

Right arm—There is a continuing decline of the supraspinatus and infraspinatus firing with a concomitant increased contribution of the subscapularis and pectoralis major. The latissimus dorsi remains approximately equal as does the deltoid component.

Left arm—there is a gradual increase in the activity of the infraspinatus and subscapularis with a minimal decline of the supraspinatus and latissimus dorsi firing. A dramatic increase in pectoralis major firing occurs equal to the firing of the right arm. The deltoids remain essentially the same with a small decrease in the posterior deltoid.

Follow-through

Right arm—There is a continued decrease in most right-handed muscles throughout the follow-through. However, the subscapularis and pectoralis major are still firing at a high level. The latissimus dorsi continues to fire at a moderate level. The deltoids increase their activity minimally.

Left arm—There is marked increase in infraspinatus activity. The subscapularis and supraspinatus maintain a moderate activity along with the latissimus dorsi. The pectoralis major is the most active of all the muscles. Interestingly, anterior deltoid activity increases to a low/moderate activity.

Observations

The participation of the deltoids is rather minimal probably due to the lack of extreme overhead activities. Also striking is the implication that the rotator cuff does not need to act in synchrony to achieve abduction. The anterior deltoid of the left arm does seem important in assisting flexion and lifting during follow-through. Unlike many sports, the supraspinatus contribution is rather minimal with golf. The lack of extreme motions into elevation and adduction explains why impingement is rather uncommon with golfers.

There appears to be a timing due to function of the pectoralis major and latissimus dorsi especially on the right. The latissimus fires first during forward swing followed by an increased activity of the pectoralis major that continues through follow-through. This difference in firing pattern is probably due to the increased demand of internal rotation during forward swing for the latissimus and the increased demand for adduction during late forward swing and acceleration for the pectoralis major.

Many golf texts of the past have emphasized that the principal power of the drive was delivered via the left arm of a right-handed golfer. Electromyographic evalu-

Table 3-7. Common Factors in Form Among Professional Golfers

1. The head remains stationary with no more than 2 inches of movement during the swing.
2. The backswing and downswing are not the same. The path is somewhat "warped." The downswing is outside of the backswing.
3. With right-handed golfers, the left arm is not straight at the top of the backswing, but flexes more than 30 degrees.
4. The "butt" of the club handle does not point down at the beginning of the downswing.
5. Weight-shift with change of club is minor. Also, the swing is essentially the same for all clubs. The backswing does vary due to the length of the club.
6. Top golfers have similar swings. Shorter golfers tend to have flatter swings than taller golfers.
7. Common errors include:
a. Stiff-leggedness leading to an excessive upright swing.
b. Ball position too far to the rear leading to player "hanging back" to the right.
c. Too much leg flexion leading to a flat swing.

(Data from Mann[88].)

ation has failed to support this contention.[85,87] It appears that golfers trying to follow the advice of these texts may predispose themselves to overload injury to the left arm. This is anecdotally confirmed by Pink et al.[85] It might be concluded that specific exercises of the rotator cuff on the left might be preventative for golfers who attempt this left-handed power drive.

Finally, Mann[88] (as reported by Carney 1986) de-

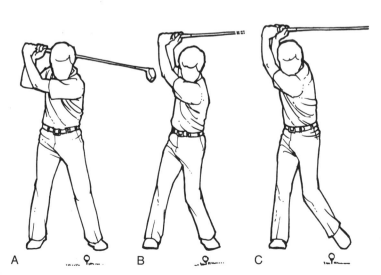

Fig. 3-30. Three golfers. **(A)** Golfer showing bent elbow and poor swinging mechanics. **(B)** Golfer showing poor weight shift and poor swinging mechanics. **(C)** Golfer showing correct swing position at top of take-away. (From McCarroll,[92] with permission.)

scribed some observations of 52 male professional golfers who were charted electronically via multiple body and golf club points in an effort to determine common positional similarities. A summary of these observations is listed in Table 3-7. Figure 3-30 illustrates some comparisons between good and poor form.

REFERENCES

1. Perry J: Anatomy and biomechanics of the shoulder in throwing, swimming, gymnastics, and tennis. p. 247. In AAOS: Symposium on injuries to the shoulder in the athlete. Clin Sports Med 2:247, 1983

2. Broer MD: Efficiency of Human Movement. WB Saunders, Philadelphia, 1969

3. Toyoshima S, Hoshikawa T, Miyashita M et al: Contribution of the body parts to throwing performance. p. 169. In Nelson RC, Morehouse CA (eds): Biomechanics IV. University Park Press, Baltimore, 1974

4. Warner JJ, Micheli LJ, Arslanian LE et al: Patterns of flexibility, laxity, and strength in normal shoulders and shoulders with instability and impingement. Am J Sports Med 18:366, 1990

5. Pappas AM, Zawacki RM, McCarthy CF: Rehabilitation of the pitching shoulder. Am J Sports Med 13:223, 1985

6. Jobe FW, Moynes DR, Tibone JE, Perry J: An EMG analysis of the shoulder in pitching: a second report. Am J Sports Med 12:218, 1984

7. King JW et al: Analysis of the pitching arm of the professional baseball pitcher. Clin Orthop Relat Res 67:116, 1979

8. Pappas AM, Zawacki RM, Sullivan TJ: Biomechanics of baseball pitching: a preliminary report. Am J Sports Med 13:216, 1985

9. Michaud T: Biomechanics of unilateral overhand throwing motion: an overview. Chiro Sports Med 4:13, 1990

10. McLeod WD: The pitching mechanism. p. 22. In Zarins B, Andrews JR, Carson W (eds): Injuries to the Throwing Arm. WB Saunders, Philadelphia, 1985

11. Kulund DN (ed): The shoulder. p. 259. In Kulund DN (ed): The Injured Athlete. 2nd Ed. JB Lippincott, Philadelphia, 1990

12. Seaver T. Lowenfish L: The Art of Pitching. Hearst Books, New York, 1984

    In Donatelli RA (ed): Physical Therapy of the Shoulder. Churchill Livingstone, New York, 1988

14. Moynes DR, Perry J, Antonelli DJ, Jobe FW: Electromyography and motion analysis of the upper extremity in sports. Phys Ther 66:1905, 1986

15. Terry GC, Hammon D, France P, Norwood L: The stabilizing function of passive shoulder restraints. Am J Sports Med 19:26, 1991

16. Harryman DT, Sidles JA, Clark JM et al: Translation of the humeral head on the glenoid with passive glenohumeral motion. J Bone Joint Surg 72A:1334, 1990

17. Atwater AE: Biomechanics of overarm throwing movements and of throwing injuries. Exer Sport Sci Rev 7:43, 1979

18. O'Connell PW, Nuber GW, Milekis RA, Lautenschlager E: The contribution of the glenohumeral ligaments to anterior stability of the shoulder joint. Am J Sports Med 18:579, 1990

19. Terry GC, Miller TK, France P: Functional anatomy of the glenohumeral ligaments. American Academy of Orthopaedic Surgeons Videotape No. 235, 1986

20. Gowitzke BA, Milner M: Scientific Basis of Human Movement. 3rd Ed. Williams & Wilkins, Baltimore, 1988

21. Sisto DJ, Jobe FW, Moynes DR, Antonelli DJ: An electromyographic analysis of the elbow in pitching. Am J Sports Med 12:351, 1987

22. Jobe FW, Tibone JE, Jobe CM, Kvitne RS: The shoulder in sports. p. 961. In Rockwood CA, Matsen FA (eds): The Shoulder. Vol. 2. WB Saunders, Philadelphia, 1990

23. Gowan ID, Jobe FW, Tribone JE et al: A comparatiev electromyographic analysis of the shoulder during pitching: professional versus amateur pitchers. Am J Sports Med 15:586, 1987

24. Braatz KJ, Gogia PP: The mechanics of pitching. J Orthop Sport Phys Ther 9:65, 1987

25. Glousman R, Jobe F, Tibone J et al: Dynamic EMG analysis of the throwing shoulder with glenohumeral instability. J Bone Joint Surg 70A:220, 1988

26. Cook EE, Gray VL, Savinag-Nogue E, Medeiros J: Shoulder antagonistic strength ratios: a comparison between college level baseball pitchers and non-pitchers. J Orthop Sport Phys Ther 8:451, 1987

27. Lombardo ST, Jobe FW, Kerlan RK et al: Posterior shoulder lesions in throwing athletes. Am J Sports Med 5:106, 1977

28. Albright JA, Jokl P, Shaw R et al: Clinical study of baseball pitchers: correlation of injury to the throwing arm with method of delivery. Am J Sports Med 6:15, 1978

29. Barnes DA, Tullos HS: An analysis of 100 symptomatic baseball players. Am J Sports Med 6:62, 1978

30. Perry J: Muscle control of the shoulder. p. 27. In Rowe CR (ed): The Shoulder. Churchill Livingstone, New York, 1988

31. Poppen NK, Walker PS: Normal and abnormal motion of the shoulder. J Bone Joint Surg 58A:195, 1976

32. Howell SM, Galinat BJ, Renzi AJ, Marone PJ: Normal and abnormal mechanics of the glenohumeral joint in the horizontal plane. J Bone Joint Surg 70A:227, 1988

33. Gainor BJ, Piotrowski G, Puhl J et al: The throw: biomechanics and acute injury. Am J Sports Med 8:114, 1980

34. Tullos HS, King JW: Lesions of the pitching arm in adolescents. JAMA 220:264, 1972

35. Adams JE: Little League shoulder: osteochondrosis of the proximal humeral epiphysis in boy baseball pitchers. Calif Med 105:22, 1966

36. Zeman SC et al: Tears of the pectoralis major muscle. Am J Sports Med 7:343, 1979

37. Richardson AB: Overuse syndromes in baseball, tennis, gymnastics, and swimming. Clin Sports Med 2:379, 1983

38. Bennett G: Elbow and shoulder lesions of baseball players. Am J Surg 98:484, 1959

39. Drez D: Suprascapulary neuropathy in the differential diagnosis of rotator cuff injuries. Am J Sports Med 4:43, 1976

40. Collins PA: Body mechanics of the overarm and sidearm throws. Master's Thesis, University of Wisconsin, Madison, WI, 1960

41. Ketinski R: How is the curve ball thrown? Athl J 5:12, 1971

42. Perry J, Glousman R: Biomechanics of throwing. p. 725. In Nicholas JA, Hershman EB (eds): The Upper Extremity in Sports Medicine. CV Mosby, St. Louis, 1990

43. Michaud M, Arsenault AB, Gravel D et al: Muscular compensatory mechanism in the presence of tendinitis of the supraspinatus. Am J Phys Med 66:109, 1987

44. Pappas AM, Goss TP, Kleinmen PK: Symptomatic shoulder instability due to lesions of the glenoid labrum. Am J Sports Med 11:279, 1983

45. Rowe CR: Tendinitis, bursitis, impingement, "snapping" scapula, and calcific tendinitis. p. 105. In Rowe CR (ed): The Shoulder. Churchill Livingstone, New York, 1988

46. Blazina ME: Shoulder injuries in athletics. J Am College Health Assoc 15:143, 1966

47. Hitchcock HH, Bechtol CO: Painful shoulder: observations on the role of the tendon of the long head of the biceps brachii on its causation. J Bone Joint Surg 2:263, 1948

48. Neer CS: Impingement lesions. Clin Orthop 173:70, 1983

49. McFarland J: Coaching Pitchers. 2nd Ed. Leisure Press, Champaign, IL 1990

50. Cahill BR et al: Little League shoulder. Am J Sports Med 2:150, 1974

51. Schneider RC, Kennedy JC, Plant ML: Sports Injuries: Mechanisms, Prevention, and Treatment. Williams & Wilkins, Baltimore, 1985

52. Ariel GB: Computerized biomechanical analysis of throwers at the 1975 Olympic javelin camp. Track Field Q Rev 76:45, 1976

53. Ariel GB: Biomechanical analysis of the javelin throw. Track Field Q Rev 80:9, 1980

54. Ariel GB: Computerized biomechanical analysis of track and field athletics utilized by the Olympic training camp for throwing events. Track Field Q Rev 72:99, 1972

55. Ariel GB: Biomechanical analysis of shotputting. Track Field Q Rev 79:27, 1980

56. Dessureault J: Selected kinetics and kinematic favors involved in shot-putting. Doctoral dissertation, Indiana University, ID, 1976

57. Ariel GB: Biomechanical analysis of the hammer throw. Track Field Q Rev 80:41, 1980

58. Doherty JK: Track and Field Omnibus. 2nd Ed. Tofnews, Los Altos, CA, 1976

59. Ryu RK, McCormick J, Jobe FW et al: An electromyographic analysis of shoulder function in tennis players. Am J Sports Med 16:481, 1988

60. Anderson MB: Comparison of muscle patterning in the overarm throw and tennis serve. Res Q 50:541, 1979

61. Miyashita M, Tsunoda T, Sakurai S et al: The tennis serve as compared with overhand throwing. p. 125. In Groppel JL (ed): Proceedings of the National Symposium on Racquet Sports. University of Illinois, Champaign, IL, 1979

62. Miyashita M, Tusnoda T, Sakurai S et al: Muscular activities in the tennis serve and overhand throwing. Scand J Sports Sci 2:52, 1980

63. Ward T, Groppel JL: Sport implement selection: can it be based upon anthropometric indicators? Mot Skills Ther Pract 4:103, 1980

64. Elliot B: Tennis racquet selection: a factor in early skill development. Aust J Sports Sci 1:23, 1981

65. Adelsberg S: The tennis stroke: an EMG analysis of selected muscles with rackets of increasing grip size. Am J Sports Med 14:139, 1976

65. Kulund D: The Injured Athlete. p. 305. JB Lippincott, Philadelphia, 1982

66. Roy S, Irvin R: Sports medicine prevention: evaluation, management, and rehabilitation. p. 220. Prentice-Hall, Englewood Cliffs, NJ, 1983

68. Nirschl RP: Arm Care. Medical Sports Publishing, Arlington, VA, 1983

69. Groppel JL: Tennis for advanced players and those who would like to be. Human Kinetics Publishers, Champaign, IL, 1984

70. Braden V, Bruns B: Vic Braden's Tennis for the Future. Little Brown, Boston, 1977

71. Beerman J, Sher L: Improve tennis service through mathematics. J Health Phys Ed Rec 9:46, 1981

72. Plagenhoef S: Fundamentals of Tennis. Prentice-Hall, Englewood Cliffs, NJ, 1970

73. Elliot BC, Wood GA: The biomechanics of the foot-up and foot-back tennis service techniques. Aust J Sports Sci 3:3, 1983

74. Elliot BC, Marsh T, Blanksby B: A three-dimensional cinematographic analysis of the tennis serve. Int J Sports Biomech 2:260, 1986

75. Van Gheluwe B, Hebbelinck M: The kinematics of the service movement in tennis: a three-dimensional cinematographic approach. p. 521. In Winter DA, Normal RW, Wells R et al (eds) Biomechanics IX. Human Kinetics Publishers, Champaign, IL, 1983

76. Van Gheluwe B: A three dimensional analysis of the tennis forehand. Unpublished manuscript. Vrije Universiteit, Brussels, Belgium, 1983

77. Ariel GB, Braden VK: Biomechanical analysis of ballistic vs. tracking movements in tennis skills. p. 105. In Groppel JL (ed): Proceedings of the National Symposium on Racquet Sports. University of Illinois, Champaign, IL, 1979

78. Hobart DJ: A cinematographic analysis of the tennis backhand using three different levels of skill. Master's thesis. University of Maryland, Baltimore, 1967

79. Holcomb DL: A cinematographic analysis of the forehand, backhand, and American twist strokes. Unpublished Master's thesis. Florida State University, Tallahassee, FL, 1963

80. Anderson JP: An electromyographic study of ballistic movement in the tennis forehand drive. Unpublished PhD thesis. University of Minnesota, Minneapolis, MN, 1970

81. Groppel JL: A kinematic analysis of the tennis one-handed and two-handed backhand drives of highly skilled females. Unpublished PhD thesis. Florida State University, Tallahassee, FL, 1978

82. Rheinhardt PT: A comparison of the accuracy of the one-handed and two-handed backhand tennis strokes. Unpublished Master's thesis. Springfield College, Springfield, MA, 1975

83. Nirschl RP: Prevention and treatment of elbow and shoulder injuries in the tennis player. Clin Sports Med 7:289, 1988

84. Jobe FW, Perry J, Pink M: Electromyographic shoulder activity in men and women professional golfers. Am J Sports Med 17:782, 1989

85. Pink M, Jobe FW, Perry J: Electromyographic analysis of the shoulder during the golf swing. Am J Sports Med 18: 137, 1990

86. Moynes DR, Perry J, Antonelli DJ et al: Electromyographic and motion analysis of the upper extremity in sports. Phys Ther 66:1905, 1986

87. Jobe FW, Moynes DR, Antonelli DJ: Rotator cuff function during a golf swing. Am J Sports Med 14:388, 1986

88. Mann R: Shattering the swing phase and other teaching myths. Golf Digest, July 1986

89. Perry J, Glousman R: Biomechanics of throwing. pp. 740–745. In Nicholas JA, Hershman EB (eds): The Upper Extremity in Sports Medicine. CV Mosby, St. Louis, 1990

90. Bryan W: Baseball. p. 465. In Reider B (ed): Sports Medicine: The School-Age Athlete. WB Saunders, Philadelphia, 1991

91. Schneider RC, Kennedy JC, Plant ML et al: Sports Injuries: Mechanisms, Prevention, and Treatment. p. 240. Williams & Wilkins, Baltimore, 1986

92. McCarroll JR: Evaluation, treatment, and prevention of upper extremity injuries in golfers. p. 884. In Nicholas JA, Hershman EB (eds): The Upper Extremity in Sports Medicine. CV Mosby, St. Louis, 1990

4
The Shoulder in Swimming

THOMAS A. SOUZA

Comparisons are often made regarding the shoulder and its use in throwing sports and swimming.[1,2] The similarities are emphasized. Although it is true that the arm is stressed in an overhead position, the similarity stops here. Swimming involves working against gravity acting at right angles to the body (this occurs mainly during recovery). Throwing sports have an axial gravity force applied; therefore, the abductors are the prime antigravity muscles. In swimming the extensors and external rotators are the antigravity muscles. The stress on the posterior decelerator musculature is much greater with throwing due to follow-through demands not found with swimming. These same muscles are needed in freestyle swimming, but they function against gravity and in a concentric rather than an eccentric mode. The forces generated in throwing are intended for acceleration of a projectile, while in swimming the body is pulled through water. The force contributions of the trunk musculature and lower extremity far exceed those made by these same muscles in swimming.[3]

Throwing requires short bursts of energy with substantial rest periods interspersed. Swimming is a continuous, unrelenting demand requiring an aerobic factor not found in throwing. Most importantly, the shoulder is in an impingement position during the most demanding phase of movement with swimming (internal rotation and adduction).[4] Throwing places the shoulder in this position only at the follow-through phase with most of the contraction occurring in the decelerators (external rotators) with less of an overhead position.[2]

Although Kennedy et al.[5] found a rather low incidence of shoulder problems in swimmers (3 percent), most studies indicate somewhere between 42 and 67 percent incidence.[6,7] McMaster[8] estimated that a competitive swimmer would swim between 8,000 and 20,000 yards per day during midseason. This would be performed usually with two practice sessions per day, 5 to 7 days per week with only a 1 to 2 month break. Some careers last between 10 and 15 years. Assuming a midrange of 10,000 y/d, 5 d/wk, 10 mo/yr with 15 individual arm strokes for each length of the pool (25-yd pool), the swimmer would log well over one million arm movements per year.[8]

PROPULSION

Twenty-five years ago there was only one concept of forward propulsion: drag propulsion. This was based on the visual and tactile assumption that forward movement in water was due to pushing water backwards. In other words, it seemed from the observer's standpoint that legs kicked back and arms pushed back against the water. The swimmer even felt this sensation of push as they moved forward. For years swimmers were encouraged to push backward as much as possible to maximize speed. Interestingly, one of the initiators of this concept, Councilman, reconsidered the theory and with Brown, investigated swimmers with stroboscopic photography.[9] Surprisingly they found that movement of the arms and legs was not backward but predominantly out and down. Other investigations followed confirming these observations.[10–13]

How then could swimmers propel themselves forward by pushing out and down? The answer lies in the concept of aerodynamic lift theory. There are essentially two components to first consider: drag and lift. Drag acts in a direction opposite to the direction an object is moving. Lift is always acting in a direction perpendicular to the direction of drag. Lift, using an airplane wing analogy, is created when faster moving air on the top surface of the wing creates a negative pressure while the slower moving air on the undersurface creates a positive pressure. The difference in speed of the air creates a difference of pressure due to the curved surface and angle of the wing. When this pressure difference exists a lift is created under the wing, acting perpendicular to the drag force of air resistance (Fig. 4-1).

Applied to swimming, this analogy must be turned on its end 90 degrees. Assuming the arms are moving downward as opposed to backward, the drag force is vertical and not horizontal to the water. First, using the hands as analogous to the airplane wing, water travels faster over the curved dorsal surface of fingers, with slower moving water under the palm. The result is a lift forward. The lift is not upward in this situation because the drag force is vertical not horizontal to the water (Fig. 4-2). Why then do the hands not simply move forward? This tendency toward forward movement of the hands is resisted by their downward movement and the stabilizing effect of the shoulders. Since the hand and arms, in effect, remain stationary, the body (freely floating) moves forward over them.

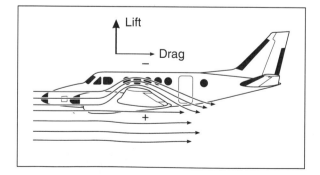

Fig. 4-1. The relationship of aerodynamic lift to flight. (Adapted from Maglischo,[17] with permission.)

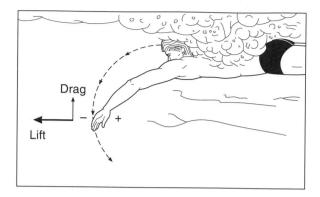

Fig. 4-2. Lift force and propulsion while swimming the front crawl stroke. (Adapted from Maglischo,[17] with permission.)

Other factors that cause the knuckleside water to accelerate are the direction and speed of arm motion, the shape of the hand, and the angle of attack.

In reality, the hands and feet act more as propeller blades than wings. Observations of world class swimmers indicate that they change direction of their hands and feet several times during a stroke. In effect, this creates "new water" to work against similar to a propeller.

SWIMMING STROKES

There are generally four major stroke patterns used. These include the freestyle (usually crosscrawl), butterfly, backstroke, and breaststroke.[6] The freestyle is often used as a training stroke substitute for the others.[14] The freestyle and backstroke use alternating arm patterns requiring body roll, whereas the butterfly and breaststroke use a simultaneous bilateral stroke.

The single arm stroke patterns rely on body roll for positioning. The use of body roll is essential in maintaining the shoulder in an efficient position of relative neutral.[15] This allows recruitment of both the pectorals (anteriorly placed adductor/internal rotators) and the latissimus dorsi (posteriorly placed adductor/internal rotator) resulting in a more powerful stroke.[16] Alteration of this position by lack of body roll or weakened/fatigued musculature will result in a less powerful propulsion with consequent overstraining of either muscle.

The hand movement through water is relatively consistent generally describing an **S** pattern (Councilman describes individual differences).[15] Observation of this movement demonstrates phases where the hand moves transversely through the water. Although at first glance this appears to be an impediment to forward movement, this position creates a lift component that helps propel the body.[17] Therefore, hand position is also crucial and is dependent on the feel of the swimmer and the efficiency of the forearm musculature. If the arm and hand pulled straight back through the water, the body would be pulled laterally decreasing the efficiency of forward movement. Schleihauf[18] compares this to the angle at which the blades of an outboard motor traverse the water (Fig. 4-3). This would be inefficient without a certain pitch to the blades, which is analogous to the angle of the hands with swimming. The more efficient swimmer pulls the body over the arm and hand as if the water was so "hard" that it acts as a solid and the athlete is climbing horizontally.

All strokes are divided into two general phases: the in-water phase called pull-through, and the out-of-water phase (the exception is the breaststroke) termed recovery. These are further subdivided based on the type of stroke. The freestyle, butterfly, and backstroke are divided into hand-entry, mid pull-through, and end pull-through subphases for in-water movement.[16] The recovery is divided into elbow lift, midrecovery, and hand-entry subphases. The breaststroke pull-through phase is divided into hand separation, mid pull-through, and rapid pull-up subphases. The recovery has no subphases; it is simply described as elbow extension/shoulder flexion.[16]

Maglischo[17] describes a separate classification system based on sweeping motions. He emphasizes four basic sweeping motions that are incorporated with different strokes and with different phases of these strokes. Even though the sweep motions are usually coupled (involving two to three components directions), Maglischo uses the dominant direction as the named pattern. The four patterns are the outsweep, the downsweep, the insweep, and the upsweep.

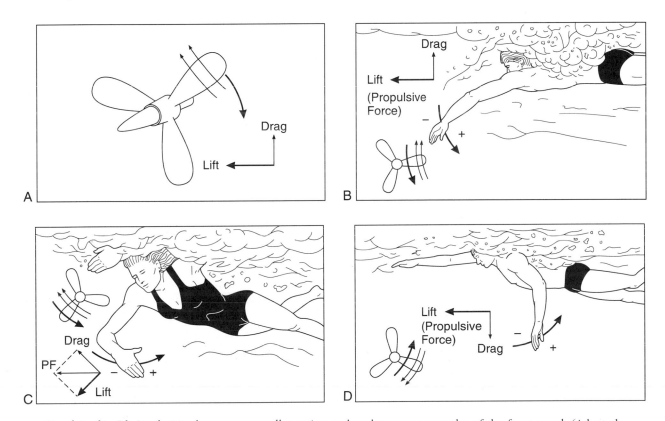

Fig. 4-3. (A–D) Similarities between propeller action and underwater armstroke of the front crawl. (Adapted from Maglischo,[17] with permission.)

The Outsweep

The outsweep (Fig. 4-4) is found in the in-water phase of the butterfly and breaststroke. It is the initial movement used with these strokes using an outward pitch of as much as 90 degrees to the horizontal. Compared to other sweep patterns, the degree of propulsion is minimal. One interesting aspect of the outsweep is the position of the fingers. The characteristic pattern is to separate the thumb from the fingers and keep the first finger slightly anterior to the rest. It is believed that this may enhance lift propulsion.[19] The angle of attack should be between 38 and 50 degrees. Beyond 50 degrees increases the drag effect.

The Downsweep

The downsweep (Fig. 4-5) is the initial in-water sweep pattern of the freestyle and backstroke. The angle of attack seems to be between 30 and 40 degrees with a cupping of the hands to improve the "aerodynamic" effect.

The Insweep

The insweep (Fig. 4-6) begins as the downsweep ends. It is part of all competitive strokes (with the exception

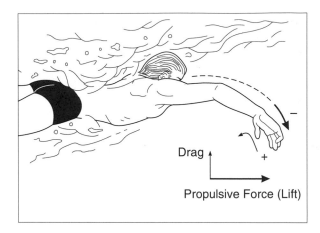

Fig. 4-5. The downsweep. Once a catch is made, the hand moves downward and outward with the palm pitched out, down, and back. Water flows upward and inward being accelerated over the knuckle side, while the water passing under the palm is deflected backward. The difference in pressure between the two surfaces exerts a lift force that propels the swimmer forward. The arrows indicate the usual distance over which the downsweep is used. (Adapted from Maglischo,[17] with permission.)

of the backstroke where it is termed an upsweep). The insweep moves up and back ending as the hand approaches the body's midline. The angle of attack appears to be between 25 and 80 degrees. The reason for this wide discrepancy is likely due to the observation that some swimmers who push back more use a smaller angle of attack. Again, angles between 30 and 50 degrees would emphasize more lift-dominated propulsion.

There is a variation in how far world class swimmers cross their hand during the insweep. Maglischo[17] recognizes three patterns based on where the hand begins in relation to the shoulder. The minimal insweep would occur if the swimmer began with the arm slightly wide of the shoulder. The midline sweep is the most common with the swimmer beginning with the hand in line with the shoulder. The crossover style starts with the hand inside the shoulder. There is disagreement as to the efficiency of one pattern over another.

The Upsweep

The upsweep (Fig. 4-7) is the final in-water movement of the front crawl and butterfly strokes. (With the backstroke it is termed a downsweep.) There are actually

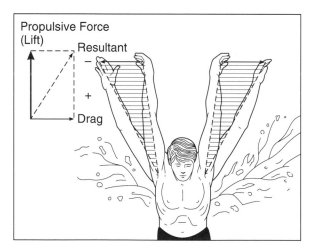

Fig. 4-4. The outsweep. The hands move outward with the palms pitched out and back. A high pressure area on the palm side, relative to an area of lower pressure on the knuckle side, creates a pressure differential that causes a lift force that propels the swimmer forward. The distance over which the outsweep is generally used is illustrated by the arrows in the stroke plot. (Adapted from Maglischo,[17] with permission.)

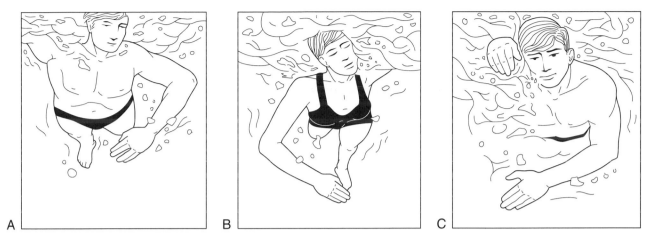

Fig. 4-6. Three insweep styles. **(A)** A minimal insweep. The swimmer's hand was wide of the shoulder during the downsweep and travels inward only to the near border of the body. **(B)** The most commonly used insweep style. The hand is brought inward to the midline. Swimmers who begin the insweep with the hand in line with their shoulder generally use this style. **(C)** The crossover style. The hand is swept inward past the midline. Swimmers who begin the insweep with the hand to the inside of their shoulder seem to prefer this style. (Adapted from Maglischo,[17] with permission.)

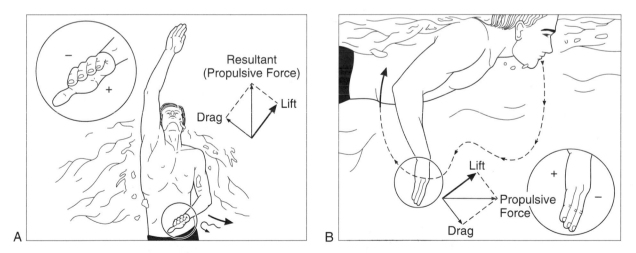

Fig. 4-7. The upsweep. The hand moves outward, upward, and backward from underneath the body to the thigh. The upsweep has two parts, as illustrated. **(A)** The outward portion of the upsweep. The hand pitch is outward and backward. Hand movement and pitch cause drag force to be exerted in an inward direction and a lift force to be exerted in a perpendicular direction. They combine to create a resultant force that propels the swimmer forward. **(B)** The upward portion of the upsweep. The hand is pitched backward and outward, the travels upward, backward, and outward. The hand movement and pitch cause drag in a downward, inward, and forward direction, and lift in a forward and outward direction. The combination of these two forces creates a resultant force that propels the swimmer's body forward. (Adapted from Maglischo,[17] with permission.)

two components: an initial out and back movement. This is followed by an up, out, and back movement. The initial component helps as a transition between the insweep and the upward portion of the upsweep. The upsweep ends as the hand approaches the anterior thigh and leaves the water. The angle of attack is similar to the previous sweep patterns.

The above movements are curvilinear and not linear. The advantages of this type of movement is minimal muscle expenditure, and maximum propulsion with less drag effect due to compensating body movements. For example, if a pure linear push is used during the pull-through phase, the body will move laterally. This tendency must be matched by muscular effort or suffer the consequences of interruption of forward movement due to the laterally exposed body. This exposure will disturb the laminar flow creating massive turbulent flow. Turbulent flow is indirectly indicated by the number of bubbles produced. Highly competitive swimmers produce fewer bubbles.

Freestyle

Freestyle (Fig. 4-8) depends mainly on the contribution of the upper extremity for forward propulsion. The pull-through phase provides this movement with use of two large muscles, the pectoralis major and latissimus dorsi, which act to move the arm through adduction and internal rotation starting from a stretched position of abduction/external rotation. The movement of the hand is specifically described by Councilman[15] as an inverted question mark pattern. This phase constitutes approximately 65 to 70 percent of the total arm cycle.[20]

Recovery allows return of the arm to the stretched starting position while the opposite arm completes its pull-through phase. Efficient recovery is based on the participation of the external rotators and body roll. Body roll must be coordinated with kicking of the legs. The kick is an alternating beat kick whose cadence depends in part on the speed of the swimmer. Six-beat kicking (three per arm stroke) provides generally a slower, smoother motion, whereas the sprint two-beat kick is more jerky.[16]

Freestyle muscle activity has been measured out of water and in water.[20] The differences have clinical ramifications regarding rehabilitation or training in or out of the pool. Since air provides less resistance than

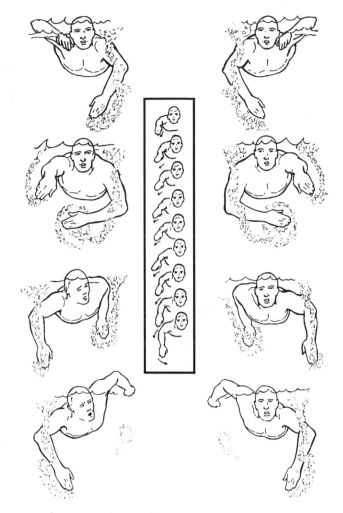

Fig. 4-8. Freestyle (crawl stroke). After the arm enters the water, the hand moves down and across before moving back and out. While the accelerating arm is performing the "power" move, the opposite arm is entering the water. The speed of both arms are different with the speed of the hand entry, much slower; too rapid an entry reduces forward speed. The elbow is bent and is slightly higher than the wrist at hand entry. Timing of the body roll is accomplished by starting the pull as the body rolls toward the forward arm. (From Colwin,[38] with permission.)

water the pull-through phase is less stressful. This results in less recruitment of the clavicular portion of the pectoralis major than occurs in water. Also body roll is more difficult to coordinate out of water, changing the contributions of the external rotators/abductors.[20]

The serratus anterior plays a role as a crucial positioner of the glenoid for proper rotator cuff function during the hand-entry subphase. To achieve a position of full elevation at hand entry, the scapula must be rotated upward and slide anteriorly (protract) on the chest wall. The upward rotation is accomplished through a force couple with the trapezius and serratus anterior. The rhomboids assist by retraction.[21] Inman[22] has demonstrated that only the upper portion of the trapezius is consistently active through flexion and abduction. This allows the serratus to abduct (protract) the scapula without the resistance of middle and lower trapezius contraction. During the last degrees of flexion the lower trapezius is active. This necessary imbalance forces the serratus to function at a near maximum output. During swimming, the serratus has been demonstrated to function at 75 percent of its maximum muscle test ability.[20] Due to the natural repetitiveness of swimming the lack of sufficient rest phases will inevitably lead to some fatiguing of the serratus. Interestingly, when looking at the potential force contributions of the serratus and trapezius, it appears that they are equal based on muscle size.[23] Glenohumeral flexion (elevation) is accomplished through the combined actions of the supraspinatus and anterior and middle deltoids.[21]

The pool electromyographic recordings confirmed the suspected need for pectorals and latissimus dorsi in the pull-through phase.[14] Again, arm position determines the relative contributions of these muscles. The pectoralis major is the initial contributor. This surge of internal rotation apparently is met by antagonistic activity of the teres minor providing an external rotation counterforce. After the humerus crosses the point at which it lies perpendicular to the body, the latissimus dorsi fires due to a newly acquired mechanical advantage. Assisting the latissimus is the subscapularis.

The serratus anterior continues to fire with the pectoralis major and latissimus dorsi through the pull-through phase. Serving two roles, the serratus anterior (through a reversal of origin and insertion) acts to propel the body over the arm while protracting the scapula.

Immediately after the latissimus dorsi stops firing, the posterior deltoid is activated. Toward the end of pull-through arm elevation is accomplished by the supraspinatus and deltoids. The scapula is positioned through the combined action of the upper trapezius, serratus anterior, and rhomboids.[21]

The supraspinatus and infraspinatus are active during recovery until hand entry. Their ability to contribute successfully is dependent on the position of the glenoid (the responsibility of the serratus anterior). Early fatigue or improper position leads to migration of the humeral head with possible impingement.

A review of a typical freestyle stroke pattern begins at hand entry when the arm is maximally elevated and externally rotated. This position is provided by contraction of the supraspinatus/infraspinatus (stabilizers), serratus anterior (scapular positioner), and deltoid (abductor) muscles. As the pull-through phase progresses, the arm adducts and internally rotates; body roll begins. Adduction and internal rotation are accomplished by the latissimus dorsi and clavicular portions of the pectoralis major. Peak activity of the latissimus is at 90 degrees of abduction with the arm rotating internally.[20] Other muscles that assist are the subscapularis and teres major (mainly internal rotators). In the mid pull-through phase body roll is at a maximum. Roll should be at the very least 40 to 60 degrees.[15] During the end of the pull-through phase the shoulder is in the impingement position of maximal adduction/internal rotation. The body is back to neutral. The triceps are needed for extension of the arm.

The recovery phase begins with elbow lift. This requires adduction (retraction) of the scapula as the shoulder begins abduction and external rotation. The rhomboids and middle trapezius retract the scapula as the infraspinatus/teres minor and the posterior deltoid externally rotate the shoulder. Abduction is performed by the supraspinatus and deltoid. The body begins to roll in the opposite direction. In midrecovery body roll is at a maximum while the arm is at 90 degrees of abduction. The serratus and upper trapezius rotate the scapula upward for stabilization. The head is turned for breathing, usually to the dominant side. At the hand-entry phase the arm is maximally elevated with neutral body roll.

The two muscles that consistently fire above 20 percent of a comparative manual muscle test (MMT) are the subscapularis and serratus anterior. If a muscle continually fires at 15 to 20 percent maximum contraction it is doomed to fatigue.[24] Clinically, this translates to specific training to prevent a tendency toward fatigue and possible pathology.

The infraspinatus and teres minor, which in the past

have been assumed to function similarly due to anatomic proximity, in fact serve separate roles with the freestyle stroke. Apparently, the infraspinatus acts as a humeral head depressor in midrecovery to offset the pull of the subscapularis. The teres minor, on the other hand, peaks in activity in concert with the pectoralis major during the pull-through phase.

Backstroke

The backstroke (Fig. 4-9) is simply a supine version of the freestyle stroke. Yet there are some significant differences in strain requirements of the shoulder. In freestyle, gravity works against the external rotators/extensors of the shoulder and the adductors of the scapula, whereas the backstroke causes the forward flexors/internal rotators of the shoulder and the abductors (protractor) of the scapula to work against gravity. At the beginning of the pull-through phase the arm is abducted and externally rotated resulting in excessive stretch to the anterior soft tissue structures of the shoulder. This requires a stabilization factor not seen in the freestyle stroke. In addition, to reverse directions, a wall turn is needed. This is performed with wall contact at the precise moment when the arm is in its maximally unstable position of external rotation and abduction.[5]

Butterfly

The butterfly (Fig. 4-10) is a slightly faster stroke pattern averaging 1.15 seconds per stroke cycle.[20] Yet the ratio of pull-through to recovery is essentially the same as freestyle (30 to 35 percent recovery time). Significant differences between the freestyle and the butterfly are the lack of body roll, the lack of head rotation for breathing, and the simultaneous movement of the arms.

As mentioned earlier, to maximize the adductor efficiency of the pectoralis major and latissimus dorsi, the shoulder must be in a neutral position. With the freestyle and backstroke this is accomplished with body roll. With the butterfly stroke this is accomplished by keeping the arms apart in the mid pull-through phase. This maintains the shoulder in a position of neutral in relation to horizontal flexion (adduction) and horizontal extension (abduction).[11]

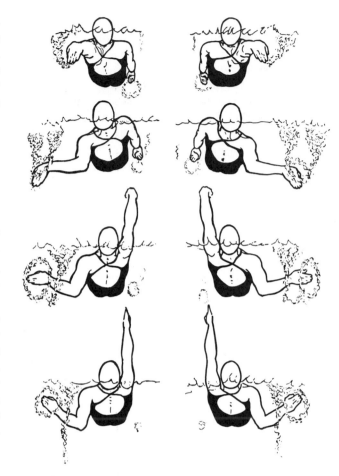

Fig. 4-9. Backstroke. The arm enters the water behind the shoulder, with the elbow straight, and the little finger first as the opposite arm completes its pull below the hips. Then the entry arm pulls down, the elbow starts to bend, and the body rolls towards the pulling arm. The recovery arm leaves the water in a vertical plane (almost directly over the shoulder) with the elbow straight. As seen in the top figures, there is a brief moment when both arms are submerged ensuring continuous propulsion. (From Colwin,[38] with permission.)

Recovery relies on the coordination of the stroke with kicking. Kicking with the butterfly is essentially bilateral flutter kicking. Timed and performed properly, this kick propels the body forward and produces upward lifting of the body allowing the arms to clear the water for recovery. It is essential that at hand entry the hands enter the water slightly outside of shoulder width to maintain neutral shoulder position allowing movement in mainly the coronal plane.

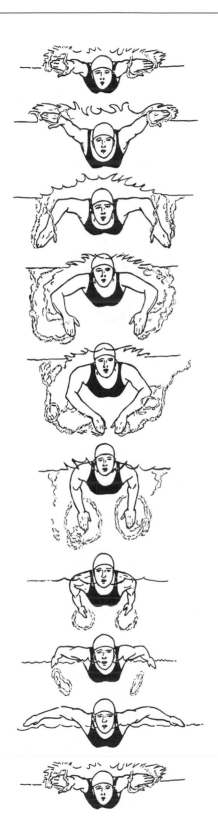

Breaststroke

The breaststroke (Fig. 4-11) is dissimilar to the other strokes for several reasons. The head must break the surface at all times while the arms must not break the surface for out-of-water recovery. In the other strokes the legs play a minor role in propulsion, whereas in the breaststroke the legs play an equal role or better.[11] The kick is described as frog-legged.

Due to the in-water recovery, the ratio between pull-through and recovery is about equal.[20] The pull-through phase is initially similar to the other strokes involving adduction and internal rotation. Councilman[15] describes the pull phase as an inverted heart pattern. The palms face diagonally outward. As the pull progresses the arms pull out, down, and back never crossing the midline. Toward the end of the pull-through there is rapid external rotation of the shoulder with elbow flexion rather than elbow extension as seen in the other strokes. The palms come together in what Richardson[16] describes as a forceful "clapping motion." This movement imparts a lift to the back of the hands dependent on the angle they form.[25] The primary muscles are again the pectoralis major and latissimus dorsi during the pull-through. However, the biceps is active during the rapid pull-up phase of pull-through. In the other strokes the triceps plays a major role in extending the arm through the latter half of pull-through. Also external rotation is crucial during the pull-up phase requiring activity from the infraspinatus/teres minor.

Recovery involves a pushing motion of the arms and elbows causing forward flexion rather than abduction to achieve full elevation. This crucial difference of achieving elevation with flexion rather than abduction spares the rotator cuff muscles from having to overcome the upward pull of the deltoid on the humeral head as in the other strokes. This lack of need for balance between the deltoid and rotator cuff is probably why shoulder impingement is less common with the breaststroke.

Fig. 4-10. Butterfly stroke. The arms enter the water almost straight just wide of the shoulders. The arms spread outward and downward. The elbows bend as the hands cut inward in a rounded action. As the hands complete the backward thrust, the mouth clears the surface for inhalation. (From Colwin,[38] with permission.)

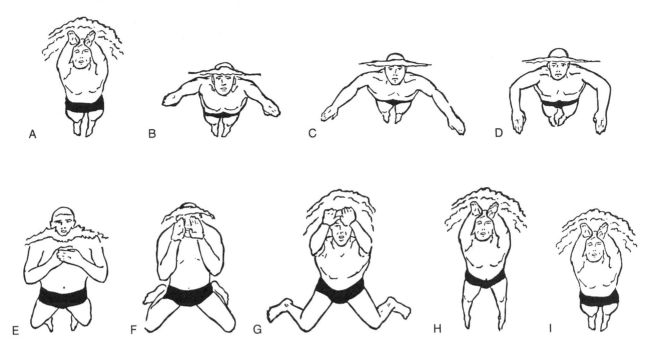

Fig. 4-11. (A-I) Breaststroke. From a streamlined position with the arms outstretched, the pull begins with the hands sculling sideways and downward. The elbows bend continuing the inward sculling of the hands. The kick starts as the hands are pushed (extended) forward. (From Colwin,[38] with permission.)

The breaststroke is mechanically the least efficient stroke. Compared to the freestyle, the breaststroke is at best only 80 percent as fast when comparing world record times. The recovery pattern of both the arms and legs act as obstruction to forward movement.[26] The average cycle time is 1.38 seconds.[20]

PATHOMECHANICS

Drag

An unmeasurable yet decisive element in successful swimming is decrease of drag. The three categories of drag include form drag, wave drag, and frictional drag.

Body position is crucial in overcoming drag, indirectly increasing the efficiency of forward propulsion. The upper body must remain above the pelvis. Additionally, any side-to-side movement of the body must be eliminated. The upper body is kept high by the lift generated in the pull-through phase of most strokes. The kick in both the butterfly and breaststroke is equally important in preventing hip drop. The side-to-side movement is a consequence of a straight arm pull-

through. If the preferable transverse movement of the hands does not occur there are two negative results: decreased lift and increased lateral body movement.[12]

Wave drag is a surface effect due to wave creation. This presents a water wall obstruction to forward movement. The wave effect increases drag by an amount equal to the velocity cubed. In other words, when swimmers double their velocity there is a drag increase by a factor of eight.[27] This can decrease speed 30 percent within 1/16 of a second. The main causative factors are (1) poor pool design or inadequate lanes, (2) smashing arm entries, and (3) excessive lateral or vertical body movement.

Frictional drag can be diminished by increasing the smoothness by which the body travels through water. This can be accomplished by decreasing the surface turbulent flow created by head and body hair and the swimsuit. Head and body hair can be shaved or a swimming cap worn. A brief, tight, lightweight swimsuit is preferred. The amount of effect is questionable, but the rituals of body shaving and the style of swimsuit are a tradition that is unlikely to be changed. Drag can also be created by faulty body positioning, body build, and body fat content. Most of these factors are alterable with training and diet.

Shoulder Position

Shoulder position determines whether muscles are allowed to function at maximum capacity. Positioning also determines whether vascularity of the muscles is patent and whether impingement occurs under the coracoacromial arch. As mentioned earlier, the efficiency of the anterior and posterior adductor/internal rotator muscles, the pectorals and latissimus, respectively, is contingent on neutral positioning of the shoulder with respect to horizontal flexion/extension. With unilateral strokes this is accomplished by body roll. With bilateral strokes it is assisted by kicking and upper body lift.

There are two crucial positions with regard to the rotator cuff musculature. The first is adduction/internal rotation. It has been demonstrated that this is the "wringing-out" position for the supraspinatus tendon.[28] It occurs during the pull-through phase of all the strokes but to a minimum with the breaststroke.

The second position is abduction/internal rotation (Fig. 4-12). With this position the humeral head (specifically the greater tuberosity) abuts into the coracoacromial space.[8] This occurs at two possible times in the stroke cycle: early and late pull-through. An added

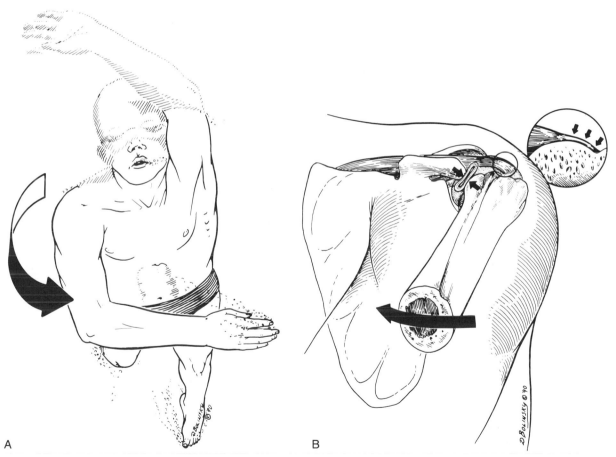

A   B

Fig. 4-12. Adduction stress in swimmer's shoulder. **(A)** Prolonged shoulder adduction due to excessive midline crossover pattern during pull-through phase. This predisposes to wringing out of the crucial vascular zone of the cuff muscles. **(B)** Excessive adduction results in bursal irritation and wringing out of the circulatory "critical" zone of the supraspinatus, infraspinatus, and biceps. (From Hammer.[37] Copyright © 1990 by David Bolinsky.)

factor is imbalance between the rotator cuff musculature and the deltoid. Due to the angle of pull of the deltoid a vertical force is generated. Without the depressive stabilizing force of the rotator cuff muscles the humeral head will migrate proximally under the unopposed pull of the deltoid. This may occur if the rotator cuff muscles are fatigued or untrained. If the serratus anterior fails to position the glenoid for proper rotator cuff function the stability of the shoulder is compromised and impingement is also a concern.

Another positional concern is the capsular straining that occurs with abduction/external rotation. Stability is dynamically provided by the subscapularis up to about 90 degrees of abduction. Beyond this point, most of the stability is capsular with some contributions dynamically from the infraspinatus/teres minor couple. The most susceptible event is the wall turn in the backstroke where a force is applied to the arm while in this vulnerable position. In a more insidious manner, the initiation of the pull-through phase of the freestyle and butterfly strokes persistently and chronically strains the anterior stabilization of the shoulder. Without previous injury or multidirectional instability from congenital or acquired sources, this type of demand would have little impact. However, if predisposed, the consequences are less assured. The more force applied, as in sprinting, the more likely problems will arise.

Muscular Imbalance

The tendency for muscular development in most sports is to build large, strong pectorals and other cosmetically rewarding musculature such as biceps, latissimus, and deltoids. This is no exception in swimming. Particularly with the hypertrophic stimulus of the high-resistance pull-through phase of most strokes it is unavoidable and desirable. Like most sports, this allows the athlete to develop strength in the primary muscles of need yet ignores musculature that is needed for fine motor control of positioning and for stability.

The mechanical consequences of this imbalance is multidimensional and interdependent. This imbalance may cause dysfunction due to strength differences, with inhibition as an added factor. The first relationship to consider is that between the pectorals and the scapular rotators.

Without specific training for the scapular musculature, fatigue is inevitable. In addition, the overdevelopment of the pectorals causes a rounded position of the shoulders leading to stretch and fatigue of the scapular stabilizers on a chronic basis. If dysfunctional, the scapula will not be rotated upward to prevent impingement as the arm is abducted. Also the lack of stabilization leads to asynchronous motion between the scapula and humerus. The rotator cuff muscles must then fire in a haphazard manner possibly leading to early fatigue, and a vicious cycle develops.

There is a natural imbalance between the adductor/internal rotation musculature and the abduction/external rotation musculature. It has been demonstrated that this imbalance is magnified in those with impingement and may even be an early prognosticator of possible impingement.[8,29,30] When the external rotators are not functioning properly internal rotation is allowed to occur during the abduction portion of recovery. As mentioned earlier, the position of abduction/internal rotation is the prime aggravator of impingement. External rotation is necessary by midrecovery or impingement is likely.

Pain

Scovazzo et al.[31] studied a number of collegiate swimmers with a complaint of shoulder pain. Comparing the normal values obtained by Pink et al.[21] several important differences were found with regard to muscle activity and the motions used. The pectoralis major, latissimus dorsi, teres minor, supraspinatus, and posterior deltoid did not show significant differences between the normal and painful group. There was, however, significant decreases with the rhomboids, upper trapezius, and middle and anterior deltoids at hand entry. Associated with this decrease was a hand entry that was more lateral compared to normal. Also the arm (humerus) was held lower (dropped elbow), which is often noted as a sign of being fatigued.

During the pull-through phase the serratus anterior activity was decreased in the painful group with an increased activity of the rhomboids. This decreased serratus anterior activity decreases propulsion and leaves the shoulder at risk for impingement. The substitution of the rhomboid firing may help prevent this. Also the increased activity of the rhomboids correlates with the early hand exit seen in the painful group.

At hand exit there was a decrease in the anterior and middle deltoids with a concomitant increase in the infraspinatus activity in the painful group. The early hand exit as compared to normals is probably an attempt to avoid the prolonged internal rotation (impingement) normally encountered; magnified by the long lever of the extended elbow. Finally, at mid-recovery the subscapularis demonstrated significantly less activity in the painful group, again in an attempt to decrease the likelihood of impingement.

Instability

Instability due to capsular laxity will always increase the demand for the dynamic stabilizers, the muscles. A study by Fowler and Webster[32] in 1982 examined swimmers and recreational athletes to determine the amount of laxity evident. Interestingly, over half of both the swimmers and the control group demonstrated significant posterior laxity. This implies that swimming was not the cause. Yet it was also evident from the data that those with posterior laxity were more likely to develop shoulder pain due to tendinitis.

Inhibition has recently been investigated in relation to supraspinatus tendinitis.[33] It appears that this would allow the unopposed pull of the deltoid to cause proximal migration of the humeral head resulting in impingement. This study demonstrated, however, that there is reflex inhibition of the deltoid. The inhibition was significant starting at 45 degrees. Theoretically, this may lead to more strain of the supraspinatus causing more damage. In general, tendinitis of any muscle will result in inhibition due to pain. This places demand on other structures to provide support. This will eventually lead to early fatigue of these muscles, continuing a vicious cycle.

Spinal Concerns

An overlooked component for swimming and other sports requiring an overhead shoulder position is the need for spinal extensor strength. The last 15 degrees of abduction require contralateral spinal extensor contraction with unilateral movements. These are found in, for example, the freestyle stroke. Bilateral abduction as required in the butterfly stroke demands lumbar spinal extensor contributions resulting in hyperextension of the low back. In addition to the obvious muscular involvement, there is a need for coupled motion in the spine for these movements to occur efficiently and pain free. Lack of normal vertebral movement must be determined and corrected to allow full painless motion. There is also the theoretical possibility of reflex inhibition of neurally related musculature.

Cervical vertebral movement is requisite for effective pain-free head turning for the breathing phase of recovery with the freestyle stroke. Neck extension is required during the breaststroke. Swimmers with neck pain, in particular due to muscle spasm and/or restricted range of motion, are likely to benefit from manipulation or adjustment of the neck and upper thoracic areas.

TRAINING

Competitive swimming involves the generation of a remarkable number of strokes (Table 4-1). Considering that the average competitor trains between 5 and 6 days a week for a 10- to 12-month period and that the average distance is between 10,000 and 20,000 y/d. Averaging[16] individual arm strokes for one length of a 25-yard pool, over one million strokes will be logged in 1 year.[8] Additionally, out-of-pool training increases the stresses considerably. These observations would lead one to believe that the more distance covered, the more likely signs and symptoms would appear. Yet it appears that long-distance swimmers are less prone to developing impingement syndrome than middle-distance and sprint swimmers.[6] So although distance is an important factor other factors must be considered (Table 4-2). The one obvious difference is in the effort exerted per unit of time. A more forceful pull-through is required, in particular, with sprinting. This theoretically will increase the chances of subacromial impingement. There may also be another factor. Disparity between the strength of the internal rotators/adductors and external rotators/abductors will more readily occur in the sprinter than the average swimmer.

A commonly used training device is the hand paddle. These are plastic extensors that increase the hand surface area. This translates into increased resistance on the pull-through phase increasing the training effort and predisposing the swimmer to impingement.[34] The mechanism is twofold. The increased resistance requires a more forceful contraction and paddles have

Table 4-1. A Summary of Swimming Strokes

Stroke	Phase	Subphase	Arm Position	Primary Muscles
Freestyle and butterfly	Pull-through	Hand-entry	Abduction/external rotation; elbow extended	Serratus anterior, rotator cuff/triceps
		Mid pull-through	Adduction/internal rotation; elbow flexing	Latissimus dorsi, pectorals, teres major
		End pull-through	Adduction/internal rotation; elbow extending	Latissimus dorsi, pectorals, teres major
	Recovery	Elbow lift	Abduction/external rotation; elbow flexed	Deltoid (mid), trapezius rhomboids, rotator cuff, serratus anterior
		Midrecovery	Abduction/external rotation; elbow flexed	Infraspinatus/teres minor, serratus anterior, deltoid
		Hand-entry	Abduction/neutral rotation, elbow extending	Deltoid, serratus anterior, rotator cuff
Backstroke	Pull-through	Hand-entry	Forward flexion, abduction, external rotation; elbow extended	Anterior deltoid, biceps, infraspinatus/teres minor
		Mid pull-through	Adduction, internal rotation; elbow flexing	Pectoralis major, teres major, latissimus
	Recovery	Elbow lift	Forward flexion, external rotation	Anterior deltoid, biceps, infraspinatus/teres minor
		Midrecovery	Forward flexion, external rotation, abduction; elbow flexed	Anterior deltoid, biceps, Infraspinatus/teres minor, serratus anterior
		Hand-entry	Forward flexion, external rotation, abduction; elbow extended	Anterior deltoid, triceps, rotator cuff, serratus anterior
Breaststroke	Pull-through	Hand separation	Adduction/internal rotation	Latissimus, pectorals
		Mid pull-through	Adduction/internal rotation	Latissimus, pectorals
		Rapid pull-up	External rotation; elbow and shoulder flexion	Infraspinatus/teres minor, biceps
	Recovery	Elbow extension	Elbow extension	Triceps, anterior deltoid, coracobrachialis
		Shoulder flexion	Shoulder flexion	

been found to increase the time of the pull-through phase. If the recovery arm is then allowed to catch up with the pulling arm there may be a decrease in body roll. Given that body roll is affected, the swimmer could increase the chances of impingement even on recovery.

Table 4-2. Factors Increasing Risk of Shoulder Injuries in Swimmers

If they are a sprint or middle distance swimmer, and
If their main stroke is freestyle, butterfly, or backstroke or
If they are a breaststroker who trains mainly with freestyle
If they suddenly increase distance or intensity or
If they train with paddles (increases resistance and decreases body roll) or
If they have poor flexibility or perform heavy weightlifting or
If they resume training too early after injury or are improperly rehabilitated

Other pool training devices include tubes and floats. Both of these are designed to decrease the contribution of the legs while increasing the contribution of the arms without sacrificing lower body buoyancy. Overutilization of such devices will have the same effects as overtraining.

Weight training for swimming involves focus on the primary muscles such as the latissimus dorsi, pectorals, deltoids, triceps, and biceps. For the pectoral group various forms of bench presses are used. This has been criticized due to the tendency toward heavy weight usage.[35] The bulking-up that may result is unnecessary for swimming and potentially harmful due to its effects on shoulder position. The rounded shoulder position that may result decreases the effectiveness of the rotator cuff and increases the chance of impingement. The incline press used for training of the deltoids is equally criticized because of the tendency toward impingement while performing the exercise. Alternative exercises include chin-ups, pull-overs (for serratus anterior), rowing, and lat pull-downs. The lat pull-down should be performed from a starting position with the shoulder in less than full elevation and the elbows bent (again to prevent impingement). With most of the exercises lighter weights should be used with an increase in repetitions, due to the fact that swimming is mainly an endurance sport.

Some specific examples of machines that have definite drawbacks are the Nautilus pull-over machine and the isokinetic swim bench. The Nautilus may subluxate the swimmer's shoulder. The isokinetic swim bench is used to help develop powerful starts and push-offs. The only significant disadvantage is that most strong swimmers can overpower the machine and need many repetitions to achieve an effective workload.[36]

The danger in disregarding specific training for the rotator cuff musculature is the lack of stabilization that will result. This becomes an important factor due to the increased likelihood of impingement and the previously mentioned observation that many swimmers have some degree of posterior instability.[32] In addition, swimmers, due to the requirements of the sport, have an imbalance between the prime movers for pull-through and those for recovery.[21] The function of the rotator cuff is not strength but fine tuning for stability. Therefore, training should focus on more proprioceptive approaches with de-emphasis of excessive strength development. Elastic tubing is ideal for these purposes. Swimming against the resistance of elastic tubing is also incorporated to increase the intensity of in-pool training.

Most authors agree that the serratus anterior is undertrained, given its high demand requirements in terms of output and endurance.[20] Emphasis on pull-overs with free weights or extended arm depressions should be included. End-range punch maneuvers in the bench press position with free weights will benefit the lower digitations.

By understanding the repetitive demands of swimming, the lack of sufficient resting periods, coupled with positional predispositions for specific disorders, a logical approach to training and rehabilitation can be developed. Initially this begins with proper swimming technique in conjunction with a specific focus on the known demands for specific muscles. Generally, these fall into several general recommendations:

1. Avoid positions that cause impingement or increase instability.
2. Maintain proper body position with body roll and/ or kicking.
3. Strengthen the rotator cuff musculature for stabilization including the serratus anterior, which functions at near full capacity.

SPECIFIC CONCERNS WITH RESPECT TO SPECIFIC STROKES

When addressing the demands of a particular stroke with regard to efficient performance or when concerned about modification of a stroke to prevent further irritation (Table 4-3), there are noted examples. The main concerns with regard to shoulder injury are impingement (with consequent bursitis or tendinitis) and/or instability. The following suggestions are aimed at increasing the efficiency of each stroke with suggested modifications to decrease the likelihood of impingement/instability.

Freestyle

On hand entry the middle fingers should enter the water first. This accomplishes the goal of neutral arm rotation increasing the efficiency of the strong internal rotators/adductors. Secondly, it decreases the tendency toward impingement that may occur when too much internal rotation is used. This would be indicated by thumb entry first. Overreaching has the effect of increasing lateral hip movement with obvious detrimental effects toward forward movement. Underreaching or smashing the hand entry will also increase resistance to forward movement.

Two concerns in the mid pull-through are to angle the arm and hand to avoid pulling straight back and avoid excessive crossover. Avoiding a straight pull-back will increase the efficiency of the pull-through by decreasing lateral body movement. By avoiding excessive crossover, the swimmer decreases the amount of adduction of the shoulder during the strenuous pull-through phase, reducing the period of hypovascularity.

Table 4-3. Ideal Use or Modification of Swimming Strokes to Avoid Injury

Stroke	Phase	Modification	Effects
Freestyle	Pull-through		
	Hand entry	Middle fingers enter water first	Avoids excessive internal rotation preventing impingement
	Mid pull-through	Angle arm and hand to avoid pulling straight back	Prevents excessive lateral body movement; early muscle fatigue
		Avoid excessive midline crossover	Prevents hypovascularity time of supraspinatus
	End pull-through	Shorten length of pull-through	Reduces time with arm adducted possibly preventing hypovascularity of supraspinatus
	Recovery		
	Elbow lift	Avoid straight arm recovery	Reduces chance of impingement
	Midrecovery	Increase elbow height mainly with increased body roll	Reduces change of impingement
		Alternate breathing sides	
In general avoid carrying head and shoulders too high causing the hips and lower extremity to drag in the water			
Butterfly	Pull-through	Arms should not enter water too far outside of shoulder width	Reduces chance of impingement
		Breath on every stroke	Keeps head up
	Recovery	Shorten follow-through	
Backstroke	Pull-through	Avoid straight arm pull-through	Less efficient causing early fatigue
Use of crossover arm modification for the wall turn to avoid excessive anterior capsular stretching			
Breaststroke	Pull-through	Avoid pulling with straight elbow	Less efficient; early fatigue
		Avoid pulling elbows into ribs	Swimmer sinks lower in water

If the swimmer is in pain or fatigued, it is suggested to shorten the pull-through phase.

Another concern is rapid extension of the elbow at the end of the upsweep, which diminishes the lift potential. Pushing the palm straight up against the surface will cause a lowering of the body and decrease forward movement.

The two factors associated with proper recovery are avoidance of straight arm elbow lift and maintaining an increased elbow height accomplished by body roll avoiding the use of predominantly muscular effort.

Another form of recovery is called the hand-swing recovery. This is a variation that involves an almost completely extended elbow lift. The hand travels above the elbow and head; it is more of a vertical lift than a lateral (horizontal) lift. The hand-swing recovery is used in two situations: sprinting and with inflexible or weakened shoulders. This position effectively changes the muscular participation and places more of a demand on body roll. The abductors are activated more against the gravity of vertical lift (abduction) with a hand-swing recovery than the usually dominant external rotators of the shoulder and adductors of the scapula found with the more common horizontal style lift.

In general, it is important to carry the head and shoulders at an angle that does not cause the hips and lower extremity to drop too low in the water increasing drag. This usually occurs when the upper body is carried too high.

Butterfly

On the pull-through phase of the butterfly it is important to avoid hand entry too far outside of shoulder width. This will help decrease the chance for impingement. Breathing on every stroke is also important in terms of proper upper and lower body alignment in the water. As with the freestyle stroke, it may be beneficial to shorten the length of the pull-through phase to decrease the forces on an already irritated tendon or muscle.

During the recovery it is crucial not to drag the arms forward or recover with too much upward movement, only enough to clear the water.

Backstroke

Common errors with the backstroke are similar to other strokes, such as pushing "backward" with the hand during the pull-through phase. Recovery errors are usually due to lifting the hand instead of the shoulder. Lifting the hand lowers the shoulder and increases drag. In the past it was also believed that a low lateral recovery was best. However, it has been found that this increases lateral hip movement to the same side again increasing drag and increasing muscular effort.

The major injury phase of the backstroke is on the wall turn. This places stress on the shoulder in a position of potential instability. The alternative is to use a crossover turn, which will eliminate the external rotation phase of the move.[32]

Breaststroke

A common mistake with the outsweep portion of the breaststroke is to use either too narrow or too wide a stroke with the hands. Schleihauf[18] demonstrated that generally a wider sweep could increase propulsive force by 5 lb. There was also an indirect effect on the subsequent insweep by starting from a wider position increasing propulsive force nearly 10 lb.

Insweep errors include moving the hands forward before the propulsive phase is complete and pitching the hands inward before they pass under the elbows. Both will decrease the amount of propulsion forward.

Other pitfalls to avoid in the pull-through phase of the breaststroke include pulling with straight elbows and pulling the elbows into the ribs. Straight arm pull-through is inefficient and leads to early fatigue. Pulling the arms into the ribs causes the swimmer to sink lower in the water. This also causes the insweep to end early.

Recovery errors include pushing the hands forward too forcefully, which actually acts as a counterforce decreasing forward velocity.

REFERENCES

1. Perry J: Anatomy and biomechanics of the shoulder in throwing, swimming, gymnastics, and tennis. Clin Sports Med 2:247, 1983
2. Richardson AB: Overuse syndromes in baseball, tennis, gymnastics, and swimming. Clin Sports Med 2:379, 1983
3. Pettrone FA: Shoulder problems in swimmers. p. 318. In Zarin B, Andrews JR, Carson WG (eds): Injuries to the Throwing Arm. WB Saunders, Philadelphia, 1985
4. Kennedy JC, Hawkins RJ: Swimmer's shoulder. Phys Sports Med 2:34, 1974
5. Kennedy JC, Hawkins RJ, Krissoff WB: Orthopedic manifestations of swimming. Am J Sports Med 6:309, 1978
6. Richardson AB, Jobe FW, Collins HR: The shoulder in competitive swimming. Am J Sports Med 8:159, 1980
7. Dominguez RH: Shoulder pain in age group swimmers. p. 105. In Erikso B, Furberg B (eds): Swimming Medicine IV. University Park Press, Baltimore, 1978
8. McMaster WC: Painful shoulder in swimmers: a diagnostic challenge. Am J Sports Med 14:108, 1986
9. Brown RM, Councilman JE: The role of lift in propelling the swimmer. p. 179. In Cooper JM (ed): Biomechanics. Chicago Athletic Institute, Chicago, 1971
10. Barthels K, Adrian MJ: Three dimensional spatial hand patterns of skilled butterfly swimmers. p. 154. In Clarys JP, Lewillie L (eds): Swimming II. University Park Press, Baltimore, 1974
11. Plagenhoff S: Patterns of Human Motion. Prentice-Hall, Englewood Cliffs, NJ, 1971
12. Schleihauf RE: A hydrodynamic analysis of swimming propulsion. In Terauds J, Bedingfield EW (eds): Swimming III. University Park Press, Baltimore, 1979
13. Schleihauf RE: A hydrodynamic analysis of breaststroke pulling efficiency. Swim Tech 12:100, 1976
14. Roodman WU: Etiologies of shoulder impingement syndrome in competitive swimmers. Chiro Sports Med 3: 27, 1989
15. Councilman JE: The Science of Swimming. Prentice-Hall, Englewood Cliffs, NJ, 1968
16. Richardson AR: The biomechanics of swimming: the shoulder and knee. Clin Sports Med 5:103, 1986
17. Maglischo EW: Swimming Faster: A comprehensive Guide to the Science of Swimming. Mayfield, Mountain View, CA, 1982
18. Schleihauf RE: A hydrodynamic analysis of swimming propulsion. In Terauds J, Bedingfield EW (eds): Swimming III. University Park Press, Baltimore, 1979
19. Schleihauf RE: The coefficient of lift and drag for human hand models as measured in an open water channel. Paper presented at the International Congress of Sports Sciences, July 25–29, 1978, University of Alberta, Edmonton, Canada
20. Nuber GW, Jobe FW, Perry J et al: Fine wire electromyography of muscles of the shoulder during swimming. Am J Sports Med 14:7, 1986
21. Pink M, Perry J, Browne A et al: The normal shoulder during freestyle swimming: an electromyographic and cinematographic analysis of twelve muscles. Am J Sports Med 19:569, 1991
22. Inman VT, Saunders JB de CM, Abbot LC: Observations on the function of the shoulder joint. J Bone Joint Surg 26:1, 1944

23. Weber EF: Ueber die Langenverhaltmisse der Fleischfasen der Muskeln im allgemeinen. Ber Verh K Sach Ges Wissensch, Math-Phys p. 63, 1851

24. Monad H: Contractivity of muscle during prolonged static and repetitive activity. Ergonomics 28:81, 1985

25. Schleihauf RE: A hydrodynamic analysis of breaststroke pulling efficiency. Swim Tech 12:100, 1976

26. Nelson RC, Pike NL: Analysis and comparison of swimming starts and strokes. p. 347. In Morehouse C, Nelson RC (eds): Swimming Medicine IV. University Park Press, Baltimore, 1977

27. Northrip JW, Logan GA, McKinney WC: Introduction to biomechanic analysis of sport. Wm C Brown, Dubuque, IA, 1974

28. Rathbun JB, Macnab I: The microvascular pattern of the rotator cuff. J Bone Joint Surg 52B:540, 1970

29. Falkel JE, Murphy TC, Murray TF: Prone positioning for testing shoulder internal and external rotation on the Cybex II Isokinetic Dynamometer. J Orthop Sports Phys Ther 8:368, 1987

30. Fowler PJ, Webster MS: Rotation strength about the shoulder: establishment of internal or external strength ratios. Presented at the American Orthopaedic Society for Sports Medicine Annual Meeting, Nashville, TN, July 1985

31. Scovazzo ML, Browne A, Pink M et al: The painful shoulder during freestyle swimming: an electromyographic cinematographic analysis of twelve muscles. Am J Sports Med 19:577, 1991

32. Fowler PJ, Webster MS: Shoulder pain in highly competitive swimmers. Orthop Trans 7:170, 1983

33. Michaud M, Arsenault AB, Gravel D et al: Muscular compensatory mechanism in the presence of tendinitis of the supraspinatus. Am J Phys Med 66:109, 1987

34. Hall G: Hand paddles may cause shoulder pain. Swimming World 21:9, 1980

35. Greipp JF: Swimmer's shoulder: the influence of flexibility and weight training. Phys Sports Med 13:92, 1985

36. Kulund DJ: The Injured Athlete. JB Lippincott, Philadelphia, 1989

37. Hammer WI: The shoulder. In Hammer WI (ed): Functional Soft Tissue Examination and Treatment by Manual Methods: The Extremities. Aspen, Rockville, MD 1991

38. Colwin CM: Swimming Into the 21st Century. Leisure Press, Champaign, IL, 1992

5

The Shoulder in Weight Training

THOMAS A. SOUZA

Although weightlifting is, in and of itself, a sport, weight training is a common thread that weaves itself throughout all sports activities. Whether for training or rehabilitative purposes, weight training is used by most athletes. It is important to understand some of the characteristics of weight training, in particular with regards to the shoulder complex. However, it is equally important to acknowledge the contribution of lower body training to upper extremity performance. Almost all throwing sports depend on a sequential transference of energy from the lower body to the upper body. Any break in this kinesiologic linkage will inevitably overload the upper body component. Conversely, lower body power development will potentially decrease the contribution of the upper extremity component, decreasing the risk of overload or overuse.

To attempt to sort out the many conflicting manufacturer-generated opinions and optimally apply the electromyographically generated data to an individual athlete it is necessary to operationally define some basic terms and clarify some generalizations that are commonly employed. In terms of clinical application it is important to understand the requirements of the sport or sports practiced by the patient. Factors such as strength, power, endurance, balance, agility, and flexibility all must be considered when prescribing or modifying a training program.

Three parameters of muscle capability are strength, endurance, and power. Strength is simply the ability to produce tension; more tension equals more strength.

Endurance is the ability to sustain this tension repetitively (repeated efforts over time). Power reflects the "explosiveness" of effort equal to unit of force over time. Torque is equal to force times the moment arm (perpendicular distance from axis of rotation to point of application). This is measured in foot-pounds and/or newton-meters. Work is the area under the torque curve (measured over time). Power in relation to torque would equal the speed at which work is completed. More power means more work performed over a shorter period of time.

The different forms of work performed have led to confusion. Past definitions of isotonic implied that there was a constant muscle tension throughout the movement. However, when applied to free weights, for example, the load remains the same, but the resistance being applied varies based on muscle length, gravity, and other variables. If the definition is simply used to contrast isometric resistance, where isotonic moves through a range and isometric involves no joint movement, then the definition is useful. Isokinetic is defined as the ability of a muscle or group of muscles to develop torque throughout a specific range of motion with the speed held constant. Both isotonic and isokinetic can then be further subdivided into concentric and eccentric contraction. Concentric occurs when the muscle is shortening against the resistance of a load. Eccentric contraction occurs when the muscle is lengthening against the resistance of a load.

It would seem logical to assume that if a muscle

was the same size as another muscle and both had a positional mechanical advantage that they would participate equally. This is not always the case.[1]

SPECIFIC MACHINE RESISTANCE

Universal

Gideon Ariel's work on *dynamic variable resistance* was used as the basis for a number of machines designed by Universal.[2] There were superiority claims made comparing Universal with free weight training and Nautilus machines. Some of the claims were based on the concept that a muscle does not perform at maximum capacity throughout the range of motion. Therefore, a rolling pivot was used to accommodate throughout the range. The rolling pivot caused changing lever-arm lengths, thereby gradually increasing the resistance as the range increased. The assumption was that this increased resistance would allow trainees to reach their maximum force production curve. Unfortunately, the ability to adjust to the different size parameters of the trainee were not met. Although Universal claims that these were averaged, one study indicated the lack of adjustability for smaller trainees.[3]

Other arguments in favor of the variable resistance approach were that multiple joints and muscle groups could be exercised and that the speed and acceleration necessary in many sports activities was in part simulated or trained by these devices. The contradiction is that the speed and acceleration factors are essentially nullified by the increasing resistance principle. Studies done by Stone and O'Bryant[4] fail to support the claim of superiority by any machine approach over free weights.

One distinct advantage of the variable resistance approach is the ease of adjusting resistance with the reduction of injury due to the obviated need for balance. Additionally, exercises with free weights such as a barbell curl or barbell chest flies require less effort as the body segments approach each other. Variable resistance ensures a constant or increasing force throughout the movement.

Nautilus

The Nautilus concept of accommodating resistance through the use of a cam or variable radius pulley wheel began in the 1970s. For optimum performance, the joint must be aligned to the axis of the cam. The belief was that through a spiral design trainees could match their maximum force production curve.[5] Independent studies have failed to support this claim.[6,7] An interesting principle of Nautilus training is to perform the exercise slowly. The rationale is that it reduces the incidence of injury and produces superior gains in strength. This apparently logical explanation seems more a rationalization of a design "flaw" in the machinery than a scientifically valid argument. Apparently, inertial effects may decrease the resistance felt during rapid movements. Also, the concept of slow movement training in an athlete who functionally needs to train for speed and acceleration seems contradictory.

Isokinetic Devices

Isokinetic simply translated means same movement or more specifically constant movement. The primary difference between variable resistance and isokinetic devices is that the velocity is held constant throughout the range of movement. Similar to the Nautilus machines, the joint is usually aligned with the axis of movement in the machine. Isokinetic devices may be controlled through hydraulics, friction, or electromechanical means. Although the velocity of movement is constant, muscles do not necessarily shorten with a constant velocity.

An example of how an isokinetic machine operates is demonstrated by the hydraulic approach. A variable hole or aperture resists the movement of a fluid that is forced through the hole by an external force applied to the lever arm. After a threshold pressure is reached, there is only a fixed amount of fluid that can pass through the hole at a fixed rate (constant velocity). One flaw with this concept is that with faster speeds, the aperture is larger allowing a longer period of time for a threshold pressure to be reached (before constant flow is reached). It has been demonstrated that at high speeds, less than half of the full range may be accomplished with a constant velocity. The beginning movement is used to reach the threshold pressure needed. This flaw has been addressed with more recent machines.

Free Weights

A distinct advantage of free weights is the need for balance and coordination. Many machines restrict movement in an attempt to isolate the contraction to the muscle or muscles desired. The secondary effect of this process is to reduce the demand for full body participation. Most free weight exercises require trunk stabilization and, if performed unilaterally, contralateral stabilization. Performed in a standing position, more demand on the lower body for balance and stabilization is required. The detrimental aspect of this increased demand is that injury may be more likely to occur. Loss of balance may lead to major injuries to the shoulder and low back.

Free weights allow considerable variation in positioning. This allows the use of rotation components excluded from the performance on most machines. As a result, more functional movement patterns may be performed.

Free weights may appear to be constant loads; however, when the variables of body position, gravity, and changing lever lengths are considered, the load does not remain constant. As a result the weight is easier to move during part of the range and harder at others. Often a "sticking point" exists with many exercises that limits the maximum weight lifted or the range of motion through which the weight is lifted. On isokinetic devices, accommodation for this limitation has been made.

When using free weights, the "sticking point" may be overcome. Through the use of "cheat" maneuvers or assisted eccentrics, this limitation may be largely eliminated. Cheat maneuvers involve a quick concentric phase contraction assisted by other muscles or body leverage allowing a full eccentric contraction. Assisted eccentrics involve assistance through the concentric phase with the opposite extremity or a partner, followed by a full range eccentric. Caution must be exercised when using these approaches.

Elastic Tubing

Although elastic tubing is not weight training per se, this common form of home and gym exercise will be discussed briefly. Various devices using elastic resistance are currently in use. The simplest device is a length of surgical tubing. The more complicated forms use varying thicknesses of elastic bands attached to machines that then simulate many of the standard free weight or variable resistance exercises (e.g., Soloflex). The variables that change the amount of tension provided by elastic tubing are the length and thickness of the tubing. Thicker tubing or a shorter length of tubing provides more resistance. Often, tubing is color coded to indicate the amount of resistance (thickness).

Advantages of tubing are the low cost and portability. The most significant disadvantage is that the amount of resistance always increases toward the end range of a concentric contraction and lessens through the eccentric phase. Another possible disadvantage is that many individuals feel that "more is better" and as a result overuse the tubing, exacerbating rather than ameliorating their problem.

Protocols for the use of elastic tubing vary; the most common rehabilitative sequence involves the use of tubing after isometrics and before free weights or machines. Some individuals recommend light free weight exercises prior to elastic tubing. An old, yet, fairly standard protocol includes a three-phased approach:

1. Facilitation—short midrange contractions to facilitate neural pathways
2. Strength—full range contractions held at concentric end range as an isometric contraction and slowly returned through the eccentric phase
3. Endurance—quick, full range of motion contractions

Another approach is to emphasize the eccentric phase by assisting the involved shoulder into the end range concentric contraction, then contracting unassisted through the eccentric phase. Although more resistance can be handled during the eccentric phase, caution should be exercised. Tubing may be used through diagonal patterns. These functional patterns involve combinations of either flexion or extension, abduction or adduction, and internal or external rotation. An extension of this functional approach is to attach the tubing to the wrist and simulate a throwing movement or attach to a sports apparatus such as a tennis racquet, bat, or golf club, and practice through a movement pattern against the resistance of the tubing. An additional proprioceptive stimulus may be added by performing any of the above exercises while balancing on a wobble board or similar device.

GENERAL PRINCIPLES

In addition to a choice of equipment, choosing the type of training and appropriate positioning for specific muscles is necessary. Elements that enter into this decision process include the intention of the exercise, the specific sport activity used, and avoidance of potentially dangerous positions.

Many of the terms used in weight training are common to the gym, but may not be known to the physician. Listed in Appendix 5-1 is a glossary of common gym terms used with weight training to assist in decoding and aid in communication with the athlete.

Intention of the Exercise

Usually a decision must be made between an emphasis on endurance or strength. This decision is dictated in large part by the type of muscle being trained. There are essentially two broad categories of muscle types. First are the slow twitch (ST) fibers (type I), which function under conditions that demand low intensity for long periods of time. The fast twitch (FT) fibers (type II) are used primarily for short intense activity. The ratio and predominance of fiber type is a genetically predetermined event; however, it appears that selective hypertrophy may be activity related.[8]

There is also the consideration of the specific demands of the individual sport or subcategory of the sport (e.g., backstroke in swimming). This principle is sometimes referred to as the SAID principle: specific adaptation to imposed demands. The above two factors are often co-dependent.

Finally, weight training as weightlifting may be divided into three sports, including Olympic lifting, power lifting, and body building. Olympic lifting is comprised of the snatch and clean and jerk. Both events require lifting of heavy barbell weights and demand both lower and upper body contribution in a balanced yet explosive performance. There is a strong upper extremity eccentric demand on the deltoids, upper trapezius, and biceps/triceps. Power lifting includes three events: the squat (lower body demand), the bench press (upper body demand), and the dead lift (combination of lower and some upper body demand).

One primary or secondary intent of weight training is cosmetic; either attempting to tone/define or enlarge specific muscles for personal aesthetic purposes or competition body building. There is a large base of anecdotal and empirical evidence suggesting that certain exercises help achieve these goals. Therefore, the assumption is that these exercises isolate the muscle that needs definition or hypertrophy. What is not appreciated by many weight training enthusiasts is that many muscles contribute to the movement and that not all muscles are superficial enough to demonstrate definition or hypertrophy. More importantly, it is not always recognized that some of these "hidden" muscles are crucial to the stability of the shoulder girdle and need specific attention to prevent injury. This attention is usually more endurance related training, which may not result in visual changes in the size of the muscle(s).

Types of Training

Energy access varies depending on the length of the activity. Therefore, if seen as a continuum of demand, energy production switches sources starting first with the "liquid asset" of phosphagens to the more "fixed asset" of glycogen. Glycogen, in relation to length of activity, is first broken down anaerobically (without oxygen). Next, with a lengthier activity, aerobic glycolysis (oxidative phosphorylation) is predominant.

From a practical standpoint, sport activities are broken down into length of the event and designated as aerobic or anaerobic. There is no clear distinction possible in many sports and each represents a combination of both systems, usually with one predominating. Short bursts of activity lasting less than 30 seconds such as the shot put, golf, and tennis swings use primarily the muscular stores of phosphagens (adenosine triphosphate and phosphocreatine). Longer activities lasting between 30 seconds and 1.5 minutes such as the 220 and 440 yard sprints, 100-yard swim, and halfbacks/fullbacks functions in football, primarily use the phosphagen source with increasing anaerobic demand. Activities between 1.5 and 3 minutes such as wrestling, boxing, and gymnastics combine both the aerobic and anaerobic sources. Finally, activities lasting continually longer than 3 minutes are primarily aerobic. With this knowledge, it is important to incorporate the type of activity demand to the type of weight training used. For example, if the predominant activity is an aerobic event, focusing on anaerobic weight training will not improve performance in that activity directly. Most weight training is primarily anaerobic; however, by using light weights for longer periods of time or using shorter rest periods between sets, emphasis is placed on the aerobic aspect. Whichever approach is taken the underlying concept of the overload principle is crucial. The principle states that to achieve gains in any of the parameters of strength, endurance, power, and hypertrophy, a muscle must work against greater loads than previously used.

PRE and DAPRE

DeLorme and Watkins[9] were the first to describe a progressive resistance exercise (PRE) program. Originally, the concept was to determine a 10 RM (resistance maximum), which is the maximum amount of weight an individual can lift 10 times. DeLorme and Watkins recommended a program using half of the 10 RM weight and doing three sets of 10. When successfully completed the athlete could move to the next highest weight. Many variations on this theme are currently in use. One such approach is the daily adjustable progressive resistance exercise (DAPRE) technique.

The DAPRE technique is a system that was devised to provide gradual development of strength while preventing injury from progressing too quickly with the amount of weight used (Table 5-1).[10] The number of repetitions is preset for the first two sets. Both use less than the full working weight. The third set with full weight uses the number of repetitions performed to determine the next set. An example follows:

1. The first set (using half of the weight used in set three) requires 10 repetitions.
2. The second set (using three-quarters of the weight in set three) requires 6 repetitions.
3. The third set uses the full working weight. In the third set as many repetitions as possible are performed; this determines the working weight for the fourth set.

4. In the fourth set as many repetitions as possible are performed; this determines the full working weight used in the third set of the next session.

Periodization

Periodization (Fig. 5-1) is a training concept that apparently developed in the Soviet Union in the 1950s. The principle was to divide an annual training plan into smaller phases or cycles. The intent was to provide a program that allows the athlete to peak during the competitive season. Through variations in intensity, volume, type of exercise, and amount of load used in the exercise, the negative aspects of acclamation to training and overtraining are hopefully avoided. Divisions may include three- or four-phased cycles. The three-phase cycle includes preseason, in-season, and postseason segments. Matveyev's program[22] consists of a four-phase cycle that includes

1. *The preparation phase:* High-volumes, low-intensity workouts are used with emphasis on proper exercise technique.
2. *The first transition:* In preparation for in-season play the emphasis shifts to power and strength workouts (if the sport is anaerobic) or high intensity with low volumes of work (if the activity is primarily aerobic).
3. *The competition:* High-intensity technique-focused exercises during short workouts are used in an effort to maintain performance without overtraining effects.
4. *The second transition:* This phase is considered one of "active rest" where an athlete is encouraged to participate in recreational sports. This approach is intended to psychologically and physiologically rest the athlete. Low volume, low to moderate exercise is performed to maintain training effects.

Table 5-1. The Daily Adjustable Progressive Resistance Exercise (DAPRE) Approach

Set	Weight	Repetitions	No. of Repetitions	4th Set	Next
1	½ working weight	10	0–2	5–10 lb	5–10 lb
2	¾ working weight	6	3–4	5–5 lb	The same
3	Full working weight	Maximum	5–6	The same	6–10 lb
4	Adjusted weight	Maximum	7–10	5–10 lb	5–15 lb
			11–...	10–15 lb	10–20 lb

(From Knight,[10] with permission.)

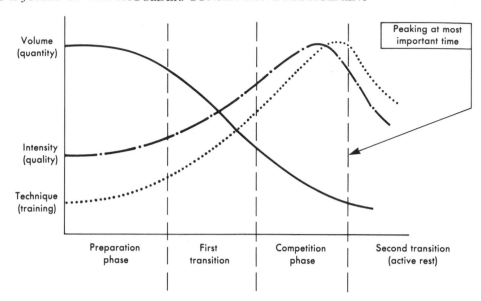

Fig. 5-1. Periodization model of Matveyev. (From Matveyev[22] as adapted in Kirkendall,[23] with permission.)

Specific periodization protocols are presented in Chapter 20 for throwing and swimming.

Eccentric

Eccentric exercise is the selective incorporation of the "negative" phase of a particular movement. The eccentric contraction occurs when the muscle is lengthening. Eccentric contraction is able to generate more force in a shorter period of time with less energy requirements. This is often observed by weightlifters and used as a means to maximally work a muscle. For example, with a biceps curl, more weight can be lowered than raised.

The interest in focused application of eccentrics centers around two important observations. First, eccentric loads seem to be a common culprit in the development of sprains and strains.[11] Secondly, isokinetic evidence indicates that patients with joint pain more often have eccentric deficits as compared to concentric testing.[12] These observations indicate to some that eccentric exercise is dangerous. However, many people feel that rehabilitation and prevention should focus on this deficit to prevent injury.

Plyometrics

An extremely important concept used in training, the stretch/shorten cycle, focuses on the ability of the ec-

centric contraction to store and release energy. This is one of the main principles of plyometric exercise. Plyometrics involve a prestretch to potentiate the following concentric contraction. In general, this is created by storage of energy in the series elastic component of the muscle and released as energy if a quick opposite movement is used or dissipated as heat if it is not. Therefore, to take advantage of this effect, there must be a quick stretch followed by a quick reversal from eccentric to concentric contraction usually within a relatively short range of motion.[13,14]

The term plyometrics was first coined by track and field coach Fred Wilt. The rationale for creation of the term is uncertain. Direct translation from the two Greek words of derivation *plyo* and *metric* is "more measure." Nonetheless, the plyometric approach has existed for many years. However, it was not until 1972 when this "new" system was incorporated into the training of Eastern bloc countries for the Olympics did it attain world recognition in the athletic community. The development of this training concept is attributed to Yuri Verhoshanski.

Examples of upper body plyometrics include rebound push-ups performed against a wall or minitramp. A rebound medicine ball toss is another method used. Lower body plyometrics usually involve jumps off of elevated surfaces with a partial squat quickly followed by a leap upward or forward. Many sports activities incorporate plyometric principles to generate force and speed. The transition from the cocking to the acceleration phase in throwing sports is an example. The quick stretch of the anterior musculature (eccentric contraction) is followed by a concentric contraction with the acceleration phase.

Isolation of a Specific Muscle

Concentrated Effort

One of the first principles of isolation is to localize the contraction. The athlete attempts to feel the contraction occurring in the muscle(s) desired. This concentrated focus probably lends some proprioceptive assistance to development of specific muscles.

Muscle on Top

The principles of proper form with weight training are based on some simple empirical and sometimes verifiable observations. One of the foremost concepts when attempting to isolate a muscle is to position the muscle "on top." This means that by placing the muscle perpendicular to gravity it must, in most situations, work harder. This may be accomplished through body positioning as well as specific variations of shoulder positioning including internal or external rotation.

Electromyographic Data

Recently, there have been several investigations into specific exercises used in rehabilitation programs.[1,15–17] These studies used either elastic tubing or light free weights; therefore direct applicability can only occur in similar prescription scenarios. With regard to the shoulder, it is not unusual, and in fact preferable to use light weights. Therefore, the electromyographic data are quite useful. However, there are many instances where much heavier weights are used, in particular with training the large pectoral or latissimus muscles. In these instances, the electromyographic data suggest which muscles are involved, but do not indicate to what degree.

Full Range/Stretch Principle

Training of an individual muscle may be limited to a small part of that muscle if a full range resistance is not incorporated. To accomplish full range resistance, the muscle should be placed in a stretched position prior to the concentric phase of movement. Additionally, most muscles have a coupled action as demonstrated by electromyographic analysis of diagonal patterns. With the use of free weights or elastic tubing exercises, these coupled patterns should be incorporated. The most obvious example is the biceps, which accomplishes mainly supination and flexion of the forearm. This combined pattern is often ignored when using heavier weights.

Avoid Recruitment

It is a natural tendency to incorporate stronger muscles when weaker muscles cannot perform an exercise. The stress to the desired muscle can be significantly decreased via synergist contraction. One method is rotation of the arm to change, for example, abduction into a more combined movement of abduction plus internal rotation. Forward flexion movement of the shoulder or forearm is often assisted by the upper trapezius evidenced by shoulder "hiking."

A common method of incorporating recruitment as a training aid is to use cheat maneuvers such as the cheat curl for the biceps. Because the eccentric phase of movement is stronger, the athlete cheats on the concentric phase with recruitment of the body or synergist muscles. Then they perform a proper form eccentric. This is often used as the athlete fatigues as a method of maximally stressing the muscle.

Positional Concerns

There are generally two positional concerns with any form of weight training. The first is any position that may overstretch or otherwise damage the capsule or labrum. The anterior capsular mechanism is at risk with maneuvers that combine a position of abduction with external rotation. Dumbbell flys are an excellent example of how the capsule is placed under considerable strain. The amount of strain may be diminished by decreasing the lever length of the arm through elbow flexion and decreasing the weight used. A similar position of concern may occur with weightlifting events where the weight is held overhead. A wide barbell grip adds to the stress applied to the anterior and inferior capsule. Examples include the snatch and clean and jerk. Finally, pull-down maneuvers with the bar brought behind the neck with a wide grip such as the lat pull-down may damage the anterior capsule or labrum.

Because of the attachment of the biceps to the superior glenoid labrum it is likely that overcontraction of the long head may induce damage. Therefore, excessive weight used with curls may be a concern.

The posterior capsule is at risk when weight is directed posteriorly as occurs with narrow grip bench press maneuvers. Individuals with posterior laxity may also have difficulty with forward flexion maneuvers such as occurs with deltoid lifts.

The second positional concern is impingement. The impingement position occurs at approximately 90 degrees abduction and is increased by internal rotation. The butterfly press for the pectorals is a common machine found in clubs and home gyms. The impinged position occurs as the arms are brought together. Impingement with this end-range position is more subcoracoid. Of more concern, however, are dumbbell raises. The forearm is usually pronated, inducing internal rotation of the humerus as the arm is forward flexed through an impingement range. The use of light weights is imperative, but more repetitions as a compensation may lead to damage. With all abduction maneuvers it is important to keep the elbow down, lower than the shoulder. A "flying" elbow or overlifted elbow induces internal rotation with increased risk of impingement.

Nontraumatic Osteolysis of the Distal Clavicle

Although a common cause of distal clavicular osteolysis is direct trauma, some authors[18-20] have suggested that repetitive movements with heavy weights will lead to osteolysis of the distal clavicle in some patients. Often referred to as weightlifter's shoulder, this disorder is radiographically indicated by subchondral bone loss with distal osteolysis of the distal clavicle (Fig. 5-2). A significant historical positive is a complaint of acromioclavicular joint pain associated with the dip, bench press, and clean and jerk.[19,20] A recent study suggests that the prevalence of nontraumatic osteolysis in competitive weightlifters may be as high as 27 percent compared with a normal (non-weightlifting) control group who had no radiographic evidence of osteolysis.[19,20] There is disagreement regarding conservative treatment. Many authors feel that resection of the

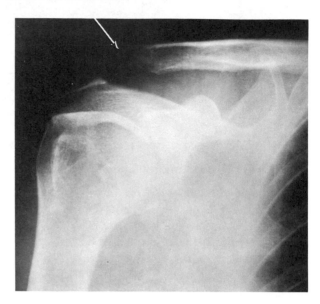

Fig. 5-2. A 25-year-old man with osteolysis of distal end of clavicle from weightlifting. (From Rowe,[20] with permission.)

distal clavicle is the only proven treatment of nontraumatic osteolysis. Haupt[21] suggests that conservative care be used first and that in his experience is often successful. Conservative care would include modification of weight training to substitute the bench press and dip maneuvers with either a narrow grip bench press, cable crossovers, and the incline and decline press. These substitute maneuvers cause less acromioclavicular joint irritation.

SPECIFIC EXERCISES FOR SPECIFIC MUSCLES

In addition to choices regarding the type of resistance applied (machine, free weights, elastic tubing, etc.), there are choices with regard to position. By combining the variables of type of resistance and position, the athlete can develop a varied routine avoiding boredom and increasing the chances of maximum development. The following discussion will focus on the main exercises used for each muscle with a brief explanation of position, positional changes to effect a division of an individual muscle, potential recruitment attempts by the athlete, and potential dangers of a particular maneuver. A list of common exercises is given in Fig. 5-

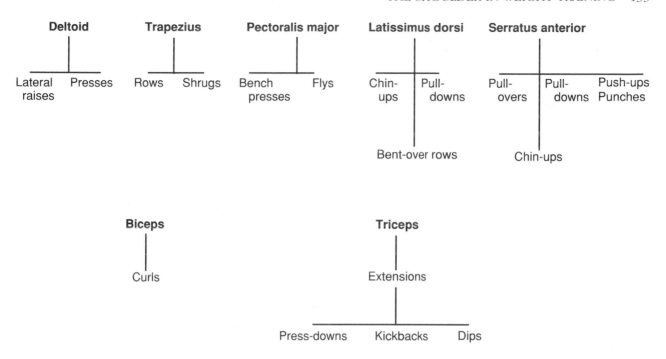

Variations include:
1. Body position: standing, seated, supine, prone, etc.
2. Type of resistance: machine (type of machine), barbells, dumbbells, bodyweight, elastic tubing, etc.
3. Type of exercise: full-range, eccentrics (negatives), PRE, DAPRE, stripping, pyramiding, etc.

Fig. 5-3. General types of exercises for specific shoulder muscles.

3 and Table 5-2 with a comparison to electromyographic-based recommendations in Table 5-3.

Deltoid

The deltoid has three divisions: anterior, middle, and posterior. The anterior and middle are involved with most elevation maneuvers such as flexion or abduction. Most throwing sports and swimming require continued use of these sections. The posterior deltoid is used more in horizontal extension and external rotation maneuvers as found concentrically in the cocking phase of throwing and the recovery phase of swimming. Eccentrically, the posterior deltoid aids in deceleration during follow-through with throwing.

The classic exercises for the anterior/middle deltoids are called raises or lifts (which represent the abduction or flexion component) (Figs. 5-4 and 5-5) and presses (abduction) (Fig. 5-6). Recruitment or cheating may occur with lateral and front raises with trunk flexion and extension, swinging the body back and forth to assist. Isolation and avoidance of trunk movement is accomplished with a seated position rather than standing. Secondly, lateral and front raises are often performed with shrugging of the shoulders, which uses the upper trapezius and de-emphasizes the deltoids.

When performing presses it is important not to fully extend the elbows at the top of the movement (Fig. 5-6). This will take some of the demand away from the deltoid. Also it is possible when using dumbbells to begin the press maneuver with the elbows down and in front of the body to initiate the contraction from a full-stretch position.

The posterior deltoid is usually emphasized with bent-over dumbbell or cable laterals (Figs. 5-7 and

Table 5-2. Commonly Used Exercises for Specific Muscles (Non-Rotator Cuff)

Deltoid
Anterior
  Front barbell raises
  Front barbell presses
  Upright rows
  Incline barbell or dumbbell presses
  Incline dumbbell flys
  Reverse overhead dumbbell laterals
Middle
  Dumbbell laterals
  Cable laterals
Posterior
  Bent-over laterals
  Bent-over cable laterals
  Bent-over barbell rows
  Seated cable laterals
  Incline bench laterals
  Side-lying laterals

Trapezius
Upper
  Upright rows
  Barbell/dumbbell shrugs
  Barbell clean and press
  Dumbbell lateral raises
Middle
  Reverse flys (prone)
  Upright rows
Lower
  Prone extensions

Pectoralis Major
Upper
  Incline bench press with barbell, dumbbell, or cable
Lower
  Decline or flat bench press with barbell, dumbbell, or cable

Serratus Anterior
Pull-overs with machines, cables, or dumbbells
Pull-downs with cable or bar
Close-grip chin-up

Latissimus Dorsi
Wide grip chin-up
Close-grip chin-up for lower trapezius (and serratus anterior)
Pull-downs behind and in front of head
Bent-over rows with barbell, T-bar, dumbbells, or cable
Pull-overs for both latissimus dorsi and serratus anterior

Biceps
Curls performed with supination are most effective
Curls performed with external rotation may develop short head more
Reverse grip curls may develop long head slightly more
Hammer curls may also develop the brachioradialis
Other curls include
  Concentration curls
  Preacher curls
  Cheat curls

Triceps
Press-downs
Kick-backs (extensions, French curls) performed standing or seated
Dips (thumbs forward)

5-8). Bending too far forward will incorporate more of the midscapular musculature. Allowing the weight to drift horizontally back will enlist the assistance of the latissimus dorsi and trapezius; too far forward enlists the other portions of the deltoid.

Latissimus Dorsi

The latissimus dorsi is a large muscle used primarily for adduction and internal rotation. Strong contraction is needed with swimming, the acceleration phase of throwing sports, and support moves in gymnastics. The commonly used exercises include pull-downs (Fig. 5-9), bent-over rows (Fig. 5-10), pull-overs (Fig. 5-11), and chin-ups (Fig. 5-12). While performing latissimus exercises two cautions must be given. For pull-downs, it is important to remember that the arms are placed in an unstable position at the initiation of the movement. The strongest concern is with bent-over maneuvers where the tendency is to use heavy weights and inadvertently incorporate the lower back muscles. This may lead to injury of the muscles or lumbar intervertebral discs.

When performing bent-over rows it is important to keep the knees slightly bent to avoid using the quadriceps for assistance. The weight should be pulled up to the abdomen and not the chest, avoiding recruitment of the biceps. Finally, no extension of the back or neck should occur in an attempt to enlist the paraspinals. When using dumbbells for bent-over rows, internal rotation of the arm with extension may isolate more the latissimus. It is also recommended to avoid any rotational trunk movements with bent-over rows.

Alternate Nautilus exercises for the latissimus include the pull-over/torso arm machine (Fig. 5-13) and the behind neck/torso arm machine (Fig. 5-14) among others.

Pectoralis Major

Like the latissimus, the pectoralis major is a power muscle used in the acceleration phase of throwing sports concentrically, and eccentrically used during the cocking phase. Concentrically, the pectorals are also extremely important for the propulsive phase of most swimming strokes. The caution, is that both sports are essentially endurance sports and may be hampered by overemphasis of anaerobic training with heavy weights.

Table 5-3. Comparison Between Typical Gym Exercise and Electomyographic-Based Exercices

Muscle	Commonly Used Exercises	Electromyographic-Based Exercises	Peak Range/Type (degrees)
Deltoid			
Anterior	Barbell raises and presses	Scaption Internal Rotation	90–150
	Upright rows	Scaption External Rotation	90–120
	Incline presses and flys	Flexion	90–120
Middle	Dumbbell/cable laterals	Scaption Internal Roation	90–120
	Involved in most anterior deltoid exercises	Horizontal abduction with Internal Rotation or External Rotation	90–120
		Flexion	90–120
Posterior	Bent-over laterals	Horizontal abduction with Internal Rotation or External Rotation	90–120
	Bent-over rows	Prone rowing	90–120
Supraspinatus	Not usually addressed or empty can position	Military press	0–30
		Scaption with Internal Rotation	90–120
		Flexion	90–120
Subscapularis	Not usually addressed or Internal Rotation arm at side	Scaption with Internal Rotation	120–150
		Military press	60–90
		Flexion or abduction	120–150
Infraspinatus	Not usually addressed or External Rotation arm at side	Horizontal abduction with External Rotation or Internal Rotation	90–120
		External Rotation	60–90
		Abduction or flexion	90–120
Teres Minor	Not usually addressed or External Rotation arm at side	External Rotation	60–90
		Horizontal abduction with External Rotation	60–90
		Horizontal abduction with Internal Rotation	90–120

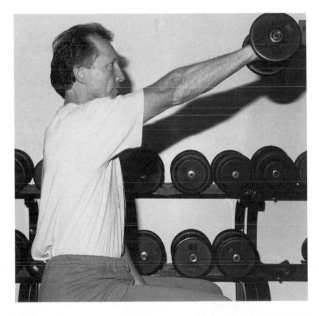

Fig. 5-4. Front raises for the anterior deltoid. It is important not to incorporate flexion or extension of the trunk to assist.

The most commonly used exercises are the bench press in various positions of inclination, flys, dips, and crossovers. The most potentially dangerous exercises are the bench press and the dip, which may cause labrum tears, aggravation of instability related pain, and atraumatic osteolysis of the distal clavicle.

To work or develop different sections of the pectorals, inclination of the bench and variation of grips are used. Narrow grips probably place more emphasis on the triceps while increasingly wider grips require more pectoral involvement (Fig. 5-15). The incline press (Fig. 5-16) and flys (Fig. 5-17) are for development of the upper pectorals. The flat and decline press are primarily used for the lower pectorals (Fig. 5-18). A narrow grip press may emphasize the inner fibers of the sternum. It is important to allow a full stretch of the pectoral fibers at the bottom of the maneuver. It is equally important to avoid overstretching of the anterior capsule and biceps. To localize the stretch to the pectoral muscles the chest should be pushed out at the bottom of the movement (Fig. 5-19). This may be assisted by slight arching of the lower back. Some individuals have a tendency to "cave in" the chest while

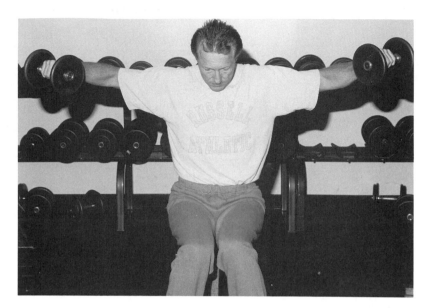

Fig. 5-5. Lateral lifts emphasize the middle deltoid. Swinging of the body to assist should be avoided.

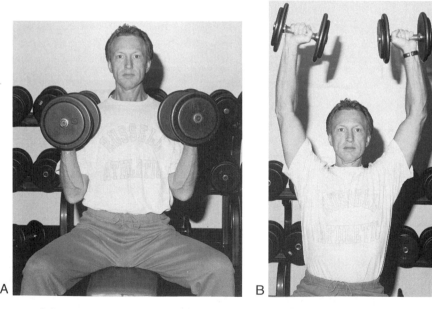

Fig. 5-6. Presses. **(A)** Beginning position with the arms at the sides. **(B)** In the lifted position avoid full extension into a locked-out position.

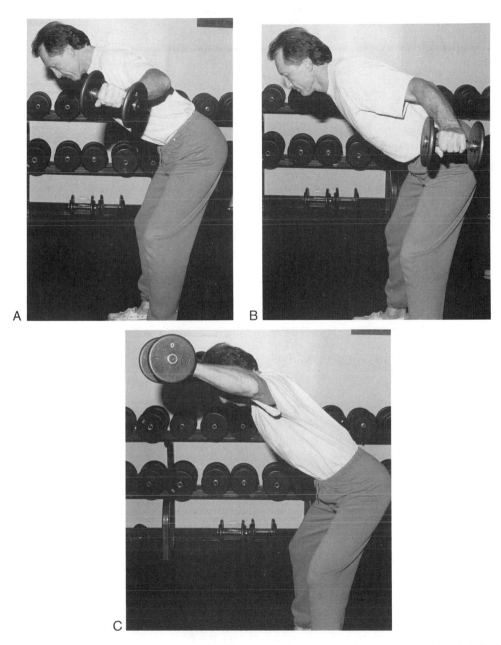

Fig. 5-7. Bent-over raises. **(A)** The bent-over raise is designed to emphasize the posterior deltoid. **(B)** The weight too far back will incorporate the latissimus and trapezius. **(C)** With the weight too far forward the other sections of the deltoids and trapezius are called into play.

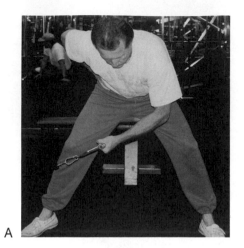 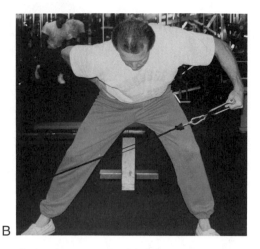

Fig. 5-8. (A & B) Cable laterals for the posterior deltoid.

performing bench maneuvers. This takes the tension off of the pectorals and onto the biceps.

There are two major phases of the bench press maneuver. The descent phase, when the weight is lowered from the stand, is primarily an eccentric event for the pectoralis and triceps. It should be performed slowly to emphasize the eccentric contraction at the same time avoiding bouncing off of the chest, which is potentially dangerous. The ascent phase, however, should be explosive in an attempt to beat the biomechanical "sticking point" that often occurs in the midrange. Interestingly, the vertical arc produced by novice lifters compared to expert lifters indicates significant differences. The novice lifters arched the weight from the chest back toward the head, whereas the expert lifters "corrected" at the top of the movement back over the chest. Elite lifters used a slower lowering rate for the barbell, a more consistent force application to the bar throughout the movement, and kept the bar closer to the shoulder (from a sagittal point of view).

An alternative exercise for the pectorals, especially for athletes who need to modify or eliminate the bench press, is the cable crossovers (Fig. 5-20). This eliminates the gravity-induced stresses to the capsule and the compressive forces to the acromioclavicular joint. Nautilus alternatives include the butterfly (arm cross) and the decline press (Fig. 5-21).

Serratus Anterior

The serratus anterior is the protractor of the scapula during elevation of the shoulder providing a stable glenoid base on which the humeral head must operate. It is maximally used in throwing and swimming. Particularly with swimming, the serratus is relentlessly required to contract. Thus, the serratus acts primarily as an endurance muscle and should be trained accordingly unless hypertrophy and definition for bodybuilding is the intent.

The traditional exercises are the pull-over (Fig. 5-11), front pull-down (Fig. 5-22), close-grip chin-ups (Fig. 5-12C) and punches. Most exercises that work the serratus also work the abdominals and either the pectoralis major and/or latissimus dorsi. Therefore, concentration is important in localizing contraction.

Trapezius

There are three divisions of the trapezius with attachments extending the length of the spinal column and insertions into the shoulder complex. Isolation exercises are performed based on some assumed differences in function. Isolation of the upper portion is usually accomplished with shrugs or upright rows (Fig. 5-23). Also, most exercises for the deltoids will inadvertently include some upper trapezius contraction.

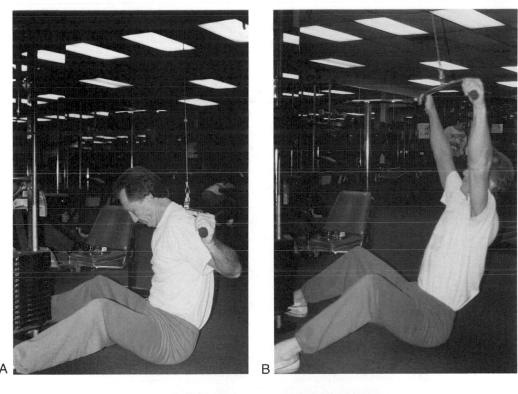

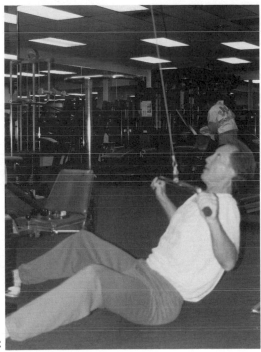

Fig. 5-9. Pull-downs. **(A)** Behind the neck pull-downs. **(B)** Front pull-downs, the beginning position. **(C)** End position. These exercises focus on the adductor function of the latissimus dorsi.

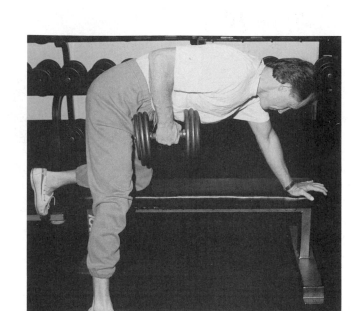

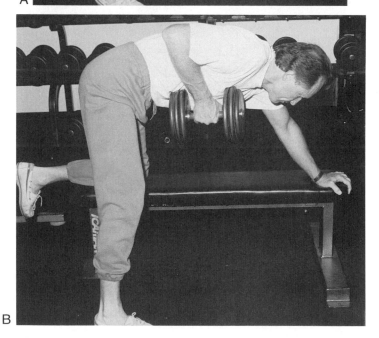

Fig. 5-10. Bent-over rows begin with the weight held below the shoulder and then **(A)** lifted back and up toward the abdominal region. **(B)** Incorrect form is demonstrated with the weight lifted straight up to the chest.

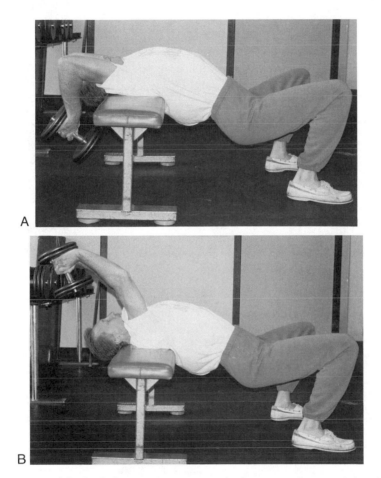

Fig. 5-11. Pull-overs are used for both the serratus anterior, the latissimus dorsi, and the abdominals. A proper stretch is obtained by dropping the buttocks toward the floor. **(A)** Beginning position. **(B)** The weight should be pulled over without bending or extending the elbows. This figure illustrates poor form with extension of the elbows incorporating the triceps.

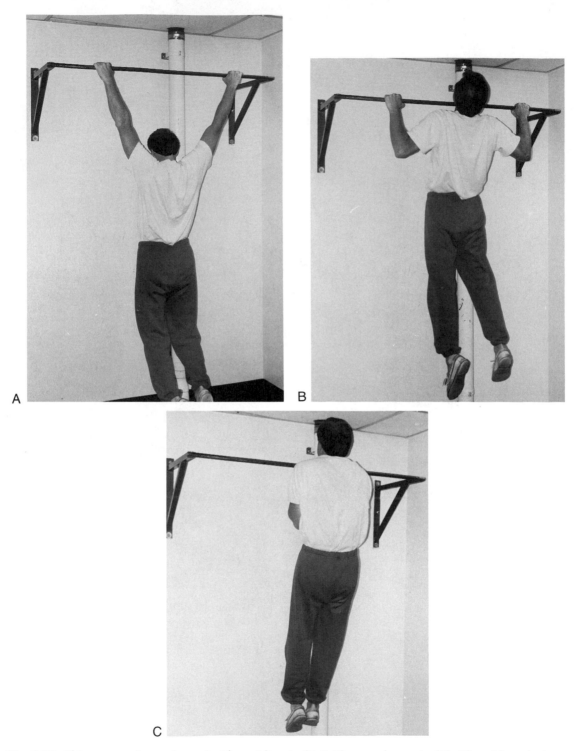

Fig. 5-12. Chin-ups may be performed with a wide grip **(A & B),** or a close grip **(C).** The wider grip is more dangerous with instability, however, but is considered an exercise to develop the latissimus dorsi fully. The close grip emphasizes the lower latissimus and serratus anterior.

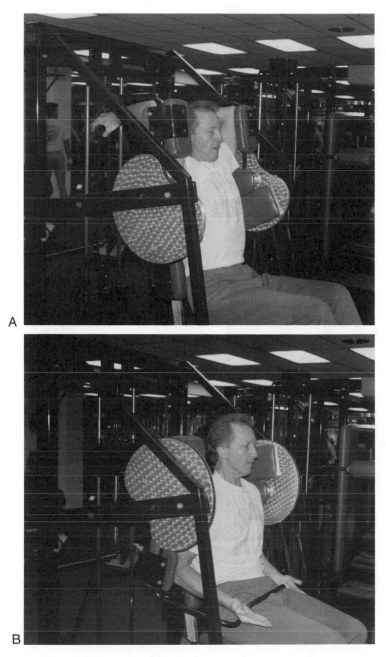

Fig. 5-13. (A & B) Pull-over/torso arm Nautilus machine for latissimus and serratus anterior. Caution in the stretched position for those with posterior instability.

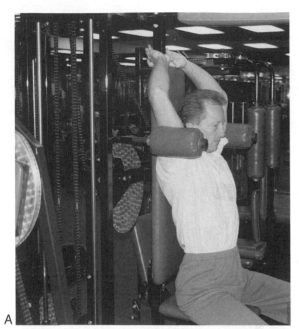

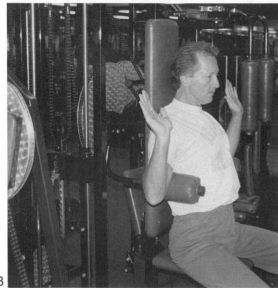

Fig. 5-14. (A & B) Behind neck/torso arm Nautilus machine for both the latissimus and serratus. Caution in the stretched position for those with instability.

Middle trapezius exercises include rows (Figs. 5-10 and 5-24) and reverse flys (Fig. 5-25). The lower portion of the trapezius is exercised with prone extension with the shoulder forward flexed (Fig. 5-26).

Biceps

Most gym exercises emphasize the flexion aspect of the biceps and largely ignore the supinator component. To incorporate the supinating aspect of biceps function the athlete should begin the curl with the palm facing in and supinate while flexing throughout the movement (Fig. 5-27). It is suggested that flexing from a fully supinated position will emphasize development of the lower biceps. Some isolation may occur with a concentration curl (Fig. 5-28). A hammer curl will switch the emphasis to the brachioradialis. Another form of isolation and avoidance of recruitment of the anterior deltoids is to use a preacher curl (Fig. 5-29) or "Arm-Blaster" to cause full extension of the elbows. The full stretched position provides a full-range contraction of the biceps. It is also suggested that barbell curls with a close grip will emphasize the outer biceps; a wide grip emphasizes the inner section.

Recruitment is often incorporated through shrugging the shoulder or use of the body to jerk the weight back into a flexed position. Many lifters use this approach as a cheat exercise where the concentric phase is accelerated via body maneuvering followed by a concentrated slow eccentric phase. Another recruitment attempt is the use of the wrist flexors. If the barbell or dumbbell cheat curl is used, it is important to keep the elbow down and at the sides in the flexed position to avoid recruitment of the anterior deltoid on the concentric phase (Fig. 5-30).

Triceps

The triceps work primarily at the elbow. They assist in extension of the elbow during the acceleration phase of throwing and the late pull-through phase of swimming. Traditional exercises used to develop the triceps include the press-down (Fig. 5-31) and extensions (Fig. 5-32) in various body positions.

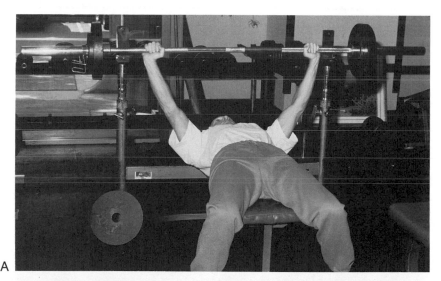

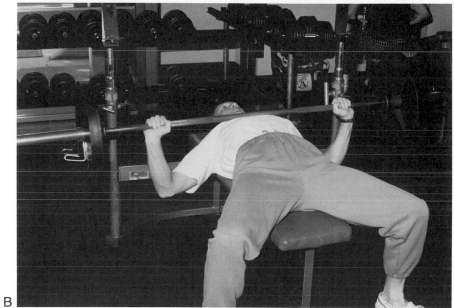

Fig. 5-15. (A & B) Wide-grip bench press. *(Figure continues.)*

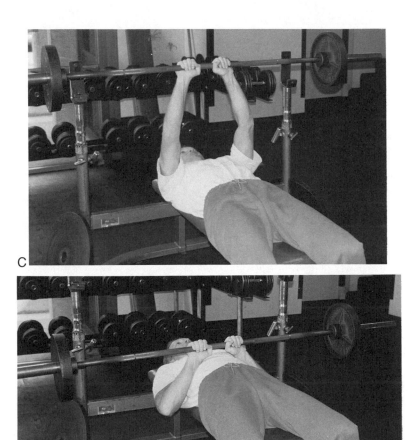

Fig. 5-15. *(Continued).* **(C & D)** Close-grip bench press.

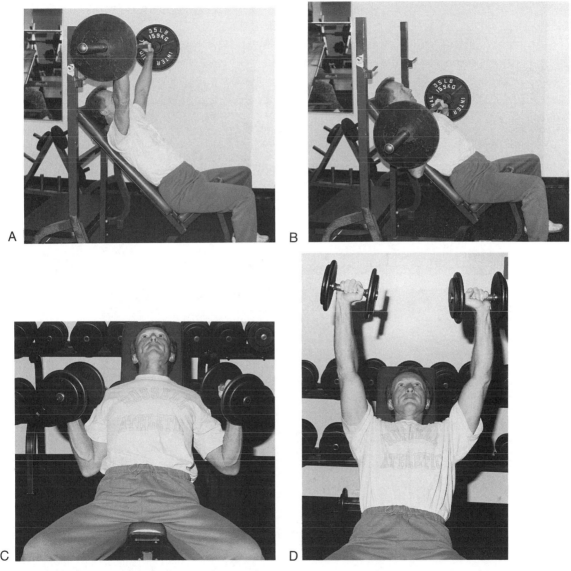

Fig. 5-16. The incline press for the upper pectorals. **(A)** Starting position for barbell. **(B)** Bottom barbell position at the upper chest. **(C)** Dumbbell starting position in full stretch. **(D)** Up position.

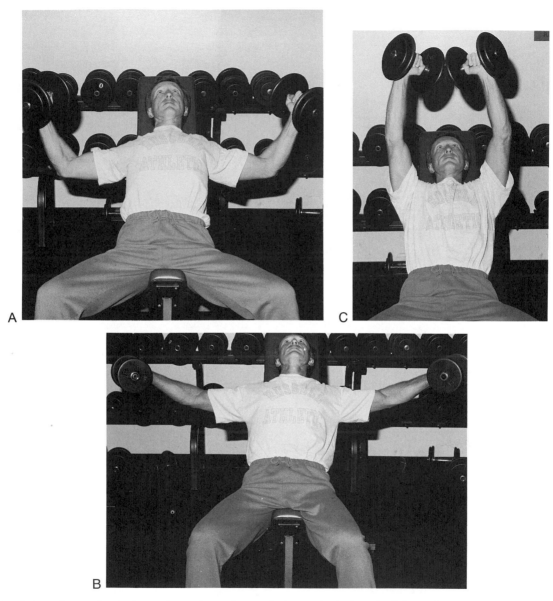

Fig. 5-17. Flys may be performed as inclines, flat, or declines. The incline fly. **(A)** The full stretch position should include elbow flexion. **(B)** With elbow extension greater tension is placed on the biceps and the increased lever arm may strain the capsule. **(C)** The up position.

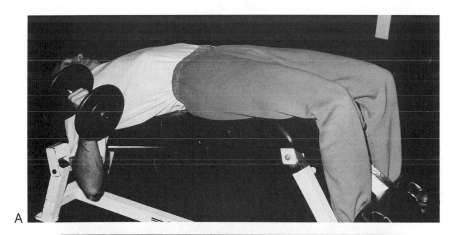

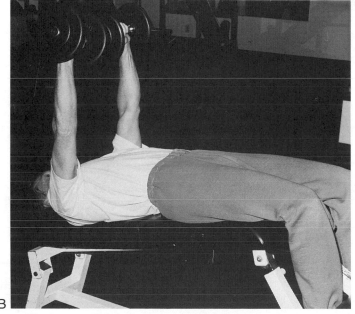

Fig. 5-18. (A & B) The decline press for the lower pectorals.

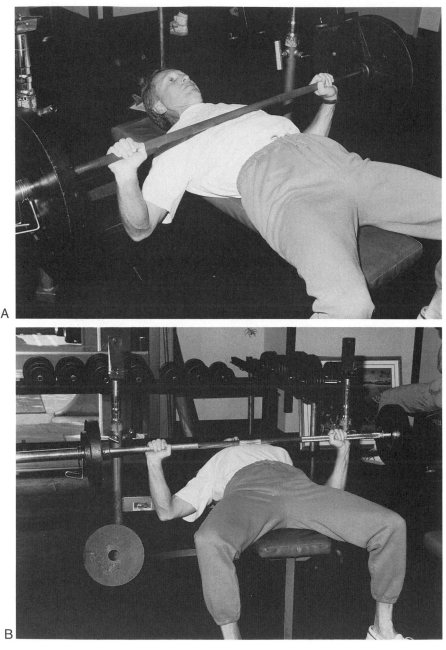

Fig. 5-19. **(A)** Bottom of bench press with chest "caved-in." This is improper technique. The focus may be more on the biceps than the pectorals. **(B)** Bottom of bench press with chest forward. This is proper technique allowing a full stretch of the pectorals. Notice that the feet do not need to be on the bench. An increase in the lumbar lordosis in the supine position is less of a concern due to the lack of a non-weightbearing (gravity influenced) position.

Dips are also a popular exercise for the triceps (Fig. 5-34). By using body weight resistance athletes attempt to lift their own weight. This exercise is used for other muscles including the latissimus dorsi and pectorals as stabilizers.

Rotator Cuff

The rotator cuff muscles are largely ignored with most weight training programs. Although they are essential to proper positioning of the humeral head on the glenoid, in particular during elevation maneuvers, most athletes ignore them during workouts. On the other hand, there are some exercises that will exercise the rotator cuff during a typical workout session. The caution is that many of these exercises use weights that are potentially damaging to the cuff.

Supraspinatus

The supraspinatus is primarily an abductor and stabilizer of the shoulder. Electromyographic evidence suggests that the supraspinatus is maximally stimulated in the first 30 degrees of a military press and with flexion and scaption with internal rotation in the range of 90 to 120 degrees.[15] Given that the 90 degree range for scaption with internal rotation can lead to impingement, it is suggested that it be substituted by flexion or the military press. The use of light weights with more of an endurance emphasis is recommended as for all rotator cuff exercises.

Subscapularis

The subscapularis is an internal rotator of the shoulder acting as often eccentrically as concentrically. Eccentrically, the subscapularis decelerates the shoulder with many external rotation maneuvers best typified during the cocking phase of throwing activities. Electromyographic evidence demonstrates maximum stimulation using scaption with internal rotation, flexion, and abduction in the range of 120 to 150 degrees. The military press between 60 and 90 degrees is also a strong stimulator. Again scaption with internal rotation and abduction through the higher ranges may risk impingement;

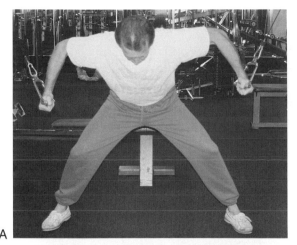

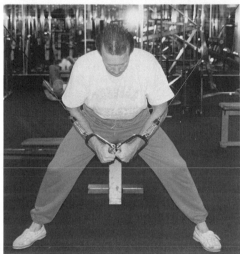

Fig. 5-20. (A & B) The cable crossover is an excellent substitute exercise for the bench press. Gravity is eliminated as a resistance in the concentric phase and compression of the acromioclavicular joint is avoided.

With both press-downs and extensions it is important to keep the arm stationary and only move the forearm to isolate the triceps. When performing supine extensions with a barbell it is important to keep the shoulder flexed slightly beyond 90 degrees and held there during forearm extension to fully stretch the triceps (Fig. 5-33). In the seated or standing one arm barbell extensions, full stretch of the triceps occurs with lowering the forearm behind the head and not the shoulder.

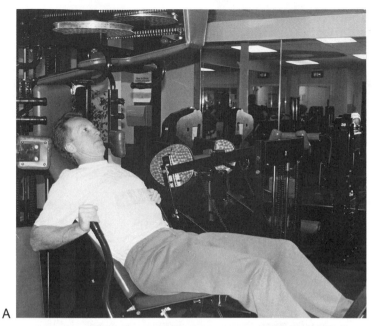

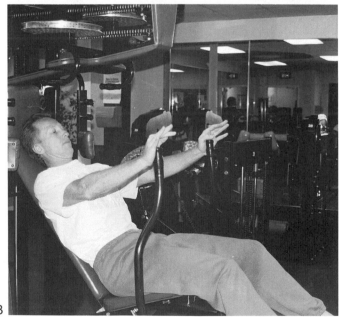

Fig. 5-21. (A & B) The Nautilus press allows a full stretch beginning position. The angle of push simulates a decline press even though the athlete is in an incline position. *(Figure continues.)*

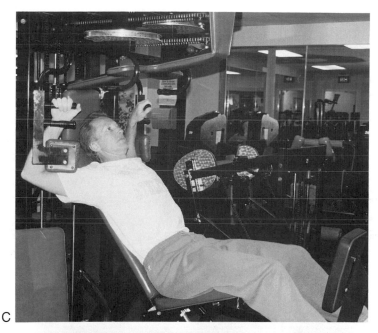

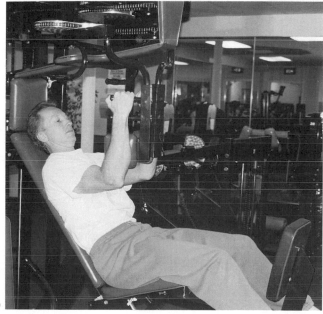

Fig. 5-21. *(Continued).* **(C & D)** The arm cross or butterfly machine simulates "flys." The beginning position allows a full stretch to the pectorals; however, the stretch to the capsule should caution the prescription of this exercise for those with anterior or multidirectional instability.

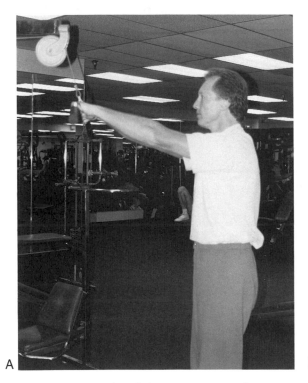
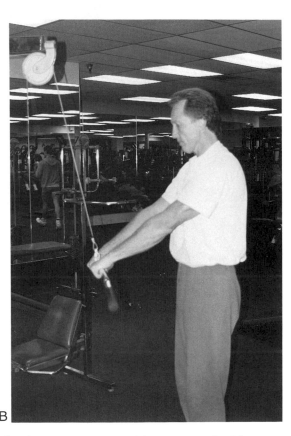

Fig. 5-22. (A & B) Pull-downs are an excellent exercise for the serratus anterior. There is considerable stress to the low back and abdominals for stabilization. The elbows must be extended to focus the contraction more to the serratus anterior and away from the triceps. Another difference from the press-down for the triceps and the pull-down is that the athlete stands away from the apparatus.

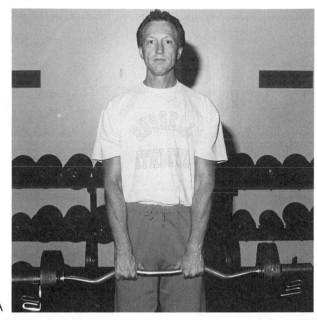

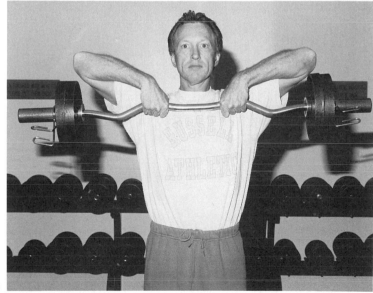

Fig. 5-23. **(A & B)** Upright rows will focus both on the upper trapezius and deltoids.

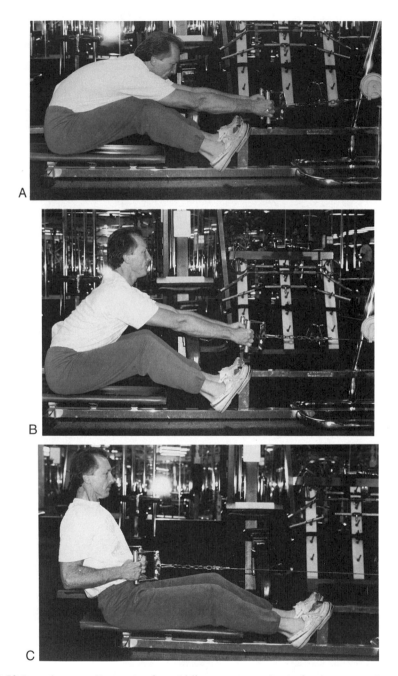

Fig. 5-24. **(A & B)** Seated rows will exercise the middle trapezius and spinal extensors and various other posterior muscles. The final portion of the maneuver **(C)** focuses more on the middle trapezius.

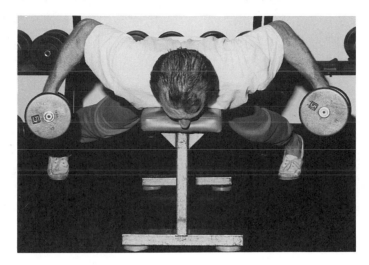

Fig. 5-25. Reverse flys. With an emphasis on scapular approximation, minimizing arm movement will focus the contraction to the rhomboids and middle trapezius.

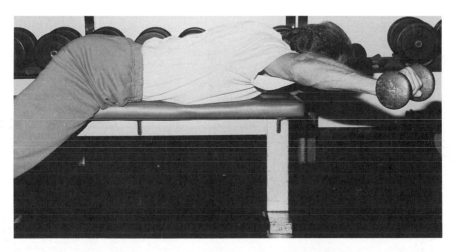

Fig. 5-26. Prone extensions for the lower trapezius and spinal extensors.

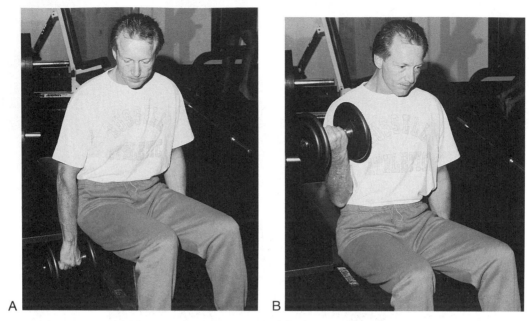

Fig. 5-27. (A) Biceps curl begins with arm pronated. **(B)** Flexion is coupled with supination for a properly executed curl.

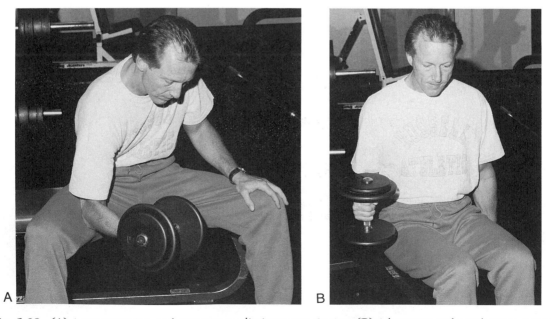

Fig. 5-28. (A) A concentration curl attempts to eliminate recruitment. **(B)** A hammer curl emphasizes more the brachioradialis.

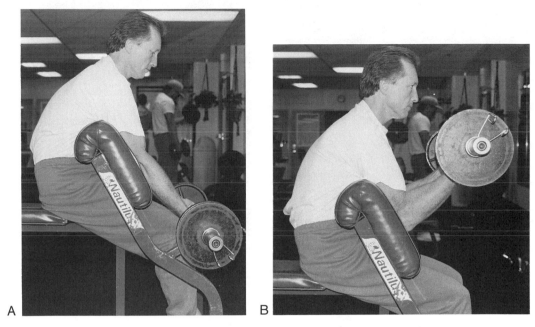

Fig. 5-29. (A & B) A preacher curl allows a full stretch of the biceps and isolates the contraction if the athlete does not hunch the shoulders during the lift.

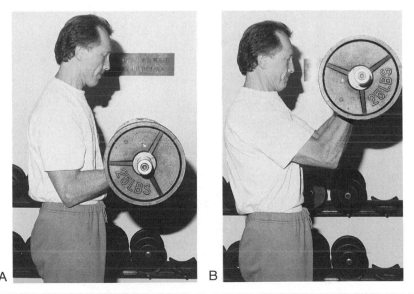

Fig. 5-30. (A) Standing curls should begin with the arms at the side. **(B)** Athlete attempts to use the deltoids to assist, reducing biceps participation.

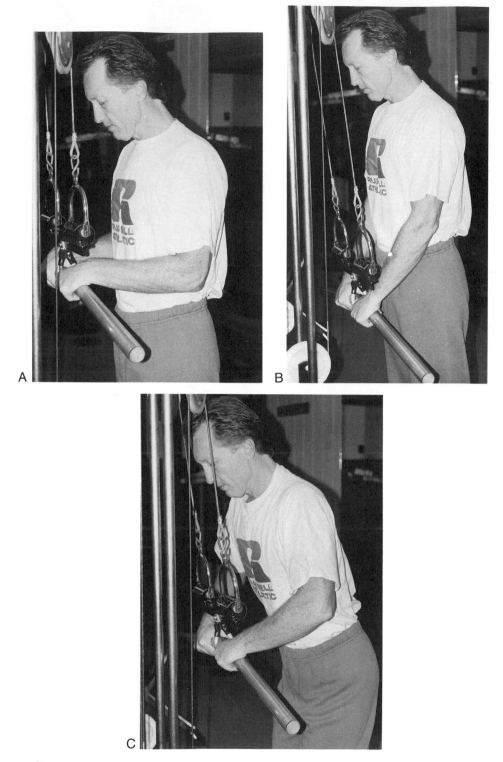

Fig. 5-31. (A & B) Triceps press-downs are effective if the arms are kept by the side. **(C)** The athlete uses incorrect form with elbow flare.

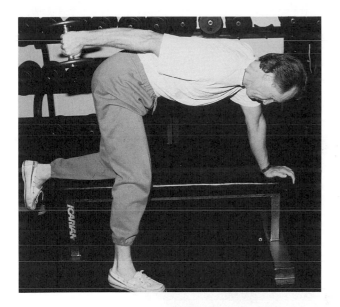

Fig. 5-32. Bent-over extensions. All elbow extensions should be performed without concomitant shoulder movement. Attempts at recruitment are evident when the shoulder extends also.

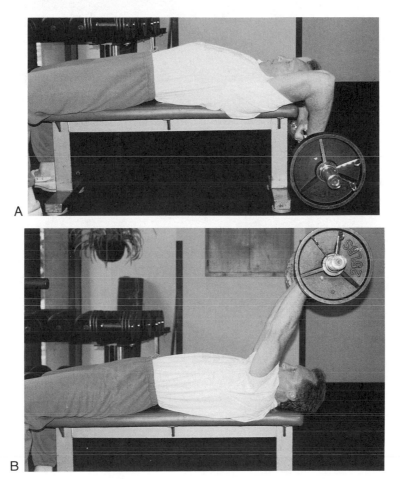

A

B

Fig. 5-33. Supine extensions should begin with the shoulder fully flexed in an attempt to pre-stretch the triceps. **(A & B)** Proper form. *(Figure continues).*

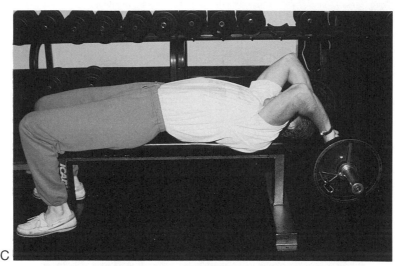

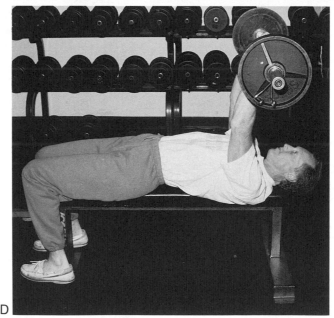

Fig. 5-33. *(Continued).* **(C & D)** Incorrect form.

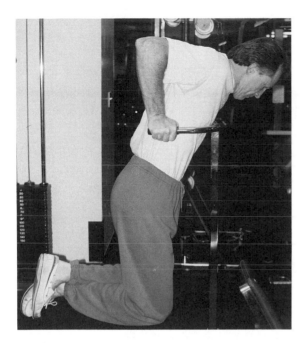

Fig. 5-34. Dips are used to exercise the triceps and other muscles. Caution is used with athletes suspected of osteolysis of the distal clavicle or acromioclavicular joint problems.

therefore, the military press and flexion may be safer exercises.

Infraspinatus

The infraspinatus is primarily an external rotator and stabilizer of the shoulder. Largely ignored, the infraspinatus and teres minor are crucial to humeral head stabilization. Exercises that maximally stimulate the infraspinatus have been demonstrated by electromyography to be horizontal abduction with external rotation with the athlete prone.[15] External rotation in most positions is also effective. Flexion and abduction between 90 and 120 degrees are other effective exercises.

Teres Minor

The teres minor is also an external rotator and stabilizer of the humeral head. Exercises that stimulate the teres minor are essentially the same as for the infraspinatus.

REFERENCES

1. Belle RM, Hawkins RJ: Dynamic electromyographic analysis of the shoulder muscles during rotational and scapular strengthening exercises. In Post M, Morrey BF, Hawkins RS (eds): Surgery of the Shoulder. CV Mosby, St. Louis, 1990
2. Ariel GB: The Effects of Dynamic Variable Resistance on Muscular Strength. Computerized Biomedical Analysis Inc, Amherst, MA, 1976
3. Hay JG, Andrews JG, Vaughan CL, Ueya K: Load, speed and equipment effects in strength-training exercises. p. 939. In Hay JG (ed): Biomechanics VII-B. University Park Press, Baltimore, 1983
4. Stone MH, O'Bryant HS: Weight Training: A Scientific Approach. Burgess Publishing, Minneapolis, 1987
5. Nautilus Sports/Medical Industries: Nautilus: a concept of variable resistance. Natl Strength Cond Assoc J 3:48, 1981
6. Flenning LK: Accomodation capabilities of Nautilus weight machines to human strength curves. Natl Strength Cond Assoc J 7:68, 1985
7. Harman E: Resistive torque analysis for 5 Nautilus® exercise machines, abstracted. Med Sci Sports Exer 15:113, 1983
8. Gollnick P, Armstrong R, Saltin B et al: Effect of training on enzyme activity and fiber composition of human skeletal muscle. J Appl Physiol 34:107, 1973
9. DeLorme TL, Watkins AL: Techniques of progressive resistance exercise. Arch Phys Med 27:645, 1945
10. Knight KL: Knee rehabilitation by the daily adjustable progressive resistance technique. Am J Sports Med 7:336, 1979
11. Garrett WE: Basic science of musculotendinous injuries. p. 42. In Nicholas JA, Hershman EB (eds): The Lower Extremity and Spine in Sports Medicine. CV Mosby, St. Louis, 1986
12. Grace TG, Sweetsser ER, Nelson MA et al: Isokinetic muscle imbalance and knee joint injuries. J Bone Joint Surg 66A:734, 1984
13. Chu D, Plummer L: The language of plyometrics. Natl Strength Cond Assoc J 6:30, 1984
14. Wilt F: Plyometrics-what it is and how it works. Athl J 55B:76, 1975
15. Townsend H, Jobe FW, Pink M, Perry J: Electromyographic analysis of the glenohumeral muscles during a baseball rehabilitation program. Am J Sports Med 19:264, 1991
16. Blackburn TA, McLeod WD, White B, Wofford L: EMG analysis of posterior rotator cuff exercises. Athletic Training 25:40, 1990
17. Moseley JB Jr, Jobe FW, Pink M et al: EMG analysis of

the scapular muscles during a shoulder rehabilitation program. Am J Sports Med 20:128, 1992

18. Cahill BR: Osteolysis of the distal part of the clavicle in male athletes. J Bone Joint Surg 64A:1053, 1982

19. Scavenius M, Iversen BF: Nontraumatic clavicular osteolysis in weight lifters. Am J Sports Med 20:463, 1992

20. Rowe CR: Acromioclavicular and sternoclavicular joints. p. 293. In Rowe CR (ed): The Shoulder. Churchill Livingstone, New York, 1988

21. Haupt HA: Strength training. p. 19. In Reider B (ed): Sports Medicine: The School-Age Athlete. WB Saunders, Philadelphia, 1991

22. Matveyev L: Periodisierang des sportichen training. Berlin, Berles & Wemitz, 1972

23. Kirkendall DT: Mobility: conditioning programs. In Gould JA III, Davies GJ (eds): Orthopedic and Sports Physical Therapy. CV Mosby, St Louis, 1990

Appendix 5-1
Glossary of Common Terms Used with Weight Training and Weightlifting

Negatives—A negative is the eccentric phase of a muscle contraction. The eccentric phase represents tension in a muscle while it is lengthening. In general, more of a load can be handled with a negative (eccentric) compared to a concentric contraction. Eccentric training is important because most muscles eccentrically will contract during a phase of movement requiring deceleration.

Cheat—Cheat maneuvers take advantage of the eccentric (negative) concept. The athlete lifts a heavy weight through a concentric contraction through the use of body movement or other muscles. In other words, with a strict technique, this weight could not be lifted. Then on the eccentric phase the athlete keeps strict form taking advantage of the stronger eccentric element.

Forced negative—An eccentric contraction can be made more difficult by the added resistance of a training partner. Any time the training partner is allowed to subjectively determine how much more weight can be lifted, there is the danger of injury.

Supersets—Supersets are an attempt at maximum training (fatiguing) of a muscle. Two to three (triset) exercises are performed without stopping, usually beginning with the more difficult and demanding exercise and progressing to the least demanding.

Stripping—Another form of maximum demand on a muscle is to begin with a heavy weight and perform a maximum number of lifts. Stripping then involves decreasing the weight slightly and performing as many repetitions as possible, continuing down to less and less weight with maximum repetitions. Another example of stripping is referred to as "running the racks." While using dumbbells the athlete starts at his maximum and performs maximum repetitions. Moving down the rack to the next lightest dumbbell, the same procedure is performed and so on.

Pyramiding—Pyramiding begins with the reverse of the stripping principle, similar to the daily adjustable progressive resistance exercise (DAPRE) or progressive resistance exercise (PRE) approach. First the athlete begins with a lighter weight, perhaps 50 percent of maximum and performs 10 to 12 repetitions. Moving to 75 percent of maximum, 6 to 8 repetitions are performed. Moving then to 100 percent maximum 4 to 5 repetitions are performed. Working down the pyramid, the reverse sequence is used.

Partial repetitions—Yet another form of maximum fatiguing is to perform maximum repetitions with a full-range motion. This is followed by half-range motions, and then quarter-range motions and so on.

Burn—The sensation of a maximally fatigued muscle is a burning sensation within the muscle. For weightlifters this is an indication of a "good" workout. Unfortunately, the same sensation may occur with a muscle tear such as a rotator cuff tear and may be difficult to distinguish from the more positive "burn" felt with fatigue.

Pumped—The perceived impression of hypertrophy, the muscle "feels" larger, is due primarily to engorgement with blood due to increased demand. This and the visual result is referred to as pumped.

"One and a half" and "platoon" methods—One method of training or emphasizing different portions of the muscle are various combinations of full range of motion with half range of motion. The "one and a half" method alternates between full and half repetitions.

Power lifting—Power lifting involves the use of three

exercises, including the squat, the bench press, and the dead lift.

Olympic lifting—Olympic lifting is comprised of the snatch and clean and jerk.

Progressive resistance exercise (PRE)—PRE is a technique devised for safety where, based on a one repetition maximum lift, a sequential group of sets is performed beginning with half the weight for a number of repetitions followed by three-quarters the maximum, and ending with the full amount.

6

History and Examination of the Shoulder

THOMAS A. SOUZA

HISTORY

Careful observation and questioning has led to a composite of specific shoulder disorders. By accessing this information in an algorithmic approach, a high level of suspicion is usually guaranteed. The history, if properly taken, should help direct the examiner in several ways:

1. Determine the nature of the disorder (what structure or structures are at fault). These may be local to the shoulder or distant; related neurologically or biomechanically.
2. Determine activities that may be causing or aggravating the condition including both occupational or "rest" activities, and sports activities involving training or competition errors. This information may then lead to recommendations as to avoidance or modification.
4. Give direction regarding further evaluation.
5. Gain information to help direct the appropriate treatment, rehabilitation, and prevention plan.

Patients may present with a variety of complaints including pain, numbness/tingling, stiffness, weakness or instability, snapping/crepitus, and swelling. These entities may be "pure" complaints or overlapping. Each should be addressed initially as separate problems. Coupled questioning then will uncover whether they are truly related.

Before specific questioning begins it is important to note that age is occasionally significant. Examples (although some are rare) include the following[1]:

Children and adolescents may have epiphysitis or osteogenic sarcoma.
Calcific deposits are more common between 20 and 40 years of age.
Chondrosarcomas usually occur after age 30.
Rotator cuff degeneration usually occurs in the 40s and 50s.
Frozen shoulder is more common in the 45 to 60 year old group.

Most athletes are aware of the difference between the true shoulder and the shoulder girdle, but it is extremely important to preface your questioning with a simple inquiry as to where the problem is. Often patients will complain of shoulder pain that in reality is upper trapezius or scapular pain. Much time and energy may be wasted by simply interpreting a shoulder complaint by the patient to mean the glenohumeral joint.

Pain Location

Pain is probably the most common shoulder complaint. It is again important to first determine location. Differentiation by location is rather nonspecific because many entities refer to common sites such as the deltoid tuberosity. Yet, if the lesion is superficial, pain location may be a helpful discriminator (Fig. 6-1; see Table 6-2 on page 203). Common location-related problems are

1. Superior shoulder—acromioclavicular problems
2. Lateral shoulder—supraspinatus, deltoid, or occa-

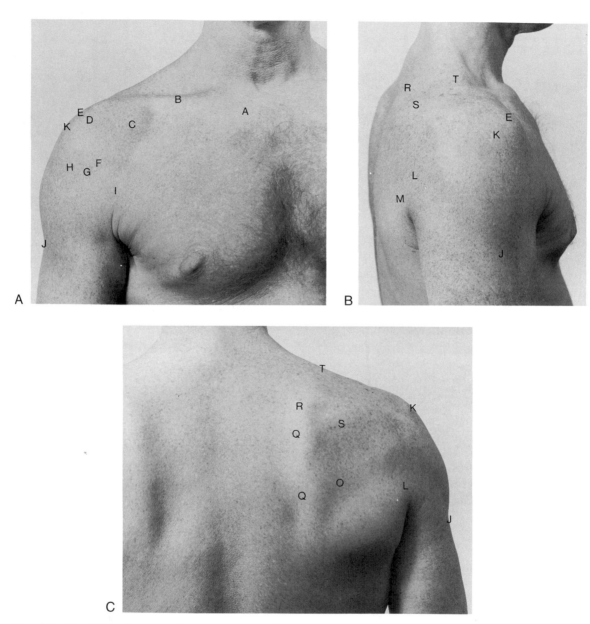

Fig. 6-1. (A–C) Tenderness indicators. *A,* sternoclavicular joint; *B,* clavicle; *C,* coracoid; *D,* between coracoid and acromioclavicular joint; *E,* acromioclavicular joint, *F,* lesser tuberosity; *G,* bicipital groove; *H,* greater tuberosity; *I,* anterior glenoid; *J,* deltoid insertion; *K,* tip of shoulder (acromion); *L,* infraspinatus/teres minor; *M,* lateral border of scapula; *O,* infraspinatus muscle; *P,* inferior border of scapula; *Q,* medial border of scapula; *R,* superior medial border of scapula; *S,* spine of scapula; *T,* upper trapezius. (See Table 6-2 on page 203 for further details.)

sionally teres minor or infraspinatus (common referral site)

3. Posterior shoulder—teres minor/infraspinatus, posterior deltoid, or capsule
4. Anterior shoulder
   a. Anterolateral—supraspinatus
   b. Anterior—subacromial bursa or biceps
   c. Anteromedial—capsule, subscapularis, pectorals
5. Deep (inside) shoulder—capsule, labrum, sometimes rotator cuff tear
6. Upper medial scapula—levator scapulae syndrome
7. Superior scapula—supraspinatus or upper trapezius

These generalizations are based on underlying anatomy and do not account for referral pain from other structures such as the neck or viscera (Fig. 6-2). It is crucial to determine whether the shoulder pain is part of a radiation from another body part or the source of radiation. The patient will often be able to clarify this distinction. Often accompanying visceral or systemic signs or symptoms will direct further investigation outside of the shoulder. The inability to mechanically reproduce the complaint will add some weight to the suspicion.

Quality of Pain

Difficulties with descriptions of pain have led to frustrations from both the patient's and doctor's perspectives. A description may have one connotation for the patient and another for the doctor. In general, several terms may be used to advantage in describing shoulder pain.

Sharp and stabbing—this is usually intermittent pain and relates to either acute injury to a muscle/bursa or deep mechanical irritation. If the pain occurs with initiation or termination of a movement a tendinitis is likely.

Boring (toothache-like)—this is neurologic pain and

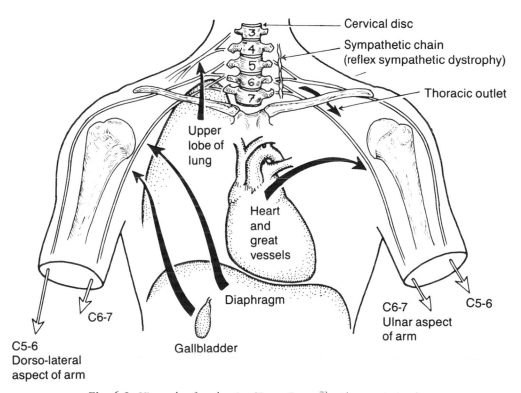

Fig. 6-2. Visceral referral pain. (From Rowe,[73] with permission.)

is usually due to neural (or neurovascular) irritation such as thoracic outlet syndrome or referred pain (usually from the cervical region).

Dull ache—this is the hallmark of muscle injury; a magnification of the "sore" muscle sensation (this is usually worse with active movement).

Burning—usually this is reported in association with referred pain from the cervical region or other forms of referral. Additionally, neurovascular pain from thoracic outlet syndrome may present similarly.

Onset

When formulating an opinion as to cause it is imperative to determine if a recent trauma, whether contact or noncontact, is evident (Fig. 6-3). If no recent event is recalled, retracing past injuries is requisite. Often detailed questioning is needed to expose a potential past or current injury if the onset is reported as insidious. Changes in training either through changes in form or equipment must be considered. When no changes are apparent, overuse due to increase in intensity or frequency must be considered. Every structure is capable of fatigue failure after an individualized threshold is reached. The most difficult scenario is found when the onset is rather acute with no obvious cause. In the older athlete it is possible to have chronic processes made acute through minor events. On the other hand, in younger individuals causes other than mechanical should be considered.

When the cause is determined to be traumatic or overuse, it is essential to elicit as much of the mechanical description as possible. There are positions, which

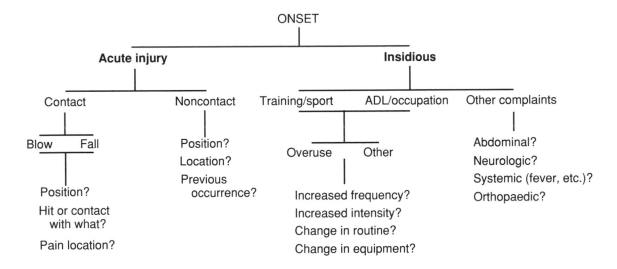

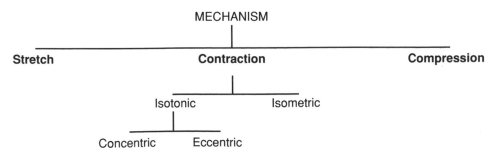

Fig. 6-3. Onset algorithm. *ADL,* activities of daily living.

when stressed by compression or exceeded by stretch, lead to predictable injury. This concept can be applied to phases of an individual activity. For example, throwing can be divided into two injury phases. The preparatory phase includes potential stretch injury to the anterior structures and compression injury of the posterior structures. Eccentric injury to the anterior structures is also a potential. The acceleration/follow-through phase involves potential contraction injury, which is eccentric for the posterior musculature and concentric for the anterior musculature. Neural stretch injury to posterior structures is also possible. Other sports have similar positionally related potentials for damage.

In general, some common examples of injury are as follows:

1. A fall on an outstretch hand—in addition to wrist injury (scaphoid fracture and dissociation), acromioclavicular separations and clavicular/humeral fractures are·possible.
2. Landing on the tip of the shoulder—this is the most common mechanism for acromioclavicular damage (separation); also a shoulder "pointer" is possible.
3. Forceful horizontal extension of the abducted/externally rotated arm—this is a common position for anterior dislocation.
4. Overhead exertion—common for impingement problems.

Specific sports-related injury patterns are described in Table 6-1. It is not enough to inquire about related sports involvement alone. Specific phases of the sports act must be included in questioning.

Next, a detailed sequential history following the injury is essential in confirming any suspicions based on mechanism. For example:

Immediate loss of strength or sense of numbness suggests the possibility of several disorders:
Dislocation/subluxation[2]
If associated with cervical trauma, a "stinger" or "burner" is suggested.[3] Additionally, central cord syndrome is a possibility especially if associated with a "burning hands" complaint.
Severe pain on top of the shoulder with an associated deformity/swelling is suggestive of acromioclavicular separation or distal clavicular fracture.

Table 6-1. Shoulder Injuries Associated with Specific Sports

Sport	Incidence (%)	Injury
Baseball		Rotator cuff lesions; impingement; anterior Glenohumeral subluxation; glenoid labrum tears; Acromioclavicular joint injuries; pot. shoulder instability; proximal humeral physeal separations; suprascapular nerve entrapment
Basketball	3	Contusions/strains; Acromioclavicular injuries
Dance	<3	Scapulothoracic joint
Diving		Anterior glenohumeral subluxation; rotator cuff injury (due to flat entry); anterior glenohumeral dislocation (due to unclasped hands)
Football	9–11	Acromioclavicular joint; brachial plexus (burner/stinger); rotator cuff; shoulder pointer; posterior/anterior/glenohumeral dislocation; myositis ossificans
Golf		Sprains; impingement syndrome
Gymnastics		Gymnast shoulder; "ringman's shoulder"; supraspinatus tendinitis
Ice hockey	8–22	Acromioclavicular joint separations; clavicular osteolysis; clavicular fracture; Glenohumeral dislocation
Martial arts	7 44 (judo)	Contusions/sprains; Glenohumeral dislocations; lacerations; clavicular fractures
Racquetball/ Squash	5	Acromioclavicular joint (impingement uncommon)
Shooting		Marksman shoulder" (coracoid bursitis); trap-shooter shoulder (coracoid stress fracture)
Snow skiing	15	Glenohumeral dislocation; fractures; Acromioclaviculor separations
Swimming	50	Impingement; anterior/posteror glenohumeral subluxation
Tennis		Impingement
Water polo		Rotator cuff tendinitis; Acromioclavicular degeneration; anterior glenohumeral dislocation; impingement
Weightlifting		Distal clavicle osteolysis; Glenohumeral dislocations; glenoid labrum tears; pectoralis rupture; impingement
Wrestling	16	Acromioclavicular joint; Sternoclaviculor joint; Glenohumeral subluxation/ dislocation

(Data from Zarins.[76])

A sensation of the joint "out of socket" followed by a "clunk" into position (usually positionally acquired) indicates subluxation or chronic dislocation.[4] Initial dislocations are rarely spontaneously reduced.

When the causative event is not obvious it is important to perform a history:

Routine daily or weekly activity
Occupational questioning is often excluded when interviewing the athlete; however, it is distinctly possible that occupational overuse injury may be the culprit or an impediment to improvement.
Changes in training
Questioning should always include any visceral complaints that might correlate with the shoulder complaint, especially a chronic history of diseases such as diabetes.

Relieving Factors

Although it is common to ask about irritating or aggravating factors, it is equally important to ask about relieving factors, such as positions assumed by the patient to relieve pain. Some common examples include

Is the pain relieved by elevation of the arm overhead? This is a unique finding that points to a cervicogenic cause (usually disc or facet).[5] This same position would be aggravating for most other shoulder problems.
Support of the elbow to relieve dependency of the shoulder is a common position of relief seen often with acromioclavicular separation and rotator cuff tears, although patients with cervicogenic or brachial involvement may use this position.
If, in addition to support, the arm is abducted and externally rotated, an anterior shoulder dislocation is considered assuming an appropriate traumatic history.
Relief by circumduction or rotation of the shoulder with an accompanying click or clunk is indicative of internal derangement or subluxation; a glenoid labrum tear or posterior subluxation are likely possibilities.
Some people obtain relief by distraction of the arm usually indicative of bursal or rotator cuff inflammation (with the exception of the supraspinatus).

It is informative to include a history of professional and/or self-treatment for the problem. Determination of effectiveness of a specific form of treatment may be indicative of a specific diagnosis. On the other hand, lack of responsiveness may suggest an erroneous working diagnosis by the previous treating physician.

Relief gained by various treatment approaches may indicate current etiology. For example, relief by cortisone injection is suggestive of impingement (depending on the location of injection).[6] Relief from an arthrogram is reported in some cases of adhesive capsulitis.[7] Relief by adjustment or manipulation of the shoulder may be suggestive of fibrous adhesions or fixation of accessory movement. Response to cervical adjusting or automated traction is suggestive of referred pain from cervical structures or nerve root compression from foraminal encroachment (sometimes an inflamed or protruded disc). Relief from specific exercises is indicative of muscle imbalance/dysfunction associated with impingement, instability, or a combination of both.

Irritating or Exacerbating Activities

With overuse injuries the whole intent of questioning is to identify activities that may irritate or exacerbate. However, even if the problem does not seem to be overuse related, similar questions should be pursued. Again, the most fruitful line of questioning is position. Of course, if positionally related, it is important to determine whether the cause of increase in pain is due to compression, contraction, or stretch of specific structures. This requires a detailed understanding of functional anatomy. Suspicions are further qualified by location of the pain complaint. Avenues of questioning include

Positions that are attained or maintained in certain phases of sports activity.
Less obvious are positions that are aggravating during work distinct from those encountered in sports activity.
Additionally, positions of irritation during rest may be helpful. Although the shoulder is a nonweight-bearing joint, it does, in fact, become compressed when lying on the affected side during sleep. In this position the upper shoulder may also be affected if not supported and allowed to roll into internal rotation. This will likely stretch posterior and compress ante-

rior shoulder structures. Location of pain or irritation should help determine which event is occurring. Head and neck positions must be identified to determine any relationship to a shoulder pain complaint.

Investigations of position should not focus only on the shoulder. There have been numerous examples in the author's experience when elbow position (sometimes unnoticed by the patient initially) was a significant contributing factor to increase in pain. This awareness should lead to questioning regarding what Rowe refers to as the flying elbow syndrome.[8] Individuals, particularly with daily living or work activities, have a tendency to use the elbows away from the body often increasing stress to the shoulder. A simple correction in posture may be dramatic.

Never to be excluded is questioning related to head and neck position. Remarkably, unless volunteered by the patient, this line of questioning is the most commonly ignored. Increase in symptoms with forward bending is probably either muscular or related to the anterior motor unit. Increase in symptoms with extension purely or coupled with rotation are often related to facet, disc, or osteoarthritic spur irritation. Lateral bending irritation, if to the same side, is probably similar to the same possibilities. Lateral bending away from the involved side is more likely due to brachial irritation or neurovascular entrapment.

Attempts at relief may result in increases in pain. These may be clues as to underlying cause. For example, if immobilization is attempted by the patient yet an increase in discomfort results, perhaps the positioning may indicate why an increase occurred. For example, taping or splinting for an acromioclavicular separation may add enough compressive force to exacerbate the patient's pain. If the immobilization was initially successful, however, and the problem has now increased, consideration of fibrous adhesions or (if prolonged) disuse atrophy (dysfunction) should be investigated on examination. If pain is increased following exposure to a "hot tub" attempt, one may suspect an acute inflammatory process (rather nondistinct). Failure or increase in pain as a result of exercise or physical therapy is not necessarily an incorrect diagnosis but may represent an overzealous attempt at a speedy rehabilitation.

Numbness and Tingling

The most important consideration with a complaint of numbness is the distinction between the patient's report and the ability to confirm this on an objective sensory examination (Fig. 6-4). The considerations with a complaint of numbness or tingling include

Neurologic—differentiate between central nervous system (CNS) or peripheral nervous system (PNS) origin
Vascular—compressive or occlusive
A *combination* of both—thoracic outlet syndrome

The most common causes are not local to the shoulder but from cervical involvement. The three most common presentations include (1) referred pain from segmentally related structures, (2) brachial plexus stretch injury ("burner" or "stinger"), and (3) cervical disc or other space-occupying lesion. The cord may be involved when instability or impingement is caused by fracture or dislocation.

Local neurologic cause may be due to local entrapment or stretch about the shoulder complex. In addition to the suprascapular nerve involved in stretch injuries in the suprascapular notch,[9] the quadrilateral space may affect the axillary nerve.[10] A common complaint associated with postdislocation or subluxation is a complaint of transient numbness and tingling.

Based on the above information it becomes apparent that a historical search for cervical trauma is mandatory. Even if a single event is not recalled, questioning regarding increase or relief of the complaint with neck or arm positions is essential. If the numbness improves with elevation there is a direct suspicion of cervical referred pain or traction on the brachial plexus. The converse is equally revealing. If the report is an increase in arm elevation (especially with continuation into the lower arm and hand) a suspicion of thoracic outlet syndrome should be investigated.

Whenever a complaint of numbness and tingling is reported, especially when unassociated with a traumatic event, it is important to question the patient regarding underlying chronic disorders or possible metabolic causes. Considerations include diabetes, chronic alcoholism, vitamin deficiency and/or associated anemia, and medications. In general, these causes will result in multiple area involvement; however, with

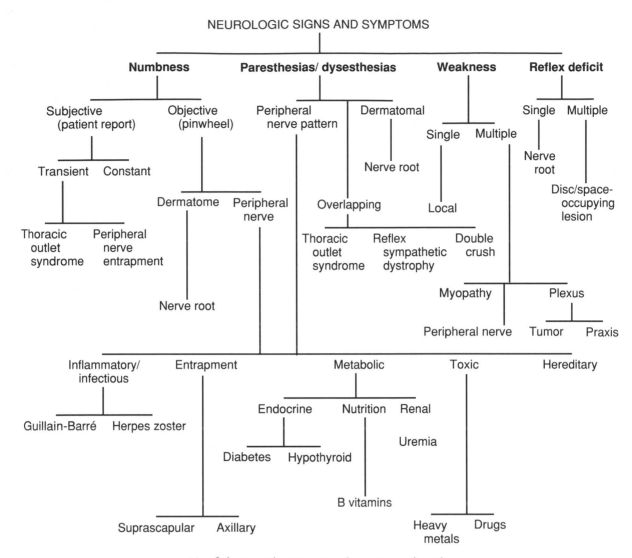

Fig. 6-4. Neurologic signs and symptoms algorithm.

early changes they may be present in a single area alone.

Weakness

A complaint of weakness is almost always associated with a complaint of pain. Often by discriminating between active, passive, and end-range pain the source of weakness will become more clear. In almost all cases a structure such as muscle/tendon, capsule/ligament, labrum, or bone is the underlying cause. Questioning should always include when the weakness is experienced and whether the patient feels it is associated with pain.

Weakness without pain but occasionally associated with numbness and tingling suggests glenohumeral subluxation or brachial plexus injury (burner/stinger). Historical questioning regarding the numbness/tingling complaint should reveal an obvious correlation based on the unique type of injury for each.

Weakness with no associated complaint is more difficult, however, and questioning should focus on differentiating between neurologic and muscular sources.

Muscular weakness may be mild to moderate and, if pure (weakness only), is associated with either disuse (atrophy) or possibly an inherent instability. Several patients have presented to the author with a complaint of inability to lift the arm above shoulder height yet with no other associated complaints. By compressing the shoulder joint the patient was able to complete the full range; this is indirect evidence of instability. In all of these cases the patient had no history of traumatic dislocation or subluxation.

When gross weakness is evident with no associated symptoms, a neurologic source must be investigated. A starting point would be to determine if there is bilateral involvement or if any other parts of the body are involved. If so a central or spinal lesion is most likely. If the weakness is isolated to a single muscle or group of muscles unilaterally, a peripheral source should be suspected. When a single muscle is involved an exception to the neurologic source is expected. For example, isolated weakness of the biceps is most likely due to rupture, which may be evident on inspection and testing of the patient. When a single nerve root is involved, decrease in muscle strength of an individual muscle is less obvious due to the common multiple root innervation. Groups of muscles accomplishing a specific movement such as wrist extension may demonstrate weakness when a single nerve root is involved. In most other cases, neurologically related muscles by peripheral nerve level will present as weakness groups. For example, if the suprascapular nerve is involved around the transverse scapular ligament, weakness or atrophy of both the supraspinatus and infraspinatus may be evident.

Stiffness

Stiffness is rarely a single pure complaint with an athlete unless the athlete is a senior. Often the complaint is phrased "stiff and sore." Therefore, most of the pain questioning presented above will reveal any underlying causes of stiffness. When stiffness is the only complaint, the most fruitful line of questioning would be onset and relationship to time of day. The majority of stiffness complaints will be following an excessively strenuous workout or practice and are often felt early morning. In the majority of these cases there is associated soreness. It develops between 24 and 48 hours after the activity and the related event should be obvious. This muscular strain should be reproducible with appropriate muscle testing.

The chronic stiffness complaint should alert the clinician to past injury and surgery questioning. In addition to the injury it is of utmost importance to determine the type of rehabilitation followed postinjury. Prolonged immobilization or lack of compliance to proper stretching postinjury or postsurgery is a common historical positive. Another consideration is the imposed increases in isolated movements with some sports activities that give an appearance of (or existence of) a decrease of reciprocal movements. For example, pitchers often have an increase in external rotation with a concomitant decrease in internal rotation. Even though the entire rotation range of motion (ROM) is within normal limits, this relative restriction may be perceived as stiffness. This adaptive "contracture" development will become most apparent at passive end range, but may not be perceived on active end-range movement.

Another misinterpretation of shoulder stiffness by the athlete may be due to elbow flexion contracture. This is not uncommon in the young pitcher.[11,12] In limiting the ability to throw, the athlete may misperceive the problem area as the shoulder. Therefore, examination of the elbow should be included if the history dictates.

A suspicion of adhesive capsulitis is suggested when a past history of myocardial infarction,[13] pulmonary disease,[14] diabetes,[15] or hyperthyroidism[16] is elicited although many cases have an unknown etiology. In addition, a reported movement restriction that includes mainly external rotation and abduction will usually confirm the suspicion. However, there are reportedly many cases of undiagnosed chronic posterior shoulder dislocations that may present with a similar restriction pattern.[17] This restriction pattern will be most evident with activities of daily living including combing hair, putting on a sweater, scratching the upper back, etc. Sports activities would include the cocking phase of throwing activities and specific stroke patterns in swimming (backstroke and butterfly) although any overhead activity would be restricted. Also osteoarthritic involvement of the shoulder may present with a similar restriction. It is important to remember that this may occur at an early age following shoulder surgery or trauma.

Diagnosis:
Aim of Procedure:
Operation:
Shoulder: right: left:
Arm Dominance: right: left:

The rating in each category can be adjusted according to the AIM of the procedure.

Patient's Name:
Hospital Unit #:
Date of Operation:
Date of Followup:
Surgeon:
Preoperative rating:
Postoperative rating:
Patient's Evaluation (circle):
Exc.   Good   Fair   Poor

Unit Rating
(circle one in each category)

I. PAIN (15)
1. None — 15
2. Slight during activity — 12
3. Increased pain during activities — 6
4. Moderate/severe pain in activity — 3
5. Severe pain, dependent on medication — 0

II. STABILITY (25)
1. Normal. Shoulder stable and strong in all positions. — 25
2. Mild apprehension in normal use of arm. No subluxation or dislocation. — 20
3. Avoids elevation and external rotation. Rare subluxation. — 10
4. Recurrent subluxations. ("Dead arm syndrome.") Positive apprehension test or recurrent dislocation. — 5
5. Recurrent dislocation. — 0

III. FUNCTION (25)
1. Normal function. All activities of daily living. Performs all work, sports/recreation prior to injury. Lifting 30 + lb. Swimming, tennis, throwing. Combat. — 25
2. Mild limitation in sports and work. Can throw, but limited in baseball. Strong in tennis, football, swimming, lifting (15–20 lb) and combat. Performs all personal care. — 20
3. Moderate limitation in overhead work and lifting (10 lb) and athletics. Unable to throw or serve in tennis. Swims sidestroke. Difficulty with body care (perineal care, back pocket, combing hair, reaching back). Aid necessary at times. — 10

4. Severe limitations. Unable to perform usual work or lifting. No athletics. Sedentary occupation. Unable to perform body care without aid. Can feed self and comb hair. — 5
5. Complete disability of extremity. — 0

Unit Rating
(circle one in each category)

IV. MOTION (25)

Abduction	151–170	15
& Forward	120–150	12
Flexion	91–119	10
	61-90	7
	31-61	5
	Less than 30	0

IR	Thumb to scapula	5
	Thumb to sacrum	3
	Thumb to trochanter	2
	Less than trochanter	0

ER	(with arm at side)	
	80°	5
	60°	3
	30°	2
	Less than 30°	0

V. STRENGTH (10) (compared to opposite shoulder) (specify method = manual, spring gauge, cybex)

Normal	10
Good	6
Fair	4
Poor	0

TOTAL UNITS — 100

Excellent	(100–85 units)
Good	(84–70 units)
Fair	(69–50 units)
Poor	(49 units or less)

Fig. 6-5. Rowe's functional evaluation form. *IR,* internal rotation; *ER,* external rotation (From Rowe,[73] with permission.)

Crepitus/Snapping

Crepitus and snapping about the shoulder are common complaints. More frequently, a complaint of crepitus on a preparticipation examination represents only a concern by the athlete as opposed to a coupled complaint with pain. In either setting, with or without pain, it must be remembered that there are multiple structures that may produce cracking and snapping of the shoulder complex. Discrimination is sometimes assisted by localization by the examiner or patient if possible. Some of the possible etiologies include the following:

Acromioclavicular joint. Crepitus is usually found through abduction or flexion, often end range induced.

Fibrous bursa. The subdeltoid (subacromial) bursa is subject to a fibrotic reaction when constantly irritated. This is common with overhead activities including swimming. The location will be similar to that of the acromioclavicular joint. Another location, found more commonly in throwers, is the scapulothoracic bursa found at the inferomedial border of the scapula.

Tendons of the teres minor/infraspinatus. These tendons have a tendency to snap or clunk when the arm is abducted, often on the descent from abduction. The location is in the posterior shoulder region about the acromion.

Biceps tendon. This is sometimes suggested as the single most common cause of a complaint of snapping. It is characteristic for this to occur on coupled movements of abduction and rotation of the shoulder. There are several orthopaedic tests that attempt to reproduce this complaint. The location is obviously anterior, sometimes perceived slightly anterolateral.

Glenoid labrum. When there is laxity of the capsule with or without a tear of the glenoid labrum, there may be a complaint of a sharp pain relieved by repositioning of the shoulder accompanied by a perceptible clunk. This may be indicative of a tear and should be further tested.

Posterior subluxation. Lifting the arm into forward flexion may cause subluxation that is not always perceived by the patient. Reduction is usually felt with posterior extension (in the flexed position) at the glenohumeral joint often causing an audible snap.

Impingement syndrome. Crepitus is often produced with the arm abducted to 90 degrees and rotated internally and externally.

Swelling

Swelling is an uncommon complaint and should add a level of concern. Distinct swelling over the acromioclavicular joint is common with separation or with fracture of the distal clavicle. This is especially true with a history of a fall onto the top of the shoulder. In the older patient with no history of immediate trauma, osteoarthritis is suspected with acromioclavicular swelling. The bursae are either relatively deep such as the subscapularis or hidden such as the subacromial. A palpable mass may be apparent at the inferomedial border of the scapula indicating scapulothoracic bursal irritation, but it is not visually evident to the athlete. Swelling is not, therefore, usually obvious and rarely alarms the patient as a visual or palpable difference. In addition to swelling associated with trauma (usually soft tissue), other causes include tumor, infection, or rheumatoid arthritis.

Swelling at the sternoclavicular joint is usually due to irritation from heavy weightlifting or excessive baseball throwing. Trauma suggests direct trauma to the joint that would warrant an investigation into dislocation if accompanied by severe pain.

Questioning of activities of daily living and occupational activities is presented in Figure 6-5. For athletes, a modification based on common requirements of the individual sport should be included to gain a full understanding of the extent of the problem. A functional approach is important for determining baseline comparisons for future evaluations. These graded approaches, although primarily used to determine disability, are often interesting when comparing objective findings with functional restrictions or lack thereof.

PHYSICAL EXAMINATION

It would be oversimplified to imply that the physical examination of the acutely injured and the chronic patient would be similar. There are the obvious emergency issues in acute trauma with the emphasis on determining immediate procedures such as reduction of a dislocation or assessment and stabilization of a possible fracture. The majority of evaluation will in most practices be in-office. Therefore, the following discussion will focus on this presentation followed by a description of "on-the-field" management.

Inspection and Observation

The most significant factor with an acute presentation in your office is the carrying position of the shoulder. Observation as to the degree of swing during normal ambulation may indicate the degree of constant pain felt by the individual. Supported or splinted positions are equally revealing and help, in some cases, to differentiate among conditions. The following are some examples:

1. Arm slightly abducted and externally rotated—common position with an anterior dislocation
2. Arm adducted and internally rotated (sling position)—found with many painful shoulder conditions including posterior dislocations
3. Arm at side, elbow supported (supported sling position)—this is commonly used to decrease traction on the shoulder or brachial plexus; seen with cervicogenic patterns, brachial irritation, or acromioclavicular separations. The extreme extension of this phenomenon with a cervicogenic cause is the overhead position of relief.

If the athlete can stand with the arm at the side, it is important to make the following observations:

1. Height of the shoulder. This is of less significance than previously thought. A low shoulder may be due to:
   a. Adaptive laxity of the capsule (sports demand)
   b. Increased weight of the dominant arm
   c. Scoliosis—appropriate tests should be performed (Adam's, etc.)
   d. Other mechanical abnormalities of the pelvis and lower extremity
   e. Soft tissue asymmetries (shortened muscles due to spasm or hypertonicity)
   Due to the marked number of benign possibilities, it is suggested that if an obvious underlying cause is not found, that overattention to this observation is probably not necessary.

2. Relationship of the palm to the body. This should clue the examiner to abnormalities in tension of the internal and external rotators. For example, normally the thumb faces anterior or slightly medial. If the dorsum of the hand faces posteriorly there may be excessive tightness of the internal rotators. Conversely, if the palm faces anteriorly, there may be tightness of the external rotators. This helps direct attention during the testing of these muscles in the examination sequence.

3. Inspect the general muscular contours of the shoulder and upper body. This inspection should help define whether the individual has any significant atrophy or possibly overdevelopment of specific musculature.

4. Winging of the scapula (Fig. 6-6). Winging is most obvious in the relaxed standing position when mechanically caused (either congenitally or through the development of a scoliosis). Further evaluation of other causes requires a wall push-up for determination of serratus anterior involvement (long thoracic nerve). If winging is due to serratus anterior dysfunction, the scapula will move proximally with the inferior angle moving medial. If the trapezius is the cause, the scapula moves down with the inferior angle moving laterally.[18]

5. Acromioclavicular deformity. Prominence of this joint should be a clue to one of three processes: acromioclavicular separation (acute or chronic), distal clavicular fracture, or acromioclavicular osteoarthritis. If related to an appropriate past or present history of separation, it can be deduced that a second or third degree separation occurred. Deformity due to arthritis is more common in the older athlete.

6. Inspection for scars. Scars are the result of past trauma either through injury or surgery. Scars due to surgery suggest a more involved pathology requiring open reduction and if not previously volunteered by the patient should be further pursued.

Observation should continue throughout orthopaedic testing.

Palpation

Palpation should not be viewed as a static process. Initially, the clinician may wish to localize the area of

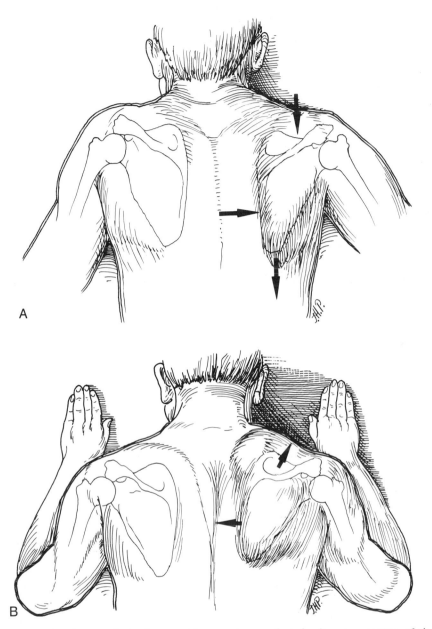

Fig. 6-6. (A) Position of right scapula is shown with trapezius paralysis leading to winging of shoulder blade. Scapula is displaced downward and outward. Upper portion of scapula is dislocated away from midline. **(B)** Position of right scapula is shown with paralysis of serratus anterior muscle. Here scapula is displaced inward and upward. Inferior angle of scapula approaches spine. (From Post,[63] with permission.)

complaint with patient input and determine other tender structures or trigger points. However, it is imperative that the palpation process proceed through the remainder of the examination to determine crepitus, changes in tenderness with maneuvers, reactive

spasm or protective recruitment, restrictions, and instabilities.

Figure 6-1 indicates common locations of tenderness related to structure. It becomes apparent that a thorough knowledge of anatomy is necessary to determine possible causes. A systematic approach is generally recommended to avoid exclusion based on a bias from the history. Many clinicians recommend starting at a point away from the presenting complaint and proceeding toward that area. It is always important to include bilateral palpation to avoid an overenthusiastic conclusion of "eureka."

Most of the bony architecture of the shoulder complex is relatively superficial, and therefore accessible to palpation. Beginning with the sternoclavicular joint, the examiner should be sensitive to any changes in contour. In particular is the importance of enlargement of the sternoclavicular joint and proceeding laterally the possibility of clavicular fracture (when a traumatic onset is present). Proceeding further laterally to the acromioclavicular joint, it is important to detect any abnormal size or shape indicating past or present separation, fracture, or osteoarthritis. Proceeding posteriorly along the acromion, the examiner may palpate the spine of the scapula. This is rarely the site of complaint or pathology. Next, palpating the medial then lateral borders of the scapula may reveal areas of tenderness, in most cases due to soft tissue tension on attachment sites. The glenoid is not directly palpable; however anteriorly and posteriorly there may be tenderness in the location of the glenoid rim with instability and with various osseous and labral lesions (Bennett's and Bankart lesions).

The coracoid lies relatively superficial, inferior and medial to the acromioclavicular joint. Serving mainly a role as an attachment site, tenderness would indicate involvement of the pectoralis minor, short head of the biceps, coracoacromial ligament, and coracohumeral ligament. A painful bursa may be detected due to repetitive trauma (marksman shoulder).[19] The coracoacromial ligament is often tender with impingement syndrome. Remember that a prominent coracoid (usually unilateral) may be suggestive of a posterior dislocation.

The humerus is relatively accessible. Starting distally it is important to palpate the medial and lateral epicondyles and proceed up the shaft noting any areas of tenderness or production of any unusual neurologic signs. Prominences of the humeral head may be palpated starting with the lesser tuberosity, progressing laterally to the bicipital groove, and finally the greater tuberosity. Again tenderness at these areas is almost always an indication of the soft tissue that finds attachment at each specific site. Further determination will be made with the appropriate challenge (contraction or stretch). At the lesser tuberosity tenderness may indicate involvement of the subscapularis. Lateral, within the groove, the biceps is implicated. However, the insertions of the pectoralis major, teres major, and latissimus dorsi may also be in close enough proximity to allow misinterpretation. Anterior greater tuberosity pain would indicate the supraspinatus, while posteriorly elicited tenderness suggests either the infraspinatus or teres minor.

By exploiting certain positional changes on structural location, the examiner may access areas not available in the static "arm by the side" position. The insertion of the supraspinatus is made more discernible by bringing the arm behind the back or other positions of mild extension.[20] The examiner then palpates anteroinferior to the acromioclavicular joint for an approximation of the insertion site (Fig. 6-7). The insertions of the infraspinatus and teres minor are brought into exposure by horizontally adducting the arm and then externally rotating.[20] Palpating posterolateral should locate more easily these sites of attachments (Fig. 6-

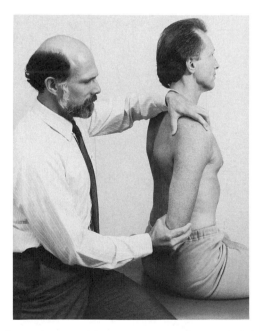

Fig. 6-7. Palpation of the supraspinatus. Moving slightly posteriorly will access the infraspinatus/teres minor insertion.

8). Lyons and Tomlinson[21] have documented accuracy in detecting full tears of the rotator cuff. They report a 91 percent sensitivity and a 75 percent specificity. The patient's elbow is bent to 90 degrees and the humeral head is palpated with internal rotation, then external rotation, followed by hyperextension. They reported being able to detect anterior supraspinatus tears with internal rotation, posterior tears with external rotation, and tears of the infraspinatus with hyperextension.

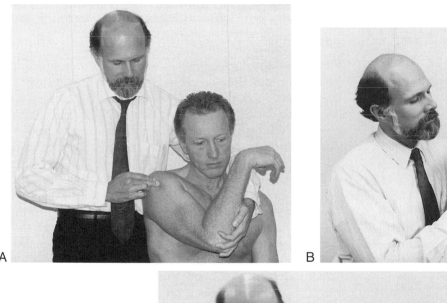

A

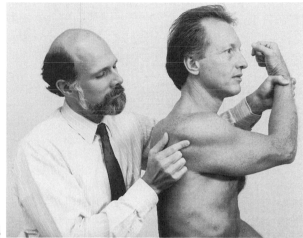

B

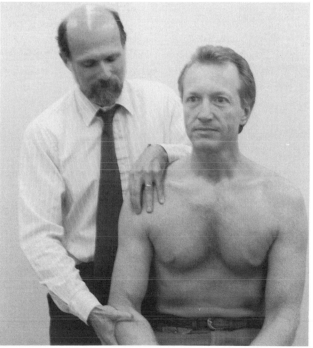

C

Fig. 6-8. **(A)** Palpation of the infraspinatus/teres minor insertions. **(B)** Palpation of the infraspinatus/teres minor tendons. **(C)** Palpation of the long head of the biceps tendon involves internal rotation of 10 degrees.

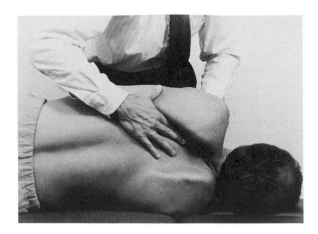

Fig. 6-9. Palpation of the medial border of the scapula.

Kulund[22] suggests that by palpating one finger-breadth lateral to the coracoid process one may access the anterior capsule. He further suggests that persistent tenderness with internal and external rotation of the arm suggests capsular involvement. In other words, other structures such as tendons and muscles move while the broad capsule remains under palpating pressure.

The biceps and bicipital groove are brought into prominence by internal rotation of the arm 10 to 15 degrees (Fig. 6-8C).[23] Care must be taken not to misinterpret the medial edge of the deltoid as the bicipital tendon.

By placing the patient supine and distracting the arm laterally, the lateral-anterior border of the scapula, and therefore the subscapularis, is more palpable. By placing patients in the lateral recumbent position and placing the arm of the patient behind their back, the examiner may access the anterior-medial border of the scapula by pushing the shoulder posteriorly (Fig. 6-9). The examiner's hand slips under the medial surface easily in this position. Palpation for rhomboid and middle trapezius involvement is the primary focus.

Prone palpation may include the belly of the supraspinatus due to the relaxation of the trapezius in this position. Additionally, the subdeltoid bursa may be palpated with passive extension of the arm. Palpation is anterior to the acromioclavicular joint (Fig. 6-10).

Soft tissue palpation includes evaluation of both contractile and noncontractile structures. As a general rule of thumb the noncontractile tissue lies deep to the contractile tissue. For example, the capsule and capsular ligaments lie under the tendinous insertions of the rotator cuff (in fact, they are blended).

In addition to direct palpation, it will be necessary to include the challenge of active and passive ROM to further clarify the causative structure or structures. Added to the complexities due to overlay there is the need to differentiate an area of localized muscle tenderness from a discrete trigger point. As a general rule, active trigger points will refer to a standard reference zone, but latent trigger points may not.

An area often overlooked on the shoulder examina-

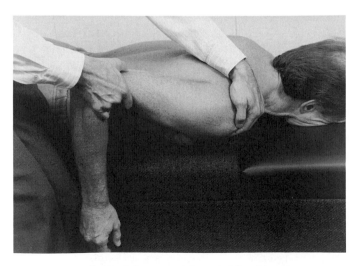

Fig. 6-10. Palpation of the subdeltoid bursa.

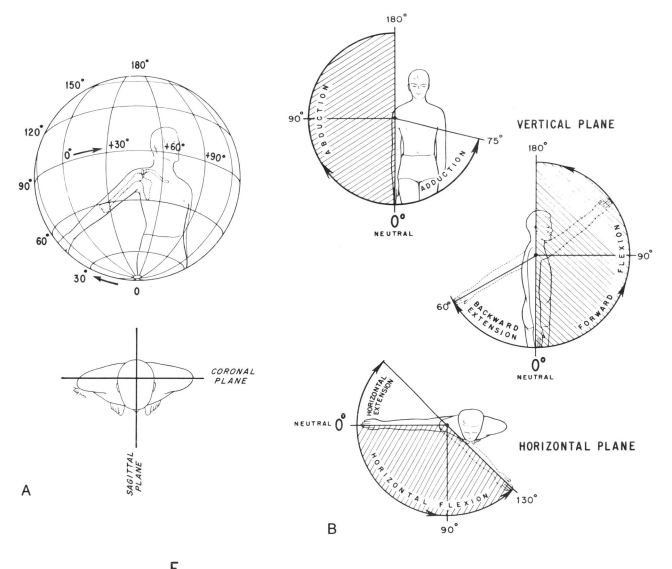

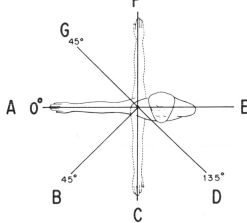

Fig. 6-11. The method of measuring and recording of joint motion as accepted by the American Academy of Orthopaedic Surgeons. **(A)** Global shoulder motion. **(B)** Vertical and horizontal motion. **(C)** Method of identifying positions of elevation of the arm. *A,* neutral abduction; *B,* abduction in 45 degrees or horizontal flexion; *C,* forward flexion; *D,* adduction in 135 degrees of horizontal flexion; *E,* neutral adduction; *F,* backward extension; *G,* abduction in 45 degrees of horizontal extension. *(Figure continues.)*

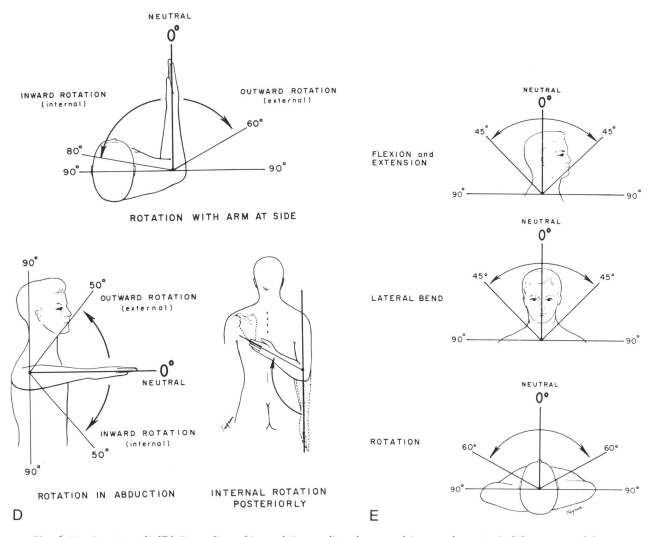

Fig. 6-11. *(continued)* **(D)** Recording of inward (internal) and outward (external rotation). **(E)** Motions of the cervical spine. *(Figure continues.)*

tion is the axilla. For most clinicians this is a "low yield" area; however, it may be helpful in determining either deep bursal irritation or lymph node involvement revealing an occasional occult process.

Range of Motion

ROM can be divided into two areas of investigation: active and passive. Each approach will individually expose specific entities, and combined, the findings help delineate more accurately which soft tissue or bony structures are involved. Beginning with active ROM to

gain a sense of restrictions before applying passive ROM is often suggested.

Active ROM

In addition to the traditional Apley's profile, active ROM should include all six glenohumeral movements and scapulothoracic movements throughout their range with additional testing of coupled movements (Fig. 6-11):

1. Flexion/extension

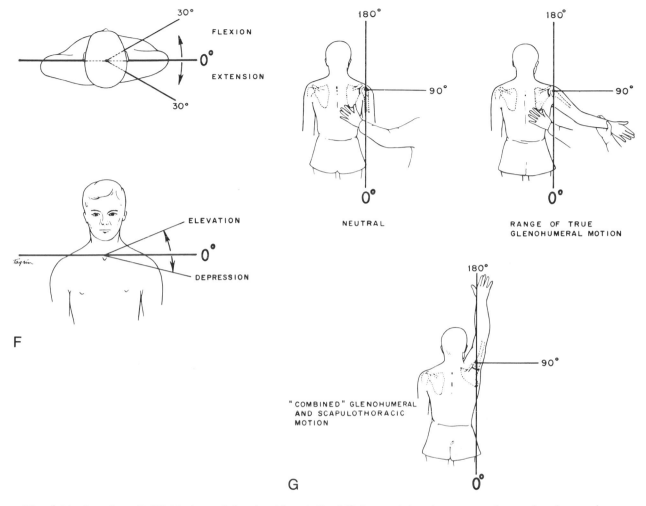

Fig. 6-11. *(continued)* **(F)** Motions of the shoulder girdle. **(G)** Determining the ranges of true glenohumeral motion and combined scapulothoracic motion. (From Rowe,[73] with permission.)

2. Abduction/adduction
3. Internal/external rotation
4. Horizontal abduction/adduction
5. Protraction/retraction of the scapula

Coupled movement such as horizontal abduction with external rotation should be evaluated (a common position for throwing sports).

The American College of Shoulder and Elbow Surgeons recommends an active ROM evaluation that is simple but accurate.[24] Forward flexion is measured as the angle between the arm and the thoracic rib cage (Fig. 6-12). External rotation is measured in two positions: arm at the side and 90 degrees abduction (same position as "crank" test for apprehension). Internal rotation is designated by the highest vertebral level that can be reached by the hand behind the back (Fig. 6-13).

Various clues can be uncovered when observing active ROM. These include

1. Painful or hesitant initiation of movement (often indicating an unstable shoulder or tendon tear)
2. Attempts at modifying movement by:
   a. Use of an altered plane of movement (e.g., scapular plane abduction when attempting coronal abduction)
   b. Recruitment of muscles not normally needed for

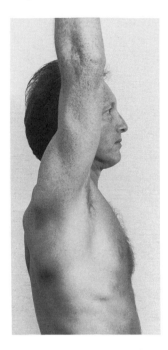

Fig. 6-12. Active forward flexion.

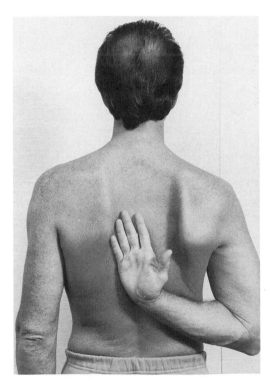

Fig. 6-13. Active internal rotation measured by highest vertebral level reached.

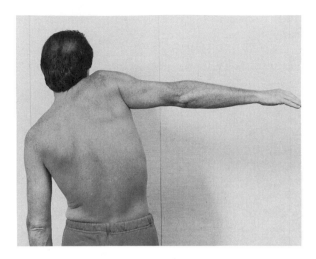

Fig. 6-14. Shoulder shrugging to accomplish elevation indicating possible frozen shoulder, rotator cuff tear, or osteoarthritic blockage of normal humeral motion.

a particular movement (e.g., upper trapezius contraction for forward flexion or abduction)
  c. Use of trunk or body substitution to simulate or acquire a particular movement (e.g., laterally bending the trunk to initiate abduction with a torn rotator cuff) (Fig. 6-14)
3. A specific mid-range arc of painful ROM; the painful arc (Fig. 6-15) indicates subacromial impingement

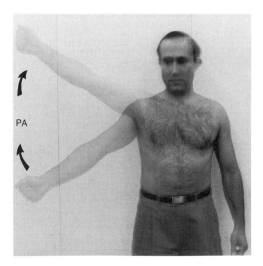

Fig. 6-15. Mid-range painful arc *(PA)* indicates impingement, whereas end-range painful arc indicates acromioclavicular joint involvement.

4. End-range restrictions and their cause; weakness, tightness, or pain

Passive ROM

Passive ROM is most revealing due not only to appreciation of restriction (or lack thereof) but also the quality of the restriction. Cyriax[25] has outlined several different abnormal end-feels with passive testing (Fig. 6-16):

1. *Bone-to-bone*—indication of fracture or severe osteoarthritis.
2. *Capsular*—a "leathery" end-feel indicative of a capsular process (in particular fibrosis) occurring short of where one would expect the "tissue stretch" feeling of normal end range.
3. *Empty*—an endpoint is reached due to pain, not a mechanical blockage. It feels incomplete and is often found without muscle spasm.
4. *Muscle spasm*—a sudden stoppage of movement elicited by the examiner's attempt at passive testing. It is often accompanied by pain. Cyriax refers to this as a *vibrant twang*.

5. *Springy*—a sensation similar to end-range tissue stretch (a normal end-feel); however, it feels more mechanically obstructed such as found with a torn meniscus on end-range knee extension.

When passive ROM (especially abduction) is limited by pain, a gentle attempt at passing through this barrier should be attempted. It is often found that the painful restriction decreases when further range is accessed (painful arc). The painful arc is an indication of an impinged structure.

Passive forward flexion is usually performed in the standing position (Fig. 6-17). Overpressure pain may indicate impingement. In the supine position, external rotation is measured at the side and with the arm at 90 degrees abduction. Internal rotation is measured at 90 degrees abduction with the scapula stabilized (Fig. 6-18). At 90 degrees abduction assessment of humeral rotation is more accurate due to the elimination of scapulothoracic movement.

Passive overpressure should be applied at various joints to determine the patient's tendency toward hyperextensibility. If the patient is able to passively bring

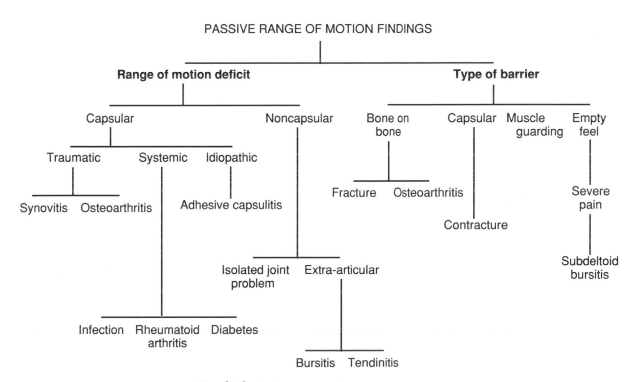

Fig. 6-16. Passive range of motion algorithm.

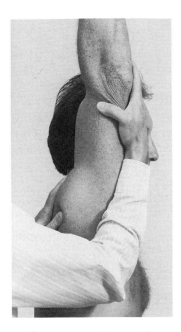

Fig. 6-17. Passive forward flexion.

the fingers to the anterior aspect of the forearm hyperextensibility is present. Other areas would include the elbow and knee. Global hyperextensibility or hyperextensibility limited to the hands and feet may indicate possible Ehlers-Danlos syndrome.[26]

Muscle Testing

A cursory evaluation of muscle strength may be helpful in detecting gross neurologic involvement; however, it hardly addresses the concerns of the athlete. Some would question whether the manual muscle testing (MMT) of an athlete can ever detect subtle weaknesses or imbalances. The manual evaluation can, in most cases, detect in a symptomatic patient the possible muscles involved due to the reproduction of a pain complaint. However, the validity of an attempt to isolate a muscle for determining its strength is doubtful. Even the most fastidious attempts at isolation of a muscle cannot eliminate other muscles from participation. The following are recommendations when manually testing muscle strength:

1. Always compare both sides.
2. Avoid resistive contact on painful or injured body parts.
3. Initially test in the midrange of a movement to eliminate overstrain or involvement of noncontractile tissues.
4. If strong in the mid-range position, test throughout the range.
5. Carefully observe for recruitment through altered position or body movement.
6. Be acquainted with the ratio of various antagonistic functional groups.

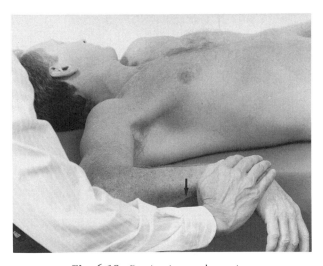

Fig. 6-18. Passive internal rotation.

Extremely valuable and enlightening is observation of the athlete during sport training and weight training.

A discussion of muscle testing for the purposes of eliciting pain and possibly weakness will be given later in the chapter.

Hand-held dynamometers (HHD) have become more popular recently. They are suggested as a superior alternative to MMT, supposedly eliminating some of the subjectiveness and offering a more discretely calibrated scale.[27,28] The HHD is stabilized against the extremity being tested. The patient attempts a maximum contraction against the dynamometer. The measurement recorded is not a direct measure of muscle strength but a force reading. If the placement site is consistent, the lever arm remains the same and the subsequent readings are relatively reliable.

There have been a number of studies on the intratester and intertester reliability.[29–31] Although results vary, reliability of both seems good. Reliabilities are apparently better with upper extremity measurements when compared to the lower extremity. To maximize accuracy and reliability it has been suggested that a more distal site of HHD application be used.[32]

Isokinetic evaluation of muscle strength is not always practical, but in some situations it is an excellent objectifiable tool for assessment. Chapter 8 discusses in detail the application of isokinetic equipment.

Combined Findings

It is important now to hypothetically take some of the possible combined findings and attempt to draw some general conclusions as to what they indicate. As an exercise in critical thinking the following examples serve a purpose; however, the physician should not assume that each represents all possible patients since the variables of onset, age, and other historical factors will not be included.

1. A patient presents with painful and restricted active abduction of the shoulder. Passive movement was free and painless. All other movements are unaffected both actively or passively. An attempt at further active abduction through the painful range was not possible. Since an active movement is the only restricted pattern and is also painful the primary muscles governing abduction must be the involved tissue. Most likely the supraspinatus or possibly the deltoid have been strained.

2. A patient presents with painful and restricted active abduction coupled with painful restricted passive abduction. The attempt at ranging through the restricted/painful range is possible, especially above 110 degrees of abduction passively. All other movements are essentially normal. This is the painful arc and represents impingement of structures under the subacromial arch. Structures that are most likely involved are the subacromial bursa or possibly the supraspinatus or biceps tendons.

3. A patient presents with restrictions and pain felt only with passive and active end-range abduction. Active resisted movement is normal in the typical mid-range testing position for all shoulder muscles tested. Since active resisted testing was essentially normal it is more likely a noncontractile such as a bursa is the involved structure and/or mechanical irritation caused by inferior acromioclavicular spur formation.

4. A patient has a severely restricted active abduction pattern with no pain. Passive abduction is full and painless. This scenario is suggestive of rupture of the supraspinatus or less possibly the deltoid. A neurologic cause of weakness is more likely and would need to be differentiated by further testing.

5. A patient presents with a chronic shoulder complaint of mainly stiffness that is evident on examination as restriction into abduction and external rotation both passively and actively. Other movements are slightly restricted. This is a classic pattern for two conditions: frozen shoulder (adhesive capsulitis) and an occult posterior dislocation.

Orthopaedic Testing

There are two primary areas of investigation when orthopaedically testing the shoulder (assuming fracture has been ruled out): is there any instability present? and are there indicators of impingement? These questions and their answers are not mutually exclusive. Both conditions may and often do coexist. The final step in the process is to determine which specific structures are involved. Many of these indicators will be exposed during the preceding testing of palpation, ROM, and muscle testing.

As with all acutely injured and/or painful joints, many orthopaedic tests may not be possible due to limitation in ROM. If serious damage must be ruled out due to a traumatic or suspicious history, specialized studies should be performed. If the etiology is not suspect, orthopaedic testing may be delayed until ROM has returned.

General Instability Testing

Stability of the shoulders is both a static and dynamic process. The dynamic process is primarily due to the rotator cuff's coordinated contraction. This cuff effect is partly due to a tightening of the static capsular component. Evaluation of the shoulder with stability testing is primarily addressing the static capsular component. However, with the exception of the apprehension position, most of the positional approaches are not end-range positions. This means that although there is a general assessment of capsular looseness, the individual portions of the capsule are not at maximum end-range tension. It is important to compare with the opposite well shoulder to distinguish between a "loose" shoulder as compared to an "unstable" shoulder. In other words, an atraumatic loose shoulder does not imply the likely possibility of labrum and capsular damage found with the traumatic unstable shoulder (although in sports it is still a possibility). Treatment approaches would be different.

There are a variety of procedures, most applying a challenge to the shoulder in a passively acquired position. There are three directions of stability that are challenged: anterior, posterior, and inferior. Although each would seem to conform to deficiency of the related direction of excessive movement there are some indications of the opposite being true. It has been demonstrated that for inferior instability to be present, for example, more than the inferior capsule must be involved.

Testing employs three principles:

1. Challenge in the direction of suspected instability (the "load and shift" test).
2. Place in a position that eliminates secondary support (the subscapularis or other muscle/tendons) and attempt a challenge for the purpose of eliciting a sensation of apprehension or pain by the patient.
3. If this is positive, attempt to externally restore stability and retest the individual to determine if the sensation of apprehension or pain is eliminated.

When testing for instability of the shoulder it is important to stabilize the scapula to localize the challenge specifically to the glenohumeral joint. Remember to begin in a position that will not inadvertently produce a subluxation or dislocation in the process. It is imperative to begin in a neutral position. In other words, by pressing medially first, the humeral head will be centered in the glenoid before attempting any translation.

Load and Shift

The load and shift tests[33] attempt to translate the humeral head in three directions. The amount of translation in normal individuals is varied, but anterior translation should not exceed about 25 percent of the glenoid surface. Posterior translation and inferior translation should not exceed 50 percent. Tested under anesthesia (or in a very relaxed individual), the following grading system is used:

Grade I—equals subluxation without dislocation. It indicates a greater than 50 percent translation of the humeral head.[34] There is no clunking sensation although grinding is noted.
Grade II—equals dislocation. A jump is noted, but the humeral head returns to position.
Grade III—equals a locked dislocation. The examiner is able to lock the humeral head over the glenoid.

Again, before evaluating the degree of laxity, keep in mind that in multidirectionally lax individuals, the starting position may begin with an already displaced humeral head anteriorly, posteriorly, or inferiorly. It is therefore important to begin with a humeral head that has been centralized by compression into the glenoid fossa guaranteeing a reduced starting position.

First, beginning with the patient standing and leaning forward 45 degrees, the arm is allowed to hang free. The examiner stabilizes the scapula (however, not too rigidly) while grabbing the humerus with the thumb posteriorly and hand anteriorly. As with similar "drawer" tests the humerus is pushed anteriorly (Fig. 6-19A). An additional inferior component is employed.

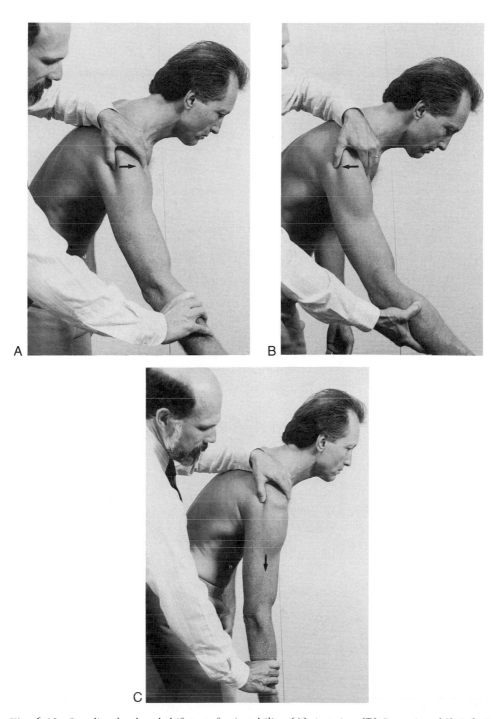

Fig. 6-19. Standing load and shift tests for instability. **(A)** Anterior. **(B)** Posterior. **(C)** Inferior.

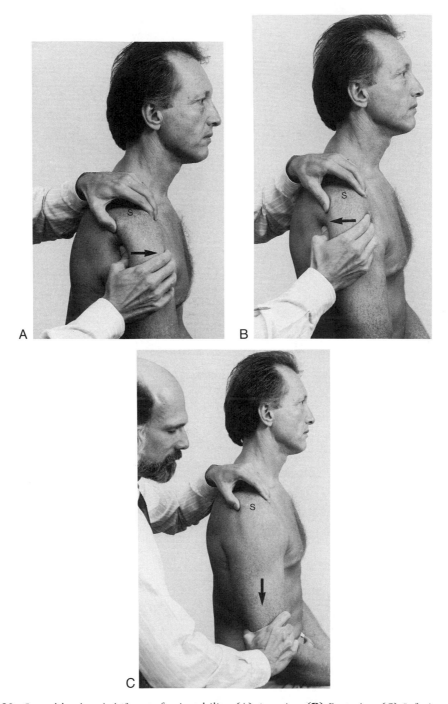

Fig. 6-20. Seated load and shift tests for instability. **(A)** Anterior. **(B)** Posterior. **(C)** Inferior. *S,* stabilize.

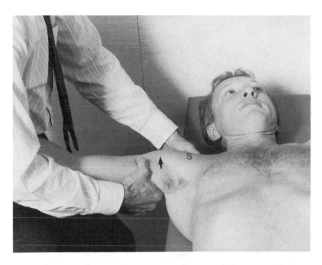

Fig. 6-21. Anterior drawer test for instability. *S,* stabilize.

Posterior stability is tested by pulling posteriorly (Fig. 19B), and inferior stability with an inferior load (Fig. 19C). A "sulcus" sign may appear seen as dimpling under the acromioclavicular joint area on inferior translation when multidirectional instability is present.[35,36] Crepitus may be palpable with these maneuvers.

With the patient seated the same challenge is performed, but the patient remains upright with the elbow at the side. Often the elbow is bent 90 degrees. Stabilization at the spine of the scapula and coracoid with one hand allows the other hand to push and pull into

anterior and posterior directions, respectively (Fig. 20A & B). Inferior stability usually involves a distracting force at the elbow (Fig. 20C). Again, the sulcus sign is an indication of not just inferior laxity but multidirectional instability.

With the patient supine, the examiner lifts the arm into 20 degrees of flexion and abduction. Loading anteriorly, posteriorly, and inferiorly is performed as above. A reminder that if the patient's shoulder is too sensitive for grasping pressure, a force may be applied distally on the arm. The sensitivity of this more distal testing is diminished significantly without direct palpation available.

Additional Load and Shift Maneuvers

Anterior Instability

An anterior drawer test[37] may be performed by placing the patient supine and abducting the arm between 80 and 120 degrees. The patient's arm is stabilized in the examiner's axilla and forward flexed 0 and 20 degrees and laterally rotated 0 and 30 degrees. Stabilizing the scapula at the scapular spine posteriorly and coracoid anteriorly, the examiner attempts forward translation at the proximal humerus with the other hand (Fig. 6-21).

Protzman[38] suggests a position very similar to the apprehension test. The examiner rests the seated patient's shoulder on the examiner's side; this should bring the shoulder to about 90 degrees abduction. The

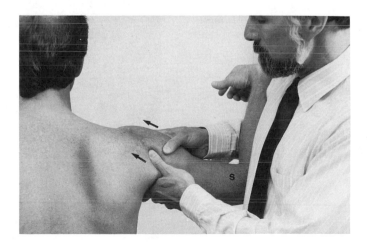

Fig. 6-22. Protzman test for anterior instability. *S,* stabilize.

examiner then pushes the posterior humeral head anteriorly while the other hand palpates for anterior movement (Fig. 6-22).

Posterior Instability

Gerber[37] describes a posterior drawer test for the shoulder performed with the patient supine. The scapula is stabilized as with other tests while the examiner flexes the elbow 120 degrees and abducts the shoulder to about 80 to 120 degrees. The shoulder is forward flexed about 20 to 30 degrees. While medially rotating the forearm the shoulder is horizontally adducted 60 to 80 degrees. At the same time the thumb that was stabilizing at the coracoid is now used to push posteriorly on the humerus (Fig. 6-23). Palpation of posterior migration or apprehension may result. The test is rarely pain producing.

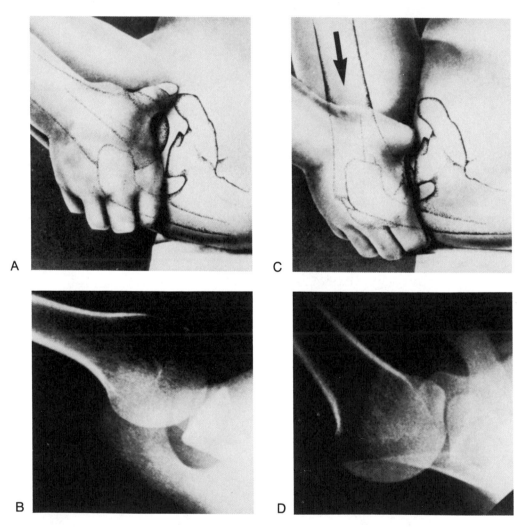

Fig. 6-23. Posterior drawer test for shoulder subluxation. **(A)** With the hand grasping the proximal shoulder and the thumb firmly over the humeral head, the elbow is supported with the other hand of examiner. **(B)** Roentgenogram of the located position. **(C)** Arm is brought into adduction and posterior pressure exerted with both the supporting hand at the elbow and the proximal hand over the humeral head. The thumb slides along the lateral aspect of the coracoid process as the head of the humerus is pushed backward. **(D)** Subluxated position is confirmed radiographically. (Modified from Gerber and Ganz,[37] with permission.)

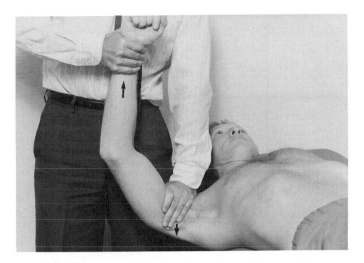

Fig. 6-24. The push-pull test for posterior instability.

Very similar tests are the push-pull test[39] and the Norwood test[40] for posterior instability. With the patient supine, the elbow is flexed 90 degrees and the arm is externally rotated and abducted 90 degrees. For the push-pull test, the examiner then horizontally adducts the arm slightly, pulling on the wrist to distract the shoulder while the other hand pushes posteriorly at the proximal humerus (Fig. 6-24). Subluxation may be felt to occur. As the arm is taken out of horizontal adduction into neutral, the head may slip back into place. The Norwood test uses the same starting position, but does not involve distraction at the wrist and employs 90 degrees of horizontal adduction (Fig. 6-25). A variation has been suggested by Cofield and Irving[41] where about 20 degrees of internal rotation is added to the end position and a posteriorly directed force is added through the patient's elbow. Apprehension is not as likely to occur as subluxation or dislocation with this maneuver.

The variation suggested above by Cofield and Irving

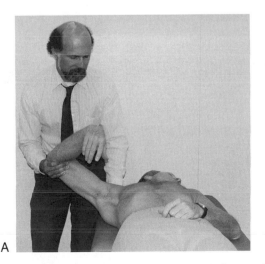

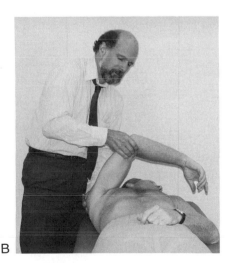

Fig. 6-25. (A & B) The Norwood test for instability involves a posterior directed force through the humerus while horizontally adducting the shoulder.

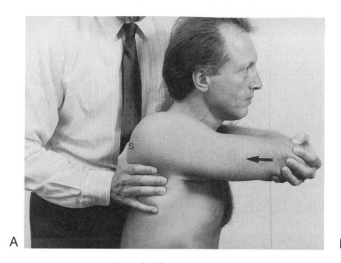

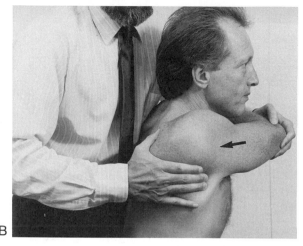

Fig. 6-26. (A & B) The jerk test is essentially a seated Norwood test. *S*, stabilize.

is performed with the patient seated. The arm is forward flexed to 90 degrees with the elbow bent 90 degrees. The examiner directs a force posteriorly through the shoulder. While maintaining the posterior load, the examiner horizontally adducts the arm (Fig. 6-26). Subluxation may occur as the humeral head subluxates posteriorly. Reduction usually occurs as the arm is taken out of horizontal adduction. This is referred to as the jerk test.[39]

Inferior and Multidirectional Instability

The Feagen maneuver as described by Norris[42] involves flexing the shoulder 90 degrees and resting the elbow on the examiner's shoulder. The examiner then uses both hands to push down on the proximal humerus in an attempt to reproduce subluxation or a palpable bounce (Fig. 6-27).

Apprehension Signs

Before adding any challenge from an external force passive positioning is attempted first to determine stability. The examiner places a hand over the shoulder with the index finger over the humeral head anteriorly, the middle finger over the coracoid, and the thumb posteriorly over the humeral head. The examiner's other hand lifts the arm from the wrist into abduction and external rotation noting any anterior movement of the humeral head determined by relative positioning of the anterior two fingers. If the index finger moves forward, anterior instability may be present

(Fig. 6-28). If on returning the arm to the neutral resting position the index finger moves back again, the test is confirmed. If the test is positive further positioning in abduction/external rotation should proceed cautiously.

Anterior.   By placing the patient's arm in 90 degrees abduction and externally rotating it, a posterior to anterior force is applied to the proximal humerus. A sense of apprehension (feels like the shoulder will slip out of place) or pain may be produced.

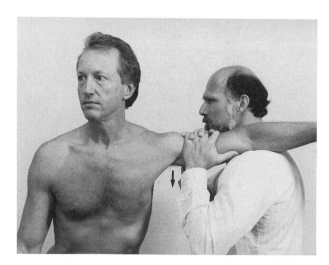

Fig. 6-27. The Feagen test for inferior and multidirectional instability.

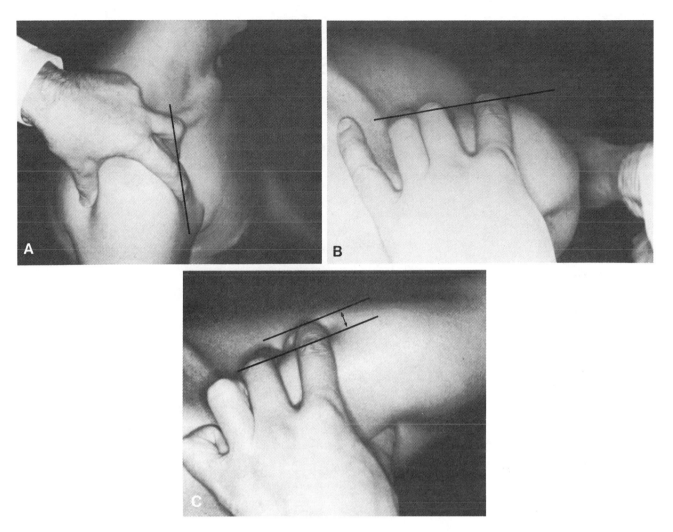

Fig. 6-28. (A–C) Anterior instability test. (From Leffert and Gumbey,[74] as adapted in Magle,[1] with permission.)

Rockwood[17] suggests performing passive external rotation with the arm at the side, and at 45, 90, and 120 degrees of abduction (Fig. 6-29). By testing the arm at 120 degrees of abduction and introducing external rotation, it is more likely that apprehension will be produced due to the lack of stability normally provided by the subscapularis below this position.

To either of the two tests above, the examiner may add a resistance to the patient's attempt to imitate a throwing motion. By applying this resistance, the throwing motion is simulated, and subtle forms of instability may be exposed.

There are a number of supine apprehension tests using slightly different contact points.

1. The crank test brings the arm to 90 degrees abduction and by contacting the elbow and wrist passive external rotation is introduced (Fig. 6-30A).
2. The fulcrum test is similar to the crank test, but it uses the posterior shoulder as the fulcrum (Fig. 6-30B).
3. Rowe suggests placing the hand behind the head while applying passive external rotation again with the fulcrum at the posterior shoulder (Fig. 6-30C).

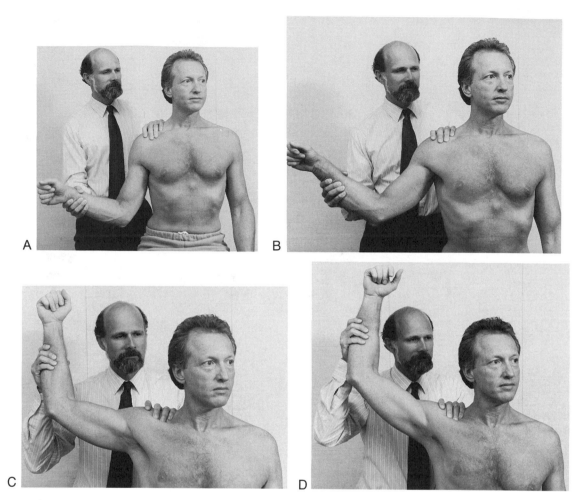

Fig. 6-29. The apprehension test is performed **(A)** by the side, **(B)** 45 degrees abduction, **(C)** 90 degrees abduction, **(D)** 120 degrees abduction. An external rotation force is applied with the outside hand while an anterior force is directed with the other.

Posterior. The posterior apprehension test is relatively unreliable. The examiner places the supine patient's arm into forward flexion with the forearm internally rotated. A posterior directed force is applied through the elbow in an attempt to elicit apprehension (Fig. 6-31).

Relocation Signs.[43] If the apprehension sign is positive, the patient is tested in the supine position. A variation of the testing maneuver is applied to determine if outward stability by the examiner alleviates a sense of apprehension or pain in this provocative position. The examiner places the shoulder in 90 degrees abduction

and externally rotates, this time applying an anterior to posterior force to the proximal humerus (Fig. 6-32). Relief of pain or apprehension is considered a positive test. An increase in pain is possible, especially in the posteriorly unstable shoulder or occasionally with impingement. Silliman and Hawkins[44] describe an extension of the relocation test called the release test. If relief is created with the posteriorly directed force of the relocation test, the posterior pressure is then suddenly released causing a sudden increase in pain.

The author has found that some patients have difficulty (without pain) with full abduction of the arm when multidirectional instability is present. By stabiliz-

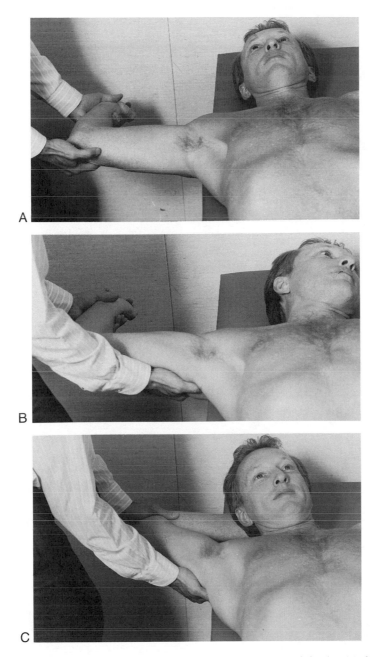

Fig. 6-30. The apprehension test performed supine with three variations. **(A)** The crank test, **(B)** the fulcrum test, and **(C)** the Rowe test.

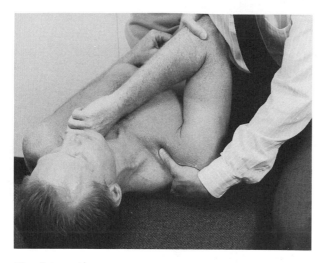

Fig. 6-31. The posterior instability test (not very sensitive).

ing the shoulder externally with both hands, the patient is sometimes able to accomplish full abduction with no sense of increased effort or weakness (Fig. 6-33).

With posterior instability, it is not uncommon for the patient to have the ability to dislocate and relocate the shoulder through voluntary contraction of various muscles. This is probably much more rewarding than many posterior stability tests in the evaluation of someone with gross posterior laxity. A maneuver that may also create subluxation/dislocation is to have the pa-

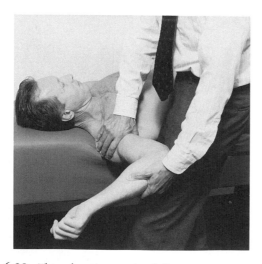

Fig. 6-32. The relocation test is a follow-up test to a positive apprehension test. A posteriorly applied force in the apprehension position reveals the original positive response.

tient raise the arm into forward flexion with supination. Often a subtle bulge will be seen posteriorly as the shoulder subluxates although the patient may be pain-free and unaware of the movement. If from this position the patient contracts the shoulder or horizontal abduction is attempted, reduction may occur with a clunk.[42]

Glenoid Labrum Signs/Tests. Although damage to the glenoid labrum may occur without damage to the capsule (due to biceps pull at its glenoid attachment), most will be found with concomitant instability. Therefore, all patients with instability positives on physical examination should be evaluated with two maneuvers, the clunk test and the Kocher maneuver. Although the sensitivity of these two tests is rather low, when positive they are an indicator for further investigation with computed tomography (CT) arthrography or arthroscopy.

The clunk test[45,46] involves abducting the shoulder in the supine patient. The examiner, similar to the apprehension test, then applies an anterior directed force to the humeral head while circumducting and/or rotating the shoulder (Fig. 6-34). A clunk or click, usually felt deep in the shoulder, is a positive response. Often there is a painful catch felt before the clunk sensation. An indicator of underlying instability may be provoked by horizontally adducting the arm. As the arm reduces into neutral a clunk or click may be heard or palpated.[47]

The Kocher maneuver,[46] although initially designed to replace an anterior dislocation, has been used recently to expose a glenoid labrum tear. The patient is seated. The examiner distracts the arm (elbow bent 90 degrees) maintaining it in the starting position of slight external rotation and abduction. Then the examiner passively adducts the arm at the elbow followed by internal rotation (Fig. 6-35). Again, a clunk or click is often felt in the presence of a glenoid labrum tear. With both tests, it must be remembered that they should be repeated several times and that the lack of a response does not exclude the possibility of a glenoid labrum tear especially if historically suggested.

Impingement Testing

Impingement occurs mainly under the coracoacromial arch. Although many etiologies have been proposed

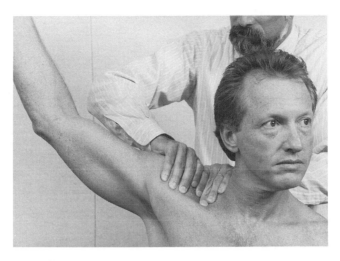

Fig. 6-33. A functional test for generalized laxity of the shoulder. If full abduction is not possible due to a sense of "weakness," outside stabilization may allow full-range movement.

the basic mechanical process is compression of the structures underlying the arch when the arm is in an overhead position. This position of impingement is increased by adding internal rotation, which jams the greater tuberosity under the arch. Testing then is based on these mechanical concepts. However, other etiologies may be detected with other portions of the examination process. For example, muscle dysfunction may be perceived with manual or isokinetic evaluation, or a hooked acromion or acromioclavicular spur may be visible on a radiograph.

General testing for impingement involves several tests:

1. *Painful arc.* This has already been addressed under passive and active ROM testing (Fig. 6-15). The painful arc is an observation of pain on passive or active abduction through a range of 70 to 110 degrees with less or no pain before and after this range.[25]
2. *Neer's test.* By passively flexing to end range the supinated arm with the elbow extended, the examiner attempts to jam the humerus under the arch (Fig. 6-36). Pain with this test is more end-range pain without the characteristic painful arc found in abduction.[48]
3. *Hawkins-Kennedy's test.* This test takes advantage of the increase in subacromial compression with

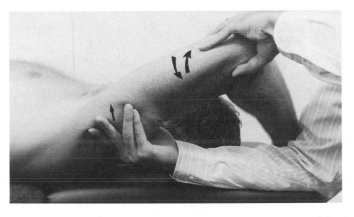

Fig. 6-34. The clunk test for glenoid labrum tears. From this position rotation of the humerus is applied to determine a deep sensation of a clunk.

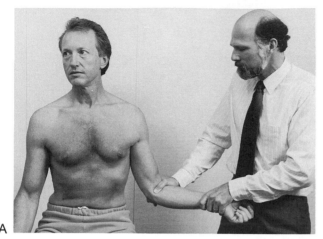
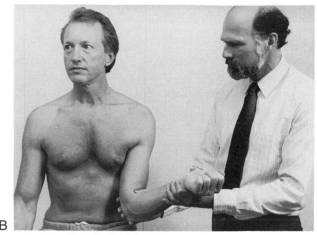
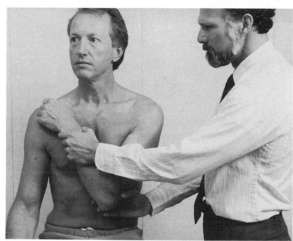

Fig. 6-35. The Kocher maneuver. **(A)** Distraction added to abduction and external rotation, **(B)** next apply adduction, followed by **(C)** internal rotation.

internal rotation of the humerus. The patient's arm is forward flexed 90 degrees with the elbow bent to 90 degrees and internally rotated so that the forearm is parallel with the floor. The examiner supports the arm at the elbow with one hand while the other imparts more internal rotation by pressure on the dorsal wrist (Fig. 6-37). This will produce more of an end-range pain felt anteriorly if impingement is present.[49] Resisted active internal rotation in the Hawkins-Kennedy's position may functionally add to the sensitivity of the test.

4. *Locking maneuver.* A fairly common test employed by physical therapists is the locking maneuver. It is performed with the patient supine. The examiner flexes the elbow to 90 degrees and then proceeds

to passively extend then abduct the shoulder. Just shy of 90 degrees abduction an almost bony lock will be felt where no more abduction is possible (Fig. 6-38). This normal end range is usually not painful, but it is with impingement.[50]

When impingement or instability are suggested by the general tests outlined above, more specific testing is necessary to further determine which structures are involved.

Specific Muscle Testing

Commonly, an orthopaedic evaluation of muscle strength involves a quick screen with shrugging of the shoulders, abduction of the arms, and an Apley's

Table 6-2. Structural and Related Tenderness Indicators

Location/Structure	Structure or Condition
A Sternoclavicular joint	Sprain or joint dysfunction
B Clavicle	Fracture
C Coracoid	Pectoralis minor; short head of biceps; coracobrachialis; coracoacromial ligament; coracohumeral ligament; marksman shoulder; bursitis
D Between coracoid and Acromioclavicular joint	Coracoacromial ligament—impingement
E Acromioclavicular joint	Separation (various grades); osteoarthritis; joint dysfunction or sprain; bursa (inferior to joint)
F Lesser tuberosity	Subscapularis
G Bicipital groove	Long head of biceps; latissimus dorsi (insertion); pectoralis major (insertion)
H Greater tuberosity	
Anterior	Supraspinatus
Posterior	Infraspinatus/teres minor
I Anterior glenoid	Capsule involement
J Deltoid insertion	Common referral zone for any shoulder condition
K Tip of shoulder (acromion)	Shoulder pointer
L Infraspinatus/teres minor	Tendinitis of infraspinatus/teres minor; teres minor trigger point; posterior capsule and triceps
M Lateral border of scapula	Infraspinatus/teres minor; teres major
N Infraspinatus muscle	Infraspinatus trigger point
O Inferior border of scapula	Bursitis
P Medial border of scapula	Rhomboids/middle trapezius
Q Superior medial border of scapula	Levator scapula syndrome
R Spine of scapula	Supraspinatus (above); infraspinatus (below)
S Upper trapezius	Upper trapezius trigger point

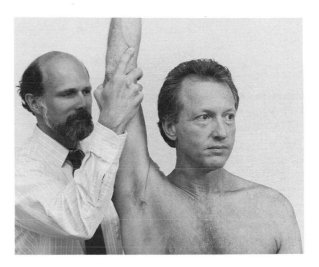

Fig. 6-36. The Neer test for impingement involves passive forward flexion with the forearm supinated.

the capsule. Next contraction throughout the range should be attempted. Some would include general testing of the shoulder through specific diagonal patterns to determine integrated function with the entire upper extremity and other parts of the body as is found with proprioceptive neuromuscular facilitation (see Ch. 20).

2. Stretching of the muscle to determine if contracture or pain is evident.

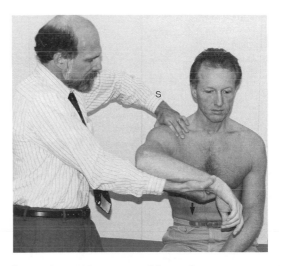

Fig. 6-37. The Hawkins-Kennedy's test for impingement involves internal rotation with the shoulder forward flexed 90 degrees with the scapula stabilized. *S,* stabilize.

scratch test. As mentioned previously, this is far from an adequate examination. Testing is really for two purposes: (1) gross evaluation of strength but more importantly, (2) determining damaged or dysfunctional muscles that may be the source of the patient's pain or dysfunction. Strength evaluation uses the standard grading approach based on the amount of resistance coupled with the patient's effort.

There are several avenues available when assessing muscle involvement. These include

1. Contraction of each muscle to determine if weakness or pain is revealed. This is performed in the midrange initially to eliminate (as much as possible) inclusion of noncontractile structures such as

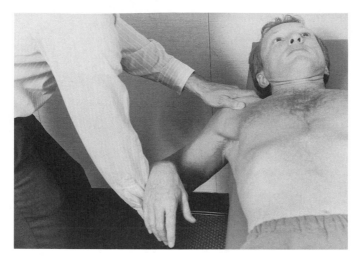

Fig. 6-38. The locking maneuver for detecting possible impingement.

3. A combination of placing the muscle in a stretched position then contracting it to expose any subtle dysfunction or pain.
4. Palpation of the muscle belly, attachment sites, and for trigger point involvement to determine localized etiology or referral pain when a complaint of radiating or distant pain is given.

Muscle testing should be integrated with the history and active/passive testing of the patient and should not be taken as a pathognomonic, isolated procedure. It must be kept in mind that there is no pure test for an individual muscle. Every test will inadvertently involve groups of muscles, some acting as synergists, agonists, and stabilizers. It is hoped that through electromyographic research each muscle may be tested in the most optimal position. However, at present there is disagreement due to conflicting data and interpretation.

Each of the major shoulder girdle muscles will now be presented with a focus on the evaluation process outlined above. The order of evaluation will be (1) palpation (with emphasis on exposing attachment sites and trigger points), (2) contraction, and (3) stretch and stretch/contraction.

Supraspinatus

The belly of the supraspinatus lies in the scapular fossa above the spine of the scapula. Due to the overlay of the trapezius, it is best to palpate the muscle belly with the patient prone. This position should relax the trapezius and make assessment of atrophy and palpation of the muscle belly more revealing. Neurologic damage should be evident with both supraspinatus and infraspinatus atrophy.

There are three potential trigger points as proposed by Travell and Simons.[51] They are located 1 inch from the medial superior border of the scapula and just proximal to the acromioclavicular joint. The third trigger point is sometimes found at the tendinous insertion into the greater tuberosity of the humerus. The reference zone is usually down the lateral arm to the area of the deltoid tubercle. Sometimes this will extend down to the lateral epicondyle or beyond. Due to the overlying trapezius, a twitch response is rarely evident with the first two supraspinatus trigger points.

Palpation of the insertion point on the greater tuberosity of the humerus is best exposed by bringing the arm behind the back (Fig. 6-7). An alternative position for the patient unable to be positioned in the previous description is to passively extend the arm. Palpation is slightly anterior and lateral to the tip of the acromioclavicular joint. It is unlikely that direct palpation is attainable, but approximation of the site is possible.

There are essentially three positions that are used to contract the supraspinatus. The first position is the traditional observation that the supraspinatus is important (and used to be believed to be isolated in function) to the first 30 degrees of abduction. The arm was abducted 20 to 30 degrees and then the patient attempted abduction in the coronal plane against the resistance of the examiner. Another similar procedure was to adduct the arm across the front of the body to the midline, forward flex approximately 20 degrees, and in this starting position have the patient attempt abduction against examiner resistance. Currently the most provocative test appears to be the "empty can" test.[52] The rationale is to have the patient attempt abduction in the plane line of the scapula. This is approximately 30 to 40 degrees forward of the coronal plane. In this plane the fibers of the supraspinatus are more aligned and the fibers of the deltoid theoretically incorporated less. The arm is maximally rotated so that the thumb points toward the ground (emptying the can) This places maximum tension on the muscle and tendon. The patient should first attempt active, unresisted abduction. If not provocative, resistance should be added, first before 90 degrees abduction, then at 90 degrees if necessary (Fig. 6-39). Garrick and Webb[53] warn of a pectoralis major recruitment pattern when the supraspinatus or other rotator cuff muscle is involved. Observation of the clavicular portion of the pectoralis major may indicate this recruitment.

Stretching of the supraspinatus is performed by drawing the arm across the back toward the opposite side. This will stretch other muscles, but resisted abduction from this position should be relatively more specific to the supraspinatus.

Teres Minor/Infraspinatus

The teres minor and infraspinatus will be evaluated as a functional group. Although their origin is separate, they have essentially a conjoined insertion onto the posterolateral greater tuberosity. The origin of the infraspinatus is off of the posterior scapula in the infra-(sub)scapular fossa. The teres minor arises from the superior lateral border of the scapula somewhat covered by the posterior deltoid muscle. The tendons of both muscles combine to insert on the posterolateral aspect of the greater tuberosity. This attachment site is best appreciated with the arm passively horizontally adducted in the 90 degree forward flexed position. Then the arm is externally rotated (Fig. 6-8A). This position should expose the attachments under the acromial arch or slightly posterior to it.[20]

There are three potential trigger points for the infra-

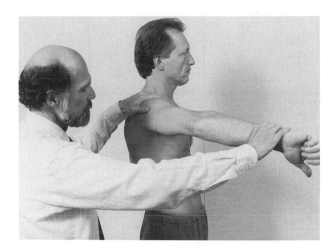

Fig. 6-39. The empty can test for the supraspinatus.

spinatus.[51] The first two are found slightly inferior to the scapular spine one-third and two-thirds distance from the medial border. They may refer pain to the lateral or anterior aspect of the arm extending as far distal as the fingertips. The third trigger point is located close to the medial border, one-half the distance inferior to the scapular spine. The referral zone is the entire extent of the medial scapular border of the involved side.

The teres minor has one trigger point, which is found about 1 inch superior to the posterior axillary crease. The referral zone is the posterior shoulder close to the insertion point for the infraspinatus/teres minor.

Optimal positioning for muscle testing of the infraspinatus and teres minor is curiously switched based on which electromyographic data are accepted.[54] For some, the infraspinatus is best tested with resisted external rotation, the arm at the side, and the elbow bent 90 degrees. This same group would test the teres minor by resisted external rotation with the arm abducted to 90 degrees and the elbow bent 90 degrees. Others use the exact opposite positions for each muscle (arm at the side for teres minor, abducted for infraspinatus). Since, in most situations, they appear to act in concert, it would seem appropriate to use both positions of testing and realize that isolation of one or the other muscle is unlikely (Fig. 6-40).

Stretching of the infraspinatus/teres minor is similar to the position used for the Hawkins-Kennedy's evalua-

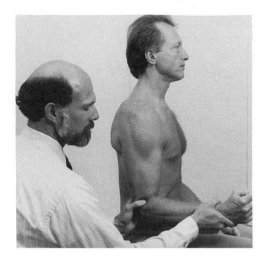

Fig. 6-40. External rotator muscle test including both the infraspinatus and teres minor.

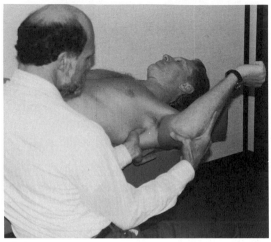

Fig. 6-41. Palpation of the subscapularis via distraction of the arm to expose the anterolateral surface of the scapula.

tion of impingement.[33] The arm is forward flexed 90 degrees and the elbow is passively supported in 90 degrees of flexion. By use of the examiner's free hand on the forearm more internal rotation is imparted (Fig. 6-37). If restriction is appreciated, testing of the well-shoulder should be used as comparison. Pain produced anteriorly by this maneuver is still suggestive of anterior impingement, whereas pain produced posteriorly is more suggestive of the infraspinatus or teres minor. If contraction is added to this position, an increase in posterior pain may be elicited with infraspinatus/teres minor involvement.

Subscapularis

The subscapularis arises from the anterior surface of the scapula. Its tendon inserts onto the lesser tuberosity of the humerus guaranteeing a strong internal rotation function. Direct palpation of the insertion point is difficult due to overlapping structures, but may be facilitated by internally rotating the arm 10 to 15 degrees and palpating slightly medial to the biceps tendon. Palpation of part of the belly is possible with the patient supine. The examiner distracts the abducted arm in an attempt to expose some of the anterior surface of the scapula. Trigger points are difficult to access; however, in the above position with the patient supine, it is possible to expose enough of the muscle belly to palpate one of the trigger points (Fig. 6-41).

Muscle testing may be performed with the arm at the side and the patient attempting internal rotation against the resistance of the examiner. Another suggested position involves abducting the shoulder 90 degrees, elbow bent 90 degrees with the palm facing the floor. From this position the patient attempts internal rotation against the resistance of the examiner (Fig. 6-42). Gerber and Krushell[55] evaluated shoulders of patients with subscapularis rupture. They used a test they call the lift-off test. Patients were asked to place

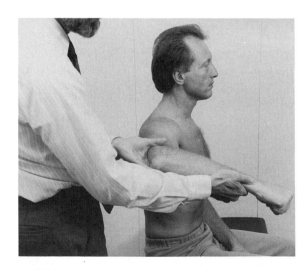

Fig. 6-42. Muscle test for internal rotation with an attempt at isolating the subscapularis.

the back of the hand of the involved side against the small of the back. Gerber and Krushell found that patients with ruptures could not lift the hand away from the back. All patients were able to perform the maneuver on the uninvolved side. Interestingly they did not experience a sensation of shoulder instability.

To stretch the subscapularis, the arm is placed in the apprehension position of abduction/external rotation.

Biceps

The biceps brachii, having two heads, has two points of origin. The long head may be approximated, yet not directly palpated, at the anterosuperior glenoid. There are multiple structures blocking this direct palpation and should caution an overenthusiastic acceptance of a positive finding when pain is elicited. Palpation is facilitated by internally rotating the arm about 10 degrees to face the biceps tendon anteriorly (Fig. 6-7). The tendon may be palpable about 3 inches below the anterior acromion. Further internal rotation will often diminish any tenderness found in the first position as the lesser tuberosity slides under the short head of the biceps and coracoid process.

The short head originates from the lateral aspect of the coracoid process. Palpation of the coracoid may reveal tenderness; however, the coracohumeral ligament may be the source. Gross palpation of the coracoid may also overlap tenderness of the pectoralis minor and the coracoacromial ligament.

Palpation of the belly is relatively obvious, made more discernible with resisted forearm flexion and supination. Lack of contour would suggest a rupture of the long head, but lack of resistance is not usually evident on MMT.

Trigger points are easily found in the medial and lateral aspects of the belly of the biceps 1 to 2 inches above the cubital fossa.[51] Referral is usually proximal to the location of the long head tendon path. Distal referral is mainly in the central cubital fossa (Fig. 6-10).

Resistive testing in the traditional manner is rather useless. Having the patient flex the forearm against resistance is nonprovocative with a torn long head of the biceps and, therefore, must be an impotent attempt at revealing pain or weakness with other forms of biceps involvement. Currently, most examiners use the Speed's test.[56,57] With the patient's elbow extended and the forearm supinated the shoulder is forward flexed to 90 degrees. The patient than attempts to resist the examiner's attempt to extend the shoulder via the forearm (Fig. 6-43). The advantage of this test is that the shoulder is in a potential impingement position at the time of the biceps contraction and is more likely to expose involvement when the underlying cause is impingement.

The Ludington's sign[58] has been used to assess tendinitis, instability of the tendon, and rupture depending on the author. Patients place their hands behind their neck so that they are in a position of abduction and

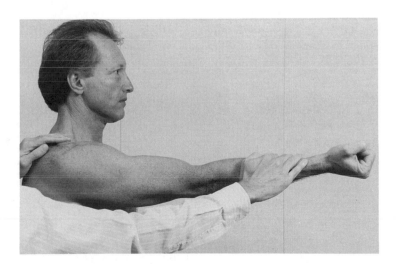

Fig. 6-43. Speed's test for the biceps. Contraction into flexion with the arm at 90 degrees.

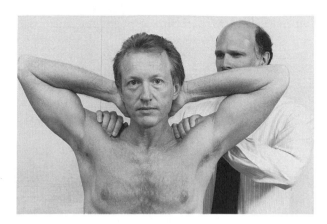

Fig. 6-44. Ludington's test for the biceps.

external rotation. The examiner places their fingers over the bicipital groove to determine if there is an increase in tenderness with an isometric contraction of the biceps or possibly snapping with instability (Fig. 6-44). If the normal contour of the biceps is not apparent, this test may be used as a rather redundant attempt at discerning a rupture of the long head.

There are two tests that challenge the supinating function of the biceps. Yergason's sign[59] is anterior shoulder pain produced by the patient's attempt at supination against the resistance of the examiner (Fig. 6-45). The patient's elbow is bent in some descriptions; in others, the patient also attempts flexion with supination. According to Post[60] the Yergason's sign is not that sensitive. He found only a 50 percent positive response in patients with primary bicipital tendinitis. Hueter's sign[61] tests not for pain but a reduction in strength of flexion with the arm supinated as compared to flexion with the forearm pronated.

The biceps brachii is unique in that, in addition to the standard approach to testing, the tendon is often evaluated for stability. There are a number of specialized tests for this purpose. Abbott and Saunders[62] describe a test where the patient's arm is abducted and externally rotated. The arm is then slowly lowered. Some authors describe lowering involving adduction only; others emphasize internal rotation. A palpable snap over the bicipital groove is supposed to indicate instability of the tendon. An augmentation of the Abbott-Saunders test is to have the patient actively go through the same maneuver holding a 5 lb weight. This is referred to as the Gilcrest sign.[63] Booth and

Marvel[64] describe a maneuver similar to the Abbott-Saunders test where the arm is abducted and externally rotated then internally rotated as the examiner palpates the bicipital groove for snapping. Finally, Lippmann test attempts to reproduce pain by displacing the tendon back and forth about 3 inches below the shoulder joint. Many feel that the deltoid is truly the structure being rolled and that often the biceps is not palpable. If the examiner feels that the biceps should always be palpable, this misinterpretation while palpating the edge of the deltoid is more likely.

It is interesting to note that the majority of the above-listed tests for the biceps were developed in the 1920s and 1930s (one as early as 1864). It is also interesting to note that when challenged as Post did with the Yergason's test, the sensitivity (and perhaps specificity) of the tests may prove inadequate.

Other Muscle Tests

Specific testing is only attempted with the understanding that many muscles are involved in any movement or resistance attempt. Following are a list of additional muscles and suggested positions for testing:

1. The deltoids are tested with the arm abducted 90 degrees. A downward force is applied with the arm in neutral for the middle deltoid, externally rotated for the anterior deltoid, and internally rotated for the posterior deltoid.

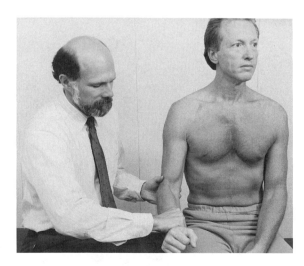

Fig. 6-45. Yergason's test requires the patient to supinate and flex against the resistance of the examiner.

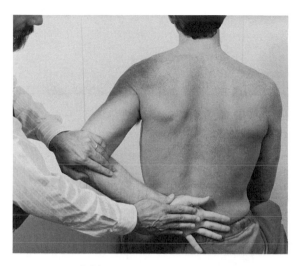

Fig. 6-46. Testing of the rhomboids.

2. The rhomboids are tested with the hand at the hip or behind the back. The patient attempts pushing the elbow back against the resistance of the examiner's hand (Fig. 6-46).
3. The serratus anterior may be evaluated by having the patient abduct the arm against the resistance of the examiner as the examiner palpates the medial border of the scapula in an attempt to detect lack of stability (Fig. 6-47). Additionally, the serratus may be evaluated by having the patient perform a wall push-up to determine winging (Fig. 6-48).

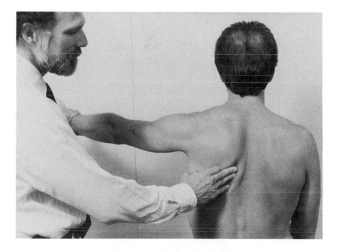

Fig. 6-47. Testing of the serratus anterior. The patient resists the downward pressure of the examiner while the examiner observes and palpates for movement of the scapula.

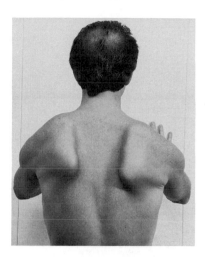

Fig. 6-48. A wall push-up may reveal winging related to serratus anterior involvement as demonstrated on the right. This specific patient created the winging intentionally to demonstrate that winging may occur due to asymetric contraction.

4. The pectoralis major may be evaluated with the patient supine. With the arm flexed and internally rotated the examiner tests the clavicular portion by directing a force outward into horizontal abduction against the patient's resistance (Fig. 6-49). The sternal portion is evaluated with an attempt by the patient mainly into more diagonal adduction.
5. The latissimus dorsi may be tested with the patient supine and the arm by the side internally rotated. The examiner attempts to abduct the arm away from the side against the resistance of the patient (Fig. 6-50).

Bursal Tests

There are a number of bursa about the shoulder; the two major bursa are the subscapularis and the subdeltoid (subacromial). The subscapularis is not palpable due to its deep location. The subacromial is sometimes palpable when irritated. The unique feature of bony positional camouflage allows a combination of palpation and movement to detect bursal involvement.

The most common test is to have the patient lie prone. The relaxed arm is extended via the distal humerus while the other hand of the examiner palpates anterior to the acromioclavicular joint (Fig. 6-9). If tenderness or a boggy structure is evident on extension,

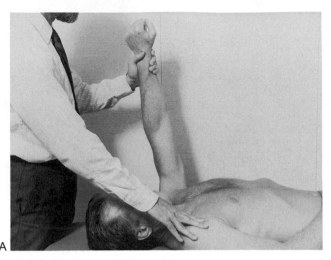
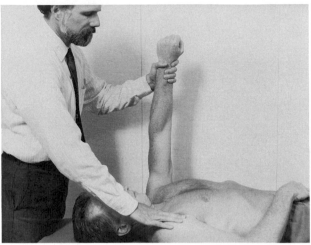

A   B

Fig. 6-49. Pectoral muscle testing. **(A)** The clavicular section, **(B)** the sternal section.

yet disappears on flexion, a suspicion of subacromial bursitis is appropriate.

Dawbarn's test is similar. The patient is palpated for tenderness lateral to the acromion. If tenderness is found, the arm is abducted. If the tenderness disappears with abduction, the bursa is implicated.

Acromioclavicular Tests

In general, the acromioclavicular joint is stressed (compressed) in most full end-range positions of elevation, forward flexion, and horizontal adduction (Fig. 6-51). The discrimination is sometimes difficult due to the other structures that are also compressed in these positions. If other structures test negative and a painful arc is not present, then full abduction pain felt in the area of the acromioclavicular joint is fairly reliable. Full passive horizontal adduction is also fairly reliable if other structures have tested clear and the pain is felt on top of the shoulder as opposed to anteriorly or posteriorly.

The Schultz test is used to feel for motion in an acromioclavicular separation or to reproduce pain if

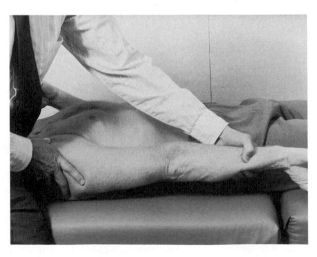

Fig. 6-50. Latissimus dorsi testing.

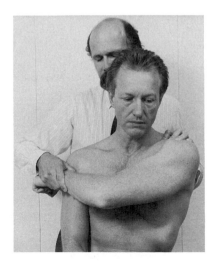

Fig. 6-51. Acromioclavicular joint compression with passive horizontal adduction.

the acromioclavicular joint is involved (especially due to osteoarthritis). The examiner supports the elbow of the seated patient with the arm at the side and the elbow flexed to 90 degrees. Upward pressure is directed along the long axis of the humerus while stabilizing the scapula (acromioclavicular joint) with the other hand (Fig. 6-52). Movement is often felt with a second or third degree acromioclavicular separation. Pain is often produced with acromioclavicular arthritis.

A squeeze test[65] for the acromioclavicular joint has been described. The examiner's hands are cupped over the involved shoulder, with one hand over the spine of the scapula and the other over the clavicle, and squeezed together approximating the acromioclavicular joint (Fig. 6-53). Pain may indicate acute inflammation or chronic osteoarthritis, whereas unusual movement or relief of symptoms may indicate an acute or chronic separation.

Thoracic Outlet Testing

Thoracic outlet syndrome is rarely a cause of isolated shoulder problems. Due to compression of the neurovascular supply to the entire upper extremity, signs and symptoms are usually also found distal to the shoulder.

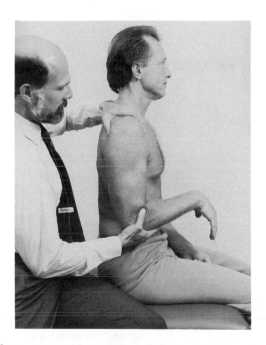

Fig. 6-52. Acromioclavicular compression test with upward force directed along the humerus with the scapula stabilized.

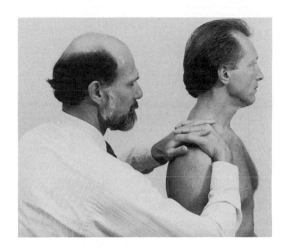

Fig. 6-53. The squeeze test for acromioclavicular joint involvement.

Testing for this syndrome is based on a search for geographic compression sites. Maneuvers have been developed to accentuate this compression and increase signs and symptoms. The pulse is monitored in these positions while the patient is monitored for an increase in symptoms. Unfortunately, these tests are not as pure as needed to confirm a diagnosis due to the overlap of normal patient positive responses. In other words, a diminished pulse or sense of paresthesias on positioning may not necessarily correlate with the patient's presenting complaint.

The standard Adson's position[66] is used to determine compression at the site of the anterior scalene muscle (Fig. 6-54A). The examiner externally rotates the arm (elbow extended). While palpating the pulse the arm is brought back into extension with slight abduction. The patient turns the head to the side of examination, takes a deep breath, and holds it. Again, positive responses are a decreases pulse or increase in pain or paresthesias.

A variation of the Adson's position is referred to as the Halstead's maneuver. With this maneuver the middle scalene is being evaluated as a possible compression site. The test is essentially the same except that long axis traction may be added to the arm and the head is extended and rotated to the opposite side of assessment (Fig. 6-54B).

Wright's test, or the hyperabduction test,[67] is probably the most common false positive maneuver. The arm is abducted to 90 degrees or more and externally

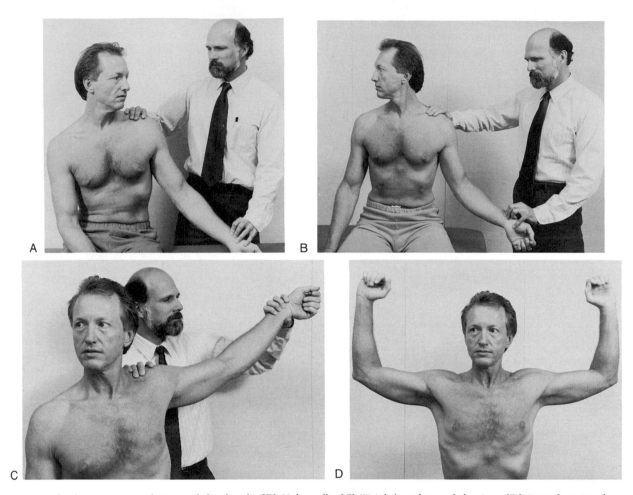

Fig. 6-54. Thoracic outlet tests. **(A)** Adson's, **(B)** Halstead's, **(C)** Wright's or hyperabduction, **(D)** Roos functional grip test.

rotated while palpating the pulse (Fig. 6-54C). Variations include turning the head to either side or holding the breath. Due to the elevated position, the pulse often diminishes in normal individuals. It is suggested that the examiner require a reproduction of the patient's symptoms before enthusiastically entering a positive response.

Eden's test, or the costoclavicular test,[68] searches for compression between these structures. The patient is asked to draw the shoulders back (military posture) and down while the pulses are bilaterally palpated by the examiner.

Roos[69] introduced a very sensible test involving a 3-minute exercise. With the shoulder abducted 90 de-grees and elbow flexed 90 degrees, the patient is asked to continually open and close the fingers slowly for 3 minutes (Fig. 6-54D). Reproduction of symptoms or inability to complete 3 minutes of exercise indicates potential thoracic outlet syndrome.

Cervical Spine Clearing Tests

The suspicion of cervical involvement is always raised when the patient complains of both cervical and shoulder problems. However, there are many instances when either the connection is not made by the patient or the cervical region remains symptom free while still being the source of shoulder pain. The two primary historical positives that help are trauma and/or osteoarthritis. Although the primary search for pathology in the allopathic community is disc lesions or foraminal encroachment, it is extremely important to consider the common entity of referred pain from structures in the neck. Unfortunately, the orthopaedic tests for the cervical region are not always effective in exposing a disc lesion or foraminal encroachment, and therefore are not very sensitive to referred pain causes. Referred pain is suspected when a complaint of radiation into the shoulder or arm does not fit a characteristic dermatomal pattern, the pinwheel examination is normal, and reflexes are intact (diagnosis by exclusion). Assist-

ing this suspicion is confirmation of restriction in cervical vertebral motion.

Standard testing of the cervical spine includes compression and distraction (Fig. 6-55A & B). Compression is performed in various positions including flexion, extension, and combined with rotation. Local positives in the neck in a patient with a radiation complaint suggest facet involvement. Radiation in a dermatomal pattern suggests nerve root compression. Relief from distraction confirms this suspicion. An increase in pain with distraction is often found with soft tissue involvement, in particular muscle splinting.

Shoulder depression is intended to stretch the nerve

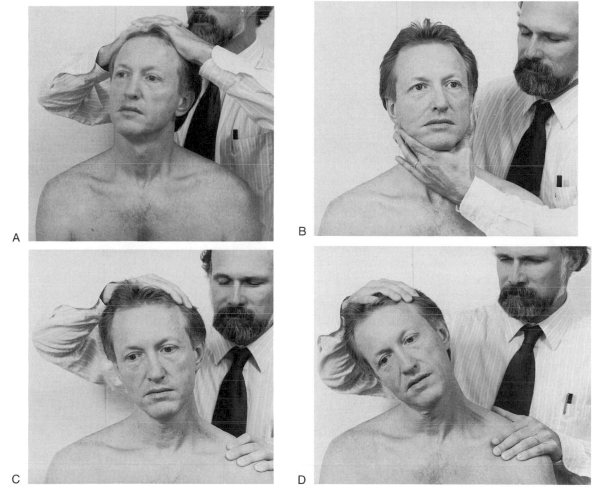

Fig. 6-55. Cervical screening tests. **(A)** Compression, **(B)** distraction, **(C)** shoulder depression without cervical lateral flexion, **(D)** shoulder depression with cervical lateral flexion.

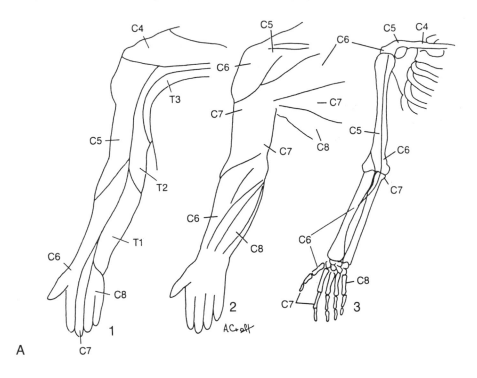

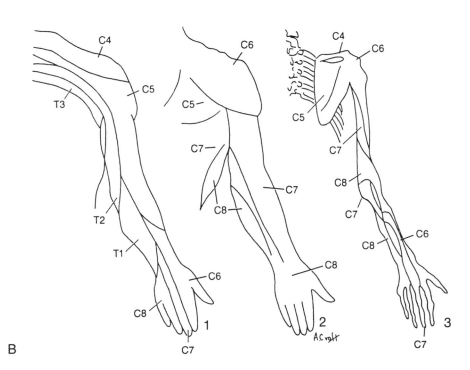

roots and their dura. If the head is neutral and the shoulder is depressed shoulder pain may be caused by cervical involvement (Fig. 6-55C). However, it is important to rule out the possibility of local pressure over the shoulder as the cause of the response. If the head is distracted away from the shoulder as it is being depressed, brachial plexus stretch is introduced (Fig. 6-55D). A positive response would be on the side of involvement. Pain on the side of cervical lateral bending is suggestive of a facet problem if local, or a nerve compression problem if radiation is produced combined with objective findings on sensory testing.

Neurologic Examination

There are several aspects to the neurologic evaluation of the shoulder. It is important to determine the following:

Is there nerve root involvement occurring at the spinal cord or cervical level?
Is there brachial plexus involvement? (identify cause: viral, mechanical, congenital, etc.)
Is there peripheral nerve involvement due to entrapment or traumatic injury?
Is there referred pain from the cervical area?
Is there CNS or spinal cord involvement by trauma or disease process? (e.g., multiple sclerosis)

Each of these possibilities are distinguished by specific orthopaedic testing of the cervical region, thoracic outlet testing, and muscle testing, which have all been described above. Further testing includes deep tendon reflex evaluation and sensory evaluation (dermatomes). More sophisticated testing may be necessary, including electromyography/nerve conduction velocity studies, CT scans, or magnetic resonance imaging.

With a complaint of numbness prior to testing, the examiner should be cautioned to the difference between subjective and objective numbness. Many patients with a true complaint of numbness have, in fact, no objectifiable numbness on pinwheel or other sensory testing. Often the described area does not fit a specific peripheral or dermatomal pattern or is diffuse. The assumption could be that the patient is misleading the examiner for some reason. However, most patients with this presentation have a referred sensation (or lack thereof) of numbness. Objectifiable numbness is not present because there is no direct compression or irritation of a nerve root or peripheral nerve or that there is early compression or transient irritation. It is beneficial to compare the patient's described zone to the mapping of Feinstein[70] and others.[71] Myotogenous and scleratogenous referral pain are also possible (Fig. 6-56).

If involved, a peripheral nerve will demonstrate rather distinct sensory loss in the peripheral sensory area of that nerve. Less specific are the dermatomes associated with nerve root involvement (Fig. 6-57). Overlap is common. The dermatomal mapping that exists was developed generally from two processes. Foerster's charts were developed through a process of elimination, sectioning the nerves above and below the level of interest. Keegan's[72] mapping was developed through sectioning of specific nerve roots and determining the altered abnormal sensory area.

Further qualification of nerve root involvement may be aided through an evaluation of several deep tendon reflexes of the upper arm. The reality, of course, is that only three are used in general evaluations, but others exist for rare cases if needed. A brief description of these extra reflexes will be given. The three standard reflexes are the biceps for C5 nerve root involvement, the brachioradialis for C6 nerve root involvement, and the triceps for C7 nerve root involvement.

The pectoralis reflex is performed with the patient's arm abducted and supported by the examiner at about 20 to 30 degrees of abduction. Placing one thumb over the distal tendon of the pectoralis, the examiner taps over this contact with the hammer. The usual response is slight adduction and internal rotation. The medial

Fig. 6-56. (A) Anterior and **(B)** posterior schematic drawings of the segmental innervation first described by Inman and Saunders in 1944. 1, Dermatomal pattern; 2, myotomal pattern; 3, sclerotomal pattern. (From Foreman and Croft,[5] with permission.)

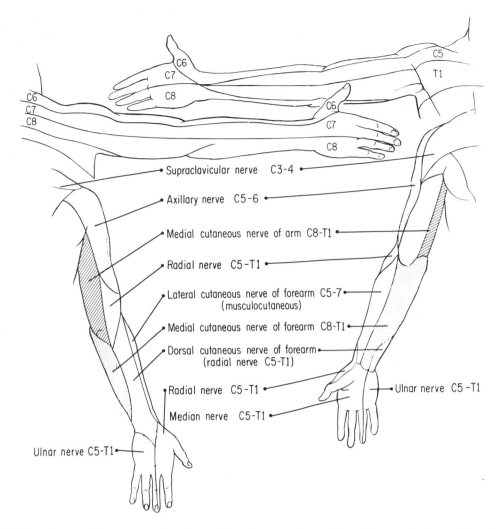

Fig. 6-57. Dermatomes of the upper extremity and the cutaneous innervation of the arm by the peripheral sensory nerves. (From Reilly,[75] with permission.)

and lateral pectoral nerves supply the pectorals with C5 to C7 supplying the clavicular and manubrial section and C8 to T1 supplying the lower sternal sections.

The scapular reflex is performed on the standing patient with the arm abducted about 15 to 20 degrees. When the inferior angle of the scapula is tapped there is a slight movement of the scapula medially due to the contraction of the rhomboids and possibly middle trapezius.

One test used to determine levels of sensitivity or irritability between the two arms is the clavicular reflex. This may be evident by tapping the lateral clavicle

and observing contraction of various muscles of the arm in a "hyper-reactive" individual (nonpathologically). *See appendices 2–4 for various exam approaches.*

On-the-Field Evaluation

Usually two scenarios occur "on-the-field" (Table 6-3). One involves a nontraumatic onset of gradual shoulder pain that becomes disabling. Often, the athlete has had previous problems or complaints that have gone unattended. A quick orthopaedic examination including

Table 6-3. On-the-Field Evaluation of the Shoulder

Observation

Mechanism of Injury

a. Fall on an outstretched hand—acromioclavicular separation, humeral or clavicular fracture

b. Fall on the tip of the shoulder—acromioclavicular separation, distal clavicular fracture, shoulder pointer

c. Forceful horizontal abduction or external rotation of the elevated arm—anterior dislocation

d. Blow to the anterior shoulder girdle—sternoclavicular dislocation, clavicular fracture, acromioclavicular separation

e. Forceful lateral flexion of the neck—"burner or stinger"

f. Forced flexion of the neck—nerve root/disc or "central cord" syndrome

Patient

Superior swelling/pain/deformity—acromioclavicular separation or distal clavicular fracture

Loss of pectorals contour—anterior dislocation

Prominent coracoid—posterior dislocation

Neuromuscular Signs and Symptoms

Sudden loss of strength associated with distal numbness/paresthesias—Dislocation/subluxation, "burner/stinger"

"Burning hands"—central cord syndrome

Discrete area of objective numbness—nerve root or peripheral nerve

Severe and distinct muscle weakness—rupture or nerve root

Unable to touch opposite shoulder—anterior dislocation

Unable to supinate forward flexed arm—posterior dislocation

Vascular Examination

Loss of distal pulse—fracture/dislocation with associated arterial damage (localize site)

---

palpation, ROM, and testing for instability and impingement will usually reveal the underlying cause. Decisions must be made regarding return to play. Follow-up should include a more thorough history and examination in the office setting.

The second scenario is the onset of sudden shoulder pain, traumatic in origin. The first historical clarifier is whether the injury was contact or noncontact. Noncontact injury would imply a less serious condition in most cases. The mechanism should be determined and an examination of the suspected structures performed.

With contact injury, it is extremely important to determine the mechanism. Either direct observation of the injury or videotape replay are ideal and are often more accurate than the athlete's description. If there is any suspicion of glenohumeral dislocation, acromioclavicular separation, or fracture, it is imperative that a vascular and then neurologic examination be performed prior to any attempts at reduction. Fractures and acromioclavicular separations should be immobilized and the athlete transported for further evaluation with radiography. Attempts at reduction of a disloca-

tion should be reserved for those cases where neurovascular status has been established and fracture is not suspected. There are various maneuvers used for the reduction attempt as described in Chapter 13.

REFERENCES

1. Magee DJ: Orthopedic Physical Assessment. WB Saunders, Philadelphia, 1987

2. Rowe CR, Zarins B: Recurrent transient subluxation of the shoulder. J Bone Joint Surg 63A:863, 1981

3. Torg JS, Vegso JJ, O'Neil MJ et al: The epidemiologic, pathologic, biomechanical, and cinematographic analysis of football induced cervical spine trauma. Am J Sports Med 18:50, 1990

4. Hawkins RJ, McCormack RG: Posterior shoulder instability. Orthopedics 7:101, 1988

5. Foreman SM, Croft AC: Whiplash Injuries: The Cervical Acceleration/Deceleration Syndrome. Williams & Wilkins, Baltimore, 1988

6. Neer CS, Welsh RP: The shoulder in sports. Orthop Clin North Am 8:583, 1977

7. Lloyd GJ, McIntyre JL, Older MWJ: The treatment of shoulder stiffness with hydrostatic manipulation. J Bone Joint Surg 60A:564, 1978

8. Rowe CR: Tendinitis, bursitis, impingement, "snapping" scapula, and calcific tendinitis. p. 112. In Rowe CR (ed): The Shoulder. Churchill Livingstone, New York, 1988

9. Ganzhorn RW et al: Suprascapular nerve entrapment. J Bone Joint Surg 63:492, 1981

10. Cahill BR, Palmar PE: Quadrilateral space syndrome. J Hand Surg 8:65, 1983

11. Gugenheim JJ et al: Little League survey: the Houston study. Am J Sports Med 4:189, 1976

12. Larson RL, Hocker JT, Horowitz M, Switzer HE: Little League survey: the Eugene study. Am J Sports Med 4:201, 1976

13. Erstene AC, Kinell J: Pain in the shoulder as a sequel to myocardial infarction. Arch Intern Med 66:800, 1940

14. Engleman RM: Shoulder pain as a presenting complaint in upper lobe bronchogenic carcinoma: report of 21 cases. Conn Med 30:273, 1966

15. Pal B, Anderson J, Dick WC, Griffiths ID: Limitation of joint mobility and shoulder capsulitis in insulin and non-insulin dependent diabetes mellitus. Br J Rheumatol 25:147, 1986

16. Oldham BE: Periarthritis of the shoulder associated with thyrotoxicosis. NZ Med J 29:766, 1959

17. Rockwood CA: Subluxations and dislocations about the shoulder. p. 722. In Rockwood CA, Green DP (eds): Fractures in Adults. JB Lippincott, Philadelphia, 1984

18. Hawkins RJ, Bokor DJ: Clinical evaluation of shoulder

problems. p. 149. In Rockwood CA, Matsen FA (eds): The Shoulder. WB Saunders, Philadelphia, 1990

19. Benton J, Nelson C: Avulsion of the coracoid process in an athlete: report of a case. J Bone Joint Surg 53A:356, 1971

20. Jackson D, Einhorn A: Rehabilitation of the shoulder. p. 103. In Jackson DW: Shoulder Surgery in the Athlete. Aspen, Rockville, MD, 1985

21. Lyons AR, Tomlinson JE: Clinical diagnosis of tears of the rotator cuff. J Bone Joint Surg 74B:414, 1992

22. Kulund DN: The Injured Athlete. JB Lippincott, Philadelphia, 1982

23. Matsen F, Kirby R: Office evaluation and management of shoulder pain. Orthop Clin North Am 13:45, 1982

24. American Academy of Orthopaedic Surgeons: Joint Motion: Methods of Measuring and Recording. American Academy of Orthopaedic Surgeons, Chicago, 1965

25. Cyriax J: Textbook of Orthopaedic Medicine. Vol. 1: Diagnosis of Soft Tissue Lesions. 8th Ed. Bailliere-Tindall, London, 1982

26. Minor RR: Collagen metabolism: a comparison of disease of collagen and diseases affecting collagen. Am J Pathol 98:225, 1980

27. Bohannon RW: The clinical measurement of strength. Clin Rehabil 1:5, 1987

28. Borden R, Colachis SC: Quantitative measurement of the good and normal ranges in muscle testing. Phys Ther 48:839, 1968

29. Agre JC, Magness JL, Wright KC et al: Strength testing with a portable dynamometer: reliability for upper and lower extremities. Arch Phys Med Rehabil 68:454, 1987

30. Bohannon RW: Test-retest reliability of hand-held dynamometry during a single session of strength assessment. Phys Ther 66:206, 1986

31. Nies Byl N: Intrarater and interrater reliability of strength measurements of the biceps and deltoid using a hand-held dynamometer. J Orthop Sports Phys Ther 9:399, 1988

32. McMahon LM, Burdett RG, Whitney SL: Effects of muscle group and placement site on reliability of hand-held dynamometry strength measurements. J Orthop Sports Phys Ther 15:236, 1992

33. Hawkins RJ, Schutte JP, Huckell GH et al: The assessment of glenohumeral translation using manual and fluoroscopic techniques. Orthop Trans 12:727, 1988

34. Norris TR: C-arm fluoroscopic evaluation under anesthesia for glenohumeral subluxations. In Bateman J, Welsh P (eds): Surgery of the Shoulder. BC Decker, Philadelphia, 1984

35. Neer CS, Foster CR: Inferior capsular shift for involuntary inferior and multidirectional instability of the shoulder. J Bone Joint Surg 62A:897, 1980

36. Warren RF, Kornblatt IB, Marchand R: Static factors affecting posterior shoulder stability. Orthop Trans 8:89, 1984

37. Gerber C, Ganz R: Clinical assessment of instability of the shoulder. J Bone Joint Surg 66B:551, 1984

38. Protzman RR: Anterior instability of the shoulder. J Bone Joint Surg 62A:909, 1980

39. Matsen FA, Thomas SC, Rockwood CA: Glenohumeral instability. In Rockwood CA, Matsen FA (eds): The Shoulder. WB Saunders, Philadelphia, 1990

40. Norwood LA, Terry GC: Posterior shoulder dislocation and subluxation. Am J Sports Med 12:25, 1984

41. Cofield RH, Irving JF: Evaluation and classification of shoulder instability. Clin Orthop Relat Res 223:32, 1987

42. Norris TR: History and physical examination of the shoulder. p. 81. In Nicholas JA, Hershman EB (eds): The Upper Extremity in Sports Medicine. CV Mosby, St. Louis, 1990

43. Jobe FW, Kvine RS: Shoulder pain in the overhand or throwing athlete: the relationship of anterior instability and rotator cuff impingement. Orthop Rev 18:963, 1989

44. Silliman JF, Hawkins RJ: Current concepts and recent advances in the athlete's shoulder. Clin Sports Med 10:693, 1991

45. Leach RE, Schepsis AA: Shoulder pain. Clin Sports Med 1:127, 1983

46. Zarin A, Andrew J, Carson M: USOC Injuries to the Throwing Arm. WB Saunders, Philadelphia, 1985

47. Walsh DA: Shoulder evaluation of the throwing athlete. Sports Med Update 4:24, 1989

48. Neer CS: Anterior acromioplasty for chronic impingement syndrome in the shoulder: a preliminary report. J Bone Joint Surg 54A:41, 1972

49. Hawkins RJ, Kennedy JC: Impingement syndrome in athletes. Am J Sports Med 8:151, 1980

50. Corrigan B, Maitland GD: Practical Orthopaedic Medicine. p. 31. Butterworths, London, 1983

51. Travell JG, Simons DG: Myofascial Pain and Dysfunction: The Trigger Point Manual. p. 368. Williams & Wilkins, Baltimore, 1983

52. Jobe FW, Jobe CM: Painful athletic injuries of the shoulder. Clin Orthop 173:117, 1983

53. Garrick JG, Webb DR: Sports Injuries: Diagnosis and Management. WB Saunders, Philadelphia, 1990

54. Basmajian JV: Muscles Alive. 5th Ed. Williams & Wilkins, Baltimore, 1985

55. Gerber C, Krushell RJ: Isolated rupture of the tendon of the subscapularis muscle: clinical features in 16 cases. J Bone Joint Surg 73B:389, 1991

56. Gilcrest EL, Albi P: Unusual lesions of muscles and tendons of the shoulder girdle and upper arm. Surg Gynecol Obstet 68:903, 1939

57. Grenshaw AH, Kilgore WE: Surgical treatment of bicipital tenosynovitis. J Bone Joint Surg 48A:1496, 1966

58. Ludington NA: Bicipital tendinitis. Am J Surg 77:358, 1923

59. Yergason RM: Rupture of the biceps. J Bone Joint Surg 13:160, 1931

60. Post M: Primary tendinitis of the long head of the biceps. Paper presented at the Closed Meeting of the Society of American Shoulder and Elbow Surgeons, Orlando, FL, 1987

61. Hueter C: Zur Diagnose der Verletzungen des M. Biceps Brachii. Arch Clin Chir 5:321, 1864

62. Abbott LC, Saunders JB de CM: Acute traumatic dislocation of the tendon of the long head of the biceps brachii: report of 6 cases with operative findings. Surgery 6:817, 1939

63. Post M: Physical Examination of the Musculoskeletal System. Year Book Medical Publishers, Chicago, 1987

64. Booth RE, Marvel JP: Differential diagnosis of shoulder pain. Orthop Clin North Am 6:353, 1975

65. Davies GJ, Gould JA, Larson RL: Functional examination of the shoulder girdle. Phys Sports Med 9:82, 1981

66. Adson AW, Coffey JR: Cervical rib. Ann Surg 85:839, 1927

67. Wright IS: The neurovascular syndrome produced by hyperabduction of the arms. Am Heart J 29:1, 1945

68. Falconer MA, Weddell G: Costoclavicular compression of the subclavian artery and vein. Lancet 2:539, 1943

69. Roos DB: New concepts of thoracic outlet syndrome: current concepts of treatment. Ann Surg 190:657, 1979

70. Feinstein B: Referred pain from paravertebral structures. p. 139. In Buerger AA, Tobis S (eds): Approaches to the Validation of Manipulative Therapy. Charles C Thomas, Springfield, 1977

71. Inman VT, Saunders JB deCM: Referred pain from skeletal structures. J Nerv Ment Dis 99:660, 1944

72. Hollinshead WH: Anatomy for Surgeons. Vol. 3: The Back and Limbs. 3rd Ed. Harper & Row, Philadelphia, 1982

73. Rowe CR: Examination of the shoulder. In Rowe CR (ed): The Shoulder. Churchill Livingstone, New York, 1988

74. Leffert RD, Gumley G: The relationship between dead arm syndrome and thoracic outlet syndrome. Clin Orthop Relat Res 223:20, 1987

75. Reilly BM: Practical Strategies in Outpatient Medicine. WB Saunders, Philadelphia, 1984

76. Zarins B, Prodromos CC: Shoulder injuries in sports. In Rowe CR (ed): The Shoulder. Churchill Livingstone, New York, 1988

7
Positional Examination

THOMAS A. SOUZA

Organization of the shoulder examination can be directed several ways. The commonly used approaches include evaluation of specific structures or suspected conditions or a combination of both. There are obvious and not-so-obvious caveats with these approaches. Many shoulder conditions are overlapping and interrelated; therefore, finding positives for one condition does not exclude another. A comprehensive appraisal is necessary. Testing by structure or condition involves a rather inexpedient use of multiple positions that may be better organized saving time and unnecessary movement by the doctor and patient. These concerns may be best addressed with a positional approach.

A caution with traditional orthopaedic testing by the novice or busy clinician is to avoid limiting the examination to "named" tests only. These are often inadequate in uncovering subtle problems in the athlete. In addition, a response not classically designated for a named test may be disregarded as insignificant. Therefore, it is important to test beyond the range of standard tests using one's knowledge of functional anatomy to further challenge suspected structures.

Any given position of the shoulder (or any other joint) will theoretically stress or potentially stress multiple structures (Table 7-1). Thus orthopaedic testing positions, test more than their intended structure. This observation accounts for the varied responses to many traditional tests. Most positions will concurrently stretch some structures, and compress others. With resistance added, multiple muscles are challenged. Therefore, any position has the potential of challenging a multitude of different structures by stretch, compression, and contraction. In most instances structures are stretched on one side while compressed on

the opposite. For example, passive horizontal adduction of the arm will compress structures anteriorly while stretching them posteriorly.

It would then seem logical to organize the examination of the shoulder by position, establishing several starting positions (Fig. 7-1) and adding modifications to fully exploit each one. Modifications include slight changes in the starting position, whether the position is actively or passively acquired, and whether resistance or stretch is incorporated.

Positional testing would potentially eliminate:

Cursory evaluation and require knowledge of functional anatomy of all potential structures that might cause a positive response to a positional challenge
Dependence on named tests
Excessive movement by the patient and doctor
Excessive time repeating positions that have already been performed
The negative aspect of bias based on historical positives

Although practical for examination purposes, charting of examination positives, at present, is best organized by structure or condition eliminating misinterpretation by outside evaluators such as insurance companies or attorneys. In other words, categorizing by structure or condition organizes findings of the positional evaluation into a diagnostically suggestive format.

Positional evaluation of the shoulder involves two aspects: body position and shoulder position. Tests can be organized by body position to avoid unnecessary (and sometimes painful) movement by the patient. Most positional testing is performed with the patient

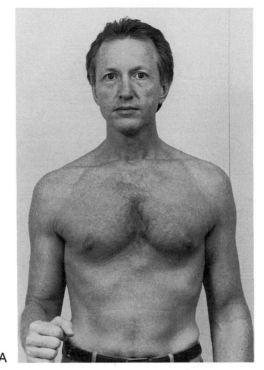

A

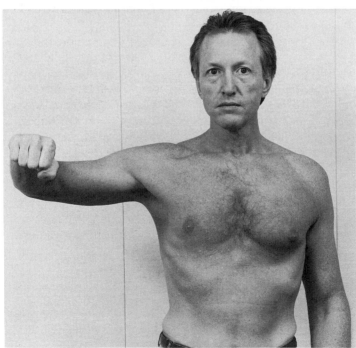

B

Fig. 7-1. Some basic starting positions that allow multiple testing with minor variations. **(A)** Arm at the side. **(B)** 90 degrees abduction. (*Figure continues.*)

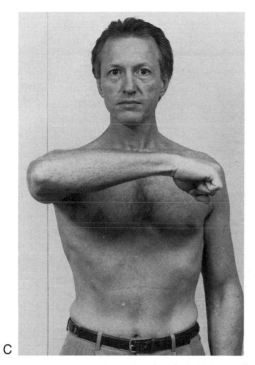
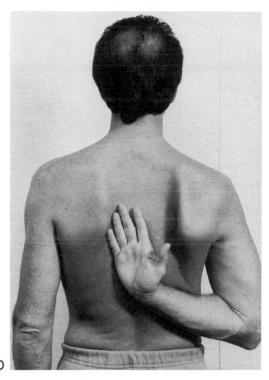

Fig. 7-1. (*Continued*). **(C)** Forward flexion 90 degrees; elbow bent 90 degrees. **(D)** Arm behind back.

Table 7-1. Possible Positional Test Responses

Position/Movement	Positives	Possible Causes
Arm distraction	Sulcus sign	Instability
	Pain	Instability or supraspinatus tendinitis
Abduction	Painful arc	Impingement
	End-range pain	Acromioclavicular joint involvement
	No glenohumeral motion	Adhesive capsulitis or cuff tear
Forward flexion		
Active	Anterior pain	Biceps
Passive (end-range)	Anterior pain	Impingement
Arm behind back with hand:		
Continuing horizontally	Inability to actively perform	Adhesive capsulitis
		Coracobrachialis trigger points
Continuing up the spine	Inability to actively perform	Adhesive capsulitis
		Infraspinatus/teres minor trigger points
Horizontal adduction	Anterior pain (compression)	Acromioclavicular joint or bursa
	Posterior pain (stretch)	Infraspinatus/teres minor or posterior capsule
90° forward flexed with passive internal rotation	Anterior pain (compression)	Impingement
	Posterior pain (stretch)	Infraspinatus/teres minor or posterior capsule
90° abduction/external rotation with a posterior/anterior force applied	Inability to actively perform	Adhesive capsulitis
	Pain or apprehension	Anterior instability

seated. Only a limited number of tests need be performed in the recumbent prone or supine position.

Organization coupled with a functional understanding of the shoulder should guarantee an expedient, yet comprehensive examination. Modification is inevitable based on patient presentation. Limitations are likely in the acute presentation, particularly on-the-field evaluation. The majority of presentations, however, allow more in-depth considerations. Integrated with a thorough history and complimented with appropriate radiographic or special imaging, the positional approach allows the examiner to gain a better understanding of overall structure and function of the individual patient.

A suggested approach is presented with the understanding that individual preference in choice of tests and sequence is best modified by each examiner (Table 7-2). The examiner may wish to include more testing or eliminate portions presented based on the individual case being evaluated. The emphasis is on the paradigm of positional examination; individualization is encouraged. The choice of whether to perform some tests seated as opposed to standing is an option. In deciding to test the patient standing as opposed to seated, the limitations of the examination table in blocking full extension of the arm, and the lower body contribution to examination findings (detrimental or supportive) should be considered. These concerns are easily eliminated with the seated patient examined close to the end of the examination table with one or both arms dependent. The sequence presented uses the seated posture in lieu of standing testing when possible. Only brief descriptions of tests are presented. The reader is referred to Chapter 6 for a detailed description and illustration. First, it is important to review the possible findings and their indications based on how the position is tested.

Table 7-2. Positional Examination of the Shoulder

Position/Movement	Test	Tested Structure(s) or Condition
Standing		
Arm at side		
Passive	Observation	Atrophy, scars, posture, winging, etc.
	Sulcus sign	Acromioclavicular separation, instability
Active	Resisted adduction	Latissimus dorsi
	Resisted abduction	Supraspinatus
Abduction/adduction		
Active	Hesitation sign	Rotator cuff
	Scapulothoracic rhythm	Frozen shoulder, rotator cuff tear
	Painful arc	Impingement (supraspinatus, biceps, or bursa)
	Codman's drop arm test	Rotator cuff tear
	Gilcrest sign	Biceps tendon
	Empty can test	Supraspinatus
	Roos test (overhead gripping)	Thoracic outlet syndrome
Passive	Painful arc	Impingement
	Wright's test	Thoracic outlet syndrome
	Overpressure (end-range)	Acromioclavicular joint
Bent forward 45°	Load and shift tests	Instability
Seated		
Arm at side		
Passive	Palpation	Soft tissue and bony structures
	Thoracic outlet tests	Scalenes and costoclavicular sources
	Cervical ortho screen	Cervicogenic shoulder pain
Arm at side/elbow bent to 90°		
Active	Resisted internal rotation	Subscapularis
	Resisted external rotation	Infraspinatus/teres minor
	Yergason's test	Biceps
Passive	Internal/external rotation ROM	Restrictive processes
	Load and shift maneuvers	Instability
	Kocher's maneuver	Glenoid labrum tear
Shoulder/elbow both flexed 90°		
Passive	Hawkins' test	Impingement
	Stretch test	External shoulder rotators
	Horizontal adduction	Acromioclavicular compression/external rotator stretch
	Jerk test	Posterior instability

(continues.)

Table 7-2. *(continued)*

Position/Movement	Test	Tested Structure(s) or Condition
Shoulder abduction 90°		
Active	Resisted abduction	Deltoid
Passive	Protzman's test	Anterior stability
Shoulder abduction/external rotation		
Active	Horizontal abduction/external rotation	Functional test for common sports position
	Wrap-around test	Active external rotator test
Passive	Apprehension testing	Anterior instability
Arm behind back		
Active	Internal rotation ROM	Restriction
	Resisted extension	Rhomboids
	Horizontal adduction	Coracobrachialis
Passive	Palpation and stretch	Supraspinatus
Supine		
Arm at side		
Active	Resisted protraction-shoulder	Pectoralis minor
Passive	Palpation	Accessory movement of shoulder girdle
	Posterior drawer test	Posterior instability
	External ROM	Restriction
Abducted 90°		
Active	Resisted horizontal flexion	Pectoralis major
Passive	Apprehension tests	Anterior instability
	Relocation test	Anterior instability
	Clunk test	Glenoid labrum tear
	Quadrant position	Capsular or pectoralis restriction
	Anterior drawer test	Anterior instability
	Norwood stress test	Posterior instability
	Internal/external rotation ROM	Restriction
Prone		
Arm relaxed		
Passive	Extension	Bursal palpation
	Palpation	Spinal
Arm behind back		
Passive	Palpation	Scapula
Abducted		
Active	Unresisted and resisted external rotation	Functional assessment for sports
Passive	Circumduction	Capsular restriction palpation

Abbreviation: ROM, range of motion

ACTIVE TESTING

The ability of the patient to actively acquire a specific position tests several parameters. First, the willingness of the patient to reach the position is evaluated. This may be limited by several factors including pain, fear of an increase in pain or instability, emotional factors, and true muscular involvement. When a muscle or muscles are the primary deterrent, there are several possibilities that may be influenced or overlapping with the above-mentioned factors, including (1) weakness of the agonists or stabilizers (potentially neurologic or disuse), (2) tightness of the antagonists or agonists, and (3) dysfunction of coordinated muscle groupings (which may be acquired due to training or protective/dysfunctional due to pathology).

There is an overlap among these three possibilities that hopefully will be differentiated by further testing. Actively acquired positions are resistive against gravity. Standard resistive testing incorporates examiner resistance.

ACTIVE RESISTIVE TESTING

Standard active resistive testing usually incorporates a mid-range isometric contraction. The intention of a mid-range challenge without movement of the joint is to isolate the interpretation of a positive finding to contractile tissue.

There have been many attempts to devise specific mid-range testing procedures for individual muscles. These are often based on electromyographic studies.[1] Although a certain amount of specificity is possible, it would be naive to assume that only a single muscle functions in any given testing position. Other means of evaluation such as palpation, stretching, and observation of stability of the scapula or glenohumeral joint must be integrated with the muscle testing finding to be assured of more specific confirmation.

As with active (unresisted) testing, active resistive testing evaluates a patient's willingness to cooperate. The examiner should look for pain, weakness, or a combination of both. If pain is the major positive, an attempt at localization should be made. Although most testing is performed in a mid-range position and therefore should implicate a specific contractile structure, it is possible to irritate other structures such as a bursa or place enough demand on the joint to irritate deeper noncontractile structures. If weakness is the chief positive, the previously mentioned possibilities under active testing should be considered.

Multiple range testing is important for a full evaluation, not necessarily to detect a specific contractile structure but to determine positionally induced problems and subtle muscular dysfunction. Eliminated is the more pure concept of mid-range testing, which attempts to eliminate other types of tissue. Testing approximately every 20 degrees is recommended using both short- and long-lever testing points.

Cautions with resistive testing are to avoid excessive initial force or trying to "overcome" the patient. Precautions should be taken not to stabilize over tender or painful areas, and any recruitment attempts by the patient (through visual cues and palpation) should be noted.

PASSIVE AND OVERPRESSURE TESTING

Naturally, passive range of motion (ROM) should always exceed active ROM. Limitations to active testing theoretically are eliminated with relaxation of the patient. This allows a more specific testing of noncontractile tissue. However, if muscle spasm is present, limitations to passive testing may also be evident. If passive ranging is markedly more than the uninvolved extremity, laxity with possible associated instability should be investigated. When passive movement is substantially more than the corresponding active range, a neural or major structural problem of the suspected muscle should be evaluated. The other possibility is severe muscle splinting, which is relieved by relaxation, particularly in a nongravity challenged position (i.e., supine or prone).

When pain is produced by stretch in one direction, the opposite direction with contraction will usually cause pain if a specific muscle is involved.

Passive testing will, at its end range, stress structures two ways: stretch and compression. Inevitably, structures on the "open" end of the movement will be stretched; those on the "closed" side will be compressed. This may seem obvious at first glance, but the distinction only becomes clinically useful when the examiner questions the patient with each maneuver regarding the location of any pain production.

Cyriax[2] felt that it was important not only to test for range of passive movement but also the quality of the end-feel. He identified several abnormal end-range palpation possibilities that he associates with particular pathologic processes:

1. Capsular—considered abnormal when reached before the end of normal ROM; described as similar to the sensation felt when stretching leather
2. Springy—a sensation of rebound at the end range of motion implicating internal derangement
3. Bone to bone—strong mechanical blockage or grating found with fractures of the proximal humerus
4. Empty—when a motion barrier is not reached due to pain restriction implying an acute process
5. Muscle guarding—restriction that is perceived as mainly muscular due to splinting

In addition to testing the shoulder complex through passive ranging with a long-lever approach, ranging may be used to evaluate the accessory range at the joint itself. Accessory motion is that movement that may be available but not under voluntary control. Standard testing does not evaluate this movement. These movements have been determined to be crucial to proper functioning of the joint as discussed later. The approach to accessory movement testing usually incorporates more a short-level testing, focusing on relaxation and palpation of only millimeters of movement at the joint. A normal joint play is considered springy. Restriction or excessive movement would be considered abnormal and addressed differently. Restriction would be eliminated through adjustment or mobilization, and excessive movement through stabilization exercises.

STANDING

Arm at the Side

The obvious starting position is with the patient standing. Note the carrying angle and position of the arm. If in a splinted position take note of which combination of internal/external rotation and abduction/adduction the patient acquires, and whether the patient feels the need to support the arm at the elbow or forearm.

Evaluation of the arm dependent at the side affords a convenient appraisal of observational positives such as atrophy, scarring, masses, and level/positioning of the shoulder girdle. Theoretically, the arm is supported mainly by ligamentous control coupled with bony and labral configuration and negative joint pressure.[3,4] Postural contributions should also be noted regarding scoliosis (with possible associated winging of the scapula), kyphosis, "rounded shoulder," or the athletic "sagging" shoulder. Checking for the position of the hand may indicate tightness or weakness of internal or external rotators.

Active resisted muscle testing can be performed with the arm at the side. Resisted adduction (with the arm internally rotated) tests the latissimus dorsi. Resisted abduction within the first 20 degrees mainly tests the supraspinatus, although the deltoid is also enlisted.

Abduction

The movement pattern of abduction, although not a single position, is a very revealing single maneuver. It is useful to divide this movement into two slightly different planes: coronal and scapular (scaption). It has been observed that many patients seek the plane of the scapula when pain or pathology exists. This is in part due to more efficient alignment of rotator cuff and capsular fibers and less tendency toward impingement. The scapular plane has been estimated to be between 30 to 45 degrees anterior to the coronal plane.[5,6] Although many muscles participate, the two major muscles include the deltoid and supraspinatus with assistance through stabilization from the infraspinatus, teres minor, and subscapularis.

Full active abduction in the coronal plane should reveal several clues to underlying pathology (Fig. 7-2):

1. *A hesitation sign.* A hesitation on initiation or ending of movement may be a subtle sign of instability or rotator cuff dysfunction.[7]
2. *Substitution of initial abduction with shoulder hiking, forward rolling, or trunk leaning.* These are all maneuvers of recruitment incorporated by the patient with a rotator cuff tear or adhesive capsulitis.[8]
3. *Scapulohumeral ratio.* The average ratio between the glenohumeral and scapulothoracic joints is 2 to 1. Therefore, for every 15 degrees of abduction, 10 occur at the glenohumeral joint and 5 at the scapulothoracic. This is an average and therefore should not be specifically applied. The first 30 degrees of abduction (and first 60 degrees of flexion) is almost purely glenohumeral representing a scapular "lag." Beyond this range the ratio becomes relatively equal so that for every 5 degrees of glenohumeral contribution there is 4 degrees of scapulothoracic. At the terminal ranges of flexion and abduction, scapular contribution again diminishes. To determine pure glenohumeral motion, the scapula should be stabilized. A reverse scapulohumeral rhythm is found with adhesive capsulitis and may result in recruitment positioning as mentioned previously.
4. *Painful arc.* Cyriax[2] noted that when a patient experienced pain mainly in the mid-range of abduction, between 70 and 110 degrees, impingement of subacromial structures was probably the underlying cause. This finding could be on active or passive ROM, but the distinctive feature is that although pain occurs at the lower level of abduction, the patient may go beyond the pain by further movement, thereby clearing the humeral head from its impinged position.
5. *End-range pain.* Pain at end range only is suggestive of acromioclavicular etiology. This is a compressive position for the acromioclavicular joint (as is horizontal adduction). The patient experi-

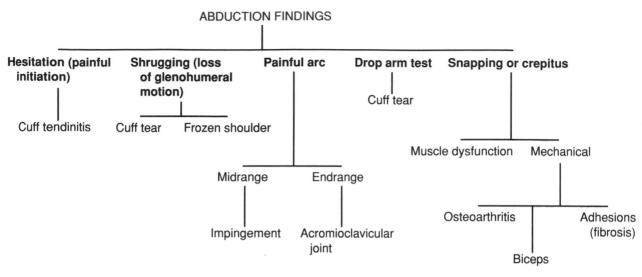

Fig. 7-2. Abduction findings.

ences anterosuperior pain if the acromioclavicular joint is involved. Due to the possibility of referred pain from subacromial osteophytes, there is a possibility of lateral arm pain (over the deltoid tuberosity).

6. *End-range weakness/numbness/tingling.* With the arm in full elevation the patient may have distal symptomatology indicating thoracic outlet syndrome or instability.

7. *Winging of the scapula.* The most common cause of winging with motion (not statically evident) involves lack of stabilization by the middle trapezius or rhomboids, which would allow for the lower border to flare out. Serratus anterior involvement would allow proximal winging.

8. *Thoracic outlet testing.* With full abduction the patient may repetitively perform clenching of the fists in an attempt to reproduce any shoulder arm symptoms (Roos test).

9. *Sudden loss of stabilization on actively lowering the arm.* This is a variation of the standard Codman's drop arm test indicating a rotator cuff tear.

10. *The "empty can" test.* With full internal rotation and elbow extended the arm is lifted 90 degrees in the scapular plane (30 degrees forward). If pain-free, the examiner applies resistance to further ab-

duction. Weakness and pain reproduction indicate supraspinatus involvement.

11. *Snapping of the biceps tendon.* Having the patient lower the arm while holding a 5 lb weight may produce a snapping sensation in the anterior shoulder. This is referred to as the Gilcrest sign.[9]

Full passive abduction may reveal the following:

1. *Painful arc.* Performed passively, abduction may reveal a painful arc more readily than with active movement given that passage past the painful range may be made more tolerable due to the lack of musculotendon participation. In other words, pain may not allow enough active range to demonstrate an involvement limited to a midrange.

2. *Dawbarn's test.* This is a questionable attempt at determining subacromial bursal involvement. The examiner palpates anterolateral to the acromioclavicular joint in an attempt to elicit tenderness. Then the arm is raised into abduction, and if the tenderness disappears it indicates that the bursa has retracted under the acromion on elevation.

3. *Performance of the Wright's maneuver.* This may be performed by palpating the radial pulse lifting the

arm above 90 degrees abduction and noting any reproduction of shoulder/arm symptoms.

4. *Snapping over the bicipital area on lowering the arm.* This finding is described by Abbott and Saunders[10] when a patient's arm is passively elevated and externally rotated. The arm is then lowered as internal rotation is introduced palpating over the anterior shoulder for a snapping tendon.

Other Tests

A functional test can be performed by having the patient perform a push-up against the wall. Note any winging of the scapula with this maneuver, which may indicate involvement of the long thoracic nerve to the serratus anterior.

By having the patient bend forward to 45 degrees the examiner can perform "load and shift" tests for anterior, posterior, and inferior stability, as described by Rowe.[11] Both posterior to anterior and anterior to posterior forces are applied to test anterior and posterior stability, respectively. Additionally, inferior stress is applied to test both inferior and multidirectional instability.

It is important to test balance, particularly with the athlete. This is an important ingredient for efficient/safe performance of many sport activities. Testing with a standard Romberg sign is essential, followed by single leg, balance with eyes open/eyes closed.

SEATED TESTING

The seated position is probably most comfortable for the patient and the doctor because it equalizes any height differences produced in the standing position. An important requisite for substitution of many standing tests to the seated position is to allow the arm to hang dependent by having the patient sit at the edge of the examining table. It is best to perform the majority of static palpation in this position. Included should be the shoulder complex and cervical region. If adjustment of the cervical spine is expected this is an appropriate position for the accessory palpation and vertebrobasilar screening.

Cervical Testing

Screening the cervical region orthopaedically is best reserved for patients with either neck and shoulder pain complaints or radicular pain involving the shoulder and arm. A brief review includes the following tests:

1. *Cervical compression in all positions.* Local pain responses suggest facet involvement on the same side as compression. On the opposite side facet or soft tissue involvement may be the cause. Reproduction of radicular pain is suggestive of nerve root compression or cervicogenic referred pain. Further testing of deep tendon reflexes, dermatomes, and muscle testing should clarify the difference in most cases.

2. *Cervical distraction.* If pain is increased with distraction the suspicion is involvement of soft tissue especially when cervical compression is negative. When cervical distraction relieves radiating pain a confirmation of nerve root involvement or cervicogenic referred pain is indicated.

3. *Shoulder depression.* Shoulder depression can be performed two ways. With only shoulder depression and no neck stretching, a positive response will occasionally correlate with nerve root testing if osteoarthritic spur involvement is present on the same side. When cervical stretching away from shoulder depression is added it is likely the patient will feel symptoms on the side inadvertently cervically compressed (the side away from shoulder depression). In this instance a reproduction of cervical compression testing is occurring and would in most cases correlate with that testing. If pain or paresthesias are present on the depressed shoulder side, it is more likely that brachial plexus stretching and irritation are the cause.

Most thoracic outlet testing can be performed in the seated relaxed position, while palpating for the radial pulse and noting any reproduction of the patient's complaint(s). Adson's test for anterior scalene compression, Halstead's test for middle scalene, and the costoclavicular test for first rib/clavicular compression can be performed.

Shoulder Testing

Arm at the Side

Palpation of the shoulder is conveniently performed with the patient in the relaxed seated position. An attempt at localization of tenderness should be made noting any areas of referral (see Ch. 6 for specific detail).

Testing of the patient should next progress to stability testing with the arm relaxed, forearm resting on the leg. A load and shift test[12] should be performed for anterior, posterior, and inferior instability (see Fig. 6-20A–C). Posterior to anterior and anterior to posterior force is applied to test anterior and posterior laxity, respectively. Distracting the arm downward tests inferior laxity evident by a sulcus sign.[13] Occasionally, this maneuver will also produce pain when the supraspinatus is involved. Release pain is often found when instability is present. When inferior instability is present, most authors feel that other directional laxity (anterior or posterior) must be present (the circle concept).[14]

Testing for apprehension with the arm at the side also evaluates passive external rotation (see Fig. 6-29A).

At this point the Kocher maneuver can be performed on the patient (see Fig. 6-35A–C). By distracting the arm inferiorly with slight abduction and external rotation, the arm is passively brought first into adduction and then internal rotation. Although this maneuver was originally designed to replace an anterior dislocation, it has been suggested as a potential test for glenoid labrum tears.[7] The positive response for a tear would include both pain and a clunk sensation.

Active testing in the dependent position includes testing of the latissimus dorsi and occasionally the supraspinatus. With the arm internally rotated and elbow extended the patient attempts adduction against the examiner's resistance to test the latissimus dorsi.[15] With the same starting position resisted abduction tests for the supraspinatus (although better tests exist).

Active resisted testing is performed with the elbow flexed 90 degrees. In this position it is possible to test for both internal rotation (mainly subscapularis) and external rotation (infraspinatus/teres minor). It is important to caution the patient against using abduction or adduction as part of the movement. This is commonly a recruitment attempt by the patient with the larger adducting muscles. The patient resists internal rotation at the forearm for the external rotators and external resistance at the forearm for the internal rotators (see Fig. 6-40).

With the arm in the same position of 90 degrees elbow flexion, the forearm should be pronated. The patient attempts to supinate and flex the elbow against the resistance of the examiner to perform one version of the Yergason's test for the biceps brachii (see Fig. 6-45).[16]

Hand Behind Back

The patient should attempt to place the hand behind the back. Although this is a gross test for the internal rotators/extensors of the shoulder, inability to perform the maneuver is most often due to tightness of the capsule or muscles rather than weakness. According to Travell and Simons,[17] inability to continue the movement of the hand horizontally across the back may indicate involvement of the coracobrachialis. Inability to raise the hand superiorly in this position may indicate tightness of the infraspinatus. This is the position recommended for measurement of active internal rotation by the American Academy of Shoulder and Elbow Surgeons.[18] The highest vertebral level the patient can achieve is noted for comparison to the well-side and for future comparison (see Fig. 6-13).

The position of the hand behind the back is considered the optimal position for palpation of the supraspinatus insertion into the greater tuberosity.[19] Some authors feel that the infraspinatus/teres minor insertion is also palpable. The location of the supraspinatus is anterolateral to the acromioclavicular joint (see Fig. 6-7).

With the hand in the initial position behind the back, the patient attempts to press the elbow backward against the resistance of the examiner. This is considered the standard muscle test for the rhomboids (see Fig. 6-46), however, some texts claim it as a test for the teres major.[20] It must be remembered, however, that the teres major is usually called into action with very strenuous activities.[21]

Forward Flexion

The patient may then rest the elbow in the examiner's hand. The examiner should then raise the arm into full forward flexion to end range (see Fig. 6-36). This test, as described by Neer and Welsh[22] is intended to reveal any signs of anterior impingement. Modification may include forward flexion with internal rotation. This may reveal subcoracoid impingement.[23]

The patient should attempt forward flexion of the arm with the elbow extended. This is a gross evaluation of the biceps brachii, the coracobrachialis, and the anterior deltoid. The ROM should be measured for future comparison.

An occult posterior subluxation tendency may be revealed by the patient forward flexing the arm slightly. A bulge may appear posteriorly with no accompanying pain. Reduction will usually occur with horizontal extension at the joint. A palpable or audible click or clunk may be felt or heard. It is also difficult for the patient to complete forward flexion with the arm internally rotated or the forearm supinated.

With the arm held parallel to the ground at 90 degrees, the patient attempts further flexion against the resistance of the examiner (see Fig. 6-43). Known as Speed's test,[24] this test should be repeated several times to determine whether overstrain or subacromial impingement of the biceps tendon may be discovered.

Forward Flexion/Elbow Bent 90 Degrees

From the Speed's position, the patient may bend the elbow 90 degrees so that the forearm is in front of the chest. The examiner then performs one maneuver to detect two possible responses. The patient rests the elbow in the examiner's hand. The examiner imparts internal rotation of the arm by pressing down on the forearm (see Fig. 6-37). The two common responses are anterior or posterior shoulder pain. Anterior compressive pain is most indicative of impingement as described by Hawkins and Kennedy.[25] Posterior pain indicates stretching of the posterior muscles, particularly the external rotators infraspinatus/teres minor and posterior deltoid.[26]

By simply externally rotating the arm from the above Hawkins and Kennedy's position, the infraspinatus and teres minor insertions become more palpable lateral and posterior (see Fig. 6-8A).[27]

Horizontal Adduction

By actively continuing the arm across the chest through horizontal adduction, the patient contracts mainly the pectoralis major. Passive horizontal adduction, especially at end range, is a compressive test for the acromioclavicular joint (see Fig. 6-51). A hard positive would be anterosuperior joint pain (unless a subacromial process is affected). If posterior pain is felt, it is likely the posterior musculature is involved such as the infraspinatus, teres minor, or posterior deltoid.

A test for posterior instability involves pushing the humerus posteriorly with the shoulder and elbow flexed 90 degrees. The posterior force is maintained while passively horizontally adducting the arm (see Fig. 6-26A & B). A positive is indicated by subluxation or dislocation posteriorly.[28]

90 Degrees Abduction Elbow Bent 90 Degrees

By moving the arm back to the coronal plane several tests can be performed. Passive testing of anterior glenohumeral laxity can be performed with the Protzman test, stabilizing the arm and directing a posterior to anterior force to the humeral head (see Fig. 6-22).[29] Testing of the inferior stability can be accomplished with the Feagen maneuver where the patient's arm rests on the examiner's shoulder. The examiner imparts a cautious inferior force with the hands (see Fig. 6-27).

Testing of the three heads of the deltoid is best evaluated in this position. First the patient attempts abduction against the resistance of the examiner to test the middle deltoid. Then the anterior deltoid can be evaluated with slight external rotation and an attempt to abduct against resistance. Finally, the posterior deltoid can be tested with slight internal rotation and resisted abduction.

Two other muscle tests, internal and external rotation, can be performed with this initial position. By supporting the patient's elbow the examiner can monitor the patient's attempt to recruit adduction or abduction into the test. The examiner then resists the patient's attempt at internal rotation of the shoulder. Resistance is best applied at the undersurface of the forearm. This tests all internal rotators with some focus on the subscapularis. The opposite procedure is used to evaluate the infraspinatus/teres minor. Again, resistance is best applied at the top (dorsal) surface of the forearm (see Fig. 6-42).

90 Degrees Shoulder Abduction with External Rotation

The patient then positions the shoulder abducted 90 degrees and rotated externally so that the forearm lies in the coronal plane. This position is often not possible when restricted by an acute inflammatory process, adhesive capsulitis, an occult posterior dislocation, and sometimes severe degeneration. Usually when a rotator cuff tear is present, the patient may find alternative movement paths to reach this position.

If the patient is able to abduct to 90 degrees with external rotation, two active tests can be added. The patient is asked to continue external rotation from this starting position, and then asked to horizontally abduct (extend). This combination of external rotation and horizontal abduction are important movement requirements for throwing and swimming. Restrictions or the production of pain is therefore functionally significant.

Apprehension testing can be performed returning to the initial starting position. The examiner pushes anteriorly on the humerus while drawing the shoulder back into external rotation/horizontal abduction. If there is no sense of apprehension (shoulder feels it will "go out of place") the examiner will repeat the test, and ask the patient to simulate a throwing movement against the resistance of the examiner's hand (see Fig. 6-29C). Sometimes subtle dysfunction will be exposed using this maneuver.[30] It is recommended to test for apprehension at various levels of abduction. It is important to test at 120 degrees of abduction if no evidence of laxity is present at 90 degrees (see Fig. 6-29D).[34]

Raising the arm slightly higher into abduction and fully flexing the elbow several evaluations can be accomplished. Having the patient contract the biceps muscle while palpating may reveal clicking or snapping of the tendon (see Fig. 6-44). This is referred to as the Ludington's test and may indicate pathology or rupture of the biceps. With the same position the examiner presses the humerus inferiorly while the patient resists. This is occasionally used as a test for the coracobrachialis muscle.

The patient can then perform the wrap-around test devised by Travell and Simons.[17] This test is intended to detect restriction in active external rotation due to functional shortening of the infraspinatus/teres minor. The patient is asked to try to touch the opposite corner of the mouth, and is allowed rotation of the head 45 degrees to assist in the motion.

SUPINE TESTING

The supine position allows some testing not available in other positions. The locking maneuver is a position that is used to test for impingement. The examiner extends the arm (with the elbow bent) and passively abducts the shoulder. A point around 90 degrees of abduction will be reached where further movement is not possible (see Fig. 6-38). The indication of impingement is pain at end range.

An anterior drawer test can be performed with the arm abducted and a posterior to anterior force directed to the humeral head (see Fig. 6-21).

Passive external and internal rotation can be measured with the shoulder abducted 90 degrees, elbow bent. An indication of capsular involvement is the inability to passively place the shoulder in abduction external rotation with the hand behind the head. Although not specific to the capsule, if this is the only restricted pattern, capsular involvement is more likely. Other soft tissue involvement can include the pectoral muscles, particularly the pectoralis minor.

This same position can be used to perform the many versions of the apprehension test (see Fig. 6-30B) and the reverse apprehension test (referred to as the relocation test). As described by Jobe and Kvitne,[32] from a patient position of abduction/external rotation the examiner directs a force anterior to posterior at the proximal humerus (see Fig. 6-32). A positive test is a reduction of apprehension or pain felt in the original apprehension position.

The clunk test can also be performed to potentially determine the presence of a glenoid labrum tear.[7] With the patient's arm left in the apprehension position, the examiner imparts an anterior force to the proximal humerus while rotating or circumducting the arm (see Fig. 6-34). A deep clicking or clunking sensation palpated or sensed by the examiner or patient is suggestive of a glenoid labrum tear.

Posterior instability testing (see Fig. 6-18) can be performed by stabilizing the scapula posteriorly and pushing through the elbow up the long axis of the humerus in a posterior direction with the shoulder flexed 20 to 30 degrees (see Fig. 6-31). This is not a very sensitive test for instability; however, the position is similar for testing posterior accessory motion and is probably more valuable in this assessment.

The Norwood test (see Fig. 6-25A & B) can be performed by flexing the elbow 90 degrees and forward flexing the shoulder 90 degrees. While palpating the posterior shoulder, the arm is passively horizontally adducted. Palpable subluxation can be perceived with this maneuver.

The supine position is ideal for performing most of the accessory motion testing. It allows relaxation of the patient with maneuverability of the upper extremity for proper position. Accessory motion is that movement available at a joint that is not normally under voluntary control. It must be passively assisted through this minimal range to what is referred to by Sandoz[33] as the paraphysiologic zone. Abrupt movement through this zone but not exceeding the physiologic limits is referred to as an adjustment of the joint.

Mennell[34] and others[26,35–37] have proposed a concept to explain why joints with limited accessory movement have joint pain but may not have obvious responses to more gross orthopaedic testing. These authors propose that without this accessory movement, the joint cannot function properly. Evaluation is based on the determination of what is often referred to as a springy end-feel. If not found, the examiner assumes restriction and attempts "impulsing" past the paraphysiologic zone to eliminate the restriction. An impulse is a short, low-amplitude, high-velocity thrusting movement that requires specialized training and experience.

An evaluation of accessory movement of the cervical spine should first be performed. Palpation is coupled with passive ranging of the cervical spine in both an attempt at detecting restrictions or reproduction of the patient's complaint.

There are essentially four shoulder joints that can be assessed. They are the sternoclavicular joint, the acromioclavicular joint, the glenohumeral joint, and the scapulothoracic (functional) joint.

There is some variation in the description of available accessory motions in the shoulder girdle. A suggested combination of these descriptions is given.

Sternoclavicular Palpation

With the patient relaxed on the table, the examiner can test anterior to posterior glide by applying pressure over the sternoclavicular joint with the palm of the hand. A normal springy sensation should be palpable. Restriction coupled with some discomfort may indicate blockage of this accessory movement. However, a past dislocation or current osteoarthritic blockage may be the cause. Proceeding with caution is then advised, using more indirect approaches to restoration of movement prior to an adjustive thrust.

All other accessory motion of the sternoclavicular joint is palpated with shoulder motion. Using active or passive movements of the shoulder the sternoclavicular joint is palpated for the accompanying accessory motion. The patient's arm is controlled with one hand while the sternoclavicular joint is palpated with the other. The movements associated with specific accessory motion are as follows:

1. Depression of the shoulder complex causes a superior glide of the medial clavicle on the sternum.
2. Elevation of the shoulder causes an inferior glide of the medial clavicle on the sternum.
3. Horizontal adduction of the shoulder causes a posterior glide of the medial clavicle on the sternum.
4. Horizontal abduction of the shoulder causes an anterior glide of the medial clavicle on the sternum.

Acromioclavicular Palpation

Acromioclavicular motion is less appreciable than sternoclavicular movement. The lateral clavicle and scapula often move more as a unit than as separate bones. In addition, contraction of surrounding musculature on active movement of the shoulder often obscures palpation. This is specifically why palpation with the patient supine is preferred. Some suggested accessory movement patterns that are coupled with shoulder movement are as follows:

1. Superior glide accompanying abduction of the shoulder
2. Inferior glide accompanying adduction of the shoulder
3. Anterior glide accompanying flexion/abduction
4. Posterior glide accompanying extension/abduction
5. Combinations of glide associated with internal and external rotation

Glenohumeral Palpation

To assess posterior to anterior glide the examiner places a hand behind the shoulder and using leverage at the elbow with the other hand, lifts the shoulder. This movement involves a downward push on the elbow with a concomitant upward push on the posterior humerus (see Fig. 19-15).

Anterior to posterior glide is best assessed by first distracting the humerus laterally. This is accomplished by leverage, again at the elbow. By stabilizing the elbow against the side, the other hand is placed high in the axilla. The axillary hand pushes laterally and inferiorly (posteriorly) (see Fig. 19-18).

Two other methods of testing anterior to posterior glide are similar to testing for posterior instability. The arm is first lifted 15 degrees. Using a contract on the elbow, the examiner pushes along the long axis of the humerus posteriorly and superiorly. The same procedure with the modification of lifting the arm 45 degrees tests another possible glide movement (see Fig. 6-31).

Inferior glide can be tested by abducting the arm 90 degrees. In this position the humerus is pushed inferiorly (anatomically) (see Fig. 19-21).

PRONE

In the prone position circumduction of the glenohumeral joint can be performed. The examiner abducts the arm to 90 degrees and stabilizes the arm between the knees. The shoulder is then rotated through circumduction with the use of both hands determining any restrictions to smooth movement (see Fig. 19-23B).

The prone position is ideal for palpation of the subacromial bursa. The examiner passively draws the relaxed arm back into extension while simultaneously palpating anterior to the acromioclavicular joint (see Fig. 6-10). Two possible indicators of involvement include either an increase in palpatory bogginess on extension or an increase in pain. This is due to the bursa sliding out from hiding under the acromioclavicular joint during extension.

By placing the patient's hand behind the back, the examiner can then control movement and palpation of the scapula. Using one hand to lift the shoulder superiorly (posteriorly) the examiner uses the other hand to slide under the medial border of the scapula for palpation (see Fig. 19-24). Restriction and tenderness may be indicative of rhomboid or middle trapezius involvement.

Static spinal palpation can be performed in the prone position adding correlative information to functional shoulder etiologies.

REFERENCES

1. Basmajian JV, DeLuca CJ: Muscles alive: their function revealed by electromyography. Williams & Wilkins, Baltimore, 1985
2. Cyriax J: Textbook of Orthopaedic Medicine. Vol. 1. Diagnosis of Soft Tissue Lesions. 8th Ed. Balliere-Tindall, London, 1982
3. Howell SM, Galiat BJ, Renzi AJ, Marone PJ: Normal and abnormal mechanics of the glenohumeral joint in the horizontal plane. J Bone Joint Surg 70A:227, 1988
4. Kumar VP, Balasubramaniam P: The role of atmospheric pressure in stabilizing the shoulder: an experimental study. J Bone Joint Surg 67B:719, 1985
5. Poppen NK, Walker PS: Normal and abnormal motion of the shoulder. J Bone Joint Surg 58A:195, 1976
6. Kondo M, Tazoe S, Yamada M: Changes in the tilting angle of the scapula following elevation of the arm. p. 12. In Bateman JE, Welsh RP (eds): Surgery of the Shoulder. CV Mosby, St. Louis, 1984
7. Andrews JR, Gillogly S: Physical examination of the shoulder in throwing athletes. In Zarin B, Andrews JR, Carson WG (eds): Injuries to the Throwing Arm. WB Saunders, Philadelphia, 1985
8. Beetham WP, Polley HP, Slocum CH, Weaver WF: Physical Examination of the Joints. WB Saunders, Philadelphia, 1965
9. Gilcrest EL, Albi P: Unusual lesions of muscles and tendons of the shoulder girdle and upper arm. Surg Gynecol Obstet 68:903, 1939
10. Abbott LC, Saunders JB de CM: Acute traumatic dislocation of the tendon of the long head of the biceps brachii: report of 6 cases with operative findings. Surgery 6:817, 1939
11. Rowe CR: The Shoulder. Churchill Livingstone, New York, 1988
12. Hawkins RJ, Schutte JB, Huckell GH et al: The assessment of glenohumeral translation using manual and fluoroscopic techniques. Orthop Trans 12:727, 1988
13. Warren RF, Kornblatt IB, Marchand R: Static factors affecting posterior shoulder instability. Orthop Trans 8:89, 1984
14. Cooper D, Warner JP, Deng X et al: Anatomy and function of the coracohumeral ligament. American Academy of Orthopaedic Surgeons, Park Ridge, IL, 1991

15. Kendall FP, McCreary EK: Muscle Testing and Function. 3rd Ed. Williams & Wilkins, Baltimore, 1983

16. Yergason RM: Supination sign. J Bone Joint Surg 13:160, 1931

17. Travell JG, Simons DG: Myofascial pain and dysfunction: The trigger point manual. Williams & Wilkins, Baltimore, 1983

18. Norris TR: History and physical examination of the shoulder. p. 72. In Nicholas JA, Hershman EB, Posner MA: The Upper Extremity in Sports Medicine. CV Mosby, St. Louis, 1990

19. Jackson D, Einhorn A: Rehabilitation of the shoulder. p. 103. In Jackson DW: Shoulder Surgery in the Athlete. Aspen, Rockville, MD, 1985

20. Walther DS: Applied Kinesiology. Vol. 1. Systems DC, Pueblo, CO, 1981

21. Broome HL, Basmajian JV: The function of the teres major muscle: an electromyographic study. Anat Rec 170:309, 1971

22. Neer CS, Welsh RP: The shoulder in sports. Orthop Clin North Am 8:583, 1977

23. Patte D: The subcoracoid impingement. Clin Orthop Relat Res 254:55, 1990

24. Leach RE, Schepsis AA: Shoulder pain. Clin Sports Med 1:127, 1983

25. Hawkins RJ, Kennedy JC: Impingement syndrome in athletes. Am J Sports Med 8:151, 1980

26. Corrigan B, Maitland GD: Practical Orthopaedic Medicine. Butterworths, London, 1983

27. Jackson D, Einhorn A: Rehabilitation of the shoulder. p. 103. In Jackson DW: Shoulder Surgery in the Athlete. Aspen, Rockville, MD, 1985

28. Matsen FA, Thomas SC, Rockwood CA: Glenohumeral instability. In Rockwood CA, Matsen FA (eds): The Shoulder. WB Saunders, Philadelphia, 1990

29. Protzman RR: Anterior instability of the shoulder. J Bone Joint Surg 62A:909, 1980

30. Kulund DN: The Injured Athlete. 1st ed. JB Lippincott, Philadelphia, 1982

31. Rockwood CA: Subluxations and dislocations about the shoulder. p. 722. In Rockwood CA, Green DP (eds): Fractures in Adults. JB Lippincott, Philadelphia, 1984

32. Jobe FW, Kvitne RS: Shoulder pain in the overhand or throwing athlete: the relationship of anterior instability and rotator cuff impingement. Orthop Rev 18:963, 1989

33. Sandoz R: Some physical mechanisms and effects of spinal adjustments. Swiss Annals 6:91, 1976

34. Mennell JM: Joint pain: diagnosis and treatment using manipulative techniques. Little, Brown, Boston, 1964

35. Kaltenborn FM: Mobilization of the Extremity Joints: Examination and Basic Treatment Techniques. Olaf Norlis Bokhandel, Oslo, 1980

36. Greenman PE: Principles of Manual Medicine. Williams & Wilkins, Baltimore, 1989

37. Paris SV: Extremity Dysfunction and Mobilization. Prepublication Manual, Atlanta, GA, 1980

8

Isokinetic Testing and Exercise*

KEVIN E. WILK
CHRISTOPHER A. ARRIGO

The glenohumeral joint is inherently unstable.[1-4] The arthrology consists of a large oval humeral head articulating with a small convex glenoid fossa, which represents a ball-and-socket type joint.[5] This type of joint geometry allows a tremendous amount of movement, but stability is compromised. The functional stability of the glenohumeral joint is accomplished by the joint's dynamic stabilizing components. The dynamic stabilizers of the shoulder complex are the rotator cuff musculature, the long head of the biceps brachii, the deltoid, and some of the scapulothoracic musculature.

The primary function of the rotator cuff muscles is one of dynamic glenohumeral stability.[1,3] These muscles function to steer the humeral head and control humeral head displacement through a co-contraction of these muscles, which results in increased joint compression forces. Secondly, the rotator cuff functions as a fine tuner during strenuous activities, especially overhead motions such as throwing, tennis, or elevated work activities. The secondary function of the rotator cuff is one of primary movement, such as with external and internal rotation of the shoulder.

It is obvious that the glenohumeral joint must rely extensively on the shoulder musculature and rotator cuff for dynamic stability during various strenuous activities. Therefore, the objective documentation of the strength, power, and endurance of the shoulder musculature is necessary to predict adequately a return to injury-free sporting activities or strenuous activities.

When a clinician refers to the assessment of muscular strength, one often thinks of the manual muscle testing (MMT) techniques. The earliest description of the MMT was by Lovett in 1912.[6] Since its conception, there have been several revisions in this technique. Two of the most popular versions of MMT have been developed by Kendall and McCreary[7] and by Daniels and Worthingham.[8] There are several inconsistencies in both the application and grading of these two techniques.[9,10] Additionally, inter-rater reliability is poor[11,12], and the grading is relatively subjective.[13,14] Wilk et al.[15] have demonstrated bilateral isokinetic knee extension deficits ranging from 23 to 31 percent in 176 arthroscopic knee patients who exhibited bilaterally equal and normal grade (5/5) MMT.[15] Lastly, MMT tells the examiner nothing regarding muscular performance parameters, such as work, power, and endurance. It determines the ability of the subject to exert force at one particular point in the range of motion.[10] Thus, the face validity of MMT for the orthopaedic and sports medicine patient may not be completely acceptable in all instances.[9,10]

Therefore, a reasonable clinical addition to MMT is the use of isokinetic testing of the shoulder. Isokinetic testing affords the clinician the ability to document objectively muscular performance in a way that is both safe and reliable using either isolated or combined movement patterns. This objectivity ensures appropriate patient progression or regression, as well as assists the clinician with the determination of functional questions such as: when can I hit a golf ball? begin throwing? begin hitting a tennis ball? or return to overhead

---

* Modified from Wilk and Arrigo,[85] with permission.

work activities? Consequently, isokinetics affords the clinician objective criteria and provides reproducible data to monitor patient function and plan patient progression.

ISOKINETIC TESTING OF THE SHOULDER

To assess the muscular performance characteristics of a shoulder joint that has sustained a repetitive microtraumatic or macrotraumatic injury, the clinician should consider the sporting/functional positions that most frequently produce this type of injury and the demands of the daily activities that are placed on the shoulder. Most commonly, the shoulder is placed at risk of sustaining a microtraumatic injury when elevation, abduction, and rotation are required while performing a wide variety of activities. Examples of these superimposed activities include throwing, tennis, swimming, volleyball, and a variety of work-related activities, such as painting and maintenance work. In these types of patients, the authors recommend testing

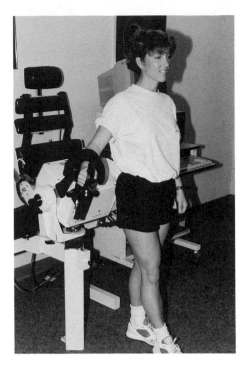

Fig. 8-2. The modified neutral position for shoulder external/internal rotation. The dynamometer is tilted 20 to 30 degrees and the shoulder is abducted approximately 20 to 30 degrees.

in the 90 degree abducted 90 degree elbow flexed position for shoulder internal and external rotation (Fig. 8-1).

In contrast, for the patient who has sustained a macrotraumatic shoulder injury involving either the capsule or rotator cuff, and engages in daily activities that do not necessitate repetitive overhead motions, testing is recommended in a less demanding position. This position is referred to as a modified neutral position.[16] (Fig. 8-2). This position or the scapular plane position (Fig. 8-3) are advised for isokinetic testing in the low-demand shoulder patient.

Wilk et al.,[17] recognizing inconsistencies in testing methodology of various published articles, have suggested a standardized isokinetic testing protocol for the shoulder. This standardized isokinetic testing protocol is referred to as the Thrower's Series.[17] The goal of a standardized testing protocol is to improve test-retest reproducibility[18] and allows the clinician to share test data.[10,17] In this chapter, we present an expansion of the Thrower's Series and explain the modi-

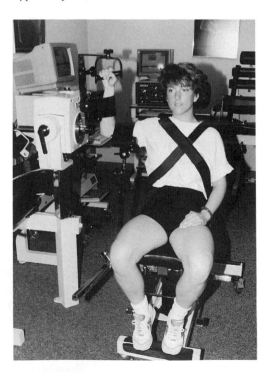

Fig. 8-1. The 90 degree abducted position for shoulder external/internal rotation.

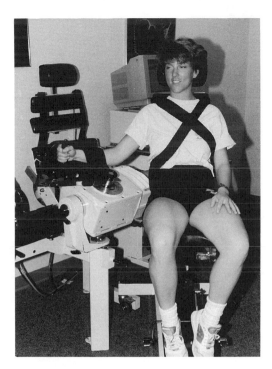

Fig. 8-3. The scapular plane position for shoulder external/internal rotation. The shoulder is abducted and flexed to 45 degrees.

Table 8-1. Standardized Isokinetic Testing Protocol

1. Planes of motion to evaluate
2. Testing position/stabilization
3. Axis of joint motion
4. Client education
5. Active warm-up
6. Gravity compensation
7. Rest intervals
8. Test collateral extremity first
9. Testing environment
   a. Standardized verbal commands
   b. Standardized visual feedback
   c Free from distractions
   d. Tester skill
10. Testing velocities used
11. Test repetitions performed
12. System calibration
13. System level/stabilized
14. Use of windowed data/semihard endstop

(From Wilk and Arrigo,[85] with permission.)

fications of this protocol to the general orthopaedic patient.

There are 14 variables that must be standardized and controlled to ensure an objective, reliable, and reproducible isokinetic evaluation of the shoulder (Table 8-1). The first variable is to evaluate the planes of motion to test. In the overhead athlete, it has been reported that the shoulder's external/internal rotators, adductors/abductors, and horizontal abductors/adductors are the most critical muscles to be tested.[17,19–25] Therefore, isokinetic testing in the Thrower's Series recommends the evaluation of the shoulder's internal and external rotators, as well as the abductors and adductors.[17] Because isokinetic testing of the horizontal abductors and adductors is performed in either the supine or prone position, these nonfunctional postures are not recommended in the testing sequence for the microtraumatically injured shoulder. In the low-demand shoulder patient, routine tests recommended include internal/external rotation and shoulder flexion/extension. The testing sequence is specifically standardized with the internal and external rotators always

evaluated first, followed by either shoulder abduction/adduction or flexion/extension.

It is necessary to test the shoulder in a position that closely resembles its position of function during activity, while isolating the specific muscle groups desired. To both approximate functional positioning and ensure muscular isolation, most testing is performed in the seated position. This position allows for normal gravitational forces acting on the trunk and upper extremities and enhances glenohumeral joint stabilization. Appropriate stabilization of the trunk, hip, and lower extremities during isokinetic testing of the shoulder is highly recommended (Fig. 8-4).

Testing of the shoulder's external and internal rotators can be performed in several test positions. These positions include the 90 degrees/90 degrees test position (Fig. 8-1), modified neutral position (Fig. 8-2), scapular plane position (Fig. 8-3), neutral position (Fig. 8-5), and/or the 90 degrees/90 degrees seated position (Fig. 8-6). Numerous authors have demonstrated significant torque value variations by altering the subjects' test position.[26–32] Greenfield et al.[27] tested external/internal rotation in both the scapular and frontal planes, and reported no significant internal rotation peak torque difference but increased external rotation torque values in the scapular plane. Walmsley and Szybbo[32] assessed external/internal rotation peak torque values in three test positions: neutral, 90 degrees abduction, and 90 degrees flexion. He found increased internal rotation torque values in the neutral

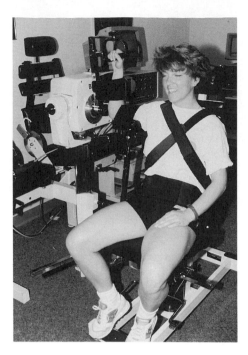

Fig. 8-4. The trunk, hip, and lower extremity are stabilized to eliminate muscular substitution during shoulder external/internal rotation.

Considering these investigations, the pathophysiology of rotator cuff injuries, and the function of the shoulder muscles, a continuum of external/internal rotation exercise positions can be developed (Figs. 8-7 and 8-8). The natural progression of this continuum is from 0 degrees abduction through the scapular plane and up to the functional 90 degrees abducted position, which maximizes the external/internal rotation length tension relationship. This position also maximally stresses the dynamic stabilizing function of the rotator cuff musculature. This exercise continuum allows for the progression of static shoulder stability from a position of maximal joint stability to one of minimal stability. As with any form of exercise, if symptoms develop at any stage, the activity is regressed to an asymptomatic level and readvanced only when appropriate. The clinician should be aware that the test results generated in any one specific position cannot be compared to test results obtained in different test positions.

position, and the highest external rotation values were exhibited in the 90 degrees flexion position. Hinton[28] reported increased torque for internal rotation in the neutral position compared with the 90 degrees abducted position, and external rotation was found to be equal in both positions.

Soderberg and Blaschek[26] tested external/internal rotation in six different test positions. They concluded that the internal rotation exhibited increased torque production in a neutral position, defined as 0 to 20 degrees of shoulder abduction; and that external rotation torque was enhanced in the 90 degrees abducted position or neutral position. Ellenbecker et al.[31] tested external/internal rotation in the plane of the scapula versus the frontal plane and reported no significant differences in torque production in either the supine or seated position. Hellwig and Perrin[30] reported no significant differences in external/internal rotation in the frontal plane compared with the scapular plane during concentric and eccentric muscular contractions.

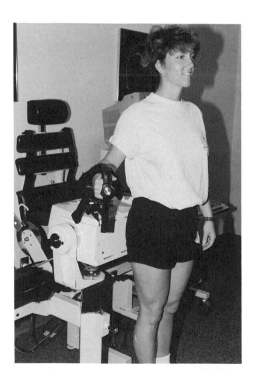

Fig. 8-5. The neutral position for shoulder external/internal rotation. The dynamometer is level, and the shoulder is abducted slightly. (From Wilk and Arrigo,[85] with permission.)

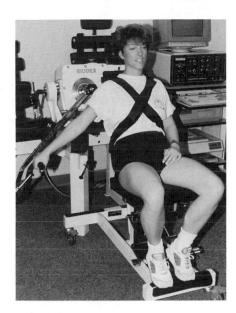

Fig. 8-6. Shoulder abduction/adduction in the seated position.

cant differences between values demonstrated in the first testing session and those of the remaining six test trials. Wilk has shown that subjects allowed one practice session prior to testing produced more consistent torque values in 83 to 88 percent of all test trials (unpublished data). Therefore, it is recommended that whenever possible clients undergo at least one isokinetic exposure prior to testing.

The fifth testing guideline is the use of an active warm-up prior to isokinetic testing. Several studies have demonstrated no direct relationship between a warm-up and increased isokinetic torque produc-

The third parameter that should be addressed is to ensure that the axis of joint motion is aligned with the axis of rotation of the shaft of the dynamometer. This alignment is necessary for accuracy in torque measurement.[10] Although not yet documented for the shoulder, changes in lever arm length of 2.5 inches or greater during knee extension/flexion testing have been shown to significantly alter torque production.[33–35] It is recommended that when testing shoulder abduction/adduction, the axis of the dynamometer be aligned 1 to 2 cm distal to the acromioclavicular joint. In testing the internal/external rotation, the axis of rotation is aligned through the center of the olecranon and the shaft of the humerus.

The next parameter ensures that the subject is informed as to the purpose and the intent of the isokinetic test. The subject should be familiarized with the testing device, how it functions, and what results will be provided. An informed client will be less apprehensive and will produce more consistent, reproducible results. Two investigators have demonstrated that subjects allowed previous isokinetic exposures demonstrate significantly favorable responses on isokinetic testing. Mawdsley and Knapik[36] have reported signifi-

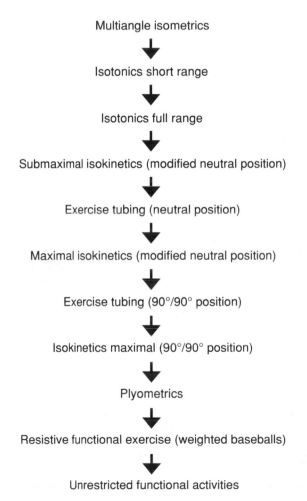

Multiangle isometrics
↓
Isotonics short range
↓
Isotonics full range
↓
Submaximal isokinetics (modified neutral position)
↓
Exercise tubing (neutral position)
↓
Maximal isokinetics (modified neutral position)
↓
Exercise tubing (90°/90° position)
↓
Isokinetics maximal (90°/90° position)
↓
Plyometrics
↓
Resistive functional exercise (weighted baseballs)
↓
Unrestricted functional activities

Fig. 8-7. Continuum of rotator cuff strengthening. (From Wilk and Arrigo,[85] with permission.)

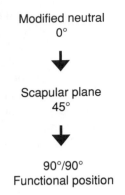

Fig. 8-8. External rotation/internal rotation rehabilitation position continuum. (From Wilk and Arrigo,[85] with permission.)

tion.[37,38] There is definite basic science research that documents the need for an active warm-up from a physiologic basis; however, this has not been found to enhance isokinetic testing.[39–42] Based on these basic exercise physiology principles, a standardized upper extremity warm-up is performed prior to isokinetic testing of the shoulder. This graded active warm-up activity includes a 5-minute upper body ergometer session (UBE) at 90 repetitions per minute at a 60 degree kg/m workload, 5 submaximal isokinetic repetitions, and 1 maximal repetition at each angular test velocity.[36]

The effects of gravity must be addressed, and therefore the authors recommend gravity compensation of the limb prior to testing. Significant differences have been demonstrated during isokinetic testing of muscle groups that were gravity compensated when compared with those that were not.[43,44] Although no specific investigations have demonstrated this fact during shoulder testing, it is generally accepted that, when gravity compensation is not used, the muscles assisted by gravity will show higher torque values, while the muscles working against gravity will demonstrate significantly smaller torque values. Also, as isokinetic angular velocities increase, so does the relative effect of gravity on torque values.[45,46] Therefore, gravity compensation should be performed prior to each test on every client.

The seventh parameter, controlling the rest interval during testing, is the next factor that must be addressed to ensure reproducibility. Ariki et al.[47] have demonstrated that the optimal period of rest between each isokinetic test speed is 90 seconds. In evaluating the

shoulder isokinetically, this time period of rest should be employed at each test speed.

Testing the uninvolved side first is the next parameter to standardize. This serves three important functions: (1) it establishes a baseline of data for the involved side, (2) it evaluates the client's willingness to be tested, and (3) it serves to decrease patient apprehension by allowing exposure to an isokinetic movement in the contralateral extremity first.[10,16]

The testing environment should be one that promotes concentration and assists in eliminating distractions. A designated room for testing is recommended to isolate the subject from interruptions, distractions, or additional activities that may impede a consistent test effort.

The verbal commands provided each client should be standardized to improve reproducibility. Johansson et al.[48] demonstrated that loud verbal commands resulted in greater isometric torque values compared with softer verbal commands. This has been empirically stated as well during manual resistance techniques.[49] Thus, it is recommended that verbal commands during isokinetic testing be consistent, encouraging, and moderate in intensity.

The subjects' knowledge of the results of torque production during testing is the third component of the testing environment to control. Several investigators have reported that knowledge of results during strength testing may enhance some parameters of performance.[50–54] Therefore, visual feedback in the form of knowledge of results can significantly influence testing performance and must be consistently used or not used during isokinetic testing. Since visual feedback has been shown to enhance torque values and promote earlier fatigue, its use is not recommended.[10,54]

The final component of the testing environment is the skill and experience of the examiner. An experienced test can greatly allay subject apprehension, improve reproducibility of testing, and maximize the efficiency and efficacy of isokinetic shoulder assessment.

The tenth guideline is the selection of the angular velocities to be used during shoulder testing. Table 8-2 illustrates the current angular velocity classifications for isokinetic testing devices. Due to the extremely high angular velocities the shoulder obtains during throwing, golf, or tennis,[19,20,25,55] testing at slow isokinetic speeds may be inappropriate and, in fact, may impart undue forces on the glenohumeral joint.[56]

Table 8-2. Isokinetic Angular Velocity Classification

15°–60°/s	60°–180°/s	180°–200°/s	300°–500°/s
Slow velocity	Intermediate velocity	Fast velocity	Functional velocity

(From Wilk and Arrigo,[85] with permission.)

Therefore, the authors recommend testing the shoulder at angular velocities of 180, 300, and 450 degrees/s.

The number of repetitions performed during isokinetic shoulder testing should be standardized. Davies[37] has previously stated that 10 isokinetic repetitions produce an optimal training effect for both peak torque and average power parameters. Based on this observation, isokinetic evaluation of the shoulder is performed using 10 repetitions at 180 degrees/s, 15 repetitions at 300 degrees/s, and 10 repetitions at 450 degrees/s. Although it has been demonstrated that peak torque for both internal and external rotation, as well as for the abductors and adductors of the shoulder, is produced during the second or third test repetition in 96 percent of all cases,[57] 10 to 15 test repetitions are used during isokinetic shoulder testing to ensure the optimal assessment of total work and average power parameters.

The twelfth parameter to consider is the significance of test system calibration. Although most manufacturers recommend calibration every 30 days to ensure validity in testing measures, the authors recommend that calibration of the testing system be performed every 2 weeks.

The next guideline is to ensure that the isokinetic system is level and stabilized to the floor. A level and stable system will minimize artifact, overshoot, and oscillation interference during testing. Each of these aberrant recordings may lead to misinterpretation of test data, especially during shoulder abduction/adduction testing.[17,58,59]

The fourteenth and final parameter concerns data collection during isokinetic testing of the shoulder. During shoulder abduction/adduction testing, there exists the potential for a tremendous amount of endstop oscillation and torque curve spiking.[58,59] These torque spikes are produced by combining the long lever arm, high test speeds, and large torque values demonstrated during testing with an abrupt terminal endpoint. Any abrupt endpoint results in the spiking of the torque curve graph far beyond the actual values produced.

The author recommends controlling this aberrant data production by using a semihard (firm) endstop and windowing the isokinetic data collection during shoulder abduction/adduction testing. An endstop is used to cushion the endrange and decelerate the lever arm during testing. A firm or semihard endstop results when the endstop control is turned one-quarter turn from the hard endpoint. This type of endstop prevents excessive deceleration produced by a soft stop or the abrupt endstop oscillation that occurs when a hard endstop is employed.[58] Endstop oscillation is also prevented by windowing the test results so that any data not obtained at the preset isokinetic test speed or at 95 percent of that speed will not be recorded.

The use of a standardized method of isokinetic assessment of the shoulder addresses one of the major pitfalls inherent in the use of isokinetic testing: not employing a standardized testing protocol with each evaluation performed. The 14 components addressed in this protocol are discussed to satisfy this limitation by outlining a clinically functional, activity-specific, and consistent means to evaluate the shoulder isokinetically. The authors feel that the overhead athlete should be tested in the 90 degrees/90 degrees seated position. The low-demand shoulder patient may be tested in a more inherently stable modified neutral or scapular plane position. The tester should use a position that places the client in the most common functional position for strenuous activities.

ISOKINETIC REHABILITATION PRINCIPLES

There are three basic categories of isokinetic exercise for the shoulder complex. These categories are (1) on-axis planes and movements, (2) scapulothoracic patterns, and (3) off-axis planes and movements. On-axis planes or movements are referred to as isolated movement patterns where the axis of rotation of the dynamometer is aligned with the axis of the joint motion. The scapulothoracic patterns are isolated movements for the scapulo-muscles, while the off-axis movements are defined as movements where the axis of the dynamometer is not aligned with the axis of joint motion.

On-Axis Planes and Movements

Shoulder Abduction/Adduction

Shoulder abduction/adduction is a movement we commonly use in the seated position (Fig. 8-6). This movement pattern attempts to isolate the shoulder abductors (deltoid, supraspinatus) and the adductors (pectoralis major, latissimus dorsi, teres major). Several authors have demonstrated a positive correlation between isokinetic shoulder adduction strength and arm velocity during throwing.[60,61] This correlation makes isokinetic exercise of this movement pattern extremely beneficial in functional strengthening of the shoulder complex.

Shoulder External/Internal Rotation

Shoulder external/internal rotation is a frequently tested movement of the shoulder. There exist numerous positions to isolate the external/internal rotation of the shoulder. These positions include neutral position (Fig. 8-5), modified position (Fig. 8-2), scapular plane (Fig. 8-3), and 90 degrees abducted position (Fig. 8-1). These positions are ranked from maximal inherent stability to minimal inherent stability. As stated previously, each position will render different torque measurements compared to another position.

Shoulder Flexion/Extension

Shoulder flexion/extension can be accomplished in several positions: seated (Fig. 8-9), prone (Fig. 8-10), supine (Fig. 8-11), and modified supine (Fig. 8-12). The supine position is frequently employed to emphasize the shoulder flexors and used to provide scapular stability (through the contact of the scapula). Conversely, the prone position is used to emphasize the shoulder extensors and to challenge the scapular stabilizing muscles.

Shoulder Horizontal Abduction/Adduction

Shoulder horizontal abduction/adduction can be employed in the supine position (Fig. 8-13). This movement is important to the overhead athlete, such as the thrower, tennis player, or racquet sport athlete, to simulate the follow-through phase. The clinician must proceed with care when using horizontal adduction

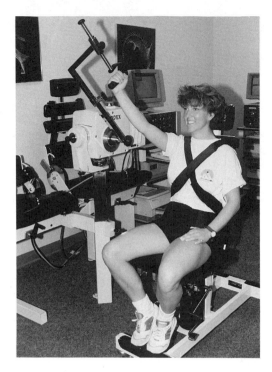

Fig. 8-9. Shoulder flexion/extension in the seated position.

because this movement can cause impingement syndrome.

Scapulothoracic Patterns

Adequate scapulothoracic muscular performance is crucial for symptom-free function of the shoulder complex. A proper exercise regimen to strengthen the scapular muscles ensures the maintenance of the normal length-tension relationship of the glenohumeral joint, a stable base from which the upper extremity can function. These three components ensure that the scapulothoracic musculature provides proximal stability for the scapula to allow distal mobility of the arm. There are two commonly used scapular patterns: scapular protraction and scapular retraction.

Scapular Protraction

A standing modified unilateral push-up activity performed isokinetically can mimic the function of the

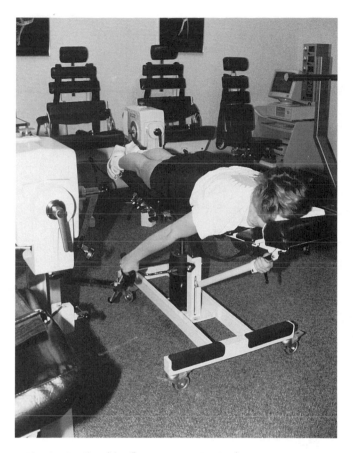

Fig. 8-10. Shoulder flexion/extension in the prone position.

serratus anterior performing a wall push-up maneuver (Fig. 8-14). It can be used both concentrically and eccentrically for serratus strengthening. The serratus anterior is an important element to scapular motion and control and must be exercised adequately to improve shoulder function.[62]

Scapular Retraction

By shortening the lever arm of motion above the elbow in the sagittal plane, the scapular retractors can be adequately strengthened isokinetically (Fig. 8-15). This motion overloads the rhomboids, middle trapezius, and posterior deltoid during scapular retraction.

Off-Axis Patterns

Supraspinatus/Scaption Exercise

As described by Jobe and others, this isokinetic exercise position approximates the muscle testing position for the supraspinatus at a 45 degree oblique plane (Fig. 8-16).[63–66] This off-axis pattern for the supraspinatus muscle can be employed for isometric or isotonic muscular contraction.

Diagonal Patterns

Diagonal combined movement patterns are exceptional exercise movements to replicate many dynamic upper extremity work and sport activities. These move-

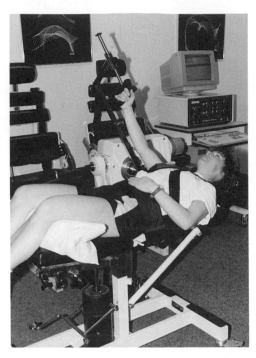

Fig. 8-11. Shoulder flexion/extension in the supine position.

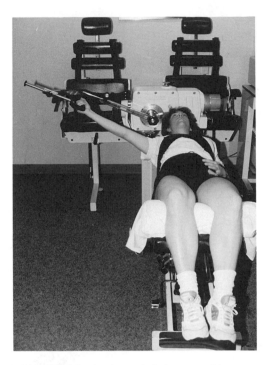

Fig. 8-13. Shoulder horizontal abduction/adduction in the supine position.

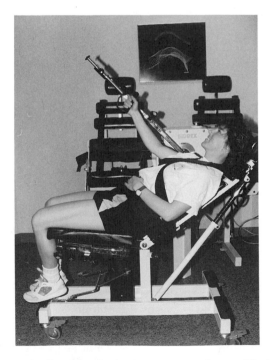

Fig. 8-12. Shoulder flexion/extension in the modified supine position; the chair is tilted approximately 45 degrees.

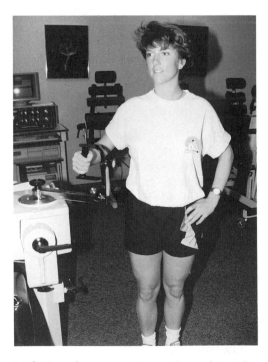

Fig. 8-14. Scapular protraction performed standing; the motion consists of a push/pull movement.

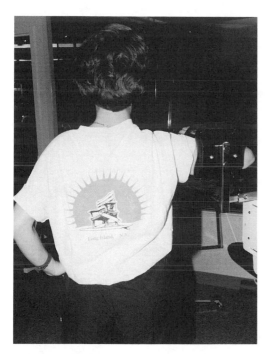

Fig. 8-15. Scapular retraction is accomplished isokinetically in the sagittal plane by shortening the knee lever arm attachment and strapping to the arm.

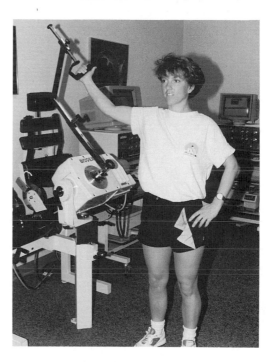

Fig. 8-17. Diagonal D_2 flexion pattern for the shoulder's abductors, flexors, and external rotators.

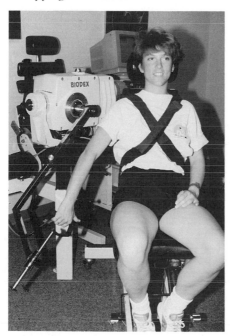

Fig. 8-16. Isolation of the supraspinatus muscle is performed in the plane of scapula. This movement is referred to as scaption.

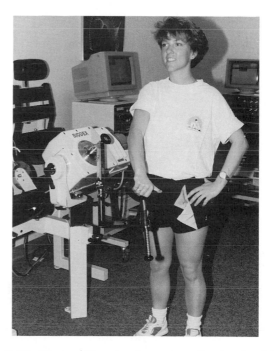

Fig. 8-18. Diagonal D_2 extension pattern for the shoulder. This movement consists of shoulder extension, adduction, and internal rotation.

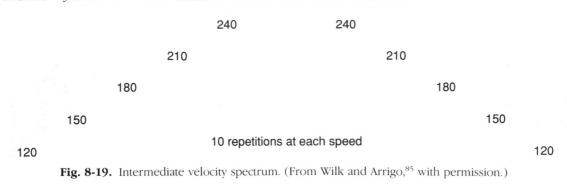

Fig. 8-19. Intermediate velocity spectrum. (From Wilk and Arrigo,[85] with permission.)

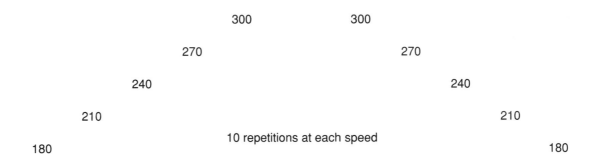

Fig. 8-20. Fast velocity spectrum. (From Wilk and Arrigo,[85] with permission.)

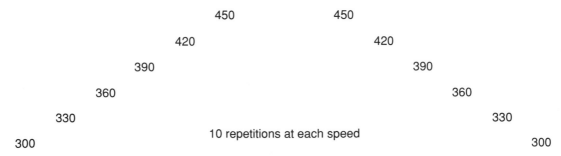

Fig. 8-21. Functional velocity spectrum. (From Wilk and Arrigo,[85] with permission.)

ments use reciprocal movement patterns and emphasize functional movements for the entire shoulder complex. The D_2 flexion pattern (abduction, flexion, external rotation) is employed to strengthen the posterior rotator cuff muscles and scapular retractors (Fig. 8-17). The D_2 extension pattern (extension, adduction, internal rotation) is used to strengthen the adductor and internal rotators of the shoulder (Fig. 8-18).

The angular velocities (isokinetic speeds) frequently used during the rehabilitation process are described in Figs. 8-19 to 8-21. These pyramids are referred to as isokinetic velocity spectrums.[16] The patient performs 10 repetitions at each of the predetermined speeds, followed by 90 seconds of rest and then 10 repetitions at the next isokinetic velocity. This process is continued until all the prescribed speeds have been performed. Figure 8-19 illustrates the intermediate velocity spectrum that is used for short movement patterns, such as shoulder external/internal rotation and scapular patterns. Figure 8-20 illustrates the fast velocity spectrum that is most often employed for larger movement patterns, such as shoulder flexion/extension and abduction/adduction. The functional velocity spectrum (Fig. 8-21) is employed for the upper extremity athletic patient and can be used for any single plane movement or diagonal pattern.

INTERPRETATION OF TEST DATA

There is a copious amount of data generated from an isokinetic evaluation of the shoulder. The data can be subdivided into topics identifying torque parameters, acceleration and deceleration characteristics, and muscular performance parameters. The remainder of this chapter will briefly define and discuss these parameters.

Torque is defined as force times the perpendicular distance from the axis of rotation. The term peak torque expresses a single repetition event that is the highest point on the graph regardless of where it occurs in the range of motion.[16] The average torque of all the test repetitions performed during one set is referred to as the mean peak torque. Mean peak torque values may prove to be more valuable information to the clinician regarding muscular performance than a single repetition peak torque value.

The test parameter referred to as time rate to torque development (TRTD) is an example of an acceleration parameter. This test parameter represents how quickly the subject can generate torque. The time rate to torque development can be expressed as a factor of time, such as TRTD at 0.2 seconds or a factor of joint position, such as at any specific joint angle or predetermined torque value. This test parameter may prove beneficial to the clinician in determining the acceleration capability of the shoulder's internal rotators.

The next test parameter to consider is the force decay rate of the torque curve or the deceleration of the muscle group. On torque curve observation it should appear straight or slightly convex. A torque curve whose force decay rate is concave indicates an inability or difficulty in producing force near the end range of motion.

The next area of data interpretation is classified as the muscular performance parameters.[67] These include total work, average power, and muscular endurance characteristics. Total work is defined as torque times an arc of movement. It represents the volume of area contained in the torque curve. The term maximum work repetition is the single repetition during which the maximum amount of work occurred. Average power is torque times an arc of movement divided by time, or work divided by time. This parameter is represented in watts. Both work and power can also be expressed in relation to body weight, such as work to body weight ratios. Additionally, work can be expressed as work in the first third and work in the last third of the repetition set. This represents the total amount of work performed in the first 33.3 percent of the test repetition set and work in the last third is the last 33.3 percent. The work fatigue percentage is the ratio of change between the first third and the last third of any test.

There exists a copious amount of data that can be produced by an isokinetic shoulder test. This vast amount of data has created a paradoxical situation for the tester. There are three commonly used parameters for data interpretation of the shoulder. These are (1) bilateral comparison, (2) unilateral data comparison, and (3) torque to body ratios. The current literature has produced significant controversy in data comparison. Some of this confusion may be attributed to the inconsistencies in the test positions used. Several investigators have demonstrated significant differences

Table 8-3. Comparison of Mean Peak Torque ± SD (Ft-Lb) between Dominant (D) and Nondominant (ND) Throwing Arms for Shoulder External/Internal Rotation[a]

Test Speed	External Rotation		Internal Rotation	
	D (ft-lb)	ND (ft-lb)	D (ft-lb)	ND (ft-lb)
180°/s	34.5 ± 6.2	36.5 ± 6.8[b]	53.9 ± 8.8	52.4 ± 9.5
300°/s	29.3 ± 5.1	30.1 ± 6.3	49.0 ± 8.5	48.0 ± 10.4

[a] n = 150.
[b] Respective pair showed statistically significant difference ($P < 0.05$).
(From Wilk and Arrigo,[85] with permission.)

Table 8-4. Mean Peak Torque ± SD (Ft-Lb) between Dominant (D) and Nondominant (ND) Throwing Arms for Shoulder Abduction/Adduction[a]

Test Speed	Abduction		Adduction	
	D (ft-lb)	ND (ft-lb)	D (ft-lb)	ND (ft-lb)
180°/s	56.1 ± 12.5	58.6 ± 9.7	68.1 ± 12.6	62.5 ± 10.5[b]
300°/s	40.3 ± 15.7	38.4 ± 14.7	61.0 ± 12.5	54.6 ± 13.2[b]

[a] n = 131.
[b] Statistically significant difference ($P < 0.05$) between respective pairs.
(From Wilk and Arrigo,[85] with permission.)

between results gathered on various testing devices.[68–72] Results of isokinetic testing cannot be compared from one device or system to results from another device or system.

In regards to bilateral comparison of peak torque of the dominant versus nondominant shoulder, Wilk et al.[73] have reported their results of isokinetic testing of 150 professional baseball pitchers. The results indicate, with regard to bilateral comparison of external/internal rotation testing, that the throwing shoulder is equal to the nonthrowing shoulder (Table 8-3). The

bilateral comparison of abduction/adduction indicated no significant differences in peak torque for the shoulder's abductors while the adductors exhibited a significant difference at both test speeds (180 and 300 degrees/s)[59] (Table 8-4). Table 8-5 illustrates the collective work of various investigators who have documented bilateral peak torque comparisons of the shoulder.

Unilateral muscle ratios express the balance between the agonist and antagonist muscle groups. Several investigators have published data regarding external/internal rotation ratios of the shoulder.[16,74–77] Ivey[78] has reported a ratio of 66 percent at 60, 180, and 300 degrees/s. Cook et al.[76] demonstrated an external/internal rotation ratio of 70 percent at 180 and 300 degrees/s on the throwing shoulder and a ratio of 83 and 87 percent at the respective speeds for the nonthrowing shoulder.[76] Davies[16] reported a ratio of 66.6 percent at 60 and 300 degrees/s. Table 8-6 represents the external/internal rotation unilateral muscle ratios for the shoulder from various investigators. The unilateral muscle ratio for the shoulder abductors/adductors has been reported to be 2 to 1 by several authors.[74,78] Wilk et al.[59] has found the abduction/adduction ratio for the dominant shoulder (throwing shoulder) to be 83 and 94 percent at 180 and 300 degrees/s. The nondominant shoulder abduction/adduction muscular ratio is 66 and 70 percent at the reported speeds.[59] Table 8-7 represents the collective work values of various authors regarding the abduction/adduction muscle ratios of the shoulder.

The last torque parameter expressed in the literature is torque to body weight ratios. Table 8-8 represents the torque to body weights ratios for the shoulder external/internal rotation and abductors/adductors.[59,73]

Table 8-5. Bilateral Comparisons

	Dominant Stronger	Nondominant Stronger	Equal Bilateral
External rotation	Brown et al.[75]	Alderink and Kuck,[74] Hinton[28]	Cook et al.,[76] Ivey et al.,[78] Jobe, Wilk et al.[73]
Internal rotation	Brown et al.,[75] Cook et al.,[76] Hinton[28]	—	Alderink and Kuck,[74] Ivey et al.,[78] Jobe,[63] Wilk et al.[73]
Abduction	—	—	Alderink and Kuck,[74] Wilk et al.[73]
Adduction	Alderink and Kuck,[74] Wilk et al.[73]	—	—
Flexion	—	—	Alderink and Kuck,[74] Cook et al.,[76]
Extension	Alderink and Kuck[74]	—	Cook et al.[76]

(From Wilk and Arrigo,[85] with permission).

Table 8-6. Unilateral Muscle Ratios

		Degrees/s						
		60	90	120	180	210	240	300
Alderink and	D	—	66	68	—	71	—	70
Kuck[74]	ND	—	70	72	—	76	—	76
Brown et al.[75]	D	—	—	—	67	—	61	65
	ND	—	—	—	71	—	66	65
Cook et al.[76]	D	—	—	—	70	—	—	70
	ND	—	—	—	81	—	—	81
Davies[16]		64	—	—	—	—	—	66.6
Hinton[28]	D	—	69	—	—	—	71	—
	ND	—	76	—	—	—	80	—
Ivey et al.[78]		66	—	—	66	—	—	—
Wilk et al.[73]	D	—	—	—	65	—	—	61
	ND	—	—	—	64	—	—	70

Abbreviations: D, dominant shoulder; ND, nondominant shoulder.
(From Wilk and Arrigo,[85] with permission.)

It should be noted that there may exist differences in isokinetic muscular performance among various types of sporting athletes, subject's age and skill, and pathologic condition. For that reason, Tables 8-9, 8-10, and 8-11 represent descriptive data from several authors regarding tennis players[79-83] and swimmers.[83,84] These data are provided to assist the reader in the interpretation of the isokinetic shoulder test data in various overhead athletic populations.

When interpreting the results of an isokinetic shoulder test, 10 key parameters have been identified for routine evaluation and interpretation. These parameters are

1. Bilateral peak torque comparison
2. Unilateral muscle ratios
3. Torque/body weight ratios
4. Bilateral work comparison
5. Bilateral average power comparisons
6. Work/body weight ratios
7. Power/body weight ratios
8. Torque at 0.2 sec for internal rotation (TRTD)
9. Endurance—work fatigue rate
10. Acceleration/deceleration parameters

There exist several pitfalls that should be avoided when performing an isokinetic shoulder test. First, the test/retest should be performed in the identical position, at the same speeds, and using the same testing protocol.[10,17,18] When the test position or protocol is altered, the test results will be significantly affected. The second pitfall is only interpreting bilateral peak

Table 8-7. Unilateral Muscle Ratios Abduction/Adduction

		Degrees/s					
		60	90	120	180	210	300
Alderink and Kuck[74]	D	—	54	54	—	50	51
	ND	—	57	57	—	52	50
Davies[16]		66	—	—	56	—	46
Ivey et al.[78]		50	—	—	50	—	50
Wilk et al.[67]	D	—	—	—	83	—	94
	ND	—	—	—	66	—	70

Abbreviations: D, dominant shoulder; ND, nondominant shoulder.
(From Wilk and Arrigo,[85] with permission.)

torque comparisons to determine patients' progress.[10,67] The review of the literature in this chapter illustrates that bilateral comparisons are inconsistent, and specifically altered by test position. Next, do not rely on torque curve shapes to determine various pathologies. The author has experienced after several hundred preoperative tests that torque curves are not consistently generated by any specific shoulder pathologies. Fourth, do not solely rely on peak torque measurements to determine a patient's status. Power, work, and time parameters must be considered to determine muscular performance. Next, realize this is not the only test. Rely on your clinical examination, functional testing, and special tests to assist in determining the condition of the shoulder. Lastly, the tester should window all test data to prevent misinterpretation.

In conclusion, the shoulder exhibits tremendous motion with inherently poor stability. The dynamic stabilizers (neuromuscular control) provide the shoulder with much needed stability during various functional activities. Due to the many imposed demands on the shoulder musculature, the clinician must routinely assess the status of the neuromuscular system in an objective, reliable, and reproducible method. Isokinetics provides the clinician with a reproducible, objective,

Table 8-8. Torque to Body Weight Ratios

Degrees/s	Abduction		Adduction		External Rotation		Internal Rotation	
	D	ND	D	ND	D	ND	D	ND
90	27	26	50	46	15	15	22	22
120	25	25	47	45	14	15	21	21
210	21	21	43	41	13	14	19	19
300	18	18	36	36	13	13	18	18

Abbreviations: D, dominant; ND, nondominant.
(From Alderink and Kuck,[74] with permission.)

Table 8-9. Isokinetic Muscular Performance Data of Collegiate Tennis Players

	Men			Women		
	60°/s	180°/s	210°/s	60°/s	180°/s	210°/s
Eccentric PT/BW ratio ER	80	80	77	46	47	46
Eccentric PT/BW ratio IR	99	91	96	56	56	57
Concentric PT/BW ratio ER	43	41	40	25	22	22
Concentric PT/BW ratio IR	59	49	50	34	27	25
ER/IR ratio concentric	59	49	50	80	82	89
ER/IR ratio eccentric	84	92	81	87	93	89
Eccentric/concentric ratio ER	202	206	202	103	107	119
Eccentric/concentric ratio IR	183	202	201	123	143	173

Abbreviations: PT, peak torque; BW, body weight; ER, external rotation; IR, internal rotation.
(From Ellenbecker,[80] wither permission.)

and safe muscular performance testing and exercise tool. The clinician is encouraged to use a standardized testing protocol to improve test-retest reproducibility. Additionally, a standardized testing protocol will allow clinicians to compare and share data, thereby opening effective communication among sports medicine practitioners.

Table 8-10. Isokinetic Muscular Performance Data of Collegiate Tennis Players

	Dominant		Nondominant	
	60°/s	300°/s	60°/s	300°/s
Internal Rotation (PT)	30	21	24	16
External Rotation (PT)	18	13	17	11
IR Torque/Body Weight	20	13	15	10
ER Torque/Body Weight	12	8	11	7
ER/IR	61	65	70	69

Abbreviations: IR, internal rotation; PT, peak torque; ER, external rotation; BW, body weight.
(From Chandler et al[81] with permission.)

Table 8-11. Isokinetic Muscular Performance Data of Scholastic Swimmers[a]

	120°/s			180°/s		
	IR	ER	ER/IR	IR	ER	ER/IR
Pretraining	36	20	57%	32	19	58%
Post 3-week training program	42	32	75%	41	30	73%

Abbreviations: IR, internal rotation; ER, external rotation.
[a] All values expressed represent peak torque in ft-lb.
(Unpublished data from Murphy TS.) (From Wilk and Arrigo,[85] with permission.)

REFERENCES

1. Inman VT, Saunders M, Abbott LC: Observations on the function of the shoulder joint. J Bone Joint Surg 26:1, 1944
2. Matsen FA, Harryman DT, Sidles JA: Mechanics of shoulder instability. Clin Sports Med 10:783, 1991
3. Saha AK: Dynamic stability of the glenohumeral joint. Acta Orthop Scand 42:491, 1971
4. Silliman JF, Hawkins RJ: Current concepts and recent advances in the athlete's shoulder. Clin Sports Med 10:18, 1991
5. Williams PL, Warwick R, Dyson M, Bannister LH: Gray's Anatomy. p. 456. 36th Ed., Churchill Livingstone, Edinburgh, 1980
6. Wright W: Muscle training in the treatment of infantile paralysis. Boston Med Surg 167:567, 1912
7. Kendall FD, McCreary EK: Muscle Testing and Function. 3rd Ed. Williams & Wilkins, Baltimore, 1983
8. Daniels L, Worthingham C: Muscle Testing: Techniques of Manual Examination. 5th Ed. W.B. Saunders, Philadelphia, 1986
9. Mayhew TP, Rothstein JM: Measurement of muscular performance with instruments. p. 57. In Rothstein JM (ed): Measurement in Physical Therapy. Churchill Livingstone, New York, 1985
10. Wilk KE: Dynamic muscle strength testing. p. 123. In Amundsen LR (ed): Muscle Strength Testing: Instrumented and Noninstrumented Systems. Churchill Livingstone, New York, 1990
11. Iddings D, Smith L, Spencer W: Muscle testing, part 2: reliability in clinical use. Phys Ther Rev 41:249, 1961
12. Wintz M: Variations in current manual muscle testing. Phys Ther Rev 39:466, 1959
13. Nicholas J, Sapega A, Kraus H, Webb J: Factors influencing

manual muscle tests in physical therapy. J Bone Joint Surg 60A:186, 1978

14. Nitz M: Variations in current manual muscle testing. Phys Ther Rev 39:466, 1959

15. Wilk KE, Arrigo CE, Andrews JR, Hinger DE: A comparison of manual muscle test results to isokinetic peak torque results in 100 ACL reconstructed knees. Presented at the Annual Conference of the American Physical Therapy Association, Denver, CO, June 15, 1992

16. Davies GJ: A Compendium of Isokinetics in Clinical Usage. 3rd Ed. S & S Publishers, Onolaska, WI, 1987

17. Wilk KE, Arrigo CA, Andrews JR: Standardized isokinetic testing protocol for the throwing shoulder: the thrower's series. Isokinet Exerc Sci 1:63, 1991

18. Byl NN, Wells L, Grady D et al: Consistency of repeated isokinetic testing: effect of different examiners, sites, and protocols. Isokinet Exerc Sci 1:122, 1991

19. Dillman CJ: Biomechanics of pitching. Presented at the 1991 Injuries in Baseball Conference, Birmingham, AL, January 25, 1990

20. Dillman CJ, Fleisig GS, Werner SL, Andrews JR: Biomechanics of the Shoulder in Sports: Throwing Activities. Post Graduate Studies in Physical Therapy, Forum Medicum, Inc., Pennington, NJ, 1990

21. Jobe FW, Tibone JE, Perry J et al: An EMG analysis of the shoulder in throwing and pitching. A preliminary report. Am J Sports Med 11:3, 1983

22. Jobe FW, Moynes DR, Tibone JE et al: An EMG analysis of the shoulder in pitching. A second report. Am J Sports Med 12:218, 1984

23. Figoni SF, Morris AF: Effects of knowledge of results on reciprocal isokinetic strength and fatigue. J Orthop Sports Phys Ther 6:104, 1984

24. Pappas AM, Zawacki RM, McCarthy CF: Rehabilitation of the pitching shoulder. Am J Sports Med 13:223, 1985

25. Pappas AM, Zawacki RM, Sullivan TJ: Biomechanics of baseball pitching. A preliminary report. Am J Sports Med 13:216, 1985

26. Soderberg GJ, Blaschek MJ: Shoulder internal and external rotation peak torque production through a velocity spectrum in differing positions. J Orthop Sports Phys Ther 8:518, 1987

27. Greenfield BH, Donatelli R, Wooden MJ, Wilken J: Isokinetic evaluation of shoulder rotational strength between plane of the scapula and functional plane. Am J Sports Med 18:124, 1990

28. Hinton RY: Isokinetic evaluation of shoulder rotational strength in high school baseball pitchers. Am J Sports Med 16:274, 1988

29. Hageman PA, Mason KD, Rydlund KW et al: Effects of position and speed on eccentric and concentric isoki-netic testing of the shoulder rotators. J Orthop Sports Phys Ther 11:64, 1989

30. Hellwig EV, Perrin DH: A comparison of two positions for assessing shoulder rotator peak torque: the traditional frontal plane versus the plane of the scapula. Isokinetic Exerc Sci 1:202, 1991

31. Ellenbecker TS, Feiring DC, Dehart RL: Isokinetic shoulder strength: coronal versus scapular plane testing in upper extremity unilaterally dominant athletes. Presented at the Annual Conference of the American Physical Therapy Association, Denver, CO, June 15, 1992

32. Walmsley RP, Szybbo C: A comparative study of the torque generated by the shoulder internal and external rotators in different positions and at varying speeds. J Orthop Sports Phys Ther 9:217, 1987

33. Johnson RJ, Wilk KE: The effects of lever arm pad placement upon the isokinetic torque during knee extension and flexion. Phys Ther 68:779, 1988

34. Siewert MW, Ariki PK, Davies GJ et al: Isokinetic torque changes based on lever arms placement. Phys Ther 65:715, 1985

35. Taylor RC, Casey JJ: Quadriceps torque production on the Cybex II dynamometer as related to changes in lever arm length. J Orthop Sports Phys Ther 8:147, 1986

36. Mawdsley RH, Knapik JJ: Comparison of isokinetic measurements with test repetitions. Phys Ther 62:169, 1982

37. Davies GJ: Cybex II isokinetic dynamometer measurements on the acute effects of direct active warm-ups and direct passive warm-ups on knee extension/flexion and power. Presented at the Annual Conference of the American Physical Therapy Association, Las Vegas, NV, June 20, 1978

38. Wiktorsson-Moller M, Oberg B, Edstrand V et al: Effects of warming up, massage and strengthening on range of motion and muscle strength in the lower extremity. Am J Sports Med 11:249, 1983

39. Asmussen E, Boje O: Body temperature and capacity for work. Acta Physiol Scand 10:1, 1945

40. Astrand PO, Rodahl K: Textbook of Work Physiology: Physiologic Basis of Exercise. 2nd Ed. McGraw-Hill, New York, 1977

41. Franks DB: Physical warm-up. In Morgan WP (eds): Ergogenic Aids and Muscular Performance. Academic Press, Orlando, FL, 1972

42. Martin BV, Robinson S, Wiogoma DC et al: Effect of warm-up on metabolic responses to strenuous exercise. Med Sci Sports Exerc 7:146, 1975

43. Caizzo VJ: Alterations in the in vivo force velocity curve. Med Sci Sports Exerc 12:134, 1980

44. Fillyaw M, Bevins T, Fernandez L: Importance of correcting isokinetic peak torque for the effect of gravity when

calculating knee flexor to extensor muscle ratios. Phys Ther 66:23, 1986

45. Nelson SG, Duncan PW: Correction of isokinetic and isometric torque recordings for the effects of gravity. Phys Ther 63:674, 1983

46. Winter DA, Wells RP, Orr GW: Errors in the use of isokinetic dynamometers. Eur J Appl Physiol 46:317, 1981

47. Ariki PK, Davies GJ, Siewert MW et al: Optimum rest interval between isokinetic velocity spectrum rehabilitation speeds, abstracted. Phys Ther 65:735, 1985

48. Johansson CA, Kent BE, Shepard KF: Relationship between verbal command volume and magnitude of muscle contraction. Phys Ther 63:1260, 1983

49. Knott M, Voss D: Proprioceptive neuromuscular facilitation. p. 84. Hoeber Medical Division, Harper & Row, New York, 1968

50. Hald RD, Bottken EJ: Effects of visual feedback on maximal and submaximal isokinetic test measurements of normal quadriceps and hamstring. J Orthop Sports Phys Ther 9:86, 1987

51. Manzer CW: The effect of knowledge of output on muscle work. J Exp Psychol 18:80, 1935

52. Pierson WR, Rasch PJ: Effect of knowledge of results on isometric strength scores. Res Q 35:313, 1964

53. Ulrich C, Burke RK: Effect of motivational stress on physical performance. Res Q 28:403, 1957

54. Figoni SF, Christ CB, Massey BH: Effects of speed, hip and knee angle, and gravity on hamstring to quadriceps torque ratios. J Orthop Sports Phys Ther 9:287, 1988

55. Bradley JP, Tibone JE: Electromyographic analysis of muscle action about the shoulder. Clin Sports Med 10:789, 1991

56. Elsner RC, Pedegana LR, Lang J: Protocol for strength testing and rehabilitation of the upper extremity. J Orthop Sports Phys Ther 4:229, 1983

57. Arrigo CA, Wilk KE: Peak torque and total work repetition during isokinetic testing of the shoulder. Isokinet Exerc Sci, 1993 (in press)

58. Wilk KE, Arrigo CA, Keirns MA: Shoulder abduction/adduction isokinetic test results: Window vs unwindow data collection. J Orthop Sports Phys Ther 15:107, 1992

59. Wilk KE, Andrews JR, Arrigo CA et al: The isokinetic abductor and adductor strength characteristics of professional baseball pitchers. Am J Sports Med, 1991 (in press)

60. Bartlett LR, Storey MD, Simons BD: Measurement of upper extremity torque production and its relationship to throwing speed in the competitive athlete. Am J Sports Med 17:89, 1989

61. Pedegana LR, Elsner R, Roberts D et al: The relationship of upper extremity strength to throwing speed. Am J Sports Med 10:352, 1982

62. Moseley JB, Jobe FW, Pink M et al: EMG analysis of the scapular muscles during a shoulder rehabilitation program. Am J Sports Med 20:128, 1992

63. Jobe FW, Bradley JP: Rotator cuff injuries in baseball: prevention and rehabilitation. Sports Med 6:378, 1980

64. Jobe FW, Moynes DR: Delineation of diagnostic criteria and a rehabilitation program for rotator cuff injuries. Am J Sports Med 10:336, 1982

65. Deluca CJ, Forrest WJ: Force analysis of individual muscles acting simultaneously on the shoulder joint during isometric abduction. J Bromech 6:385, 1973

66. Townsend H, Jobe FW, Pink M, Perry J: Electromyographic analysis of the glenohumeral muscles during a baseball rehabilitation program. Am J Sports Med 19:264, 1991

67. Wilk KE: Isokinetic testing and exercise for the shoulder complex. Presented at Annual Conference Biodex Corporation, Ft. Lauderdale, FL, October 3, 1991

68. Francis K, Hoobler T: Comparison of peak torques of the knee flexor and extensor muscle groups using the Cybex II and Lido 2.0 isokinetic dynamometers. J Orthop Sports Phys Ther 8:480, 1987

69. Wilk KE, Johnson RJ: A comparison of peak torque values of knee extensors and flexor muscle groups using the Biodex, Cybex, Kin-Com isokinetic dynamometer. Phys Ther 67:789, 1987

70. Wilk KE, Johnson RJ: A comparison of peak torque values of knee extensor and flexor muscle groups using the Biodex, Cybex, and Lido isokinetic dynamometer. Phys Ther 68:792, 1988

71. Thompson MC, Shingleton LG, Kegerreis ST: Comparison of values generated during testing of the knee using the Cybex II + and Biodex mode B-2000 isokinetic dynamometers. J Orthop Sports Phys Ther 11:108, 1989

72. Gross MT, Huffman GM, Phillips CN, Wray JA: Intramachine and intermachine reliability of the Biodex, Cybex for knee flexion and extension peak torque and angular work. J Orthop Sports Phys Ther 13:329, 1991

73. Wilk KE, Andrews JR, Arrigo CA et al: The internal and external rotator strength characteristics of professional baseball pitchers. Am J Sports Med 21:61, 1993

74. Alderink GJ, Kuck DJ: Isokinetic shoulder strength of high school and college aged pitchers. J Orthop Sports Phys Ther 7:163, 1986

75. Brown LP, Niehues SL, Harrah A et al: Upper extremity range of motion and isokinetic strength of the internal and external shoulder rotators in major league baseball players. Am J Sports Med 16:577, 1988

76. Cook EE, Gray VL, Savinor-Nogue E et al: Shoulder antagonistic strength ratios: a comparison between college-level baseball pitchers. J Orthop Sports Phys Ther 8:451, 1987

77. Williams M: Manual muscle testing, development and current use. Phys Ther Rev 36:717, 1956

78. Ivey FM, Calhoun JH, Rusche K et al: Normal values for isokinetic testing of shoulder strength, abstracted. Med Sci Sports Exerc 16:274, 1988

79. Ellenbecker TS: Eccentric and concentric isokinetic strength characteristics of the rotator cuff: presented at the 1991 Annual Conference of the American Physical Therapy Association, Boston, MA, June 20, 1991

80. Ellenbecker TS: A total arm strength profile of highly skilled tennis players. Isokinet Exerc Sci 1:9, 1991

81. Chandler TJ, Kibler WB, Stracener EC et al: Shoulder strength, power, and endurance in college tennis players. Am J Sports Med 20:455, 1992

82. Kibler WB, McQueen C, Uhl T: Fitness evaluations and fitness findings in competitive junior tennis players. Clin Sports Med 7:403, 1988

83. Ng LR, Kramer JS: Shoulder rotator torques in female tennis and non-tennis players. J Orthop Sports Phys Ther 13:40, 1991

84. Falkel JE, Murphy TC, Murray TF: Prone positioning for testing shoulder internal and external rotation on the Cybex II isokinetic dynamometer. J Orthop Sports Phys Ther 8:368, 1987

85. Wilk KE, Arrigo CA: Isokinetic exercise and testing for the shoulder complex. In Andrews JR, Wilk KE (eds): Athlete's Shoulder. Churchill Livingstone, New York, 1993

9
Radiography

JOAN DAVIS

The osseous structures that comprise the bony architecture of the shoulder girdle include the proximal humerus and humeral head, body of the scapula, glenoid process, acromion and corocoid processes, and clavicle. The anatomic arrangement of these structures allows for a greater degree of motion than in any other joint in the body. Stability of the joint is compromised as a result of the small size of the glenoid fossa relative to the large articular surface of the humeral head. The contiguous soft tissue structures include the joint capsule, ligaments, muscles, and tendons, all of which contribute to the stability of the joint. However, the shoulder remains susceptible to trauma.

While nonathletic shoulder injuries occur frequently, sports injuries to the shoulder are the result of a particular pattern of motion or combination of motions causing injuries that are sport specific. The clinician treating sports injuries encounters a wide variety of shoulder conditions. Awareness of specific injury patterns allows the clinician to perform a more revealing physical examination as well as determine the most appropriate projections to include in the radiographic examination. Indications for specific radiographic examinations of the shoulder (Table 9-1) and a discussion of the more frequently occurring sports-related injuries of the shoulder and their radiographic diagnosis are presented in this chapter.

ROUTINE AND OPTIONAL RADIOGRAPHIC VIEWS

For most radiographic examinations, it is essential that a minimum of two projections at right angles to one another be obtained. The size and shape of an object cannot be fully appreciated from a single view. Complete examinations of extremities usually consist of frontal and lateral projections and frequently an oblique projection as well. Anything else constitutes an incomplete and legally indefensible examination.

The objective of the radiographic examination of the shoulder should be considered prior to x-ray examination. The examination should be tailored to rule out or confirm the suspected condition. Potential subtle radiographic findings related to specific sports injuries may contribute to the decision.

There are a number of radiographic projections that can be utilized in the evaluation of the shoulder girdle; however, there is some variability in what is considered the routine radiographic examination. Most views are taken at a focal film distance of 40 inches unless otherwise specified. Most projections will fit on 8 × 10 cassettes unless otherwise specified.

Glenohumeral Projections

Anterior Posterior Projection

In most instances the shoulder is evaluated by the anterior posterior (AP) view obtained with the humerus in both internal rotation and external rotation (Fig. 9-1). In the past these views were taken with the patient's back against the bucky, which in reality gave an oblique view of the glenohumeral joint due to the angulation of the scapula between 30 and 45 degrees forward. At present, most facilities take these views in the plane line of the scapula by rotating the patient 30 to 45 degrees.[1] These views demonstrate the proximal hu-

Table 9-1. Radiographic Projections: Structures Demonstrated and Findings

Projection	Structures Demonstrated	Radiographic Findings
AP neutral	Proximal humerus	Proximal humeral fracture
	Glenohumeral joint	Clavicular fracture
	Scapula	Scapular fracture
	Acromioclavicular joint	Anterior glenohumeral dislocation
	Distal clavicle	Calcific tendinitis
		Osteolysis of distal clavicle
AP with 30° caudad tilt	Acromioclavicular joint	Spur formation, acromial morphology
AP internal rotation	Proximal humerus	Lesser tuberosity fracture
	Lesser tuberosity	
AP external rotation	Proximal humerus	Humeral head compression fracture
	Greater tuberosity	
Transthoracic	Proximal humerus	Posterior glenohumeral dislocation
	Glenoid fossa	
Anterior oblique	Scapula	Proximal humeral fracture
		Posterior glenohumeral dislocation
Posterior oblique	Glenohumeral joint	Posterior glenohumeral dislocation
	Glenoid fossa	
AP axial	Glenohumeral joint	Posterior glenohumeral dislocation
Apical oblique	Glenohumeral joint	Hill-Sachs lesion
		Bankart lesion
Stryker	Posterior superior humeral head	Hill-Sachs lesion
West Point	Anterior inferior glenoid fossa	Bankart lesion
Tangential	Bicipital groove	Fracture of tuberosities
	Axial acromioclavicular joint	
AP acromioclavicular	Acromioclavicular joint	Acromioclavicular sprain/separation
	Acromion process	Osteolysis distal clavicle
	Distal clavicle	Distal clavicular fracture
PA clavicle	Clavicle	Clavicular fracture
AP scapula	Scapula	Scapular fracture
Lateral scapula		
Y view	Proximal humerus	Posterior dislocation
Serendipity view	Clavicle, sternoclavicular joint, manubrium	Sternoclavicular dislocation
Hobb's view		
PA sternoclavicular joints		
Oblique sternoclavicular joints		

merus, humeral head and tuberosities, glenohumeral joint, clavicle, acromioclavicular joints, and scapula. They are sufficient to demonstrate gross trauma in most instances as well as most osseous pathologies and limited soft tissue abnormalities. The posterior oblique or Grashey's projection is essentially the same as the true AP with internal rotation. In the athlete 40 years of age and older and in the smoker, the apex of the ipsilateral lung should be included to rule out rib and/ or lung pathology as the etiology of pain[2] (Fig. 9-2).

The transthoracic lateral projection provides a view tangential to the AP and demonstrates the proximal humerus and its relationship to the glenoid fossa. This view is technically difficult to obtain and as a result is often inadequate. It also superimposes the ribs and other structures over the humerus.

Anterior Oblique (Y) Projection

The anterior-oblique (Y) projection, although not truly tangential to the AP, is useful in demonstrating proximal humerus fractures as well as posterior humeral head dislocations that may be easily overlooked on the AP view. In addition, the scapula is well demonstrated. This view does not require painful positioning of the patient (Fig. 9-3).

Axial Projections

Routine radiographic examination of the shoulder may include an axial projection. Axial projections provide tangential visualization of the glenohumeral joint and margins of the glenoid process with minimal superimposition of adjacent bony structures and are useful in

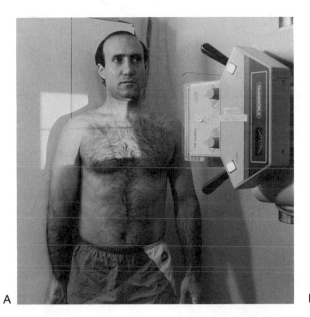 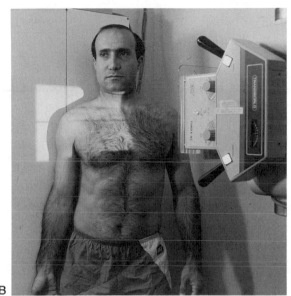

Fig. 9-1. True AP view of the shoulder taken with 30 to 45 degrees angulation of the patient into the scapular plane. **(A)** Internal rotation, **(B)** external rotation.

the detection of both anterior and posterior humeral head dislocations. There are several variations of the axial projection. These include the standard axial view with an abducted humerus, the AP inferosuperior axial projection (Lawrence method, Fig. 9-4), and the posterior anterior (PA) inferosuperior projection (West Point projection, Fig. 9-5), all of which necessitate painful and/or impossible abduction of the humerus. Axial projections that do not necessitate abduction of the humerus are the Velpeau (Fig. 9-6) and the Stripp pro-

jections. The Stripp projection is similar to the Velpeau, but the beam is directed superiorly with the cassette held above the shoulder. The Hermodsson view is a modification of the Stripp projection with the beam angled 30 degrees (Fig. 9-7).

Apical Oblique Projections

The apical oblique projection is extremely useful in the demonstration of glenohumeral dislocations and the Hill-Sachs and Bankart lesions, which frequently

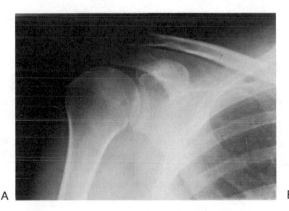 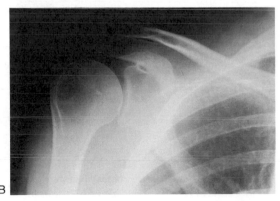

Fig. 9-2. **(A)** Internal rotation, and **(B)** external rotation views of the shoulder including the apex of the lungs.

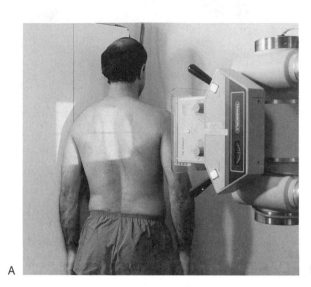

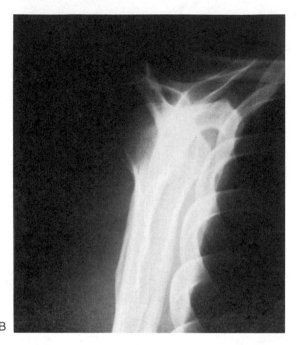

A   B

Fig. 9-3. (A) Positioning for the anterior oblique (Y) view is with the patient angled so that the spine of the scapula is perpendicular to the film. This is usually between 30 and 35 degrees. **(B)** Y projection.

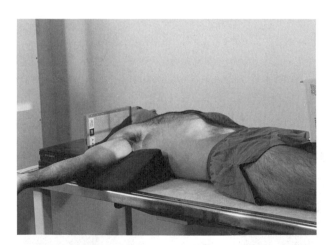

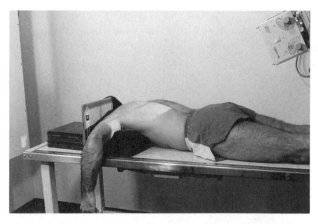

Fig. 9-4. The Lawrence axillary view is positioned with the patient supine with the shoulder abducted and externally rotated. It should be elevated 2 to 3 inches from the table. The head is turned away from the involved side. The beam is essentially horizontal and directed medially about 25 degrees. If the tube does not rotate, the patient or table may need to be turned to acquire this medial angulation.

Fig. 9-5. The West Point view is performed with the patient prone, the shoulder abducted about 90 degrees. Elevation is accomplished with padding. The beam is angled 25 degrees caudad and 25 degrees medial. If the tube does not allow medial angulation, changing the position of the table or patient may simulate this position.

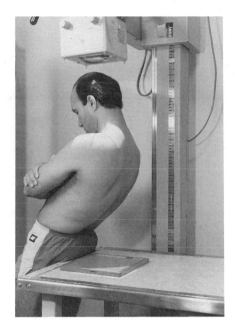

Fig. 9-6. The Velpeau axillary view is more accessible for acute patients. The patient leans back about 30 degrees.

accompany dislocation (Fig. 9-8). Similar to a true AP view the beam is then angled 45 degrees caudad. Another version is referred to as the Didiee view. This is essentially a posterior oblique projection with the beam angled superiorly (Fig. 9-9).

Stryker (Notch) Projection

The Stryker notch projection demonstrates the superior posterior aspect of the humeral head tangentially and as a result is valuable in the diagnosis of Hill-Sachs lesions (Fig. 9-10).

Tangential (Fisk) Projection

The tangential projection is primarily intended for evaluation of the bicipital groove, but it also provides an axial projection of the acromioclavicular joint (Fig. 9-11). The bicipital groove may be superimposed by the acromion process.

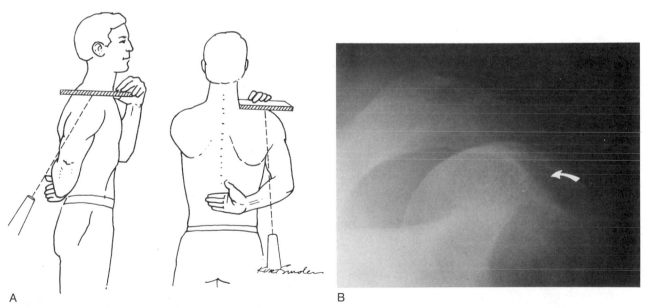

A   B

Fig. 9-7. **(A)** The Hermodsson view is performed with the patient standing holding the cassette above the shoulder parallel to the floor with the uninvolved hand. The involved arm is placed behind the back. The beam is angled superiorly with an angulation of 30 degrees. **(B)** Hill-Sachs defect *(arrow)*. (Fig. **A** from Resnick and Niwayama,[39] with permission; Fig. **B** from Rafii et al,[38] with permission.)

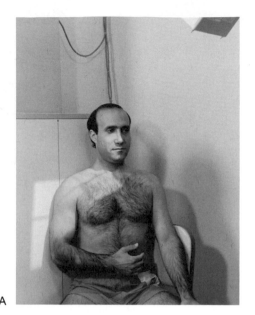

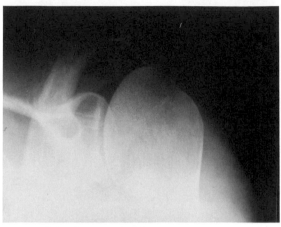

Fig. 9-8. (A) The apical oblique projection is accomplished by positioning the patient for a true AP projection while angling the tube 45 degrees caudad. **(B)** Although giving a distorted view of the humerus, this view is sensitive for glenoid defects and Hill-Sachs lesions. This is a normal view.

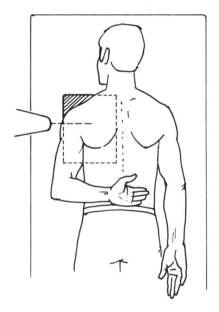

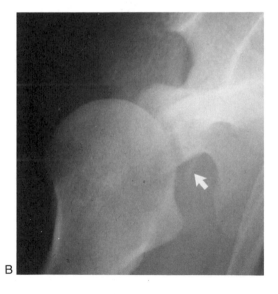

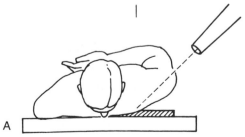

Fig. 9-9. (A) The Didiee view is performed with the patient prone and arm behind the back. The tube is angled 45 degrees. **(B)** Anterior instability. Osseous Bankart lesion is visualized *(arrow)*. (Fig. **A** from Resnick and Niwayama,[39] with permission; Fig. **B** from Rafii et al,[38] with permission.)

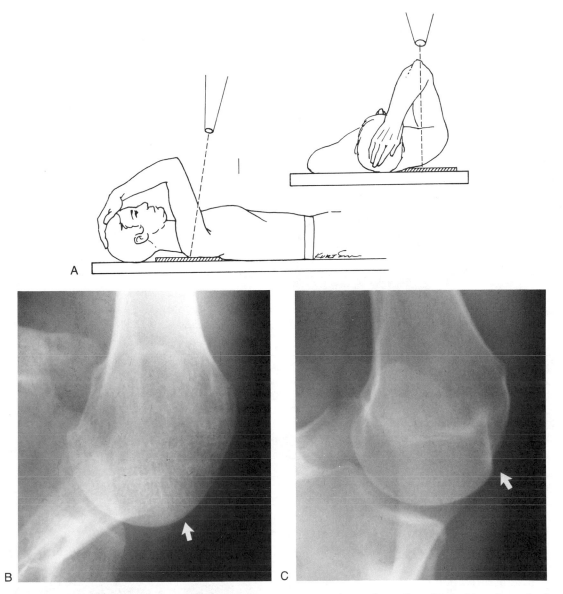

Fig. 9-10. (A) The notch view is taken with the patient supine and arm elevated so the patient places the hand behind the head. In the traditional view the tube is angled 10 degrees cephalad. The Stryker notch view angles the tube 45 degrees. **(B)** The posterosuperior aspect of the humeral head seen in profile *(arrow)*. **(C)** Anterior instability. Hill-Sach's defect is visualized *(arrow)*. (Fig. **A** from Resnick and Niwayama,[39] with permission; Figs. **B** & **C** from Rafii et al,[38] with permission.)

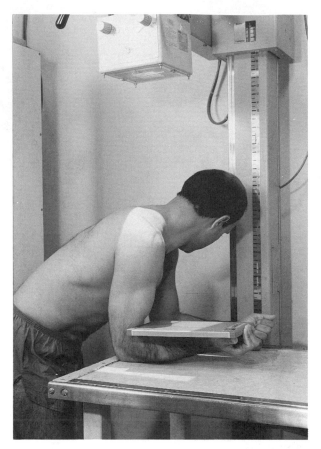

Fig. 9-11. The bicipital groove (Fisk) projection is performed by positioning the patient leaning forward to align the bicipital groove with the tube supporting the cassette on the forearm.

Acromioclavicular Projections

AP Acromioclavicular Projection

Although the acromioclavicular joint is demonstrated on the AP projection of the shoulder, the technique used will usually overpenetrate the acromioclavicular joint. A unilateral projection should be taken with a 10 to 15 degree tube tilt (Zanca projection [Fig. 9-12]). This will allow better visualization of the joint clear of overlap. The radiographic examination of this joint consists of bilateral weighted and nonweighted AP projections. Ten to fifteen pound weights are used for the weighted views. The weights should be strapped to the wrist or lightly held without firmly grasping the hands, which will potentially contract the shoulder muscle

resulting in a false negative film. These views are useful in the demonstration of acromioclavicular joint sprain and dislocation (Fig. 9-13).

Outlet View and 30 Degree Caudad Tilt View

Two views used in the detection of abnormal structure are the outlet view and the 30 degree tilt view. The outlet view is described in various ways, but the standard approach is to take a true scapulolateral view (Y view) with between 10 and 40 degrees of caudal tube tile (Fig. 9-14). The 30 degree tilt view is positioned just as the true AP projection, but the tube is angled caudad 30 degrees (Fig. 9-15). Both views allow the acromion and underlying acromioclavicular space to be better visualized compared to other views.

PA and AP Clavicle Projection

Radiographic examination of the clavicle routinely consists of PA and PA axial projections obtained with a 10 to 30 degree caudal tube tile (Fig. 9-16). If the patient cannot be placed in a prone position because of pain, AP and AP axial views obtained with a 10 to 30 degree cephalad tube tilt are an alternative. The views are taken with full inspiration to aid in elevation of the clavicles.

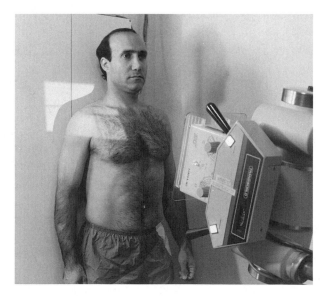

Fig. 9-12. Unilateral acromioclavicular joint projection with 10 to 15 degree tube tilt.

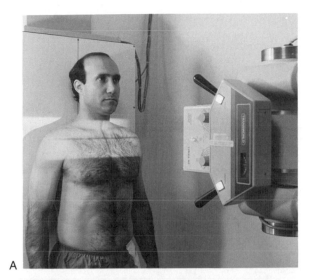

A

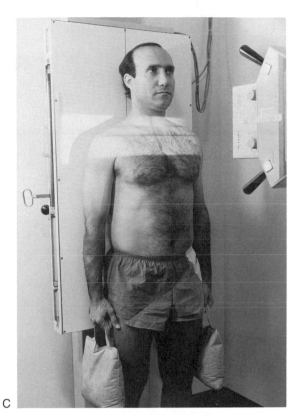

C

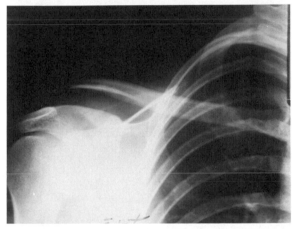

B

Fig. 9-13. (A) Nonweighted view usually positioned for a bilateral view. **(B)** Nonweighted view of third degree separation. **(C)** Weighted view.

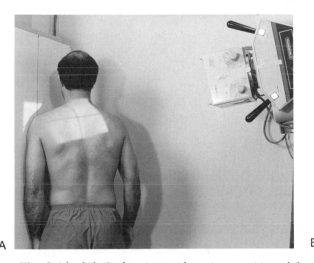

A

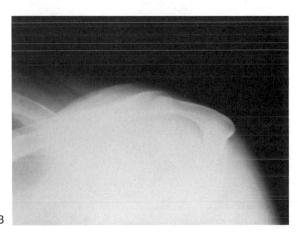

B

Fig. 9-14. (A) Outlet view with patient positioned for lateral scapular view with 10 to 40 degrees tube tile. **(B)** Normal outlet view.

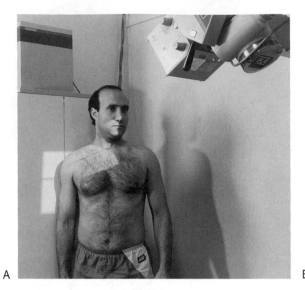
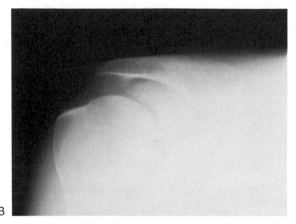

Fig. 9-15. (A) 30 degree tilt view taken as a true AP of the shoulder with 30 degree caudad tube angle. **(B)** Normal tilt view.

Scapular Projections

Radiographic examination of the scapula consists of the AP and lateral projections. The AP projection demonstrates the scapula with the lateral aspect of the scapula body free of superimposition by the adjacent ribs. The lateral projection is the tangential to the AP projection and is essentially the same as the Y view for the glenohumeral articulation. The focus is on the scapula, which necessitates a slightly lower target area along the middle scapula. A modification of this view is referred to as the Alexander view. Essentially the only difference between a true lateral scapular view and the Alexander view is that the patient is reaching around

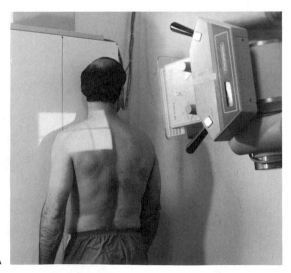
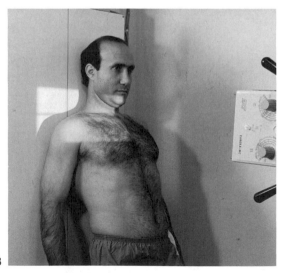

Fig. 9-16. (A) PA clavicular projection. Patient is flat against bucky. **(B)** AP clavicular projection with patient leaning back against bucky. The tube in angled between 10 and 30 degrees depending on the degree of patient angulation.

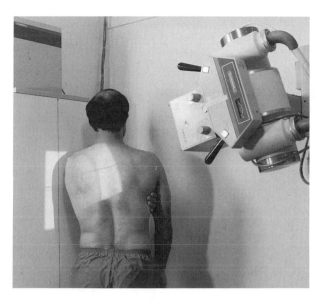

Fig. 9-17. The Alexander view positions the patient and tube similar to the lateral scapular view, but the patient reaches around to grasp the chest causing a more slumped posture.

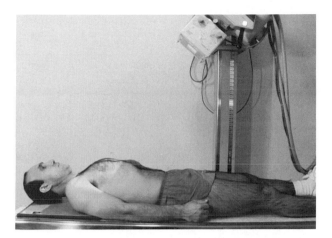

Fig. 9-18. Serendipity view for the sternoclavicular joint. Patient is supine with large cassette placed behind head and upper back. The tube is angled 40 degrees cephalad. The distance is 60 inches in adults and 40 in children.

to grasp the opposite side of the chest causing more shoulder depression (Fig. 9-17). This view was designed to demonstrate posterior displacement of the clavicle, which may occur with acromioclavicular injuries.

Sternoclavicular Projections

The sternoclavicular joints are examined in the PA and PA oblique projections. The PA projection demonstrates the sternoclavicular joint as well as the medial aspect of the clavicles. The PA oblique views are performed as right anterior oblique and left anterior oblique projections. These views are technically very difficult to obtain, and as a result computed tomography (CT) is often necessary for adequate visualization.

Serendipity and Hobb's Projections

In instances in which CT is unavailable the serendipity view is useful in distinguishing between anterior and posterior dislocation of the sternoclavicular joint (Fig. 9-18). Dislocation is detectable by drawing a horizontal line through the unaffected clavicle and determining superiority related to the line (anterior dislocation) or inferiority related to the line (posterior dislocation).

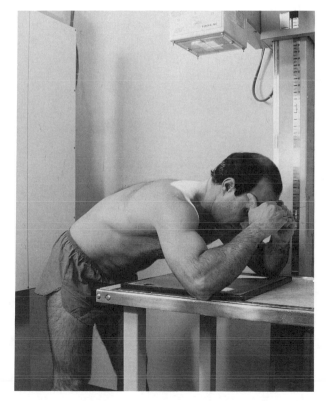

Fig. 9-19. Hobb's view. The patient leans over the cassette resting on the forearms. The tube is targeted through the lower cervical spine.

Table 9-2. The Efficiency of Various Radiographic Views in Evaluation of Hill-Sachs and Bankart Lesions[a]

View	Hill-Sachs	Bankart
45 degree craniocaudal	22/27	10/10
Stryker notch	25/27	1/10
Didiee	7/27	Not reported
Frontal (AP)	7/27	Not reported
Hermodsson	12/27	0/10
Axial	0/27	2/10

Commentary: 45 degree craniocaudal view has high yield for both lesions. Stryker notch view excellent for Hill-Sachs.

Recommendations: Do craniocaudal view first, and if defect is not seen, do Stryker notch view. West Point and Didiee views may be added to see Bankart lesion.

[a] Twenty-seven shoulders, with recurrent anterior dislocation Hill-Sachs defect seen in 26; Bankart defect seen in 10.
(From Rozing et al,[35] as adapted in Rafii et al,[38] with permission.)

Table 9-3. The Efficacy of Various Radiographic Views in Evaluation of the Hill-Sachs Lesion[a]

View	Result
AP external rotation	1/15
AP internal rotation 45 degrees	15/15[b]
Axillary	7/15
AP internal rotation 20 degrees	4/15
PA external rotation 45 degrees	10/15
PA internal rotation 45 degrees	12/15[b]
Stryker notch	14/15[b]
Modified Didiee	12/15[b]

Recommendation: Take three views to show Hill-Sachs: AP (or PA) in 45-degree internal rotation, Stryker notch, and Didiee.

[a] The Hill-Sachs lesion in 15 patients with anterior shoulder dislocation.
[b] Views that are particularly efficacious.
(From Danzig et al,[36] as adapted in Rafii M et al,[38] with permission.)

Medial clavicular fractures are also evident with this view. The serendipity is probably the most accurate projection. Additionally, some authors recommend the Hobb's projection. The patient leans over a cassette with the beam directed through the cervicothoracic spine (Fig. 9-19).

Other nonroutine views of the shoulder as well as their effectiveness are displayed in Tables 9-2 to 9-6.

LINES AND ANGLES OF MENSURATION

Various lines and angles can be applied to radiographs of the glenohumeral joint. These lines and angles may be useful in establishing bony relationships of the joint; however, it must be cautioned that tube angulation and/or patient positioning can geometrically alter the image thereby invalidating findings.

Glenohumeral Joint Space

The glenohumeral joint space is best assessed utilizing the AP external rotation projection. The superior, middle, and inferior aspects of the joint are measured. The average joint space should measure between 4 and 5 mm. An increase in the joint space could be the result of posterior dislocation (Fig. 9-20).

Table 9-4. The Efficacy of Various Radiographic Views in Evaluation of Hill-Sachs and Bankart Lesions[a]

View[a]	Hill-Sachs (%)	Bankart (%)
Internal rotation	92	15
External rotation	32	65
Axillary	44	66
West Point	51	70
Stryker Notch	92	11
Didiee	35	71

Commentary: Maximal yield in diagnosing the lesions of anterior instability are achieved with three combined views: anterior posterior internal rotation, Stryker notch, and either West Point or Didiee.

Percentages of Lesion by Type[b]				
Bankart or Hill-Sachs (%)	Hill-Sachs and Bankart (%)	Isolated Hill-Sachs (%)	Isolated Bankart (%)	Normal
82	16	61	5	18

Type of Instability and Lesion Incidence[b]		
	Hill-Sachs (%)	Bankart (%)
	(with or without each other)	
Subluxations	66	40
Dislocations	77	15
Combined	87	20

Commentary: Isolated Hill-Sachs occurs much more often than isolated Bankart. One or the other is often present, but they occur together infrequently. The type of instability bears upon defect incidence.

[a] A study of 83 patients with unilateral anterior shoulder instability.
[b] (From Pavlov and Freiberger,[26] as adapted in Rafii et al,[38] with permission.)

Table 9-5. The Efficacy of Various Radiographic Views in Evaluation of Acute Trauma of the Shoulder

Trauma	AP External Rotation	AP External and Internal Rotation	Anterior Oblique	AP Internal Rotation and Anterior Oblique
Anterior dislocation	0	0	0	8
Humeral head fracture	2	0	*1	4
Acromioclavicular separation	0	0	0	5
Clavicle fracture	0	0	0	3
Scapular fracture	0	1	3	2

Note: 60-degree anterior oblique = Y view.

Commentary: In this series four fractures (*) would have been missed with an anterior oblique projection. It may be obtained at 45 degrees or 60 degrees and requires no movement of the humerus.

(From DeSmet,[37] as adapted in Rafii et al,[38] with permission.)

Axial Relationship

The axial relationship of the shoulder is determined by utilizing the AP external rotation projection. A line is drawn parallel to and bisecting the shaft of the humerus. A second line is drawn extending from the superior margin of the greater tuberosity to the lateral margin of the junction of the head of the humerus and proximal humeral diaphysis. This angle measures approximately 60 degrees in normal males and approximately 62 degrees in normal females (Fig. 9-21).

Acromioclavicular Joint Space

The acromioclavicular joint space is evaluated by utilizing the AP neutral shoulder projection. The joint space is measured superiorly and inferiorly and these measurements are averaged. The average measurement is 3 mm with 2 to 3 mm or less difference between the right and left joints. An increase in this measurement is seen in acromioclavicular separation and in post-traumatic osteolysis (Fig. 9-22A).

Acromiohumeral Joint Space

The acromiohumeral joint space is evaluated on the AP shoulder radiograph by measuring the distance between the inferior margin of the acromion process and

Table 9-6. The Efficacy of Various Radiographic Views in Evaluation of Traumatic Shoulder Abnormalities

Abnormality	No.	Anterior Posterior (%)	Lateral (%)	Y View (%)	Apical Oblique (%)
Humerus fracture	56	100	70	68	93
Glenohumeral dislocation	34	100	94	91	100[a]
Clavicle fracture	22	100	9	68	73
Glenoid rim fracture	7	39	0	11	94[b]
Acromioclavicular separation	14	100	14	21	14
Hill-Sachs lesion	5	42	8	8	100[c]
Scapular fracture	9	90	30	50	50

Commentary: Twenty of 161 abnormalities would have been missed in a study of 511 traumatized shoulders if an apical oblique (45 degree posterior oblique with 45 degree caudal angulation) view was not performed. It is a good view to show posterior glenohumeral dislocation,[a] glenoid rim fractures,[b] and Hill-Sachs lesions.[c]

(From Kornguth and Salazar,[9] as adapted in Rafii et al[38] with permission.)

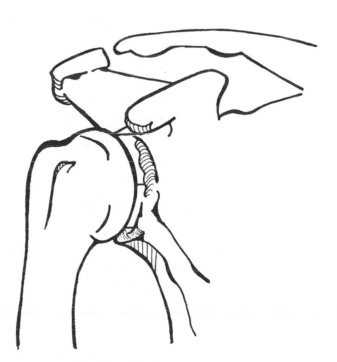

Fig. 9-20. Glenohumeral joint space.

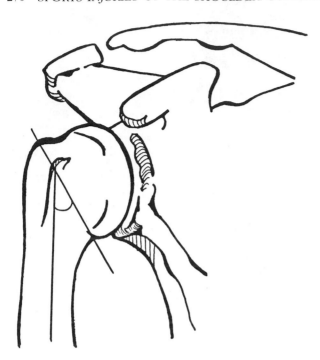

Fig. 9-21. Axial relationship of shoulder.

the superior articular surface of the humeral head. The average joint space measures approximately 9 mm. A measurement of less than 7 mm indicates a chronic rotator cuff tear. A measurement of 11 mm or greater may indicate dislocation of the humeral head (Fig. 9-22B).

Coracoclavicular Interval

The coracoclavicular interval is the distance from the superior margin of the coracoid process of the scapula to the inferior margin of the clavicle. This distance measures 1.1 to 1.3 cm in the normal population. An increase in measurement is indicative of disruption of the coracoclavicular ligament (Fig. 9-22C).[3]

INJURIES TO THE SHOULDER GIRDLE

Activities frequently resulting in injury to the shoulder include swimming, baseball, tennis, football, and gymnastics. These injuries can be classified as intrinsic injuries (resulting from repetitive activity or overuse) or extrinsic injuries (resulting from direct force). Intrinsic and extrinsic injuries frequently coexist.

Shoulder Dislocations

The most frequently dislocated joint of the body is the shoulder. Approximately 85 percent of all shoulder dislocations involve the glenohumeral joint, of which approximately 95 percent are anterior dislocations and approximately 3 percent are posterior dislocations.[2] Acromioclavicular joint separations/dislocations account for approximately 12 percent of all shoulder girdle dislocations and sternoclavicular joint dislocations comprise approximately 3 percent.

Anterior Dislocations

Anterior glenohumeral joint dislocation typically is a result of falling with the arm abducted and externally rotated. Forceful hyperextension and abduction of the arm and direct posterior blows are less commonly implicated mechanisms. Football players are vulnerable to this type of injury as a result of blocking and tackling. Skiers are also vulnerable because of falling injuries and less commonly by striking an outstretched arm or ski pole on a fixed object.

As anterior dislocation occurs, the humeral head impacts the inferior margin of the glenoid process. This impact can result in a compression fracture of the relatively soft cancellous bone of the humeral head along its posterolateral aspect. This fracture is referred to as both a hatchet defect and a Hill-Sachs lesion. Hill and Sachs initially reported this fracture (Fig. 9-23A) as occurring in up to 75 percent of those patients with anterior glenohumeral dislocations, although other investigators have reported it as occurring with virtually all anterior dislocations. As the humeral head impacts the glenoid fossa, there may be concomitant fracture of the inferior glenoid rim or avulsion of the fibrocartilaginous glenoid labrum. These injuries are called Bankart lesions. Approximately 10 percent of all anterior glenohumeral joint dislocations are also associated with avulsion fractures of the greater tuberosity (Fig. 9-23B) as a result of forceful traction by the supraspinatus tendon. The clinician must be alert for associated potential brachial plexus injury, specifically injury to the axillary nerve.

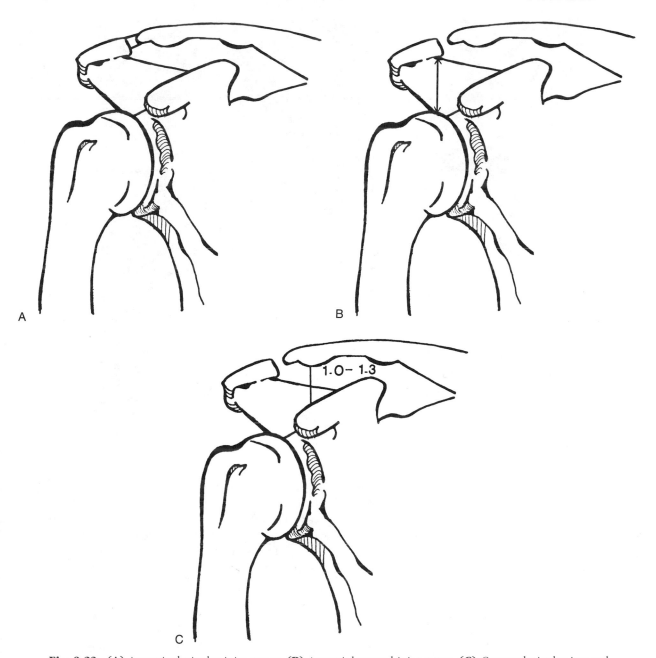

Fig. 9-22. **(A)** Acromioclavicular joint space. **(B)** Acromiohumeral joint space. **(C)** Coracoclavicular interval.

If the initial dislocation occurs in athletes 20 years of age or younger, there is an 80 to 90 percent incidence of recurrence. Recurrence in those athletes who experience initial dislocation at 40 years of age or older has a 10 to 15 percent incidence.

Most anterior glenohumeral dislocations are easily diagnosed on the AP shoulder projection by inferomedial displacement of the humeral head relative to the glenoid fossa. Hill-Sachs lesions are best visualized on the AP internal rotation projection as a **V** shaped

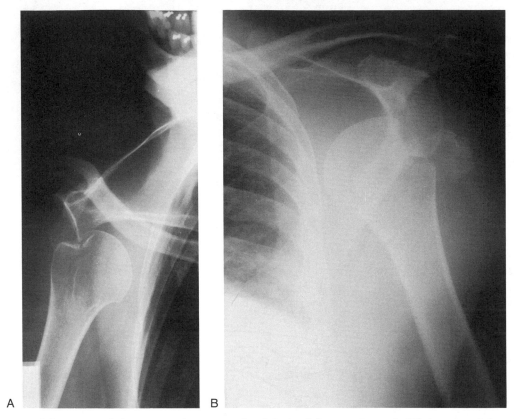

Fig. 9-23. (A) Anterior dislocation with associated Hill-Sachs deformity *(arrow)*. **(B)** Anterior dislocation with avulsion fracture of greater tuberosity.

deformity of the humeral head. Osseous Bankart lesions are best demonstrated on specialized views as a separate bony fragment lying within the soft tissue immediately inferior to the inferior glenoid rim or ectopic bone formation of the glenoid rim. Fibrocartilaginous Bankart lesions require either CT or magnetic resonance imaging (MRI) for demonstration. The Bankart lesion is considered pathognomonic for instability.[4,5] Avulsion fractures of the greater tuberosity are seen best on the AP external rotation projection as a separation of the greater tuberosity away from the shaft of the humerus (Table 9-7).

Due to the difficulties in positioning the traditional axillary view (Alexander) in an acute patient and the overlap found on the transthoracic view, it is recommended to attempt one of a variety of modified axillary views. The Velpeau view by Vastamaki and Solomen[6] allows the arm to remain immobilized while taking the radiograph (Fig. 9-6). The difficulty for the patient

may be leaning back for proper positioning. The apical oblique view reveals both Hill-Sachs lesions and Bankart lesions without the difficulty of West Point or Stryker notch positions. The Stripp axial view by Horsefield and Jones[7] is an option; however, it may not be possible depending on the mobility of the particular x-ray unit being used, requiring an upward shot through the shoulder.

Posterior Dislocations

Posterior dislocations of the glenohumeral joint are the result of direct anterior to posterior trauma to the shoulder or falling on an outstretched arm (Fig. 9-24 and 9-25). As the humeral head moves posteriorly it may impact the glenoid process resulting in a compression fracture of the anteromedial humeral head margin. This compression defect is referred to as the trough sign[8] (Fig. 9-26). Avulsion fractures of the lesser tuberosity may be seen as well.

Table 9-7. Radiographic Findings of Specific Shoulder Conditions

Anterior shoulder dislocation
    Inferomedial displacement of humeral head relative to glenoid fossa
    Possible compression fracture of posterolateral humeral head (Hill-Sachs lesion)
    Possible fracture of inferior rim of glenoid rim (osseous Bankart lesion)
Posterior shoulder dislocation
    Humeral head posterior to glenoid fossa
    Possible trough lesion
Acromioclavicular joint injury
    Type I
        No alteration in width of joint space
    Type II
        Inferior displacement of acromion process relative to distal clavicle
        20 to 25 percent increase in width of coracoclavicular joint space
    Type III
        Inferior displacement of acromion process relative to distal clavicle
        Widening of coracoclavicular joint space
Impingement syndrome
    Acromiohumeral joint space measures less than 6 mm
    Erosion of inferior margin of acromion process
    Cephalad migration of humeral head
    Flattening of greater tuberosity

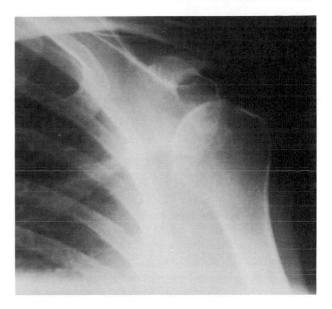

Fig. 9-25. Posterior dislocation of glenohumeral joint.

Posterior glenohumeral joint injuries may be difficult to diagnosis on radiographic examination. The AP shoulder projection is generally unrevealing, with signs of dislocation being subtle, if present at all. Normally on the AP view the head of the humerus superimposes the glenoid fossa and results in an elliptical overlap shadow. In posterior dislocations the elliptical overlap shadow is distorted (Fig. 9-27). The transthoracic projection, while technically difficult to obtain, will reveal the humeral head to lie directly posterior to the glenoid fossa. However, Kornguth and Salazar[9] have demonstrated that the transthoracic view is poor in detecting Hill-Sachs lesions and glenoid rim fractures.

The Y view (true lateral scapular) is one of the best views for patient comfort and the ability to detect a

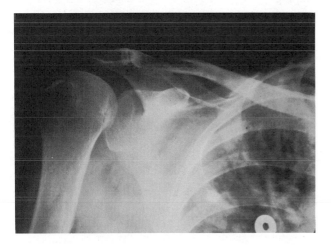

Fig. 9-24. Posterior dislocation of glenohumeral joint.

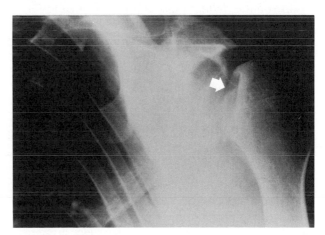

Fig. 9-26. Trough sign (arrow).

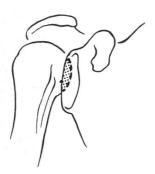

Fig. 9-27. With a posterior dislocation there may be an "empty glenoid" sign with no overlap of the humeral head or, alternatively, minimal overlap in the subspinous position. With this dislocation the inferior one-third of the glenoid is empty of overlapping shadow. (From Reid,[41] with permission.)

posterior dislocation.[10] Centering of the humeral head on the glenoid is readily visible if positioning is correct. Additionally posterior rim and lesser tuberosity fractures are also visible. Another patient-conscious view mentioned previously is the Velpeau view. Axial views are beneficial in making this diagnosis as well as in demonstrating the trough lesion. In addition, the West Point and Stryker views nicely demonstrate this lesion. The AP external rotation view demonstrates the avulsed lesser tuberosity to lie in a position separate from the shaft of the humerus (Table 9-7).

Multidirectional Instability

Patients with multidirectional instability may have signs visible on the standard instability views. In addition, it is recommended that a stress view be taken. This is accomplished by having the patient hold a 10 to 15 lb weight (preferably strapped to the wrist) while taking an AP projection. Inferiority of the humerus is often apparent.

Acromioclavicular Joint Injury

Acute trauma to the acromioclavicular joint is a common sports injury. Various forces may result in acromioclavicular joint injury but the most common are a downward blow to the lateral aspect of the shoulder, which drives the acromion process caudally, or traction of the arm, which pulls the shoulder away from the chest shoulder away from the chest. Falling onto

an outstretched arm or a flexed elbow can also result in injury to this joint. The type of force involved is directly related to which soft tissues will be affected. The acromioclavicular ligament, joint capsule, and coracoclavicular ligament may be injured.[11] Acromioclavicular joint injuries are very common in football and are the most common hockey injuries.

Rockwood[1] describes six types of acromioclavicular joint injuries, designated as types I, II, III, IV, V, and VI. Types I, II, and III acromioclavicular joint injuries are clinically referred to as mild, moderate, and severe sprains, respectively (Table 9-7). Type I is described as a partial tear of the acromioclavicular ligament with no displacement of the acromion process or distal clavicle and no alteration of joint space. Plain film examination is unrevealing (Fig. 9-28A). Type II represents a complete rupture of the acromioclavicular ligament and capsule with a partial tear of the coracoclavicular ligament (Fig. 9-28B). This results in slight inferior displacement of the acromion process relative to the distal clavicle. AP radiographs of the acromioclavicular joint will also demonstrate the coracoclavicular distance to be increased by 25 to 50 percent of its normal measurement (1.0 to 1.5 cm). Type III is described as rupture of the acromioclavicular ligament and the coracoclavicular ligament. The acromion process is displaced inferiorly relative to the distal clavicle and coracoclavicular joint space is significantly widened (Fig. 9-28C). The diagnosis of type IV, V, and VI acromioclavicular joint injuries is often based on physical examination findings in conjunction with radiographic findings. In type IV injuries, the distal end of the clavicle is displaced posteriorly, this may rupture the trapezius muscle (Fig. 9-28D). In type V injuries, there is marked superior displacement of the distal clavicle relative to the acromion process (Fig. 9-28E). Type VI injuries are very rare and involve injury to the sternoclavicular joint as well as the acromioclavicular joint. In this injury the distal aspect of the clavicle is displaced inferiorly relative to the coracoid process (Fig. 9-28F).

Post-traumatic Osteolysis of the Distal Clavicle

A relatively uncommon but potential sequela of acromioclavicular joint injury is post-traumatic osteolysis of the distal clavicle.[2] This condition is also encountered in weightlifters without history of trauma secondary to chronic stress and repeated microtrauma. The mecha-

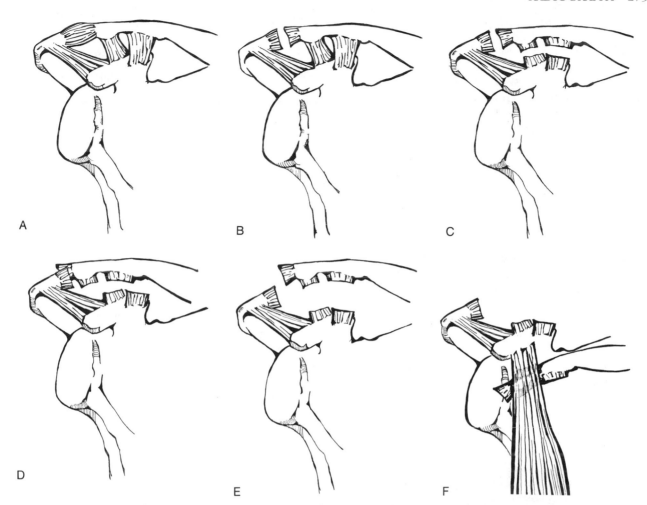

Fig. 9-28. Rockwood's classification of acromioclavicular injuries. **(A)** Type I: partial tear of acromioclavicular ligament without displacement. **(B)** Type II: complete rupture of acromioclavicular ligament and partial tear of coracoclavicular ligament. **(C)** Type III: rupture of acromioclavicular ligament and coracoclavicular ligament. **(D)** Type IV: distal clavicle is displaced posteriorly. **(E)** Type V: marked displacement of the distal clavicle relative to the acromion. **(F)** Type VI: distal clavicle is displaced inferiorly relative to the coracoid process. (Modified from Rockwood and Green,[40] with permission.)

nism of post-traumatic osteolysis is not entirely understood. A slight degree of bone loss secondary to trauma occurs commonly; however, in cases of post-traumatic osteolysis bone resorption is excessive. Bone resorption of the distal clavicle can begin to occur as early as 2 weeks postinjury or as late as several years. It is frequently seen in conjunction with erosion of the articular surface of the acromion process and concomitant soft tissue swelling and dystrophic calcification. Repair generally occurs over a 4 to 6 month period;

however, when complete the acromioclavicular joint can remain permanently widened. The diagnosis of post-traumatic osteolysis of the clavicle must be considered in instances of persistent post-traumatic distal clavicle pain.[12–14]

Nontraumatic osteolysis is documented as occurring with increasing frequency in weightlifters working with heavy to moderate weight.[15] These are usually Olympic and competition level athletes (see Ch. 15). Partial resolution occurs if the activity is discontinued.

Sternoclavicular Joint Injury

Sternoclavicular joint dislocation is a relatively uncommon but severe injury involving the clavicle and sternum. The joint may dislocate anteriorly (presternal dislocation) or posteriorly (retrosternal dislocation). The incidence of presternal dislocation to retrosternal dislocation is approximately 3 to 1. Sternoclavicular joint dislocations are poorly demonstrated on plain films. However, if CT is not available the serendipity view may be helpful.[1] Rockwood[1] also suggests the Hobbs[16] view as an option. CT or conventional tomography are the imaging modalities of choice in the evaluation of this type of injury. Traumatic dislocation of the sternoclavicular joint requires a direct or indirect force of great magnitude, but most are the result of indirect force.[11] Direct force applied to the anteromedial aspect of the joint results in retrosternal dislocation. Indirect force transmitted to the sternoclavicular joint from the shoulder, as in various contact sports, can result in either presternal or retrosternal dislocation. Of critical significance is the fact that in retrosternal sternoclavicular joint dislocation, the clavicle can cause injury to the trachea, esophagus, great vessels, or major nerves.

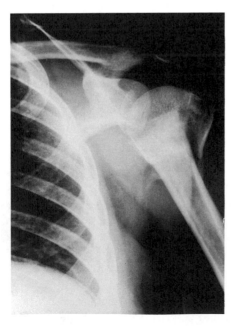

Fig. 9-29. Proximal humeral fracture.

Fractures of the Shoulder

Proximal Humeral Fractures

Fractures of the proximal humerus comprise approximately 4 to 5 percent of all fractures and are uncommon in the athlete. Those that do occur among athletes typically are found in middle-aged or older skiers and equestrians of any age, as a result of falling on an outstretched arm. Less frequently, proximal humerus fractures can result from torque placed on the humerus during throwing in the unconditioned athlete. The cause is biceps and triceps strength that is inadequate to counteract the rotational forces during throwing. A direct blow to the lateral aspect of the arm, as in many contact sports, may also result in proximal humerus fractures (Fig. 9-29).

Neer[17] originally described a classification system for proximal humeral fractures based on the locations and the relationships of four major fragments: the articular surface proximal to the anatomic neck, the lesser tuberosity, the greater tuberosity, and the humeral shaft as well as the presence or absence of significant displacement of the fracture fragments (Fig. 9-30A). A nondisplaced fracture of the proximal humerus is classified as a two-part fracture (Fig. 9-30B). There is no significant displacement of the fracture due to fragments being held together by the rotator cuff musculature, periosteum, and joint capsule. Displacement of one fragment is also classified as a two-part fracture (Fig. 9-30C & D). The displacement is defined as a separation of the fracture fragments by 1 cm or 45 degrees of angulation. These fractures are generally unstable due to injury of the rotator cuff.

A three-part fracture is a fracture with displacement of two fragments. The surgical neck is often fractured with rotation of the humeral head. If the greater tuberosity remains attached to the humeral head the rotator cuff muscles rotate the humeral head anteriorly (Fig. 9-30E). If the lesser tuberosity remains attached the humeral head is rotated posteriorly by the external rotator muscles (Fig. 9-30F). The humeral shaft is displaced anteromedially due to action of the pectoralis major muscle. A four-part fracture is a fracture of the anatomic neck of the humerus as well as displacement of the lesser and greater tuberosities (Fig. 9-30G).

The radiographic evaluation of the post-traumatic humerus consists of two views obtained at right angles to one another. In most instances, these views include

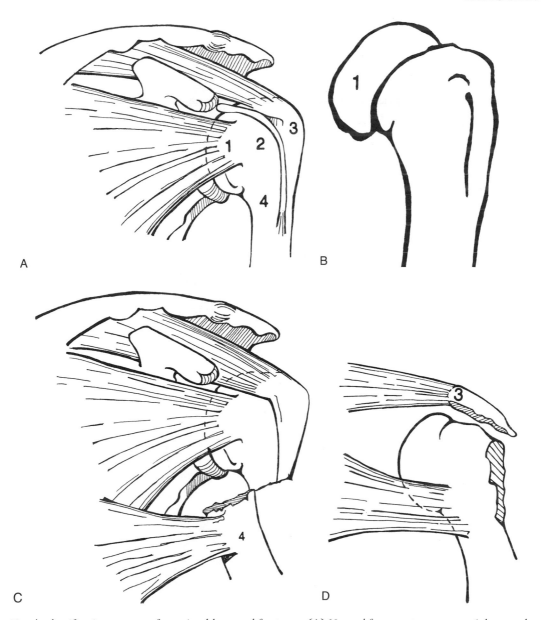

Fig. 9-30. Neer's classification system of proximal humeral fractures. **(A)** Normal four-part segments: *1,* humeral head; *2,* lesser tuberosity; *3,* greater tuberosity; *4,* shaft of humerus. **(B)** Two-part fracture of anatomic neck. *(1).* **(C)** Two-part fracture resulting in displacement of shaft *(4).* **(D)** Two-part fracture resulting in displacement of greater tuberosity *(3).* (*Figure continues.*)

an AP and a lateral view, or in more severely injured patients, an AP and a transthoracic lateral projection. Rockwood[1] recommends a "trauma series," which consists of two projections of the proximal humerus obtained with the patient in a posterior oblique posi-tion with the scapula parallel to the x-ray table, one of which is perpendicular to the plane of the scapula and the other is parallel with the plane of the scapula. These may be obtained with the patient standing, sit-ting, or lying.

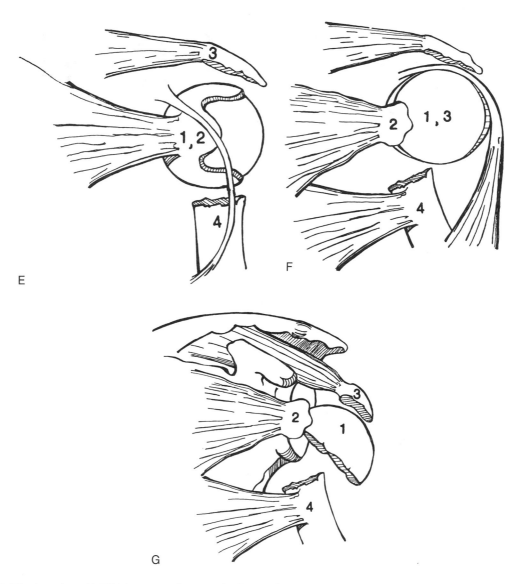

Fig. 9-30. *(continued)* **(E)** Three-part fracture displacing the greater tuberosity *(3)*, with rotation of the humeral head *(1,2)*. The shaft is displaced relative to the humeral head *(4)*. **(F)** Three-part fracture in which the lesser tuberosity *(2)* is detached and displaced. The humeral head faces anteriorly. **(G)** Four-part fracture in which the humeral head *(1)* is detached from the tuberosities *(2,3)*. (Modified from Rockwood and Green,[40] with permission.)

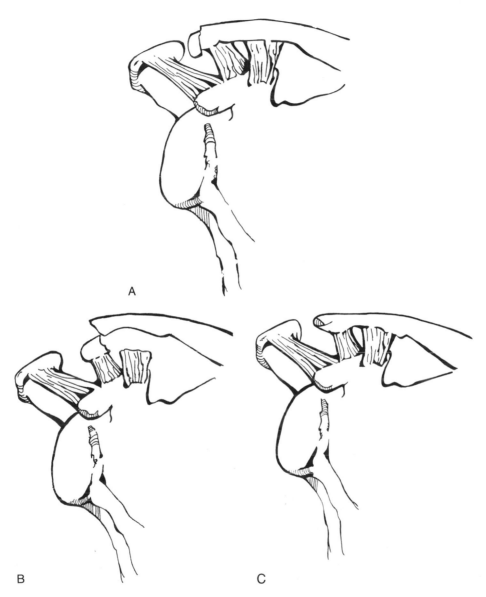

Fig. 9-31. Classification of distal clavicle fractures. **(A)** Type I: nondisplaced fracture with intact ligaments. **(B)** Type II: coracoclavicular ligaments are detached from proximal segment. **(C)** Type III: fracture of articular surface. (Modified from Greenway et al,[32] with permission.)

Clavicular Fractures

The most common fracture involving the shoulder girdle is fracture of the clavicle. The middle third of the clavicle is fractured with a frequency of approximately 80 percent. The reason for this is that the clavicle is an S shaped bone and lateral forces result in a shearing force on the middle third. The distal third of the clavicle is fractured with a frequency of approximately 15 percent and the proximal third with a frequency of approximately 5 percent. Clavicle fractures are typically the result of indirect trauma such as falling on an outstretched arm or direct trauma such as that occurring in skiing, football, rugby, hockey, and lacrosse. Football injuries are responsible for most sports-related clavicle fractures (Table 9-8).

Neer[18] classifies fractures of the distal clavicle into three categories: type I, type II, and type III. In type I fractures, the fragments demonstrate minimal displacement and the ligaments are intact (Fig. 9-31A). In type II fractures (Fig. 9-31B) the ligaments are detached from the proximal fragment, the proximal fragment is tractioned superiorly by the force of the sternocleidomastoid muscle, and the distal fracture fragment is tractioned inferiorly by the weight of the arm and inward by the force of the pectoralis major and latissimus dorsi muscles (Fig. 9-32). A type III fracture involves the distal articular surface of the clavicle[19] (Fig. 9-31C).

Radiographic examination of the clavicle consists of PA and PA axial projections. AP and AP axial projections will suffice in the acutely injured patient. The integrity

Table 9-8. Sport Specific Shoulder Injuries

Sport	Injury	Mechanism(s)
Football	Anterior glenohumeral dislocation	Blocking, tackling
	Acromioclavicular joint sprain/dislocation	Blocking, tackling, fall
	Sternoclavicular joint sprain/dislocation	Fall on shoulder
	Clavicle fracture	Fall, blow to shoulder
Skiiing	Anterior glenohumeral dislocation	Fall on outstretched arm, striking ski pole on fixed object
Hockey	Acromioclavicular joint injury	Fall, blow to shoulder
	Clavicle fracture	Fall, blow to shoulder
Weightlifting	Post-traumatic osteolysis distal clavicle	Chronic stress and microtrauma
Equestrian	Proximal humeral fracture	Fall on outstretched arm
Baseball	Subacromial impingement syndrome	Repetitive motion of arm above horizontal plane
	Proximal humeral fracture	Torque forces in unconditioned athlete
Swimming	Impingement syndrome	Repetitive motion of arm above horizontal
	Bursitis	Same as above
	Tendinitis	Same as above
Tennis	Impingement syndrome	Repetitive motion of arm above horizontal plane
	Rotator cuff tear	Repetitive motion of arm above horizontal plane
Golf	Impingement syndrome	Repetitive motion of arm above horizontal plane
Gymnastics	Tendinitis	Overuse from high and parallel bars

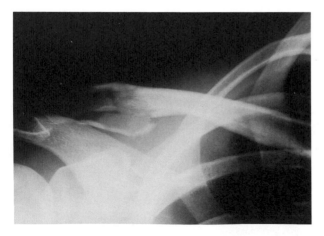

Fig. 9-32. Type II clavicular fracture.

of the coracoclavicular ligament can be assessed by AP weight-bearing and non-weight bearing projections utilizing 10 lb weights. The coracoclavicular distance will widen with weight-bearing in those instances of coracoclavicular ligament rupture.

Scapula Fractures

The scapula is well protected by a large surrounding muscle mass and as a result scapula fractures are uncommon in the athlete (as in the general population), comprising only approximately 5 to 7 percent of all shoulder girdle fractures. The most common site of scapula fracture is the body followed by the neck.

Other potential fracture sites include the glenoid process, articular surface, head, scapular spine, acromion process, and coracoid process. Contact sports such as football and rugby can result in comminuted fractures of the scapula. Fractures of the neck of the scapula can occur from indirect forces such as a fall onto the shoulder or an outstretched arm. Coracoid fractures are most likely associated with acromioclavicular joint dislocations. Glenoid process fracture can occur in association with dislocations of the shoulder.

Radiographic evaluation of the scapula consists of an AP projection obtained with the scapula parallel with the table and a lateral projection obtained with the scapula perpendicular to the table.

Impingement Syndrome

The impingement syndrome is one of the most common causes of shoulder pain and disability in the athlete. Impingement syndrome results from repetitive placement of the arm above the horizontal plane. Clinically, the patient presents complaining of shoulder pain and inability to abduct the arm. Athletes most commonly manifesting impingement syndrome participate in baseball, swimming, and tennis although impingement syndrome is by no means limited to these sports.

Factors predisposing the athlete to the development of impingement syndrome have been identified. These include the shape and slope of the acromion process, which can potentially limit the amount of space available within the coracoacromial outlet through which the rotator cuff must pass. Degenerative change presenting as hypertrophic bone formation along the inferior aspect of the acromioclavicular joint is an additional frequent cause of coracoacromial outlet narrowing. Less frequently, a persistent, unfused acromial process epiphysis may be implicated. In those athletes predisposed to impingement syndrome, the condition becomes a repetitive cycle of irritation and injury. The musculotendinous structures of the rotator cuff consist of four intrinsic muscles: the subscapularis, the supraspinatus, the infraspinatus, and the teres minor. The tendons of these muscles converge to insert into the anatomic neck and tuberosities of the humerus. The muscles of the rotator cuff along with the deltoid muscle function to secure the humeral head in the glenoid fossa. Neer[17] developed a four-stage system useful in describing rotator cuff injury.

Stage I impingement is present when the initial injury causes acute changes in the intact rotator cuff. Edema and hemorrhage occur. These changes are transient and reversible. Stage II impingement syndrome is a result of repetitive irritation that produces fibrosis and chronic tendinitis. MRI can reveal incomplete rotator cuff tears. Stage III impingement results from chronic rotator cuff irritation that produces irreversible degenerative changes in the rotator cuff as well as the subacromial/subdeltoid bursae, the acromial arch, and the humeral tuberosities. Complete, full-thickness tears of the cuff occur that allow communication between the glenohumeral joint space and the subacromial/subdeltoid bursa. These manifest on both MRI and arthrography. There may be retraction of the musculotendinous junction. In stage IV impingement, full-thickness tears of the rotator cuff are present in conjunction with retraction of the muscles. Frequently biceps tendon rupture will be associated. Although plain film findings of rotator cuff may not always be specific, there are often indirect indicators (Table 9-7).

While shoulder MRI is the most sensitive and specific imaging modality for the evaluation of impingement syndrome, plain film findings may be present in later stages (Table 9-7). Commonly these findings are not present because disability associated with impingement syndrome prohibits participation in causative activities. Those findings that can be demonstrated on AP shoulder projections include an acromiohumeral space measuring less than 6 mm, erosion of the inferior margin of the acromion process secondary to the cephalad migration of the humeral head, and irregularity of the contour of the greater tuberosity including flattening and atrophy. This is the result of lack of traction stress normally provided by the rotator cuff. In addition, the AP projection of the acromioclavicular joint obtained with a 10 to 15 degree cephalic tube tilt may demonstrate hypertrophic bony proliferation along the acromion process at the site of coracoacromial ligament attachment as a result of increased tension within this ligament. A lateral projection of the scapula with 10 to 40 degrees angulation (outlet view) can be useful in demonstrating the size and contour of the coracoacromial outlet.[19] As mentioned previously an additional helpful view is the 30 degree caudad tilt view, which is a modification of the true AP view of the shoulder.

Finally, a profile view is suggested by Andrews et al.[20] A difficult view in standard practice, this view takes a superiorly directed shot through the shoulder with the patient supine. The cassette is place above the shoulder held at an angle of 20 degrees away from the head (as if the head were laterally flexed 20 degrees). The tube is angled perpendicular to the cassette. Abnormal acromial architecture is fairly evident with these views.

MISCELLANEOUS CONDITIONS OF THE SHOULDER

Calcific Tendinitis

Calcium hydroxyapatite (HA) crystals can be deposited in periarticular soft tissues. Various theories have been postulated to explain the etiology of HA deposition. Repetitive trauma and microtrauma is implicated as the cause of the initial lesion with HA crystal deposition occurring in the injured and necrotic tissue. It is established that relatively avascular tissues are more common sites of crystal deposition. Alterations in local pH and/or decreased CO_2 tension within the tissue can also be contributing factors. The resulting deposition of the crystals, commonly referred to as calcific tendinitis, can occur in any of the periarticular soft tissues of the shoulder. The most common site, however, is within the supraspinatus tendon, often at its insertion into the greater tuberosity. The right shoulder is involved with greater frequency than the left, an obvious result of the predominance of right-handed individuals. Calcific tendinitis at the site of supraspinatus tendon attachment into the greater tuberosity is best demonstrated on the AP external rotation projection of the shoulder because the AP internal projection will often project the humeral head superimposing the calcific deposits, thereby obscuring them.

Ringman's Shoulder

This uncommon entity was originally described by Fulton[21] as an area of benign bony hypertrophy occurring at the site of insertion of the pectoralis major and latissimus dorsi muscles on the humerus. This lesion, which is without clinical significance, has been identified exclusively in male gymnasts and is associated with the gymnastic use of rings. The lesion is demonstrated

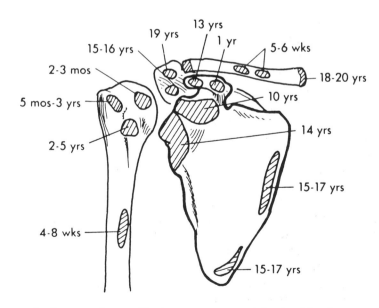

Fig. 9-33. Fusion times for the secondary ossification centers around the shoulder. (From Reid,[41] with permission.)

on radiographs as being cortico-desmoid in appearance.

SPECIAL CONSIDERATIONS IN THE YOUNG ATHLETE

The skeletally immature athlete is subject to unique sports-related shoulder injuries by virtue of the presence of incompletely fused epiphyseal plates. The epiphyseal plate is a cartilaginous structure that is responsible for longitudinal bone growth. Injuries to the epiphyseal plates are of particular significance because of potential disturbance of the rate of bone growth. Knowledge of the normal locations and variable radiographic appearance of epiphyses is necessary for accurate radiographic interpretation (Fig. 9-33). Normal epiphyses can be mistakenly diagnosed as fractures by

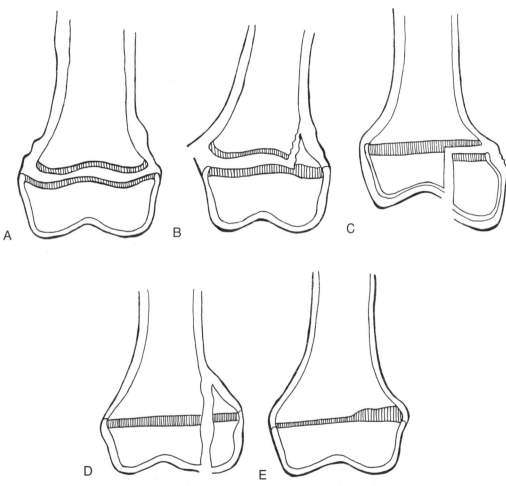

Fig. 9-34. Salter-Harris type fractures. **(A)** Type I: split of the growth plate. **(B)** Type II: split of the growth plate with fracture producing triangular metaphyseal fragment. **(C)** Type III: a vertical fracture through the epiphysis that enters the epiphyseal plate. **(D)** Type IV: a fracture extending across the epiphysis, epiphyseal plate, and metaphysis. **(E)** Type V: compression of a portion of the epiphyseal plate. (Modified from Resnick and Niwayma,[39] with permission.)

the nonradiologist. Likewise, fractures involving the epiphyses can be subtle and as a result go unrecognized. The epiphyseal centers of the humeral tuberosities appear at approximately 7 months of age; the epiphysis of the humeral head appears at approximately 2 years of age; and those of the distal clavicle, acromion process, and corocoid process appear at approximately 8 years of age. The closure of these growth centers occurs relatively late. Some may remain open until the age of 25 years.

Salter-Harris Fractures

Acute injury to the growth plates is most commonly described according to the classification system of Salter and Harris as types I, II, III, IV, and V injuries. Types I, II, and III have a good prognosis. Six percent of all epiphyseal injuries are type I and the proximal humerus is the most common site for this type of injury. In type I injury there is an epiphyseal separation that is typically the result of shearing or avulsive forces (Fig. 9-34A).

Type II injury is the most common epiphyseal injury, accounting for approximately 75 percent of all epiphyseal injuries. This type of fracture occurs most commonly within the distal radius, distal tibia, distal fibula, and distal ulna in order of decreasing frequency. Type II injuries are generally the result of a shearing or avulsion force that splits the growth plate and enters the metaphysis producing a metaphyseal fragment (Fig. 9-34B).

Type III injuries account for approximately 8 percent of epiphyseal injuries. This type of injury occurs in the distal tibia and less commonly in the proximal tibia and distal femur. In these types of injuries, the fracture line extends vertically through the epiphysis and epiphyseal plate resulting in an epiphyseal fragment (Fig. 9-34C).

Type IV injuries comprise approximately 10 percent of all epiphyseal injuries and are most commonly encountered in the distal humerus and distal tibia. Type IV injuries result from a vertical splitting force that results in a fracture that extends across the epiphysis, epiphyseal plate, and metaphysis with an epiphyseal metaphyseal fragment (Fig. 9-34D).

Type V injuries are very rare, accounting for only approximately 1 percent of epiphyseal injuries. They occur as a result of compressive force as in a crushing injury to the distal portion of a tubular bone (Fig. 9-34E).

Little League Shoulder

Little League shoulder is a condition of the skeletally immature throwing athlete. It is considered to be either a stress-related condition or a subacute type I Salter-Harris injury. Clinically, the patient presents complaining of pain involving the dominant throwing shoulder. Healing normally is complete within 4 to 6 weeks following restriction of all throwing-related activity. The AP and lateral projections of the proximal humerus may demonstrate widening of the proximal humeral epiphyseal plate.

Acromioclavicular Joint Injury

Acromioclavicular injuries are uncommon in the skeletally immature athlete. When present, they are typically type I or II injuries. Radiographic examination and evaluation is identical to that of adult patients.

Post-Traumatic Osteolysis

Post-traumatic osteolysis of the distal clavicle is sometimes seen as a late sequela of type I and type II acromioclavicular joint injuries in the young athlete. The radiographic examination and radiologic appearance is identical to that of adult patients.

Clavicular Fractures

The most common fracture involving the shoulder in young athletes is the clavicular fracture. The usual mechanism is a direct trauma sustained in a football injury. As in the adult patient, the middle third of the clavicle is most frequently the site of injury. Radiographic examination and radiologic appearance are identical to that of the adult patient (Fig. 9-35).

Pathologic Fracture

Underlying pathology can predispose the skeletally immature athlete to fracture. Simple bone cysts (unicameral bone cyst) are a relatively common benign lesion of childhood seen with relative frequency in the proximal humerus. This lesion is present in young males with a ratio of 2 to 1 relative to young females.

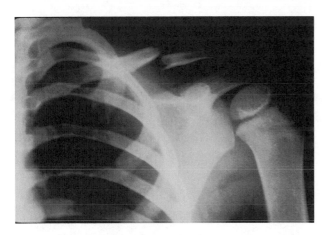

Fig. 9-35. Clavicular fracture.

SPORT SPECIFIC INJURIES

Most forms of athletic activity are associated with specific types of sports injuries. Shoulder injuries are particularly common in swimming, baseball, tennis, football, and gymnastics (Table 9-8).

Swimming

Freestyle swimming, the butterfly stroke, and the backstroke are all implicated in anterolateral shoulder pain. This pain is believed to be the result of a combination of impingement syndrome complicated in many cases by instability.

Baseball

Anterior shoulder problems, common in pitchers, are believed to be due to subacromial impingement. Ossification of the posterior glenoid cavity occurs and possibly is due to pinching during the cocking phase or excessive distraction of the tissues during follow-through.

Tennis

The tennis serve can be a cause of shoulder pain and it is thought to be related to subacromial impingement. In older tennis players a rotator cuff tear is a possibility. In the younger athlete early impingement syndrome may be present.

Football

Football results in both direct and indirect trauma to the shoulder. Direct trauma includes acromioclavicular or sternoclavicular joint sprain or dislocations as well as clavicular and humeral fractures. Indirect injuries include shoulder dislocations and fractures of the proximal humerus.

Gymnastics

Overuse tendinitis syndromes can develop from the high bar and parallel bars. Rings cause subacromial bursitis or instability syndromes. Another entity referred to as Ringman's shoulder is apparently an overuse reaction described in detail previously.

SPECIALIZED IMAGING

Fluoroscopic Evaluation (Cineradiography)

Fluoroscopic evaluation has been recommended for the detection of subtle instability in patients with recalcitrant undiagnosed shoulder pain.[22] The examination is performed under anesthesia. A recent study suggests that the specificity for determining instability was 100 percent and the sensitivity was 93 percent.[23] It would seem apparent that this tool should be used only in cases where other less expensive and invasive procedures have failed to provide a diagnosis.

Arthrography

Conventional arthrography was used as early as 1933 in the evaluation of capsular injuries. Evaluation of rotator cuff tears (Fig. 9-36), capsular lesions, and labrum tears are the most common applications. Distension arthrography is used in the evaluation of frozen shoulder. Two general techniques employed include single and double contrast studies.

Single contrast studies use injection of a contrast agent (60 percent meglumine diatrizoate). Routine views of the shoulder are performed prior to injection. Views include anteroposterior, internal/external, axillary, and bicipital groove positions. After injection, these views are repeated. If a complete tear is not evident, another repeat series is performed after exercise

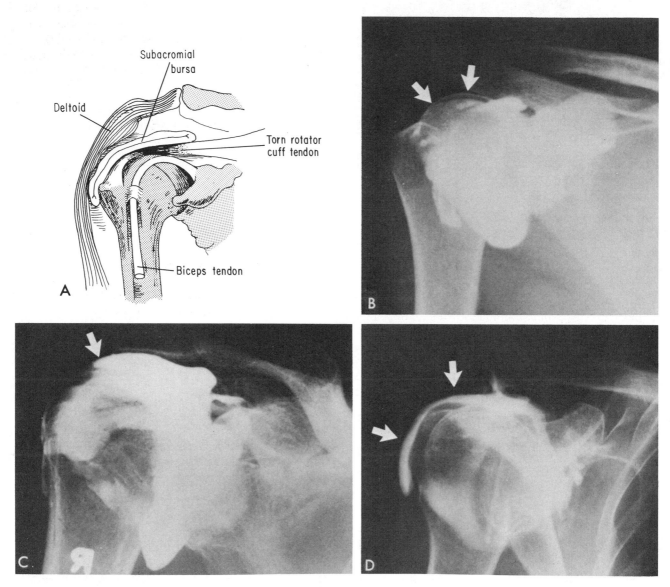

Fig. 9-36. Rotator cuff tear. **(A)** Tear of the tendons of the rotator cuff muscles will cause inflammation of the overlying subacromial (subdeltoid) bursa or communication of the glenohumeral joint space with the bursa or both. **(B)** The normal arthrogram demonstrates dye filling the glenohumeral joint (where the dye is injected) but not communicating into the subdeltoid bursa *(arrows)*. **(C & D)** This patient sustained a fall on his outstretched arm and complained of inability to use his shoulder. Examination revealed normal passive range of motion but markedly impaired active abduction. The arthrogram reveals extravasation of dye into the suprahumeral space *(arrow)* and dye outlining the entire subdeltoid bursa *(arrows)*. Surgical repair was successful. (From Reilly,[33] with permission.)

of the shoulder in an attempt to distribute the contrast material.[24]

Double contrast studies use a mixture of 4 ml contrast medium, 1/3 ml of 1/1,000 epinephrine, and 12 ml of room air. Anteroposterior views are taken after injection. The patient is upright with 5 to 10 lb strapped to the wrists. An axillary view is taken in the supine position. Using the same protocol and rationale as with the single contrast study, the radiographic series is repeated after exercise of the shoulder.

Given that the contrast material will not be capable of penetrating the substance of a tendon, incomplete tears (intratendinous and those on the superior surface) are not visualized.[25] Tears that have sealed are also undetected. Inadequate distribution of contrast material will also lead to false negatives. False positives can occur with inadvertent injection into an enlarged bursa, which may be misinterpreted as a full-thickness tear of the rotator cuff.

Comparison of single versus double contrast studies indicates that double contrast arthrography is better at delineating the quality and extent of the tear.[26] However, Cofield[27] feels that single contrast is sufficient for the diagnosis of a tear and will usually result in fewer false negatives. Regarding the clinical importance of distinguishing between partial and full-thickness tears, a study by Calvert et al.[28] demonstrated leakage in patients who had amelioration of their symptoms with surgical repair. This indicates that finding leakage on arthrography may not be as significant in determining need for surgical intervention given that patients can be asymptomatic with leakage. Also patients with full-thickness tears do respond well to conservative care. When surgical intervention is necessary, Neviaser[29] suggests an outside window of 2 to 3 weeks for successful repair due to the tendency for retraction of the edges, which makes surgical repair more difficult.

CT–Arthrography

CT–arthrography (Figs. 9-37 to 9-39) is considered the tool of choice for visualization of capsular and labral lesions.[30] The study is simply an addition to a routine double contrast study. The addition of the CT scan adds approximately 15 minutes. The patient is supine and usually has the arm in a neutral position (palm against the side). Others use internal or external rotation positions; however, external rotation may allow some de-

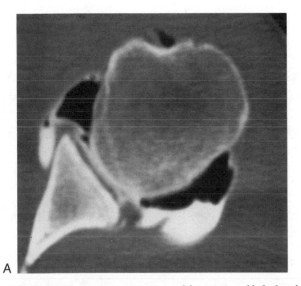 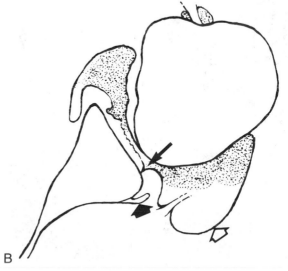

Fig. 9-37. Recurrent posterior subluxations of left shoulder in a high school football player. **(A)** CT image, zone C; **(B)** line drawing. There is a tear and outpouching of the posterior capsule *(hollow arrow),* and the posterior labrum is torn *(long solid arrow).* A bony ridge formed along the glenoid margin is identified *(short solid arrow).* (From Rafii et al,[34] with permission.)

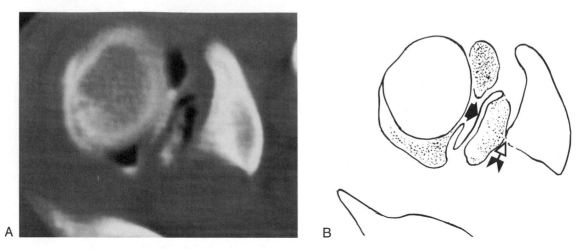

Fig. 9-38. Superior labral detachment of right shoulder in a recreational tennis player. **(A)** CT image, zone A; **(B)** line drawing. The superior labrum *(solid arrow)* is detached and separated from the glenoid margin *(hollow arrow)*. (Fig. **A** from Rafii,[42] with permission; Fig. **B** from Rafii et al,[34] with permission.)

gree of misinterpretation. On the other hand, some centers use external rotation to aid in the visualization of the posterior labrum.[31]

Labrum tears, whether isolated without instability or associated with instability, are well visualized with CT-arthrography. These isolated tears are found more commonly with repetitive throwing activities such as pitching. They are often found anterosuperior. Signs of instability are often not present. The next most common location with this non-instability presentation is a middle anterior labral lesion.

Comparing CT-arthrography to arthrotomography,

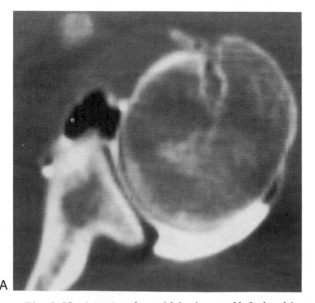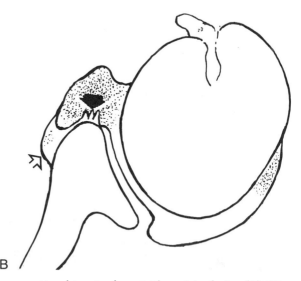

Fig. 9-39. Anterior glenoid labral tear of left shoulder in a recreational tennis player without joint laxity. **(A)** CT image at the junction of zones B and C; **(B)** line drawing. The anterior labrum is irregularly torn *(solid arrow)*. The smaller collection of contrast media is in the inferior margin of the subscapularis bursa *(hollow arrow)*, which was better visualized on the proximal image (not shown). (From Rafii et al,[34] with permission.)

it appears that arthrotomography offers no significant advantages. Arthrotomography is more difficult to position, involves more radiation, and requires more time. Compared to arthroscopy, a CT-arthrogram is not as diagnostic. There are distinct advantages and disadvantages for both approaches dictated, in large part, by the suspicion of the underlying process and potential need for surgical intervention.

In evaluating the unstable shoulder, one of the caveats is that large capsular recesses may be misinterpreted as the sine qua non of instability. However, large recesses may represent a normal variant. More importantly, it is important to search for evidence of either a more distal capsular insertion (on the neck rather than the glenoid), glenoid detachment or stripping, and capsular widening or redundancy.

Labral lesions are commonly found with either recurrent dislocation or subluxation. Labral lesions also occur on the opposite side of instability (i.e., posterior labral tear with anterior instability or vice versa).

Magnetic Resonance Imaging

MRI of the shoulder is rapidly replacing arthrography as the modality of choice in demonstrating soft tissue injuries. While plain films remain the first modality in shoulder imaging, MRI should be considered when plain films are unrevealing and significant soft tissue injury is clinically suspected. MRI is discussed in detail in Chapter 11.

REFERENCES

1. Rockwood CA, Szalay EA, Curtis RJ et al: X-ray evaluation of shoulder problems. p. 178. In Rockwood CA, Matsen (eds): The Shoulder. WB Saunders, Philadelphia, 1990
2. Arndt J: Posterior dislocation of the shoulder. Am J Radiol 94:639, 1965
3. Bowerman J: Radiology and Injury in Sports. Appleton-Century-Crofts, East Norwalk, CT, 1983
4. Bankart ASB: The pathology and treatment of recurrent dislocation of the shoulder joint. Br J Surg 26:23, 1938
5. Pavlov H, Freiberger RH: Fractures and dislocations about the shoulder. Semin Roentgenol 13:2, 1978
6. Vastamaki M, Solomen KA: Posterior dislocation and fracture dislocation of the shoulder. Acta Orthop Scand 51:479, 1980
7. Horsefield D, Jones SM: A useful projection in radiography of the shoulder. J Bone Joint Surg 69B:338, 1987
8. McLaughlin H: Posterior dislocation of the shoulder. J Bone Joint Surg 34A:584, 1952
9. Kornguth PJ, Salazar AM: The apical oblique view of the shoulder. Am J Radiol 149:113, 1987
10. Gambrioli PL, Maggi F, Randelli M: Computerized tomography in the investigation of scapulo-humeral instability. Intal J Orthop Traumatol 11:223, 1985
11. Greenspan A: Orthopedic Radiology. A Practical Approach. JB Lippincott, Philadelphia, 1988
12. Jacobs P: Post-traumatic osteolysis of the outer end of the clavicle. J Bone Joint Surg 46B:705, 1964
13. Levine AH, Pais MJ, Schwartz EE: Post-traumatic osteolysis of the distal clavicle with emphasis on early radiologic changes. Am J Roentgenol 127:781, 1976
14. Madsen B: Osteolysis of the acromial end of the clavicle following trauma. Br J Radiol 36:822, 1963
15. Scavenius M, Iversen BF: Nontraumatic clavicular osteolysis in weight lifters. Am J Sports Med 20:463, 1992
16. Hobbs DW: Sternoclavicular joint: a new radiographic view. Radiology 90:801, 1968
17. Neer CS II: Fractures about the shoulder. p. 679. In Rockwood CA, Green DP, Bucholz RW (eds): Rockwood and Green's Fractures in Adults. 3rd Ed. JB Lippincott, Philadelphia, 1991
18. Neer CS II: Fractures of the distal third of the clavicle. Clin Orthop 58:43, 1968
19. Bigliani LU, Morrison D, April EW: The morphology of the acromion and its relationship to rotator cuff tears. Orthop Trans 10:228, 1986
20. Andrews JR, Byrd JW, Kupperman SP, Angelo RL: The profile view of the acromion. Clin Orthop Relat Res 263:142, 1991
21. Fulton M: Cortical desmoid like lesion of the proximal humerus and its occurrence in gymnastics (Ringman's shoulder lesion). Am J Sports Med 7:57, 1979
22. Maki NJ: Cineradiographic studies with shoulder instabilities. Am J Sports Med 16:362, 1988
23. Papilion JA, Shall LM: Fluoroscopic evaluation for subtle shoulder instability. Am J Sports Med 20:548, 1992
24. Rafii M, Minkoff J, DeStefano V: Diagnostic imaging of the shoulder. p. 91. In Nicholas JA, Hershman EB (eds): The Upper Extremity in Sports Medicine. CV Mosby, St. Louis, 1990
25. Kilcoyne RF, Marcove RC, Freiberger RH: Shoulder arthrography. Am J Radiol 103:658, 1968
26. Pavlov H, Freiberger RH: The roentgenographic evaluation of anterior shoulder instability. Clin Orthop 194:153, 1985
27. Cofield RH: Tears of rotator cuff. Mayo Clin Proc 258, 1980

28. Calvert PT et al: Arthrography of the shoulder after operative repair of the torn rotator cuff. J Bone Joint Surg 68B: 147, 1986

29. Neviaser RJ: Tears of the rotator cuff. Orthop Clin North Am 11:295, 1980

30. Singson RD, Feldman F, Bigliani L: CT arthrographic patterns in recurrent glenohumeral instability. Am J Radiol 149:749, 1987

31. Deutsch AL Resnick D, Mink SH, Berman JL: Computed and conventional arthrotomography of the glenohumeral joint: normal anatomy and clinical experience. Radiology 153:603, 1984

32. Greenway GD, Danzig LA, Resnick D, Haghighi P: The painful shoulder. Med Radiog Photography 58:42, 1982

33. Reilly BM: Practical Strategies in Outpatient Medicine. 1st ed. WB Saunders, Philadelphia, 1984

34. Rafii M, Minkoff J, Bonamo J, Firooznia H: Computed tomography (CT) arthrography of instabilities in athletes. Am J Sports Med 16:356, 1988

35. Rozing PM, de Bakker HM, Obermann WR: Radiographic views in recurrent anterior shoulder dislocation. Acta Orthop Scand 68:479, 1967

36. Danzig LA, Greenway G, Resnick D: The Hill-Sachs lesion. Am J Sports Med 8:328, 1980

37. DeSmet AA: Anterior oblique projection in radiography of the traumatized shoulder. Am J Radiol 134:515, 1980

38. Rafii M, Minkoff J, DeStefano V: Diagnostic imaging of the shoulder. p. 91. In Nicholas JA, Hershman EB (eds): The Upper Extremity in Sports Medicine. CV Mosby, St. Louis, 1990

39. Resnick D, Niwayma G: Diagnosis of Bone and Joint Disorders. WB Saunders, Philadelphia, 1988

40. Rockwood CA, Green DP, Bucholz RW (eds): Rockwood and Green's Fractures in Adults. 3rd ed. JB Lippincott, Philadelphia, 1991

41. Reid DC: Sports Injury Assessment and Rehabilitation. Churchill Livingstone, New York, 1992

42. Rafii M, Finoznia H, Bonamo JJ et al: Athlete shoulder injuries. Radiology 162:559, 1987

10
Sonography

JOSEPH H. INTROCASO

Diagnostic ultrasound is playing an increasing role in the noninvasive evaluation of musculoskeletal injuries. Its greatest application is in the examination of the shoulder. Sonographic evaluation of joints began as a noninvasive means of detecting Baker cysts. This soon progressed to the detection of full-thickness tendon injuries, principally of the rotator cuff of the shoulder and Achilles tendon. Recent improvements in transducer technology have allowed greater definition of anatomic structures and broadened the scope of musculoskeletal sonography. We can now accurately evaluate partial thickness rotator cuff tears, detect tiny joint effusions, and diagnose subtle fractures missed on conventional radiographs. Abnormalities of the periarticular structures, such as muscle ruptures, can also be detected.[1]

Ultrasound examination has many advantages over other modalities. The most significant advantages are accessibility, real-time dynamic examination, and cost. Ultrasound machines are small compared with other pieces of medical imaging equipment and are easily transported to outpatient clinics. This allows performance of the imaging examination on the same day as the patient's first clinic appointment. Long waiting lists for ultrasound examinations are almost nonexistent. Legislative restrictions on the availability of magnetic resonance imaging (MRI) equipment have resulted in waiting times of several weeks at most institutions. The ability to examine a joint throughout its range of motion in real-time is unique to ultrasound, when compared with computed tomography (CT) and MRI. The lack of ionizing radiation and much greater soft tissue contrast make ultrasound far superior to CT and fluoroscopy. The cost of an ultrasound examination is a small fraction of the cost of CT and MRI examinations,

making it by far the most cost-effective diagnostic modality for the shoulder. This makes serial follow-up examinations economically feasible.

EXAMINATION TECHNIQUE

It is impossible to describe fully a technique for sonographic examination of the shoulder within the limitations of this chapter. However, certain principles can be emphasized. The use of linear array transducers is essential in musculoskeletal imaging. This is due to the strong anisotropic properties demonstrated by muscles and tendons. Curved array and sector scanning transducers will produce images that demonstrate artifactually decreased echogenicity peripherally, leading to an incorrect diagnosis. Another consideration in transducer selection is frequency of the sound beam. Higher frequency transducers produce images with greater spatial resolution at the expense of the depth of penetration. Clearly, the best transducer for musculoskeletal imaging is one having the highest frequency that will penetrate to the area of interest. This is usually a 7.5 MHz linear array for shoulder examinations. In obese patients it may be necessary to utilize a 5 MHz linear array for greater penetration. Examination of superficial structures, such as tendons of the fingers, can be performed using 10 MHz linear array transducers.

One final point to be emphasized in examination technique is the concept of sonographic palpation. Sonographic palpation is the technique of applying gentle but firm pressure with the transducer during the examination to elicit the point of maximal tenderness. This allows the examiner to direct the examination to the point of greatest clinical interest. In addition, it helps the examiner to distinguish between symptomatic and asymptomatic lesions. In this manner musculoskeletal sonography is an interactive examination. This advantage over other imaging modalities should not be ignored.

SHOULDER PATHOLOGY

Tendons

Tendons of the rotator cuff of the shoulder (supraspinatus, infraspinatus, subscapularis, and teres minor) and the long head of the biceps are easily evaluated sonographically. Normal tendons are homogeneous echogenic structures of uniform thickness with regular striations corresponding to the collagen bundles of the tendon (Fig. 10-1).[2,3] Tendonitis, tendon subluxation/

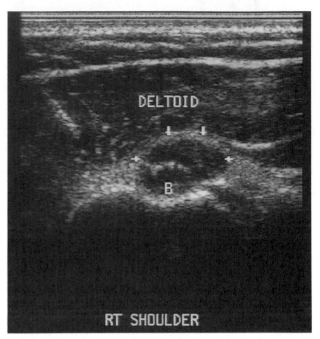

Fig. 10-2. Biceps tendonitis—transverse sonogram. This patient is a tennis player who had recently experienced increasing right shoulder pain. Note the hypoechoic fluid collection *(arrows)* surrounding the biceps tendon *(B)*. No fluid was seen in the posterior joint recess, consistent with the diagnosis of biceps tendonitis.

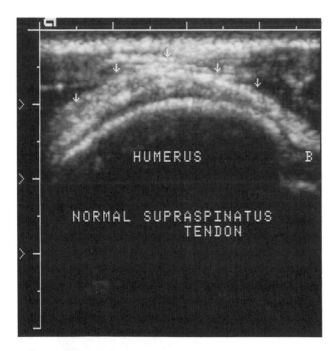

Fig. 10-1. Normal rotator cuff—transverse sonogram. The patient is a normal 31-year-old man. The tendon of the long head of the biceps muscle *(B)* is seen at the right. Arrows indicate the substance of the supraspinatus portion of the tendons of the rotator cuff. Note the uniformly echogenic appearance of this tendon and its uniform thickness. The hypoechoic band deep to the tendon is the articular cartilage of the humeral head.

dislocation, partial rupture, and complete rupture are entities that can be diagnosed sonographically.

Thickening and decreased echogenicity of the tendon are classic sonographic findings in cases of tendonitis and shoulder impingement syndrome. When tendonitis involves a tendon having a synovial sheath increased fluid will be seen within the sheath (Fig. 10-2). When examining the tendon of the long head of the biceps muscle it is important to remember that its tendon sheath is in communication with the joint space of the shoulder. Therefore, a joint effusion will also be seen within the biceps tendon sheath. To confirm that fluid in the tendon sheath is related to biceps tendonitis rather than a joint effusion the posterior recess of the joint must be examined. The posterior recess of the shoulder joint is the most sensitive region for detection of joint effusion (Fig. 10-3). An increase in joint fluid of as little as 1 ml can be detected sonographically.[4] Detection of a joint effusion is essential because

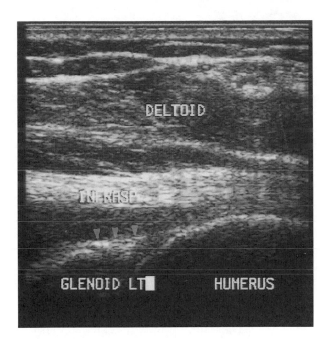

Fig. 10-3. Posterior joint recess—transverse image. The posterior recess of the shoulder is the most sensitive location for detection of joint effusion. This demonstrates the normal anatomy of the posterior joint recess. Note that the infraspinatus muscle and tendon lie in close proximity to the bony glenoid, fibrocartilaginous labrum *(arrowheads)*, and the humeral head.

this is a good indicator of intra-articular pathology, such as septic arthritis or avascular necrosis. If an effusion is detected in the posterior recess, but no fluid is present around the biceps tendon, septic arthritis should be at the top of the list in the differential diagnosis (Fig. 10-4). Ultrasound guided aspiration is indicated whenever there is clinical suspicion of septic arthritis. Sonographic guidance eliminates the possibility of false negative or "dry" taps.

In the shoulder, tendon subluxation or dislocation may involve the long head of the biceps. This tendon is secured within the bicipital groove by the transverse ligament. Rupture of the transverse ligament can occur with trauma or as a sequella of rheumatoid arthritis. This allows subluxation or frank dislocation of the biceps tendon, which usually is displaced medially (Fig. 10-5). Often it is found deep to the subscapularis muscle. Tendon luxation may also be seen in the hand, wrist, and foot.

Partial tendon rupture may be seen as a hypoechoic cleft extending into the tendon or as focal thinning of the tendon (Fig. 10-6). Careful examination in two planes may be necessary to detect subtle lesions. Rarely, incomplete tendon ruptures may appear as hyperechoic clefts interrupting the normal tendon architecture. It is felt that the hyperechoic material represents granulation tissue within the defect.

Full-thickness tendon ruptures will present as a hypoechoic defect separating the two torn ends (Fig. 10-7). Acute traumatic tears tend to be associated with small joint effusions, making sonographic examination easier. However, if imaged very close to the time of injury, the effusion may be isoechoic relative to the tendon due to its hemorrhagic nature. In these cases gentle compression applied with the transducer will express the fluid from the defect, revealing the torn

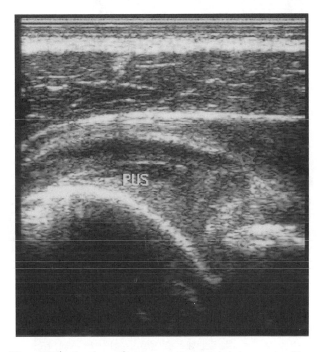

Fig. 10-4. Septic arthritis—posterior joint recess. Two weeks prior to this examination the patient had received an intra-articular injection of steroids for an exacerbation of his rheumatoid arthritis. He presents now with increasing pain in the shoulder. This image demonstrates a large joint effusion with abundant internal echos consistent with a septic arthritis. The infraspinatus *(arrows)* is elevated away from the glenoid *(G)*. The joint was drained surgically and *Staphylococcus aureus* was cultured.

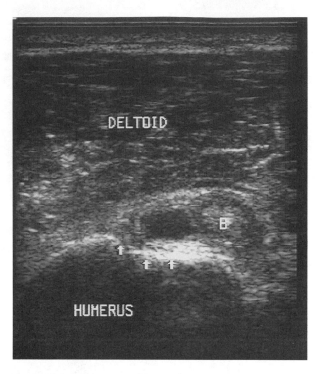

Fig. 10-5. Biceps tendon luxation—transverse sonogram. Fluid is demonstrated within the bicipital groove *(arrows)* and the biceps tendon is dislocated medially, beneath the subscapularis tendon. This is the most common pattern of biceps tendon luxation.

ends of the tendon. When assessing complete tears of the rotator cuff it is important to measure the extent of the tear. This is most accurately performed using ultrasound.

Muscles

A patient's complaint of shoulder pain may also be the result of muscle injury involving the biceps, deltoid, and pectoralis, as well as the muscles of the rotator cuff. Sonography can detect muscle rupture, muscle hernias, ischemia, infarction, and infection.[1] Ultrasound provides superb detail of the pennate structure of muscles.[5] The muscle bundles composed of regularly arranged actin and myosin filaments appear hypoechoic. Fibroadipose septae are hyperechoic struc-

tures that separate muscle bundles (Fig. 10-8). These septae contain fat, arteries, veins, and nerves. Disruptions in this highly organized pattern can be easily detected sonographically.

Muscle ruptures can be divided into two groups: compressive and distraction. Compressive muscle ruptures are usually seen as the result of contact sports or motor vehicle accidents. They are the result of a forceful blow to the body, compressing the muscle between the external object and the underlying bone. This causes extensive tissue injury with shearing of muscle fibers, blood vessels, and nerves. Large hematomas tend to accumulate within the defect. Ultrasound will easily demonstrate these lesions, which appear as hypoechoic cavities with shaggy borders. Echogenicity of the fluid is determined by the time interval between injury and examination. In the subacute stage a hematocrit level may also be observed within the hematoma.

Distraction muscle ruptures are the result of sudden forceful contraction of a muscle with separation of muscle fibers primarily along interstitial planes.[6] This

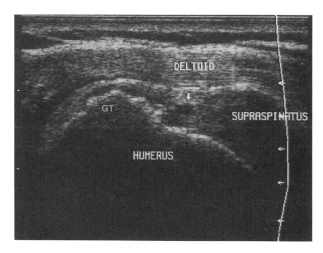

Fig. 10-6. Partial thickness tear of the rotator cuff—transverse sonogram. This baseball player presented with a complaint of increasing pain with throwing over the past two weeks. This image of the supraspinatus tendon as it inserts on the greater tuberosity *(GT)* shows a focal hypoechoic defect *(arrow)* along the inner portion of the tendon with thinning of the tendon in this region. The defect does not extend through the entire thickness of the tendon; therefore, arthrography will not demonstrate leakage of contrast material into the subacromial-subdeltoid bursa.

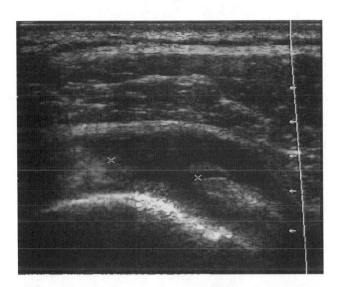

Fig. 10-7. Full thickness rotator cuff tear—transverse image. A full thickness tear *(X)* is demonstrated in the supraspinatus portion of the rotator cuff of this weightlifter. He experienced a sharp painful snap during a workout. Fluid is seen separating the torn ends of the supraspinatus tendon and fills the subacromial-subdeltoid bursa. The extent of the tendon injury can be accurately measured using ultrasound; the defect measures 11 mm in width in this case.

is seen as a hypoechoic cleft within the muscle filled with hematoma. Often free ends of torn muscle fibers can be identified floating within the hematoma, referred to as the "bell clapper" sign.[5]

The role of ultrasound in both compression and distraction muscle ruptures is more than simply establishing a diagnosis. Ultrasound will accurately evaluate the extent of injury, estimate size of the associated hematoma, and provide a reliable means of following healing to determine when it is safe to resume a normal level of activity. Estimation of the size of the hematoma is very important. Large hematomas increase the likelihood of myositis ossificans and scar formation. Therefore, ultrasound guided aspiration of the hematoma can be performed to obtain the best possible clinical outcome, when surgical repair is not indicated. In some cases, ultrasound guided placement of a percutaneous drain is indicated to prevent reaccumulation of the hematoma.[1]

Infection, ischemia, and infarction of muscle can also be detected sonographically. Edema within mus-

cle results in increased echogenicity of muscle bundles, which will disrupt the normal pennate architecture of the muscle observed sonographically. In severe cases, relative echogenicity of muscle architecture will be reversed. Muscle bundles will appear hyperechoic and the fibroadipose septae will be hypoechoic. Cases of ischemia and infarction can be further evaluated using duplex and color flow Doppler flow techniques. Compartment syndromes can also be diagnosed noninvasively using ultrasound.[1]

Bone and Cartilage

Ultrasound is very valuable in the detection of lesions involving cortical bone and cartilage, but it cannot evaluate trabecular bone and the medullary cavity. It is a multiplanar tomographic modality, giving it considerable advantage over conventional radiographs in the

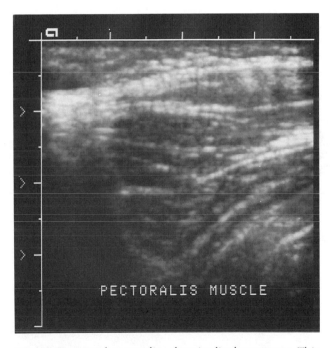

Fig. 10-8. Normal pectoralis—longitudinal sonogram. This longitudinal image of the pectoralis muscle of a normal patient demonstrates the pennate structure of the muscle. Muscle bundles are hypoechoic and are separated by hyperechoic fibroadipose septae.

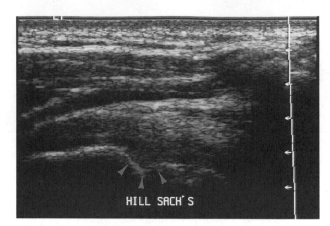

Fig. 10-9. Hill-Sachs defect—coronal sonogram. The patient had experienced multiple shoulder dislocations in the past. Conventional radiographs were normal. A moderate Hill-Sachs defect is demonstrated *(arrowheads)* in the contour of the cortical bone of the humeral head. Ultrasound is more sensitive for detection of these lesions than conventional radiographs because it is a multiplanar tomographic imaging modality.

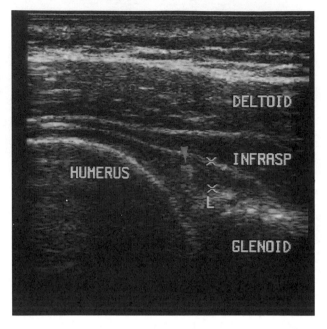

Fig. 10-10. Glenoid labrum tear—transverse sonogram. A discontinuity is demonstrated in the fibrocartilaginous labrum *(L)* of this 30 year old woman. The distal fragment of the labrum *(arrowhead)* is well visualized. A tiny joint effusion is present in the posterior recess.

evaluation for marginal erosions in cases of inflammatory arthritis. Nondisplaced fractures that are radiographically occult can be diagnosed using ultrasound. The tiny cortical discontinuity will be seen in association with subperiosteal hematoma. This technique is very valuable when clinical suspicion of fracture remains high despite negative conventional radiographs. Hill-Sachs fractures, which may be occult on conventional radiographs are easily observed sonographically (Fig. 10-9).

In children, cartilaginous ossification centers are poorly evaluated on conventional radiographs. Sonography provides an excellent means of evaluating joints in children. The unossified epiphysis can be easily visualized and their relationship to other joint structures observed throughout the full range of motion. Thus, dislocations and Salter-Harris type I and type V fractures are easily diagnosed without the use of ionizing radiation.[7]

Serial measurements of cartilage thickness have proven valuable in the follow-up of arthritis in adults. This gives rheumatologists a quick noninvasive means of assessing the degree of success of therapy.[8] Cartilage

edema, surface pitting, and osteochondritis dissecans can also be detected. Disruption of the fibrocartilaginous labrum of the glenoid can be seen in its posterior extent (Fig. 10-10).

Diagnostic ultrasound can be a very powerful tool in the evaluation of shoulder pain. Its scope extends beyond that of simply evaluating for tears of the rotator cuff. Three-dimensional reconstruction of ultrasound images of the shoulder, now under investigation, will further enhance the utility of ultrasound.

REFERENCES

1. van Holsbeeck M, Introcaso J: Musculoskeletal Ultrasound. Sonography of Muscle. p. 13. Mosby-Yearbook, Chicago, 1991
2. Fornage BD, Rifkin MD, Touche DH et al: Sonography of the patellar tendon: preliminary observation. 143:179, 1984

3. Fornage BD: Achilles Tendon: US Examination. Radiology 159:759, 1986

4. van Holsbeeck M, Introcaso J: Musculoskeletal Ultrasound: Sonography of the Shoulder. p. 265. CV Mosby, St. Louis, 1991

5. Fornage BD, Touche DH, Segal P et al: Ultrasonography in the evaluation of muscular trauma. J Ultrasound Med 2:549, 1983

6. Bouvier JF, Chassain AP, Veyriras E: Place de l'echo—Tomographie dans les accidents musculaires des membres inferieurs du footballeur. Cinesiologie 21:274, 1982

7. Dias JJ, Lamont AC, Jones JM: Ultrasonic diagnosis of neonatal separation of the distal humeral epiphysis. J Bone J Surg 70B:825, 1988

8. Aisen AM, McCune WJ, McGuire A et al: Sonographic evaluation of the cartilage of the knee. Radiology 153:781, 1984

11

Magnetic Resonance Imaging

HOWARD R. UNGER, JR.
CHRISTIAN H. NEUMANN
STEVE A. PETERSEN

The clinical evaluation of the injured shoulder can be challenging. Imaging techniques such as arthrography, frequently combined with computed tomography (CT), provide a means of evaluating rotator cuff integrity, and may demonstrate findings suggestive of instability. These procedures are invasive, however, and expose the patient to ionizing radiation. Ultrasound can identify some rotator cuff tears, but this modality is very operator dependent and has certain imaging limitations as well.

Magnetic resonance imaging (MRI) is now being used with frequency. It provides diagnostic information not readily available with other modalities. Its advantages are based on multiplanar imaging capability and superior soft tissue contrast, in a noninvasive format that includes lack of ionizing radiation.

MRI TECHNIQUE

MRI is a safe procedure. However, because the patient is subjected to a strong magnetic field, certain precautions are required. Patients with intraocular metallic foreign bodies, cardiac pacemakers, certain intracranial aneurysms and hemostatic clips, and several other devices[1] pose a contraindication to entering the magnetic field. Relative contraindications include recent (4 to 6 weeks) surgery with metallic implants in place prior to formation of adequate scar tissue, and patients requiring close monitoring, depending on the monitoring capabilities of the facility being utilized.

Because even a small amount of movement can de-grade images, patients must be able to hold still for extended periods of time. Children under 6 years of age generally require sedation or light anesthesia. Claustrophobic or agitated patients are administered anxiolytics or sedatives before entering the relatively small bore magnet.

The typical MRI examination of the shoulder takes approximately 45 to 55 minutes, although this can be reduced to 30 minutes or less with use of the new fast spin-echo techniques. The patient is placed into the magnet supine with the arm of interest in a neutral to slightly externally rotated position along the side. A surface coil is placed over the shoulder, centered over the humeral head. Many specialized surface coils are now available that provide the necessary signal-to-noise ratio. The more commonly used include a single anterior coil, paired coils in a Helmholtz configuration,[2] and a loop-gap resonator design.[3] New phased-array and quadrature coils are now being marketed (Fig. 11-1).

Many different types of imaging methods can be utilized with MRI. Spin-echo imaging is the most commonly employed. In classic spin-echo sequences, a burst of radio-frequency energy is delivered to the patient in such a manner as to realign some of the un-bound protons within the body or scan volume in a perpendicular direction to the main magnetic field. This is called a *90 degree pulse.* This is followed by a 180 degree pulse, which has a refocusing effect on the signal, allowing collection of a radio-frequency signal, or *echo,* a short time later. The time between administration of the 90 degree pulse and collection of the echo is called the *echo time,* or TE. The time between

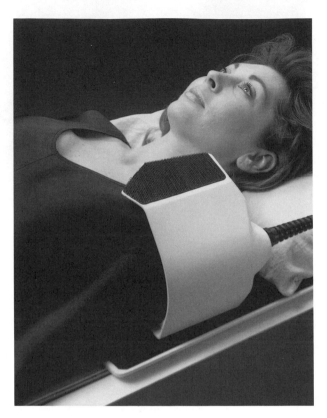

Fig. 11-1. Prototype of a new quadrature shoulder surface coil, with a shell molded to the anatomy of the shoulder placed on a volunteer in the scanning position. (Courtesy of MRI Devices Co., Hartland, WI.)

successive 90 degree radio-frequency pulses is the *repetition time,* or TR. Three orthongonal magnetic gradients are superimposed upon the main magnetic field during this time, thus providing the ability to select the desired imaging plane and slice, as well as allowing

for spatial localization of the signal. An image can be T_1-weighted by using a short TE and short TR, intermediate-weighted or proton-density weighted by using a short TE with a long TR, and T_2-weighted by using a relatively long TE and long TR. A variant of traditional spin-echo, now increasingly employed, is *fast spin-echo.* This uses multiple 180 degree refocusing pulses, or an echo train, in a single TR. Typically the pulses are delivered in such a manner as to produce T_2-weighted images. Excellent results can be obtained by this method in only a fraction of the time needed for traditional spin-echo imaging.

Gradient-echo imaging is also commonly used in shoulder imaging. This technique substitutes rapid reversal of the gradients for the 180 degrees radio-frequency pulse used in spin-echo imaging. It is considerably faster than standard T_2-weighted images performed with the spin-echo technique, but it suffers from a relatively poor signal-to-noise ratio.

With the recent introduction of fast spin-echo technology, many centers are reevaluating their traditional imaging protocols. The protocol now used at San Francisco Magnetic Resonance Center (SFMRC), which takes advantage of the time savings available from fast spin-echo technique, is shown in Table 11-1.

Proper selection of the optimal scan plane (Fig. 11-2) is performed by first obtaining a coronal ''scout,'' then aligning the axial images to cover the glenoid fossa. Coronal images are chosen from the axial images in a plane parallel to the long axis of the supraspinatus tendon, and the sagittal oblique images perpendicular to the former, parallel to the glenohumeral joint.

Axial images (Fig. 11-3A & B) are best for evaluating the anterior and posterior glenoid labrum, the relationship between the humeral head and glenoid cavity,

Table 11-1. Magnetic Resonance Imaging Protocol Currently Used at San Francisco Magnetic Resonance Center[a]

Plane	TR/TE/NEX	Slice/Gap (mm)	Flip Angle	Matrix (256×)	FOV	Comments
Coronal scout	300/min/1	10/5	—	128	24	
Axial	700 min/2	4/1	—	192	12–14	
Axial	400/15/4	4/0	20	192	12–14	MPGR
Coronal oblique	1,000/min/2	5/0.5	—	192	12–16	CSMEMP
Coronal oblique	4,000/102/2	5/1	—	256	14	FSE
Sagittal oblique	3,000/102/2	6/2	—	192	16	FSE

Abbreviations: TR, repetition time; TE, echo time; NEX, number of excitations; FOV, field of view; MPGR, multiplanar gradient-recalled acquisition steady state, a multislice gradient-echo technique; CSMEMP, technique to acquire closely spaced multiple echo multiplanar spin-echo images using a rectangular-shaped pulse profile to avoid noise from cross-talk; FSE, fast spin-echo.
[a] Based on the 4.7 software capability of the GE-Signa scanner, using conventional and fast spin-echo technique. The average examination time is 30 to 35 minutes.

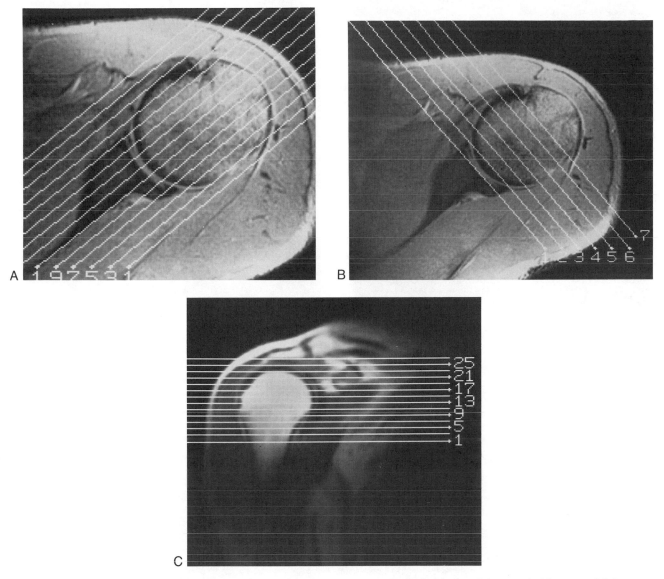

Fig. 11-2. "Localizer" images demonstrating placement of the **(A)** coronal oblique, **(B)** sagittal oblique, and **(C)** axial sequences, in relation to shoulder anatomy. The coronal oblique sequences are obtained in a plane parallel to the long axis of the supraspinatus muscle, and perpendicular to the glenohumeral joint. The sagittal oblique sequences are obtained in a plane parallel to the glenohumeral joint, and perpendicular to the coronal oblique images. The axial sequences are obtained in such a manner as to cover the entire glenohumeral joint.

the subscapularis muscle and its insertion into the lesser tuberosity, the subscapularis bursa in the presence of joint fluid, and the anterior and posterior joint capsule (also best evaluated in the presence of joint fluid). The long head of the biceps, including its course within the bicipital groove, and the infraspinatus muscle and tendon are also well seen in the axial plane.

Coronal oblique images (Fig. 11-3C & D) are optimal for evaluating the supraspinatus muscle and tendon, the subacromial/subdeltoid bursa, and the superior and inferior glenoid labrum. The infraspinatus and subscapularis muscles and tendons can be seen on these images, although not always to best advantage. Sagittal oblique images are good for evaluation of

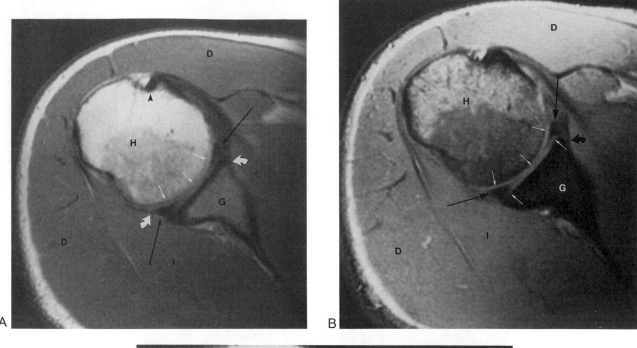

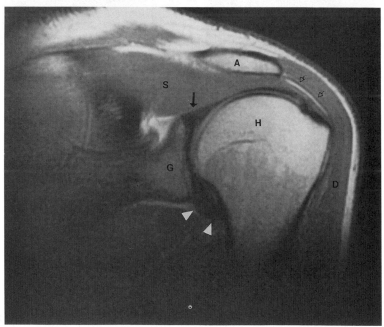

Fig. 11-3. Normal anatomy. **(A)** Axial proton density (TR/TE 1,800/25) and **(B)** multiplanar gradient-recalled (MPGR) (TR/TE flip angle 700/10/20) images taken through the midportion of the glenohumeral joint. **(C)** Coronal oblique proton-density (TR/TE 1,800/25) and **(D)** T₂-weighted (TR/TE 1,800/80) images taken through the midportion of the supraspinatus muscle and tendon. **(E)** Sagittal oblique T₁-weighted image (TR/TE 700/10) taken through the midhumeral head. *G,* bony glenoid; *H,* humerus; *A,* acromion; glenoid labrum *(straight black arrows);* type II anterior capsular insertion and type I posterior capsular insertion *(curved arrows);* hyaline cartilage *(straight white arrows); D,* deltoid muscle; *S,* supraspinatus muscle; *I,* infraspinatus muscle and tendon; long head of biceps tendon *(black arrowheads);* subdeltoid fat *(open arrow);* axillary recess *(white arrowheads). (Figure continues.)*

302

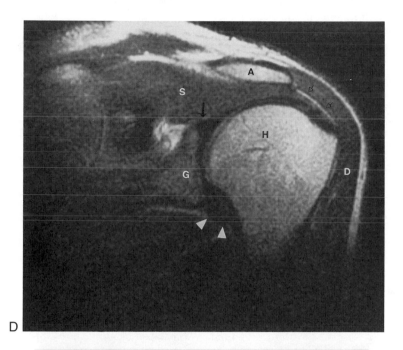

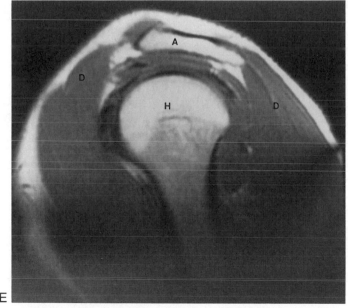

Fig. 11-3. (*Continued*). (**D**) and (**E**)

the osseous-acromial outlet, formed by the osseous ligamentous coracoacromial arch, which includes an assessment of the shape and appearance of the acromion itself, as well as its relationship to the supraspinatus tendon and humeral head (Fig. 11-3E).

SHOULDER ANATOMY

The humeral head articulates with the shallow glenoid fossa, in a multiaxial ball and socket type relationship. Static stability is provided by the capsule and glenohumeral ligaments, with dynamic stability largely supplied by the muscles and tendons of the rotator cuff. The glenohumeral joint is surrounded by a complex array of muscles, tendons, bones, and bursae that serve mechanical, protective, and supportive functions.

The rotator cuff is composed of four muscles and their tendons, which blend with the fibrous capsule. The supraspinatus, infraspinatus, and teres minor muscles all originate from the dorsal aspect of the scapula and insert on the greater tuberosity of the proximal humerus. They function in abduction and external rotation. The supraspinatus tendon inserts on the promontory or highest point of the greater tuberosity, the infraspinatus tendon on the posterior, and the teres minor tendon on the posterior-inferior portion. The musculotendinous junction of the supraspinatus usually coincides with the 12 o'clock position of the humeral head.[4] The fourth muscle of the rotator cuff is the subscapularis, which functions primarily in adduction and internal rotation. It originates from the ventral aspect of the scapula and inserts on the lesser tuberosity and transverse ligament of the bicipital groove.

Typically, normal rotator cuff tendons are of low signal intensity on all sequences. Intermediate signal intensity on T_1-weighted and proton-density images has been observed, however, in many asymptomatic patients.[4] This may be secondary to subclinical inflammation, degeneration, or partial tearing, or simply be related to normal aging. Other causes of intermediate or even high signal intensity within normal rotator cuff tendons will be discussed in the section *Pitfalls of MRI*.

The subacromial/subdeltoid bursa is a potential space, located above the rotator cuff and below the acromion and deltoid muscle, lined by fine, filmy areolar tissue. It facilitates gliding between the deltoid and teres major muscle, and the rotator cuff muscles. A peribursal fat plane partially invests this bursa, and can be visualized as a thin band of high signal intensity on T_1-weighted images. It may be absent or obscured in patients with rotator cuff tears, although this finding by itself is of poor predictive value on MRI.[4] Communication with the joint cavity occurs only if a tear involving the full thickness of the musculotendinous rotator cuff opens into the floor of the bursa.

The subscapularis bursa is normally not seen, unless an effusion is present. It can then be identified as a fluid-filled pouch underlying the coracoid process. It may communicate with the joint through a variable access in the superior-anterior capsule and anterior labrum.

The coracoacromial arch is a strong bony and ligamentous structure that protects the humeral head and rotator cuff tendons from direct trauma. It also limits the space available to the rotator cuff tendons during abduction. It is composed of the acromion and the acromioclavicular joint, the coracoid process, and the coracoacromial ligament. The shape of the acromion has been classified by Bigliani et al.,[5] with frequency of occurrence recently documented by Farley et al.[6] A type I acromion (47 percent) has a flat undersurface, while a type II (39 percent) undersurface is concave. Type III (11 percent) acromions are concave or flat inferiorly, with an anterior hook or spur, the latter being associated with an increased incidence of rotator cuff pathology. Farley et al.[6] also reported a type IV (3 percent) acromion, distinguished by its concave superior surface.

The glenohumeral joint is enveloped by a low signal intensity capsule that extends distally to line the bicipital groove. Superiorly, the capsule encroaches on the base of the coracoid process and inserts in the supraglenoid region, thus including the long head of the biceps tendon within the joint. Laterally and inferiorly the capsule inserts into the anatomic neck of the humerus. Medially, the insertion is quite variable. It can attach directly into the labrum, or more medially along the scapular neck.

Anteriorly, the capsule thickens to form the superior, middle, and inferior glenohumeral ligaments. They arise from along the anterior aspect of the glenoid labrum and insert on, or adjacent to, the lesser tuberosity. The superior glenohumeral ligament is relatively small and difficult to distinguish as a distinct structure on MRI studies. The middle glenohumeral ligament is usually seen, and appears to have a variable attachment medially on the anterior-superior labrum or glenoid neck. The inferior glenohumeral ligament reinforces the capsular area between the subscapularis and the origin of the long head of the triceps. On MRI it may appear merely as diffuse thickening of the anterior-inferior capsule.

According to Moseley and Overgaard,[7] the anterior capsule may attach on the tip or outer surface of the anterior labrum (type I), on the adjacent glenoid rim (type II), or more medially along the scapular neck (type III). The type I and II attachments anteriorly are normal, while type III may indicate capsular stripping. Posteriorly, the capsular attachments are similarly defined, but much less variable. Only the type I attachment is normal posteriorly.

The glenoid labrum is a fibrous structure and imaged as a signal void. It is continuous with the glenoid articular cartilage, which, in contrast, is of high signal. Normal variation of the anterior and posterior labrum has been documented on CT[8] and MRI.[9] The anterior labrum, although commonly having a triangular configuration (45 percent), can be variable. It can be rounded (19 percent), cleaved (15 percent), notched (8 percent), flat (7 percent), or even absent (6 percent) (Fig. 11-4). The posterior labrum generally appears triangular (73 percent), although it can be rounded (12 percent), flat (6 percent), or absent (8 percent). The superior and inferior labrum will usually be triangular in appearance.

The tendon of the long head of the biceps brachii muscle, surrounded by a synovial sheath, lies anteriorly in the intertubercular or bicipital groove, between the greater and lesser tuberosities. It is secured within the groove by the transverse humeral ligament, which passes between the tuberosities over the synovial sheath of the tendon. It also serves as part of the attachment of the tendon of the subscapularis. The long head of the biceps tendon extends over the anterior aspect of the humeral head and attaches to the supraglenoid tubercle, which lies immediately above the glenoid cavity, as well as to the superior aspect of the anterior and posterior labrum.

The normal biceps tendon will be of low signal intensity on all imaging sequences. The biceps tendon sheath communicates with the joint. Fluid within this structure is commonly seen in normal patients, and does not necessarily indicate pathology.

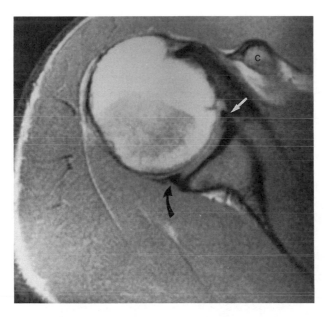

Fig. 11-4. Axial proton-density (TR/TE 1,800/20) image at the level of the coracoid process *(C)*. The anterior labrum *(white arrow)* has a "cleaved" appearance, with high signal hyaline cartilage extending partway through its base. The posterior labrum *(curved arrow)* is triangular and of homogeneous low signal intensity.

IMPINGEMENT SYNDROME/ ROTATOR CUFF DISEASE

Rotator cuff disease can occur in a wide variety of individuals, including young athletes, laborers, and in many older patients. Occasionally, an acute traumatic event can be the cause, although chronic insidious trauma is more common. Two predominant theories exist regarding the etiology of tendon disease. One considers extrinsic compression the culprit, which Neer[10] described as the impingement syndrome. The other theory holds that intrinsic tendon degeneration is the primary pathology, with rotator cuff tears occurring when the intrinsically weakened tendon is subjected to trauma. Ozaki et al.[11] suggest that pathologic changes in the undersurface of the acromion such as trabecular irregularity, sclerosis, hypertrophy, and/or cystic changes, occur as a secondary event. This is supported by their observation that acromial changes occur with partial tears on the bursal side of the joint and in all patients with complete rotator cuff tears, but not with partial tears on the articular or undersurface of the rotator cuff.

Rotator cuff disease is often not an isolated disorder, as it may coexist with instability. Many believe that the presence of anterior instability predisposes a patient to rotator cuff impingement.[12] This situation arises in younger patients who engage in repetitive high-velocity throwing motions. Chronic microtrauma may adversely affect the stabilizing mechanisms of the glenohumeral joint, leading to anterior subluxation of the humeral head. Recurrent subluxation, in turn, can result in a secondary impingement phenomenon, with the humeral head pushing up against the overlying rotator cuff. This may cause eventual cuff tearing, as well as biceps tendon damage.

Neer's theory of the impingement syndrome[10] suggests that abnormalities within the rotator cuff tendons are secondary to chronic trauma from an impinging acromion and adjacent structures. As described in the section on anatomy, a certain shape of acromion is associated with impingement and subsequent rotator cuff disease. Impingement can occur against the anterior edge and undersurface of the acromion, the coracoacromial ligament, and the acromioclavicular joint. This is the rationale for surgical decompression of the rotator cuff, which includes anterior acromioplasty, generally in conjunction with coracoacromial ligament resection. Resection of the distal clavicle and subacromial bursectomy may also be accomplished. If the impingement is thought to be secondary to instability, then capsular strengthening exercises or surgical correction of the instability should be performed.

Impingement is a clinical diagnosis, often supported by a history of overuse. A positive impingement sign is pain that develops when the arm is raised in forced forward elevation with a fixed scapula. This is present in all stages of the impingement syndrome, but is nonspecific. It can also occur with calcific tendonitis, glenohumeral instability, and arthritis. These entities can usually be differentiated by the impingement test, which involves injection of an anesthetic agent underneath the acromial arch. Marked improvement of symptoms after the injection constitutes a positive test.[10]

Neer[10] also proposed a classification scheme for rotator cuff disease (Table 11-2). Treatment for stage 1 disease is conservative, as is the initial therapy for stage 2 disease. Conservative treatment may include nonsteroidal anti-inflammatory drugs, cortisone injection, or strengthening exercises in a nonprovocative position. Refractory cases may be surgically treated. Treatment for stage 3 disease is generally operative, except in those chronic cases where successful repair is deemed unlikely, such as when MRI demonstrates a torn, retracted tendon, with muscular atrophy. MRI can also be helpful in planning the surgical approach, specifically arthroscopy versus open surgery. Unfortunately, it is

Table 11-2. Neer's Classification of Rotator Cuff Disease with MRI Correlation

Stage	Clinical	Pathology	MRI Correlation
1	Young (<25 yr); history of overuse	Reversible edema and hemorrhage	T_1, PD, proton-density: intermediate signal tendon; T_2: low to intermediate signal tendon
2	25–40 yr; chronic history of shoulder pain	Fibrosis and tendonitis	Tendon appearance similar to stage I
3	Older (>40 yr)	Degeneration and rupture	Discontinuous tendon with intervening fluid; ± retraction of the musculotendinous junction, muscular atrophy

difficult to distinguish stage 1 from stage 2 disease with MRI. In addition, this classification does not distinguish partial tears as a separate entity, although clinically they may be treated as such.

Magnetic Resonance Imaging

The signs and symptoms of impingement and rotator cuff disease can be nonspecific; therefore, MRI can help support or refute the diagnosis. It can help evaluate all of the soft tissue abnormalities associated with the impingement syndrome, as well as the offending structures above the bursa and tendon. MRI may actually identify the source of impingement, such as a hypertrophic acromioclavicular joint, inferior spurring, or a type III acromion. Impingement is a dynamic process, however, with the greatest compression often occurring when the arm is in abduction. Therefore, standard MRI with the arm positioned along the patient's side has its limitations.

Classification schemes for rotator cuff injury have been developed that are applicable to MRI. In a recent study by Farley et al.,[13] a modification of the classification scheme of Zlatkin et al.[14] was presented. In this classification, staging is based on the appearance of the supraspinatus tendon on proton-density and T_2-weighted images (see Table 11-3). The hallmark of a

Table 11-3. Supraspinatus Tendon Signal Patterns

Type	Proton-density	T_2	Clinical Interpretation
0	Signal void	Signal void	Normal
I	Focal, linear, or diffuse intermediate signal	Signal void or faint signal less than fat and water	Normal[a] Degeneration[a]
II	Focal, linear, or diffuse intermediate signal	Focal, linear, or diffuse increased signal equivalent to water; less than full thickness	Partial tear, possible full tear[a]
III	Focal, linear, or diffuse intermediate signal	Focal linear increased signal equivalent to water extending through the full thickness of tendon	Full tear

[a] Secondary corroborating findings such as large amounts of bursa fluid, musculotendinous retraction, or atrophy may indicate more severe disease.
(Data from Farley et al.,[13] and Zlatkin, Dalinka, and Kressel.[14])

tear is fluid, seen as high signal intensity on T_2-weighted images, passing through the full thickness of one of the rotator cuff tendons. This most commonly occurs within the distal 1 cm of the supraspinatus tendon, adjacent to its insertion into the greater tuberosity. This region of the tendon, the *critical zone,* is relatively avascular and subsequently more susceptible to the effects of acute and chronic trauma and degeneration (Fig. 11-5). Not all tears, however, are complete or full-thickness. Partial tears, arising from either the humeral or acromial surface, can also be detected (Fig. 11-6).

In the assessment of a possible rotator cuff tear, other structures besides the actual cuff tendon assume importance. The most sensitive finding for a full-thickness tear is actually fluid in the subacromial/subdeltoid bursa, although this is rather nonspecific. Its absence, however, renders a full-thickness tear highly unlikely. Interruption of tendinous continuity, musculotendinous junction retraction, and muscular atrophy are the most specific findings[9] (Fig. 11-7).

Several investigators[2,13,15,16] have reported statistics for the detection of rotator cuff tears by MRI (see Table 11-4). For all tears of the rotator cuff, including both full and partial thickness, the sensitivity of MRI generally falls in the 80 percent to 90 percent range. If only complete tears are considered, the statistics would naturally be slightly more favorable. The specificity has a mean near 90 percent. In addition, linear regression analysis has shown excellent correlation between preoperative MRI assessment of the size of rotator cuff tears and their actual measurement at surgery ($r = .95$).[13] Finally, a recent study[17] indicates that performing an MRI arthrogram increases the likelihood of diagnosing a partial tear on the humeral surface of the tendon, although this then becomes an invasive study, and partial tears on the acromial surface may still be missed.

Comparison with Other Modalities

Conventional radiographs are useful in the assessment of osseous abnormalities. The presence of inferiorly directed osteophytes or a downsloping or anteriorly hooked acromion or subacromial cortical erosion supports a diagnosis of impingement. Radiographs can also help exclude pathology that can clinically masquerade as rotator cuff disease, such as fractures, bone tumors, and masses within the lung apex. Plain films

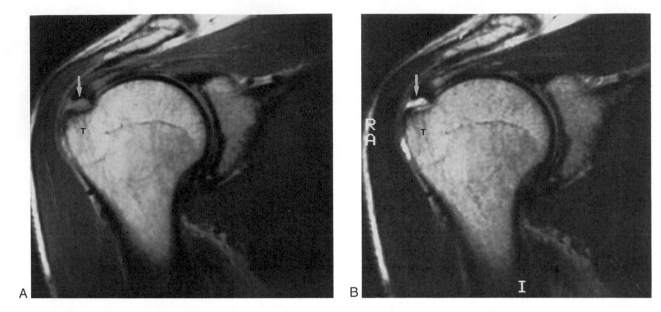

Fig. 11-5. Full-thickness tear of the supraspinatus tendon in the "critical zone." **(A)** Proton-density (TR/TE 1,800/25) and **(B)** T$_2$-weighted (TR/TE 1,800/80) coronal oblique images. On the proton-density image a band of intermediate signal intensity *(arrow)* courses, through the entire thickness of the distal supraspinatus tendon, adjacent to its attachment to the greater tuberosity *(T)*. This band becomes bright on the T$_2$-weighted image, consistent with fluid.

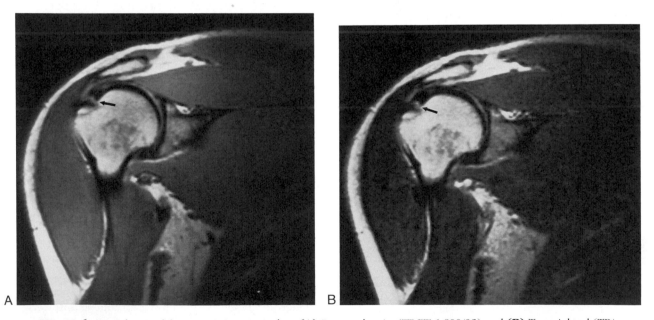

Fig. 11-6. Partial tear of the supraspinatus tendon. **(A)** Proton-density (TR/TE 1,800/25) and **(B)** T$_2$-weighted (TR/TE 1,800/80) coronal oblique images. On the proton-density image, a band of intermediate signal intensity *(arrow)* appears to extend across the full thickness of the distal supraspinatus tendon. On the T$_2$-weighted image, the tear can be seen to extend only part way through the tendon, as opposed to the full tears shown in Figures 11-5 and 11-7.

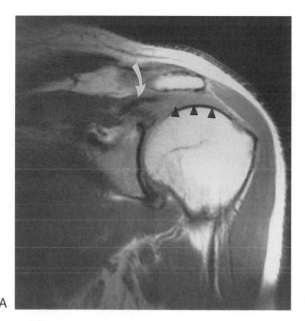
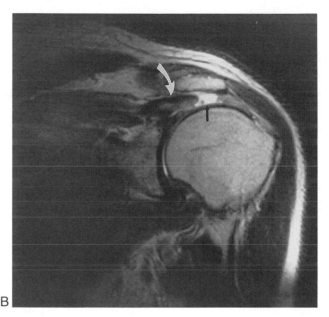

A   B

Fig. 11-7. Full-thickness tear of the supraspinatus tendon, with retraction of the musculotendinous junction. **(A)** Proton-density weighted image demonstrates diffuse intermediate signal intensity in the expected position of the distal supraspinatus muscle and tendon *(arrowheads)*. **(B)** T$_2$-weighted image. Focal fluid accumulation is present *(black arrow),* filling the space vacated by the retracted supraspinatus tendon *(curved arrow)* and allowing communication of the subacromial space with the joint.

are not helpful in evaluating subtle soft tissue findings, however, and thus can only suggest a diagnosis of impingement fairly late into its course.

Arthrography is quite sensitive in the diagnosis of full-thickness rotator cuff tears, but because it relies on the visualization of contrast extending outside the normal confines of the joint, it is less sensitive in the detection of partial tears and tendonitis.[18–20] Although the accuracy of arthrography in detecting full-thickness

Table 11-4. Evaluation of Rotator Cuff Tears by Magnetic Resonance Imaging

Study	Sensitivity (%)	Specificity (%)	PPV (%)	NPV (%)	Accuracy
Zlatkin et al.[2]	91[a]	88[a]		47[a]	91[a]
Farley et al.[13]	89[a]	77[a]	60[a]	95[a]	81[a]
Burk et al.[15]	92[b]	100[b]			
Evancho et al.[16]	69[a]	94[a]			84[a]
	80[c]	94[c]			89[c]

Abbreviations: PPV, positive predictive value; NPV, negative predictive value.
[a] Statistics for all tears (partial and complete).
[b] All but one of the surgically proven tears were full thickness.
[c] Statistics for complete tears only.

tears has been reported to be as high as 98 percent to 99 percent,[20] a study that considered both partial and complete tears reported a sensitivity of only 71 percent for arthrography.[2] MRI can, at times, even diagnose full-thickness tears not detected by arthroscopy (Fig. 11-8). In a study by Burk et al.[15] of 38 patients, MRI detected 22 of 22 tears, and 14 of 16 intact cuffs, as determined by arthrography. In 16 surgically proven cases (12 tears), MRI and arthrography showed identical results, with a 92 percent sensitivity and a 100 percent specificity. Attempts have been made to improve the accuracy of arthrography via injection of contrast into the subacromial bursa (subacromial bursography), but this is not commonly done.

Ultrasound is a relatively inexpensive, noninvasive method for evaluating the rotator cuff, and has many advocates. In a study by Hodler et al.,[21] the sensitivity of ultrasound was 100 percent, with a specificity of 75 percent, giving an overall accuracy of 92 percent. They also found sonography useful for estimating the size of the tear. Ultrasound, like MRI, has the advantage of scanning adjacent structures, and has been reported to be superior to arthrography in detecting bicipital

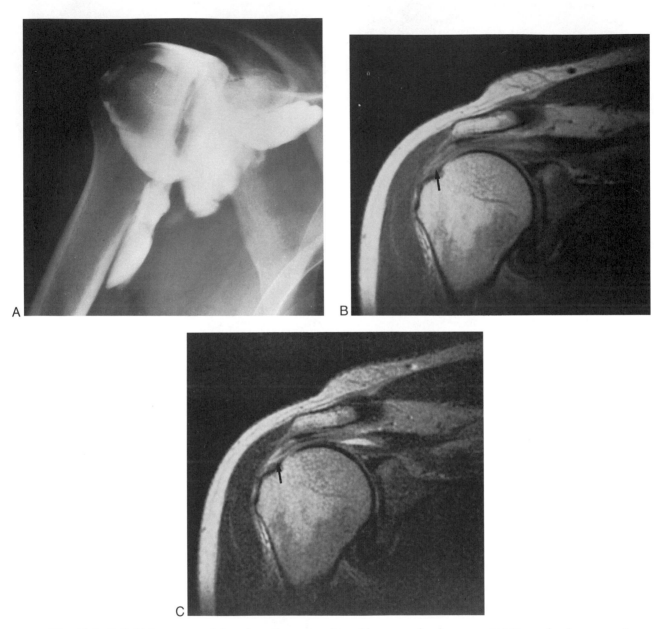

Fig. 11-8. Full-thickness tear of the supraspinatus tendon with a normal arthrogram. **(A)** Normal arthrogram of the right shoulder, followed by **(B)** proton-density (TR/TE 1,800/25) and **(C)** T$_2$-weighted (TR/TE 1,800/80) images from a magnetic resonance imaging study. Intermediate signal intensity on the proton-density image, with corresponding high signal intensity on the T$_2$-weighted image passing through the full thickness of the supraspinatus tendon, demonstrating the tear *(arrow)*. The false negative arthrogram was due to an intact synovial lining under the subacromial space, as found during surgery.

tendon abnormalities.[22] In a recent study, Hodler et al.[23] directly compared MRI with sonography in diagnosing rotator cuff tears. Sonography was 93 percent sensitive, as compared with 67 percent for MRI. This study, however, used arthrography as a gold standard and only full-thickness tears were taken into account. A larger series with surgical correlation would be helpful for further evaluation. As with all ultrasound examinations, however, the study is operator dependent and not all investigators report such favorable statistics. Brandt et al.[24] compared 38 shoulder sonograms with subsequent surgery and found a sensitivity of only 57 percent, with a specificity of 76 percent. In addition, because of problems with acoustic impedance and visualization, ultrasound cannot adequately evaluate the subacromial portion of the rotator cuff and the osseous abnormalities associated with impingement.

Computed arthrotomography (CT-arthrography) is excellent in the evaluation of labral abnormalities, as will be described later, but is less sensitive in the evaluation of the rotator cuff. In a study by Callaghan et al.,[25] 30 patients who underwent double contrast CT-arthrography prior to shoulder arthroscopy were evaluated. Only 50 percent of the proven rotator cuff tears were detected by CT-arthrography, which is a sensitivity far below that commonly reported for arthrography, sonography, and MRI. Habibian et al.[26] studied 18 patients who underwent conventional double-contrast arthrography, CT-arthrography, and MRI. MRI was comparable to conventional arthrography in the evaluation of the rotator cuff, and also allowed evaluation of tendonitis, which could not be accomplished with conventional arthrography. In most cases, information from MRI equaled or exceeded that obtained from conventional arthrography and CT-arthrography.

Pitfalls of MRI

The postoperative shoulder can be difficult to assess by any imaging modality. The usual diagnostic criteria may not be valid. Evaluation by arthrography may be impaired, because there is often persistent communication of the joint with the subacromial/subdeltoid bursa following successful rotator cuff repair. On ultrasound, the postoperative rotator cuff is usually abnormally echogenic, which can be difficult to distinguish from a rotator cuff tear.[27] Some investigators, however,

report success in the postoperative evaluation of the rotator cuff by sonography.[28]

Despite certain difficulties (obscuration of anatomic planes, persistent signal in the rotator cuff tendons, and artifacts), evaluation of the postoperative rotator cuff by MRI is often helpful. The thickness of the supraspinatus and other rotator cuff tendons can be noted. Persistent postsurgical continuity of the tendon or graft, and its attachment site may be demonstrated. A fluid-filled gap within the tendon, or retraction of the musculotendinous junction or muscular atrophy may be identified, suggesting recurrent tearing. As always, comparison with prior studies is invaluable.

Several other common pitfalls in the interpretation of shoulder MRIs exist. One of the more common involves mistaking the relatively high signal intensity of the articular cartilage of the humeral head for a signal within the cuff tendons.[29] This error can usually be avoided by careful attention to detail: the signal from the articular cartilage actually lies beneath the cuff tendons, and is continuous medially with the cartilage along the surface of the humeral head. Another pitfall is the "anterior interval pitfall", and occurs as a result of the space between the superior border of the subscapularis and the inferior border of the supraspinatus.[29] This interval is seen on anterior images in the coronal oblique plane, at the level where the supraspinatus, subscapularis, and biceps tendons are all visualized together. As the anterior aspect of the distal supraspinatus tendon can curve anteriorly here, images may demonstrate some suspicious intermediate signal on T_1- or proton-density weighted sequences just proximal to it, coming from membranous tissue within the rotator interval. This can be distinguished from true pathology by noting its typical location and the absence of high signal on T_2-weighted images.

The "muscle in place of tendon" pitfall occurs in patients whose supraspinatus tendon inserts more anteriorly than usual, and the infraspinatus more posteriorly.[29] Midcoronal oblique sections may demonstrate intermediate signal intensity from muscle in these patients, in the expected location of signal void from cuff tendons. This situation can be distinguished from a tear by the subsequent low signal seen on T_2-weighted images. Careful study of the most superior axial images and the location of the tendinous insertions might suggest this possibility.

Another potential pitfall has recently been described. Intermediate or even increased signal intensity within the tendon may at times result from an imaging artifact caused by the orientation of the tendon in relationship to the static magnetic field, with increased signal occurring at a "magic angle" of 55 degrees.[30] This area will be of low signal intensity on T_2-weighted images, which should help differentiate it from significant pathology.

Intermediate to increased signal within the rotator cuff on T_1-weighted and proton-density images can also occur in asymptomatic volunteers, as mentioned in the earlier section on anatomy. This, along with the other pitfalls described, makes a thorough knowledge of the appearance of normal and normal-variant anatomy on MRI mandatory for reliable interpretation of studies.

INSTABILITY

The glenohumeral joint is both the most mobile and the most frequently dislocated in the human body, largely because only a small part of the humeral head is in contact with the bony glenoid at any given time. Although glenohumeral instability often follows trauma, many patients with instability cannot recall a specific traumatic episode. Anterior dislocations of the glenohumeral joint account for approximately 95 percent of all shoulder dislocations. When the initial event occurs before age 35, as it most commonly does, the dislocations are more likely to become recurrent or habitual.

Almost all anterior glenohumeral dislocations occur when the humerus is abducted and externally rotated. As the humeral head dislocates anteriorly, the postero-lateral surface of the humeral head impacts against the inferior glenoid rim, often resulting in a wedge-shaped fracture known as the Hill-Sachs lesion (Fig. 11-9). Tears of the anterior glenoid labrum, separation of the capsule from the anterior glenoid rim (capsular stripping), or fractures of the glenoid rim (Bankart lesion) may occur at the same time. Posterior glenohumeral dislocations are far less common than anterior ones. When they occur, the anteromedial surface of the humeral head impacts the posterior glenoid, and frac-

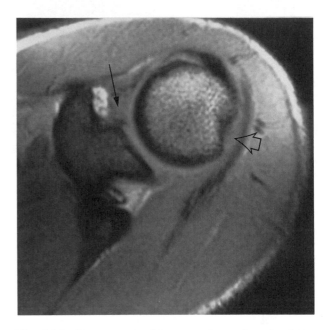

Fig. 11-9. Torn anterior labrum with a Hill-Sachs defect. Axial multiplanar gradient-recalled (MPGR) (TR/TE/flip angle 700/10/20) image demonstrates the torn and detached anterior labrum *(thin arrow)*. The wedge-shaped compression fracture along the postero-lateral aspect of the humeral head is seen *(open arrow)*.

tures of these bony surfaces can occur, as can tears of the posterior labrum and capsule.

Previously Bankart believed that the essential lesion in instability was a labral abnormality.[31] Today the most widely accepted theory holds that a labral tear is a result of glenohumeral instability rather than the primary etiologic factor.[32–34] Instability generally involves injury to or laxity of the capsular mechanism, described by Townley in 1950.[35] The capsular mechanism provides the majority of stability to the glenohumeral joint, and consists of the rotator cuff muscles and tendons, the joint capsule and synovial membrane, the glenohumeral ligaments, and the fibrous glenoid labrum.

Abnormalities of the capsular mechanism and associated structures occur predominantly in patients with a history of recurrent subluxations and dislocations. The spectrum includes Hill-Sachs and Bankart lesions, capsule and labral tears and detachments, formation of a large anterior pouch, and laxity or tear of the subscapularis muscle and tendon. Documenting these abnormalities can be helpful in differentiating patients with recurrent subluxation/dislocation (and thus laxity) from other entities that might present with similar symptoms and signs.

The diagnosis of occult instability of the glenohumeral joint remains a significant challenge. Because of its similar clinical presentation, recurrent shoulder instability can be confused with disorders of the rotator cuff or biceps tendon, and may coexist with these disorders. Failure to identify the causative pathology can result in inaccurate diagnosis and treatment. MRI can be particularly helpful in these patients.

Table 11-5. Magnetic Resonance Imaging in Evaluation of the Glenoid Labrum

Study	Sensitivity (%)	Specificity (%)	Accuracy (%)	PPV (%)	NPV (%)
Gross et al.[38]	91	69	83	85	79
Neumann et al.[39]	85	90	88	90	85
Garneau et al.[40]	61	67			
Legan et al.[41]	95[a]	86[a]	92[a]		
	75[s]	99[s]	95[s]		
	8[p]				
	40[i]				

Abbreviations: PPV, positive predictive value; NPV, negative predictive value. [a], anterior labral tears; [s], superior labral tears; [p], posterior labral tears; [i], interior labral tears.

MRI Findings

Tearing of the labrum is demonstrated by its absence, detachment, truncation, fragmentation, or reactive enlargement (Fig. 11-10). Focal or diffuse increased signal within the labrum, particularly if only seen on T_1-weighted images, is more difficult to interpret and may well be the normal variant rather than intrasubstance degeneration. If the high signal intensity within the labrum persists on T_2-weighted images degeneration is likely. If it appears to extend through the full thickness of the structure, then actual tearing is likely. Surface fraying or irregularity suggests degeneration.[32,36,37]

MRI can also depict other abnormalities associated with instability, including capsular stripping (separation of the joint capsule from the scapula), Hill-Sachs deformities (Fig. 11-9), Bankart lesions (Fig. 11-10), and disruption of or increased signal within the subscapularis tendon.

The reported sensitivity of MRI in detecting tears of the glenoid labrum has been variable, ranging from 61 to 95 percent in recent studies[38-41] (Table 11-5). It is most reliable in detecting tears of the anterior and superior labrum.[41] Comparatively, CT-arthrography detects labral pathology with a sensitivity reported to range from 66[39] to 100 percent.[42] Perhaps more importantly, direct comparisons of MRI to CT-arthrography for evaluation of the glenoid labrum have been performed. One study reported equal efficacy for the two modalities.[36] Our study group found superior sensitivity (85 percent) and accuracy (88 percent) for MRI

when compared with CT-arthrography (66 and 78 percent, respectively) in the evaluation of the anterior and posterior labrum, wherein both had specificities of 90 percent.[39] While neither MRI nor CT-arthrography was proficient in evaluation of the shoulder capsule in that latter study, MRI was slightly better. In addition, MRI provides better visualization of the glenohumeral ligaments. This can help in differentiating the superior or middle glenohumeral ligament from a detached torn labrum, and in evaluating capsular laxity.

Pitfalls of MRI

The anterior labrum in particular, as described in the anatomy section, tends to be variable in appearance. These variations can be difficult to distinguish from a tear on both CT and MRI. Partial volume averaging can also pose a problem. In addition, when a part of the superior or middle glenohumeral ligament is seen adjacent to the anterior labrum, differentiation from a tear can be difficult. Another problem with the evaluation of instability with MRI concerns the depiction of the anterior capsular insertion. The type of insertion can be particularly difficult to demonstrate in the absence of an effusion. Injection of gadolinium into the joint prior to the study (an MRI arthrogram) can, in selected cases, be helpful and improve visualization of the joint capsule as well as of the glenohumeral ligaments, synovium, and the subscapularis bursa.[37] This procedure, however, increases the time and cost

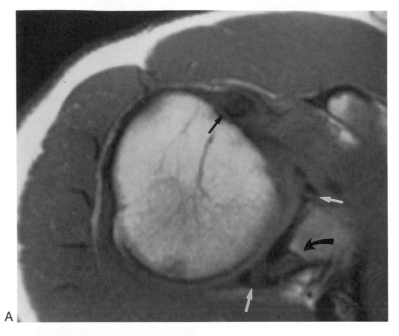

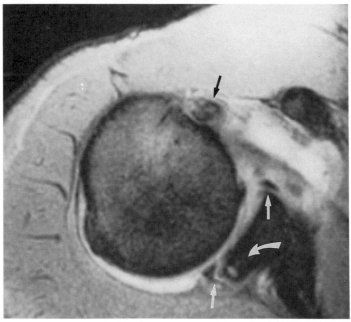

Fig. 11-10. SLAP (superior labrum anterior and posterior) injury, with anterior, superior, and posterior labral tearing, with associated biceps tendon inflammation. **(A)** Axial proton-density (TR/TE 1,800/20) and **(B)** multiplanar gradient-recalled (MPGR) (TR/TE/flip angle 700/10/20) images demonstrate anterior and posterior labral tears *(white arrows)*. The long head of the biceps tendon is enlarged and of increased signal, although it still lies within its normal position within a shallow bicipital groove *(black arrow)*. **(C)** Coronal oblique proton-density (TR/TE 1,800/25) and **(D)** T$_2$-weighted (TR/TE 1,800/80) images show the tear of the superior labrum *(black arrowhead)*. Posterior-superior Bankart lesion *(curved arrow)*, joint effusion *(open white arrow)*. *(Figure continues.)*

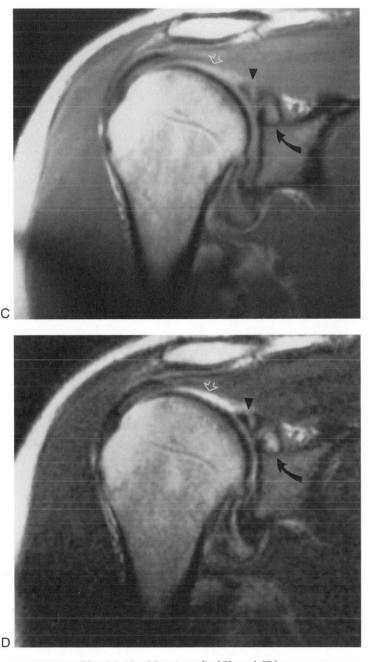

Fig. 11-10. (*Continued*). **(C)** and **(D)**

of shoulder MRI, turns it into an invasive procedure, and may decrease its specificity.

BICEPS TENDON AND RELATED PATHOLOGY

The normal long head of the biceps tendon is seen on MRI scans as a low signal intensity cylindrical structure within the bicipital groove. Complete tendon rupture, generally diagnosed clinically, should be suspected when the tendon is either not visualized or appears discontinuous. The tendon can also be dislocated, usually medially. When the dislocation occurs anterior to the subscapularis, then an isolated tear of the transverse ligament should be suspected. When the dislocation is deep to the subscapularis, then a concomitant tear of the subscapularis tendon should be diagnosed, as some of its fibers insert on the transverse ligament, which keeps the biceps tendon within the bicipital groove. The biceps tendon sheath communicates with the joint, and may be fluid filled in the presence of a joint effusion. Even isolated fluid surrounding the biceps tendon does not necessarily indicate tendon disease, particularly if the tendon retains its normal size and signal intensity (although it can be an early sign of tenosynovitis).

The long head of the biceps tendon is continuous with the superior aspect of the glenoid labrum, and may be a cause of tearing of the labrum, particularly in throwing athletes.[43] Snyder et al.,[44] in a study of 27 arthroscopies, combined with a retrospective review of over 700 others, described a specific pattern of injury to the superior labrum that begins posteriorly and extends anteriorly, stopping at or before the mid-glenoid notch, and including the "anchor" of the biceps tendon to the labrum. The most common mechanism of injury involved a compression force to the shoulder, with the shoulder positioned in abduction and slight forward flexion at the time of impact. He called these SLAP (superior labrum anterior and posterior) lesions (Fig. 11-10).

The significance of SLAP lesions was evaluated by Rodosky et al.,[45] using a dynamic shoulder model in cadaver dissections in which the muscle forces were replicated by pneumatic cylinders. They concluded that the long head of the biceps contributes to anterior stability by resisting external rotatory forces in the abducted, externally rotated position. This is consistent with electromyographic studies in throwing athletes that show that the biceps is most active in the late cocking phase of pitching and is increased during this phase in pitchers with anterior instability. The implication is that for a given external torque, the long head of the biceps is able to reduce the amount of external rotation, thus preventing an increase in inferior glenohumeral ligament strain. Using similar techniques, in the same study, Rodosky et al.[45] also concluded that a lesion involving the superior aspect of the glenoid labrum, particularly in the region of the long head of the biceps, can also contribute to anterior instability.

OTHER PATHOLOGY

Trauma

Plain films are the primary imaging modality for trauma. In some situations, however, further imaging is required. Plain film tomography and CT allow adequate visualization of most fractures, and will generally suffice. If necessary, however, MRI can demonstrate fractures, dislocations, hematomas, and other sequelae of trauma. MRI provides better assessment of the soft tissues than does CT and can show evidence of bony contusion not evident on other modalities. MRI can also demonstrate occult fractures difficult to detect with other studies (Fig. 11-11), and can play a complimentary role with nuclear medicine in the evaluation of stress fractures.

MRI can help grade the severity of acromioclavicular joint injuries, using the classification of Allman.[46] A grade I injury involves the tearing of only a few fibers of the acromioclavicular ligament and capsule, and results in no instability of the joint. This will usually have a normal appearance on MRI. A grade II injury involves a rupture of the capsule and acromioclavicular ligament, and is often associated with a subluxation. The coracoclavicular ligament is not ruptured, although the coracoclavicular interspace can be up to 25 percent greater than on the contralateral shoulder. The MRI may show fluid within the joint, as well as the subluxation. A grade III injury usually results from a severe force with rupture of the acromioclavicular and coracoclavicular ligaments and associated dislocation. The coracoclavicular interspace is typically 25 to 100 percent greater than the opposite side. More severe injuries are grade IV, which can involve a severe complete dislocation with possible fracture of the clavicle itself.

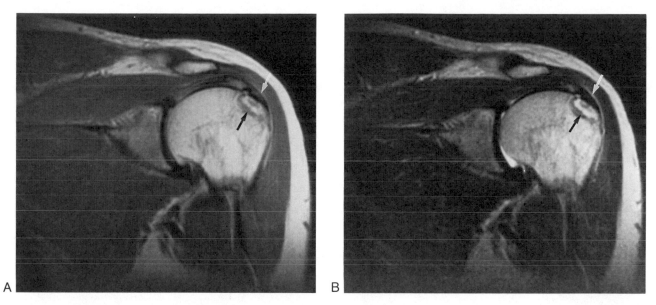

Fig. 11-11. Previously undiagnosed fracture of the greater tuberosity. Plain radiographs were normal. **(A)** Coronal oblique proton-density (TR/TE 1,800/25) and **(B)** T$_2$-weighted (TR/TE 1,800/80) images demonstrate a minimally displaced fracture of the greater tuberosity *(black arrow)*, at the attachment site for the supraspinatus tendon *(white arrow)*. The fracture fragment is surrounded by fluid.

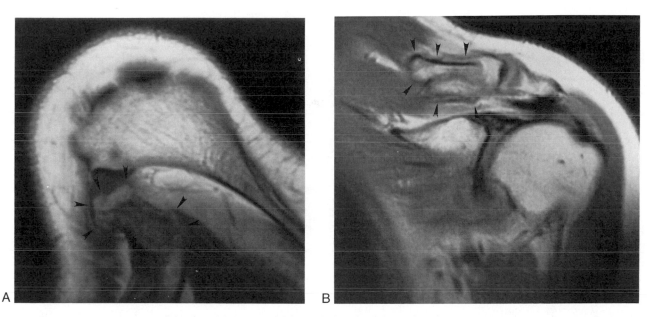

Fig. 11-12. Comminuted displaced fracture of the distal clavicle. **(A)** Axial multiplanar gradient-recalled (MPGR) (TR/TE/flip angle 700/10/20) and **(B)** coronal oblique proton-density (TR/TE 1,800/25) images. The fracture of the distal clavicle with its surrounding callous formation *(arrowheads)* protrudes inferiorly, resulting in compression of the underlying supraspinatus muscle and tendon.

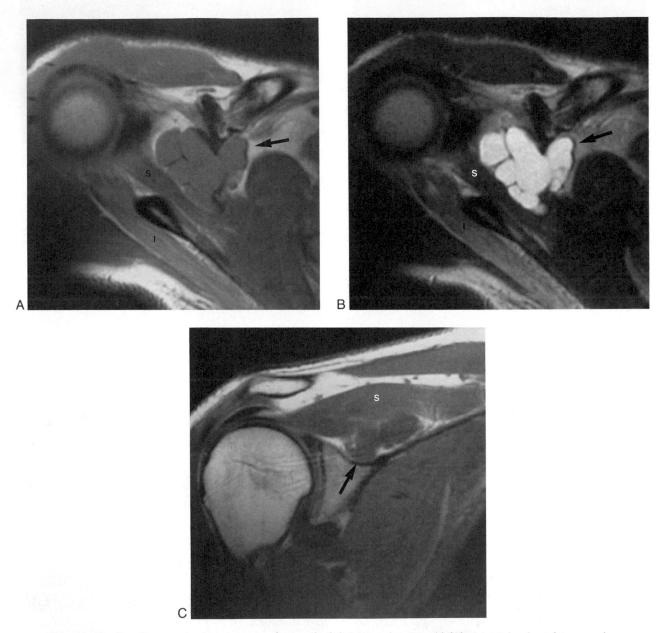

Fig. 11-13. Ganglion cyst in the suprascapular notch. **(A)** Proton-density and **(B)** T₂-weighted axial images show a large multiloculated mass *(arrow)* lying adjacent to and along the undersurface of the supraspinatus muscle *(S)*. It extends anteriorly and posteriorly over the neck of the scapula, causing impingement of the suprascapular nerve and atrophy of the infraspinatus *(I)*, and to a lesser degree, the supraspinatus muscle. **(C)** T₁-weighted sagittal oblique image confirms the position of the lesion.

The coracoclavicular space may be displaced, but can appear the same as the normal shoulder. Generally included in this category are any injuries to the joint associated with an avulsion fracture of the coracoclavicular ligaments, severe tear, or other injury to the soft tissue envelope about the lateral aspect of the clavicle. Unusual types of injury would include posterior displacement of the lateral clavicle, classified as grade V, and inferior displacement, or grade VI.[47] The effect of fragments of the clavicle on the surrounding soft tissue can also be delineated (Fig. 11-12).

Osteonecrosis

Osteonecrosis, or avascular necrosis, of the humeral head often follows trauma, particularly fractures of the anatomic neck. It may also be idiopathic, or occur in association with steroid use, alcoholism, sickle cell disease, or caisson disease. MRI is more sensitive than other imaging modalities, even radionuclide imaging, as shown in the early detection of osteonecrosis of the hip,[48] and has similar potential in the shoulder. The earliest change seen on MRI is a loss of the normal high signal of fatty marrow within the postero-superior aspect of the humeral head on T_1-weighted images.

Progression of the disease can also be documented. The symptoms and signs of avascular necrosis can be very nonspecific, and therefore the MRI study may occasionally be the first to suggest the diagnosis.

Miscellaneous Lesions

In the work-up of shoulder pain, MRI may detect the unsuspected. Benign lesions such as simple bone cysts, enchodromas, osteochondromas, and ganglion cysts are easily identified (Fig. 11-13). Malignant neoplasms may occasionally be found.

MRI is playing an increasing role in the staging of neoplasms, often replacing other imaging modalities such as CT. Within the shoulder, malignant tumors occurring in the scapula and the proximal end of the humerus are most commonly metastatic lesions or multiple myeloma. Less commonly, primary osseous lesions such as osteosarcoma, chondrosarcoma, osteochondroma, and Ewing and synovial sarcomas may be found.

MRI can also detect arthritis or synovial disease in patients thought to have impingement or instability (Fig. 11-14). Joint effusions, loose bodies, and bony erosions can all be identified. If a joint effusion does

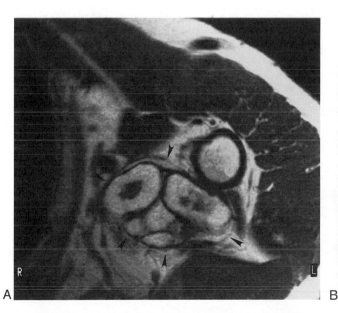
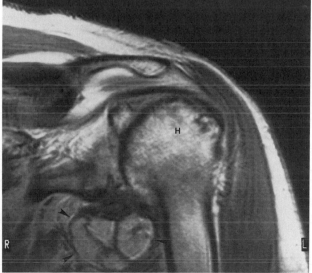

Fig. 11-14. Synovial osteochondromatosis. **(A)** Axial T_1-weighted (TR/TE 300/10) and **(B)** coronal oblique proton-density (TR/TE 1,800/25) images demonstrate multiple well-circumscribed osteochondral fragments within the axillary sheath *(arrowheads)*. Associated degenerative change of the humeral head *(H)* is present, indicating that the osteochondromatosis is a secondary process.

not have signal characteristics of simple fluid, then an infectious or hemorrhagic process should be suspected.

MRI offers a comprehensive diagnostic imaging approach to the shoulder joint, combining the evaluation of soft tissue structures, bone, and articular surfaces. It provides valuable information in patients with suspected instability or impingement, as well as other differential diagnostic considerations, in a single test. It is generally of comparable or better diagnostic value than other imaging methods, in addition to its noninvasiveness, and has therefore become the imaging procedure of choice for many clinicians, after the initial plain radiograph.

REFERENCES

1. Shellock FG, Swengros Curtis J: MR imaging and biomedical implants, materials, and devices: an updated review. Radiology 180:541, 1991

2. Zlatkin MB, Iannotti JP, Roberts MC et al: Rotator cuff tears: diagnostic performance of MR imaging. Radiology 172:223, 1989

3. Kneeland JB, Carrera GF, Middleton WD et al: Rotator cuff tears: preliminary application of high-resolution MR imaging with counter rotating current loop-gap resonators. Radiology 160:695, 1986

4. Neumann, CH, Holt RG, Steinbach LS et al: MR imaging of the shoulder: appearance of the supraspinatus tendon in asymptomatic volunteers. AJR 1992 (in print)

5. Bigliani LU, Morrison D, April EW: The morphology of the acromion and its relationship to rotator cuff tears. Orthop Trans 1:228, 1986

6. Farley TE, Neumann CH, Steinbach LS, Petersen SA: MR evaluation of the subacromial outlet of the shoulder (submitted).

7. Moseley HF, Overgaard B: The anterior capsular mechanism and recurrent anterior dislocation of the shoulder. J Bone Joint Surg 44B:913, 1962

8. McNiesh LM, Callaghan JJ: CT arthrography of the shoulder: variations of the glenoid labrum. AJR 149:963, 1987

9. Neumann CH, Petersen SA, Jahnke AH: MR imaging of the labral-capsular complex: normal variations. AJR 157:1015, 1991

10. Neer CS: Impingement lesions. Clin Orthop 173:70, 1983

11. Ozaki J, Fujimoto S, Nakagawa Y et al: Tears of the rotator cuff of the shoulder associated with pathologic changes in the acromion. A study in cadavers. J Bone Joint Surg 70A:1224, 1988

12. Jobe FW, Kvitne RS: Shoulder pain in the overhand or throwing athlete: the relationship of anterior instability and rotator cuff impingement. Orthop Rev 18:963, 1989

13. Farley TE, Neumann CH, Steinbach LS et al: Full thickness tearing of the rotator cuff of the shoulder: diagnosis with MR imaging. AJR 158:347, 1992

14. Zlatkin MB, Dalinka MK, Kressel HY: Magnetic resonance imaging of the shoulder. Magn Reson Q 5:3, 1989

15. Burk DL, Karasick D, Kurtz AB et al: Rotator cuff tears: prospective comparison of MR imaging with arthrography, sonography, and surgery. AJR 153:87, 1989

16. Evancho AM, Stiles RG, Fajman WA et al: MR imaging diagnosis of rotator cuff tears. AJR 151:751, 1988

17. Hodler J, Kursunoglu-Brahme S, Snyder SJ et al: Rotator cuff disease: assessment with MR arthrography versus standard MR imaging in 36 patients with arthroscopic confirmation. Radiology 182:431–6, 1992

18. Kneeland JB, Middleton WD, Carrera GF et al: MR imaging of the shoulder: diagnosis of rotator cuff tears. AJR 149:333, 1987

19. Goldman AB, Ghelman B: The double-contrast shoulder arthrogram: a review of 158 studies. Radiology 127:655, 1978

20. Mink JH, Harris E, Pappaport M: Rotator cuff tears: evaluation using double-contrast shoulder arthrography. Radiology 157:621–3, 1985

21. Hodler J, Fretz CJ, Terrier F, Gerber C: Rotator cuff tears: correlation of sonographic and surgical findings. Radiology 169:791–4, 1988

22. Middleton WD, Reinus WR, Totty WG et al: Ultrasound of the biceps tendon apparatus. Radiology 157:211, 1985

23. Hodler J, Terrier B, von Schulthess GK, Fuchs WA: MRI and sonography of the shoulder. Clin Radiol 43:323, 1991

24. Brandt TD, Cardone BW, Grant TH et al: Rotator cuff sonography: a reassessment. Radiology 173:323, 1989

25. Callaghan JJ, McNiesh LM, Dehaven JP et al: A prospective comparison of double contrast computed tomography (CT) arthrography and arthroscopy of the shoulder. Am J Sports Med 16:13, 1988

26. Habibian A, Stauffer A, Resnick D et al: Comparison of conventional and computed arthrotomography with MR imaging in the evaluation of the shoulder. J Comput Assisted Tomography 13:968–5, 1989

27. Crass JR, Craig EV, Feinberg SB: Sonography of the postoperative rotator cuff. AJR 146:561, 1986

28. Mack LA, Nyberg DA, Matsen FR III et al: Sonography of the postoperative shoulder. AJR 150:1089, 1988

29. Zlatkin MB. Anatomy of the shoulder. p. 21. In Zlatkin MB (ed): MRI of the Shoulder. Raven Press, New York, 1991

30. Erickson SJ, Cox IH, Hyde JS et al: Effect of tendon orientation on MR imaging signal intensity: a manifestation

of the "magic angle" phenomenon. Radiology 181:389, 1991

31. Bankart ASB: The pathology and treatment of recurrent dislocation of the shoulder-joint. Br J Surg 26:23, 1938

32. Seeger LL, Gold RH, Bassett LW et al: Shoulder instability: evaluation with MR imaging. Radiology 168:695, 1988

33. Turkel SJ, Panio MW, Marshall JL, Girgis FG: Stabilizing mechanisms preventing anterior dislocation of the glenohumeral joint. J Bone Joint Surg 63A:1208, 1981

34. Rose CO, Patel D, Southnayd WW: The Bankart procedure. J Bone Joint Surg 60A:1, 1978

35. Townley CO: The capsular mechanism in recurrent dislocation of the shoulder. J Bone Joint Surg 32A:370, 1950

36. Kieft GH, Bloem JF, Rosing PM et al: MR imaging of recurrent anterior dislocation of the shoulder: comparison with CT arthrography. AJR 150:1083, 1988

37. Zlatkin MB, Bjorkengren AF, Gylys-Morin V et al: Cross-sectional imaging of the capsular mechanism of the glenohumeral joint. AJR 150:151, 1988

38. Gross ML, Seeger LL, Smith JB et al: Magnetic resonance imaging of the glenoid labrum. Am J Sports Med 18:229, 1990

39. Neumann CH, Petersen SA, Jahnke AH et al: MRI in the evaluation of patients with suspected instability of the shoulder joint including a comparison with CT-arthrography. Röfö 154:593, 1991

40. Garneau RA, Renfrew DL, Moore TE et al: Glenoid labrum: evaluation with MR imaging. Radiology 179:519, 1991

41. Legan JM, Burkhard TK, Goff WB II et al: Tears of the glenoid labrum: MR imaging of 88 arthroscopically confirmed cases. Radiology 179:241, 1991

42. Wilson AJ, Totty WG, Murphy WA et al: Shoulder joint: arthrographic CT and long-term follow-up, with surgical correlation. Radiology 173:329, 1989

43. Andrews JR, Carson WG, McLeod WD: Glenoid labrum tears related to the long head of the biceps. Am J Sports Med 13:337, 1985

44. Snyder SJ, Karzel RP, Del Pizzo W et al: SLAP lesions of the shoulder. J Arthrop Relat Surg 6:274, 1990

45. Rodosky MW, Rudert MJ, Harner CD et al: The role of the long head of the biceps and superior glenoid labrum in anterior stability of the shoulder. Paper presented at the American Academy of Orthopedic Surgery Annual Meeting, New Orleans, 1990

46. Allman FL Jr: Fractures and ligamentous injuries of the clavicle and its articulation. J Bone Joint Surg 49:774, 1967

47. Post M: Current concepts in the diagnosis and management of acromioclavicular dislocations. Clin Orthop Relat Res 200:234, 1985

48. Mitchell DG, Kundel JL, Steinberg ME et al: Avascular necrosis of the hip: comparison of MR, CT, and scintigraphy. AJR 147:67, 1986

12
Arthroscopy

WARREN D. KING

With the advent of arthroscopy a new era of shoulder evaluation and treatment has arrived. Direct visualization of the shoulder has allowed a more comprehensive understanding of the types of lesions associated with the athlete and provided an opportunity for immediate correction or more accurate planning for open repair. Arthroscopy has increased the diagnostic armamentarium and at the same time provided a surgical option for many conditions with the combined advantages of decreased morbidity and rehabilitation time, both crucial to the athlete. Another advantage of arthroscopy is a magnification effect, which allows better visualization than even open procedures.

Most overuse and nontraumatic shoulder conditions will usually respond to a trial of extended conservative care comprised of physical therapy and sport specific rehabilitation. This period of time may be as long as 6 months. Further evaluation may then be necessary with a choice of magnetic resonance imaging (MRI), computed tomography (CT)–arthrography, sonography, and isokinetic testing. When conservative approaches fail and/or when other imaging or testing fails to reveal a clear etiology, arthroscopy serves as a useful aid for both diagnosis and often surgical correction. Although initially a diagnostic tool, advances in arthroscopy have allowed the treatment of a number of conditions previously requiring open procedures. Some of the most common procedures include subacromial decompression, repair of partial rotator cuff tears and labral pathology, removal of loose bodies, and stabilization.

TECHNIQUE OF SHOULDER ARTHROSCOPY

The equipment used with arthroscopy includes the arthroscope, the arthroscopic pump, and various cannula-guided surgical tools. The arthroscope is connected to a video recorder to document evaluation for future reference. Andrews et al.[1] and others have established the standard protocols for shoulder arthroscopy. The patient is usually under general anesthesia and placed in either a semi-seated[2] (beach-chair) or lateral recumbent position. In the lateral recumbent position, the torso of the patient is supported by a padded bean-bag vacupack and an axillary roll (Fig. 12-1A). Padding is provided over all bony prominences. The patient is rolled posteriorly approximately 30 degrees and the arm is suspended with a Buck's traction device and tractioned with about 10 lb. The arm is abducted about 70 degrees with forward flexion between 15 and 20 degrees. This position is changed to only 10 to 15 degrees abduction when viewing subacromially and the weight is increased to 15 lb. It is important that no more than 20 lb of traction be used because of the increased risk of musculocutaneous or ulnar nerve damage.[1]

Installation of the arthroscope and tools is provided through a series of portals (Fig. 12-1B). Although there are a variety of portals recommended by various authors, there are generally three standard portals in use with some minor variations. Before the portals are created bony landmarks are identified with a marker.

323

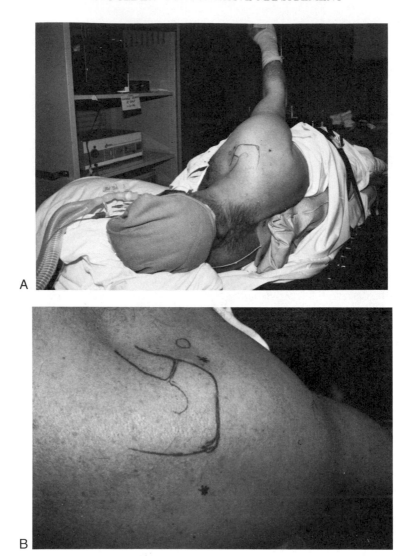

Fig. 12-1. (A) The landmarks for entering the shoulder arthroscopically are the acromioclavicular joint and the coracoid process, seen outlined here. The anterior and posterior portals are drawn as black dots. **(B)** A closer view of the anatomic landmarks for the anterior and posterior portal. The posterior portal orientation is to enter posteriorly and aim anteriorly and medially approximately 25 degrees toward the coracoid process. The anterior portal is just lateral to the line between the coracoid process and the acromion. Both of these portals can be used secondarily for arthroscopic approaches to the subacromial bursa. (From Wilkes,[23] with permission.)

These include the anterolateral and posterolateral borders of the acromion, the coracoid process, the distal clavicle, and the posterior glenohumeral joint. The posterior portal is the primary diagnostic portal. It is located about 2 to 3 cm inferior and 1 to 2 cm medial to the posterolateral corner of the acromion. Andrews et al.[1] refer to this as the "soft spot" of the posterior shoulder corresponding to the space between the infraspinatus and teres minor muscles. Using a spinal needle, saline solution is injected to distend the joint. Then a small incision is made to allow entrance of a cannula and finally the arthroscope. An anterior portal is created through the posterior portal from the inside out. This second portal is generally in between the coracoid and anterolateral edge of the acromion. Mathews et al.[3] describe an "intra-articular" or "safe" triangle bordered by the humeral head, glenoid, and biceps tendon, which constitutes an area of decreased risk to neurovascular structures. The advancement is made anteriorly through this triangle and an incision is made. Accessory anterior portals or a superior portal may be needed to aid in irrigation or provide a specific advantage with specific surgical techniques.

The anterior and posterior are the two primary portals used for evaluation and treatment. They may be switched depending on the structures evaluated. The posterior portal has a wider range of view and is used as the primary visualization portal.[4]

Other portals include anterolateral and posterolateral portals, which may be used when viewing the subacromial space.[5] These portals are inferior to the anterolateral and posterolateral edge of the acromion.

Standard landmarks include the articular surface of the glenoid, the articular surface of the humeral head, the biceps tendon, and the tendon of the subscapularis (Fig. 12-2). Using the tendon of the biceps as a reference point, location of the superior labral attachment point, the superior supraspinatus tendon, and posteriorly the infraspinatus tendon can be made. Using the subscapularis (which runs at approximately 90 degrees to the glenoid) the capsular ligaments can be located.

Variations in normal anatomy that can lead to misdiagnosis or confusion include a normally occurring humeral head sulcus that is essentially bare bone. It is located between the capsular insertion and the edge of the humeral head articular cartilage. This area may increase in size due to normal aging and does not represent pathology.[6] This area is not the same as a Hill-Sachs lesion, which does represent pathology of the humeral head resulting from shoulder dislocation. Superior labral detachments in the older individual may represent a normal aging process and not repre-

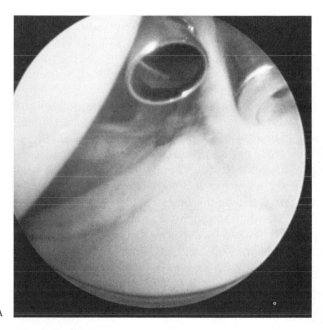
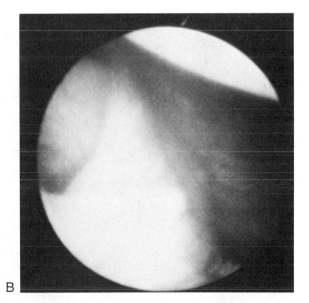

Fig. 12-2. (A) To the upper left is the humeral head. Between the two metallic instruments is the biceps tendon; the anterior labrum is seen coursing from the attachment of the biceps tendon along the anterior glenoid, and the surface of the glenoid is shown toward the bottom of the figure. **(B)** Anteriorly and inferiorly is the inferior glenohumeral ligament coursing away from the anterior glenoid labrum. The humeral head is at the upper right. (From Wilkes,[23] with permission.)

sent a source of symptomatology.[6] Another variant is a double-headed biceps and intracapsular biceps both represented rarely.[6]

SPECIFIC CONDITIONS

Impingement and Rotator Cuff Tears

Impingement syndrome is often an overlap diagnosis usually with supraspinatus or biceps tendon/muscle involvement and subacromial bursal pathology (Fig. 12-3). The overlap occurs with instability and acromioclavicular degeneration, both of which may allow an accentuation of the problem of subacromial compression with abduction and internal rotation of the shoulder. This position acquired repetitively in many sports will result in damage to the occupying structures of the subacromial area. Compression is either from the acromion, the coracoacromial ligament, and some suggest the coracoid itself.

Clinical evaluation involves standard orthopaedic tests that attempt to recreate typical positions of impingement and reproduce the patient's complaint. The

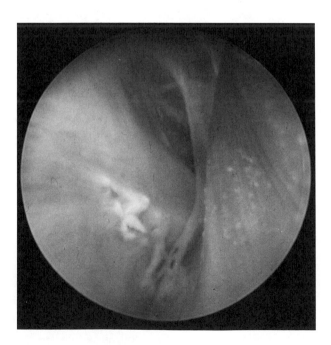

Fig. 12-3. Arthroscopic view, right subacromial bursa, showing coracoacromial ligament attachment to acromion process. (From Zarin and Boyle,[24] with permission.)

Neer sign is the production of pain when the arm is forward flexed maximally by the examiner. The Hawkins–Kennedy's test involves passive internal rotation with the arm and elbow flexed to 90 degrees. The patient may also complain of a "painful arc" of motion. Pain is felt in the midrange of abduction yet not before or after this range. Further confirmation is possible with a lidocaine injection (impingement test) subacromially. Impingement signs becoming painless after the injection is an indication of impingement. In younger patients, especially overhead athletes, primary instability can cause secondary impingement. These patients will have positive apprehension signs and a positive relocation test. The relocation test popularized by Jobe et al.[7] attempts to duplicate the pain produced by instability. It is performed by placing the patient in the supine position with the involved arm abducted to 90 to 100 degrees. As the arm is externally rotated maximally the patient experiences pain. The examiner then places a hand behind the patient's arm and gently pulls forward. This should increase the pain reported by the patient. The examiner then pushes downward on the arm with relief reported by the patient. If all three parts of the test (pain with abduction/external rotation, increased pain with anterior pull, and decrease pain with posterior push) are present, then the patient likely has a primary anterior instability with a secondary impingement.

Rotator cuff tears can be a complication of later stages of impingement or exist as separate entities. The patient with a tear may complain of inability to raise or lower the arm coupled with resting pain, especially at night. However, many partial tears are relatively asymptomatic. If a complete rotator cuff tear is suspected, then the diagnosis should be confirmed with MRI or arthrography. If painful, then early surgical repair should be performed.

Arthroscopy may be necessary to distinguish between the various types of partial tears possible with the rotator cuff. Tears can be bursal-sided or articular-sided, each representing a different etiology. Bursal-sided tears are believed to represent more of a compressive insult via subacromial impingement. This may occur due to a "hooked" or type III acromion,[8] degenerative spurs, a thick coracoacromial ligament, or an os acromiale. The "inside-out" tear or articular-sided tear probably represents more of a tensile overload process found commonly in athletes.[9] Instability is a secondary cause of rotator cuff tears that may overlap with the above primary causes.

The first type or compressive tear is often associated with stage II impingement as described by Neer.[10] This classification system recognizes a progression of changes associated with subacromial impingement. Stage I is reversible and involves inflammation of the underlying bursa and tendons. Stage II involves more of a fibrotic reaction in these same tissues and surrounding tissues. Stage III represents degenerative tears and osseous changes reflecting this long-term process. Stages I and II usually respond to conservative care; however, some stage II cases are nonresponsive even after 6 months to a year. These cases may progress to arthroscopic decompression when significant acromioclavicular involvement is found. Complicated stage II and most stage III lesions are still treated with open procedures, but this is changing.

Snyder[11] suggests the use of a classification system to allow better communication, recording for research, and decision making for rotator cuff repair. He suggests a system based on the location of the lesions. The first designation is whether the lesion is bursal-sided or articular-sided. The designation of a complete tear indicates connection of the articular and bursal surfaces. Location is more specifically designated by relationship to the supraspinatus tendon, infraspinatus tendon, rotator cuff interval, and subscapularis tendon.

Arthroscopy is more commonly used for debridement of partial tears (Fig. 12-4). Full-thickness tears are more commonly repaired using open procedures or arthroscopic assisted "mini-open" repairs. Compressive partial-thickness tears on the bursal side are treated usually with an anterior acromioplasty removing about 8 mm of the anterior acromion and debridement of the partial tear to healthy, bleeding tissue. Any accompanying bursal adhesions can be debrided also.

Tensile lesions that are partial and on the undersurface (articular-sided) can be debrided to healthy, bleeding tissue using a motorized shaver. This is performed by switching the arthroscope to the anterior portal and the shaver introduced through the posterior portal.

If instability is felt to contribute to rotator cuff pathology, exercise and rehabilitation are the first course of treatment. Failure of a conservative approach for at least 6 months may result in the requirement for surgical repair. Most procedures would include both labral

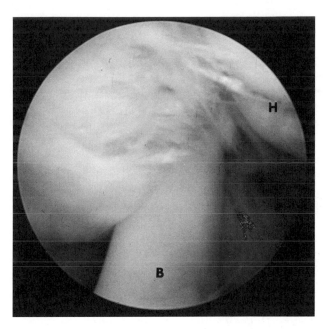

Fig. 12-4. Arthroscopic view of right shoulder showing frayed inferior surface of supraspinatus tendon insertion. This is a partial thickness tear of the inferior surface of the rotator cuff. *B,* biceps tendon; *H,* humeral head. (From Zarin and Boyle,[24] with permission.)

and capsular correction of laxity. Arthroscopic stabilization may be the procedure of choice in the future.

Instability

Instability can be caused by dislocation/subluxation as a result of contact injury or may preexist as a congenital or acquired looseness of the shoulder. Most traumatic instability results in anterior-inferior instability with associated damage to the anterior-inferior labrum. Posterior instability can be traumatically induced or be due to inherent looseness of the shoulder allowing the individual to voluntarily dislocate. Multidirectional instability is usually an indication of generalized capsular laxity often found bilaterally, often in an individual with no report of trauma. Treatment of these various types of instability varies. Conservative treatment is recommended in individuals who have inherent looseness of their shoulders.[12] Conservative care involves stabilization of the humeral head with a graded exercise program focusing on the rotator cuff and scapular stabilizing musculature. Traumatically induced anterior or posterior dislocation may require surgery.

Instability is still mainly a clinical diagnosis most of the time. Findings of pain or instability with the apprehension test, load and shift tests, and relocation test are suggestive of instability coupled with the patient's history. Arthroscopy can be helpful diagnostically in difficult cases where instability or labral pathology is suspected yet the clinical exam or ancillary testing is equivocal. Arthroscopic evaluation is preceded by an anesthetized examination for instability bilaterally. Then arthroscopically a search for labral and capsular pathology is performed via visualization and probing. Secondary evidence of instability is found with the demonstration of Hill-Sachs and Bankart lesions.

Arthroscopy is still in its infancy with regard to stabilization procedures. Various Bankart repairs have been developed. Johnson[13] developed a technique suing staple capsulorrhaphy. The glenohumeral ligaments are attached via a staple to a new bone bed. The recurrence rate has been reported to be as high as 21 percent compared with about 3 percent with open procedures in those patients with recurrent dislocations.

Arthroscopic stabilization should be offered to those high-risk younger patients with an acute first-time dislocation. Arthroscopic stabilization using suture, absorbable tacks, or staples, repairs the torn inferior labrum-ligamentous complex and results in a very low recurrent dislocation rate. Acute arthroscopic stabilization of first-time high-risk dislocations also avoids the necessity of two separate rehabilitations. Double-contrast arthrotomography can be helpful in identifying the types of capsular pathology that offer sufficient reattachment capabilities.

Other procedures include the Caspari[14] technique of reattachment of the labrum with sutures that are advanced through osseous tunnels posteriorly and fixed with a Steinman pin. With this technique the posterior portal is used for the arthroscope while the anterior portal is the operative access. Whereas in most procedures a 30 degree angle scope is used, a 70 degree angle scope is used with this procedure to allow better visualization of the anterior glenoid. Finally, a screw fixation procedure of the anterior capsule has been described. This is not considered a recommended technique in most instances due to the higher risk of complications.[15] Patients with inferior or multidirectional instability are not good candidates for ar-

throscopic repair. Again, absorbable tacks, staples, and suture anchor devices have been developed to perform successful arthroscopic stabilization procedures if necessary.

A 4 percent recurrence rate and one-time resubluxation rate were reported at the American Academy of Orthopaedic Surgeons meeting in 1989 with regard to arthroscopic Bankart repair.[16] There was also a report of 90 percent good or excellent results. Many surgeons are still not comfortable with this approach to repair and will use it selectively.

Labrum Tears

The diagnosis of labrum pathology is clinically difficult. Although the sensitivity of CT–arthrograms is quite high,[17] many authors feel that arthroscopy is still often needed for a definitive diagnosis.[18] Tears that are inferior are either detachments from the glenoid (Bankart lesion) or substance tears. Associated findings include glenoid erosion or fracture. Superior lesions are commonly degenerative in older individuals and the result of tension overload in the young throwing athlete. Tears can be similar in presentation to the menisci in the knee. Longitudinal tearing produces a bucket-handle type while radial tears with a longitudinal component are flap tears (Fig. 12-5).

The cause, degree, and location of labral pathology determine the appropriateness of arthroscopic repair. Throwing athletes without signs of instability but who present with mechanical signs may respond well to labral debridement. These patients often present with no signs of instability, but have "functional instability." When a labral fragment is caught between the articular surfaces, mechanical symptoms are possible similar to a torn meniscus. These lesions are most often found with the anterior-superior quadrant of the glenoid and are associated with overcontraction of the tendon of the long head of the biceps during deceleration maneuvers.[19] These have been called "SLAP" lesions (superior labral anterior to posterior). Andrews et al.[19] found that 83 percent of throwing athletes with labral tears had a superior tear associated with the biceps tendon. There may also be a tearing of the biceps near the glenoid that should be debrided. It is important to note that if the tear extends to the middle or inferior glenohumeral ligaments, debridement would only

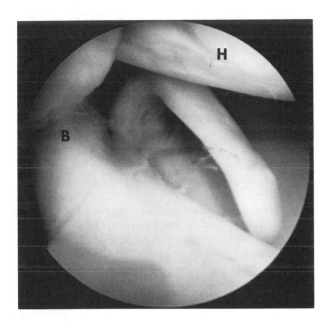

Fig. 12-5. Posterior arthroscopic view of right shoulder. The patient has a large superiorly based flap tear of the anterior glenoid labrum. *H,* humeral head; *B,* biceps tendon. (From Zarin and Boyle,[24] with permission.)

lead to instability, and therefore surgical repair is recommended.

One precaution should be noted with debridement. Resection of labral fragments should be performed only if the integrity of the glenohumeral ligaments and labral rim is intact. Excessive resection may lead to instability. A labral debridement is analogous to a partial meniscectomy.

Bennett's Lesions

With throwing athletes the development of an exostosis posteriorly at about the eight o'clock position of the glenoid represents a reaction to repeated microtrauma to the posterior and inferior capsule. Referred to as a Bennett's lesion,[8] this entity is arthroscopically managed with a synovial resector using the posterior portal and a 70 degree angle arthroscope.

Osteolysis of the Distal Clavicle

Weightlifters may develop a poorly understood reaction in the distal clavicle that results in nontraumatic lysis. This is considered an overstress reaction due to

excessive weightlifting. The bench press and dip have been found to be some of the most common causative maneuvers.[20] Conservative treatment including rest followed by modification of lifting and exercise selection is usually helpful. However, many cases still require arthroscopic debridement of the joint with decompression of both the acromion and clavicular aspects of the joint.

A similar traumatic event can occur following partial or complete acromioclavicular separations. Treatment is the same.

COMPLICATIONS OF ARTHROSCOPIC PROCEDURES

Arthroscopy is generally a very safe procedure. Ogilivie-Harris and Wiley[21] reported only a 3 percent complication rate consisting of massive fluid leakage, abrasion of articular cartilage, sepsis, and nerve palsy, all of which resolved without sequelae. A specific technique, anterior staple capsulorrhaphy, however, has been reported to have a 5.3 percent complication rate. Subacromial decompression has the lowest at 0.76 percent.[22]

Neurologic concerns consist of damage due to creation of the portals and secondly from tractioning of the arm during the surgical procedure. Careful selection of portals and correct positioning of the arm will obviate these transient complications.

POSTSURGICAL MANAGEMENT

Most arthroscopic procedures are followed by ice and rest for 24 to 48 hours. The arm is placed in a sling for 3 to 5 days. For diagnostic procedures or simple debridement, exercise (beginning with isometrics and mild range of motion) can begin as soon as the patient feels capable; care should be taken to avoid extreme ranges or excessive exercise.

A large bandage used to collect postsurgical drainage should be changed after 36 hours and then bandages placed over the wounds. The patient can then be allowed to shower. For most procedures other than those used for diagnosis only or debridement, heavy activity and exercise is avoided for a minimum of 2 weeks. For stabilization procedures, this period of relative immobilization extends to as much as 1 month. Mild isometrics can begin close to the side within the first week. Mild to moderate isometrics (away from the side but not beyond 90 degrees elevation) and gentle stretching can begin after 2 to 3 weeks.

Goals for rehabilitation involve return of full motion initially, followed by strengthening, and finally return to functional activities. Reeducating the synchronous motions and firing of the shoulder muscles during sport specific activities is the final goal of rehabilitation. Recommendations for rehabilitation and specifically arthroscopic repairs are given in Chapter 20.

REFERENCES

1. Andrews JR, Carson WG, Ortega K: Arthroscopy of the shoulder: technique and normal anatomy. Am J Sports Med 12:1, 1984

2. Skhar MJ, Altcheck DW, Warren RF: Shoulder arthroscopy in the seated position. Orthop Rev 10:1033, 1988

3. Mathews LS, Vetter WL, Helfet DL: Anterior portal selection for shoulder arthroscopy. J Arthroscopy 1:33, 1985

4. Rojvanit F: Arthroscopy of the shoulder joint—a cadaver and clinical study. I Cadaver study. J Jpn Orthop Assoc 58:1035, 1984

5. Nottage WM: Shoulder arthroscopy: portals and surgical techniques. Tech Orthop 3:23, 1988

6. DePalma AF: Surgery of the Shoulder. 3rd Ed. JP Lippincott, Philadelphia, 1983

7. Jobe FW, Tibone JE, Jobe CM et al: The shoulder in sports. p. 961. In Rockwood CA, Matsen FA (eds): The Shoulder. WB Saunders, Philadelphia, 1990

8. Bigliani LU, Morrison DS, April EW: The morphology of the acromion and its relationship to rotator cuff tears. Orthop Trans 10:216, 1986

9. Andrews JR, Angelo RL: Shoulder arthroscopy for the throwing athlete. p. 79. In Paulos LE, Tibone JE (eds): Operative Techniques in Shoulder Surgery. Aspen, Rockville, MD, 1991

10. Neer CS II: Impingement lesions. Clin Orthop 173:70, 1983

11. Synder SJ: Rotator cuff lesions: acute and chronic. Clin Sports Med 10:595, 1991

12. O'Brien SJ, Warren RF, Schwartz E: Anterior shoulder instability. Orthop Clin North Am 18:395, 1987

13. Johnson LL (ed): Shoulder arthroscopy. In: Arthroscopic Surgery: Principles and Practice. CV Mosby, St. Louis, 1986

14. Caspari RB: Arthroscopic reconstruction for anterior shoulder instability. p. 57. In Paulos LE, Tibone JE (eds): Operative Techniques in Shoulder Surgery. Aspen, Rockville, MD, 1991

15. Zuckerman JD, Matsen FA III: Complications about the glenohumeral joint related to the use of screws and staples. J Bone Joint Surg 66A:175, 1984

16. Yahirso MA, Mathews LS: Arthroscopic stabilization procedures for recurrent anterior shoulder instability. Orthop Rev 18:1161, 1989

17. Singson RD, Feldman F, Bigliani L: CT arthrographic patterns in recurrent glenohumeral instability. Am J Radiol 149:749, 1987

18. Altcheck DW, Warren RF, Skyhar MJ: Shoulder arthroscopy. In Rockwood CA, Matsen FA (eds): The Shoulder. Vol. 1. WB Saunders, Philadelphia, 1990

19. Andrews JR, Carson WG, McLeod WD: Glenoid labrum tears related to the long head of the biceps. Am J Sports Med 13:337, 1985

20. Scavenius M, Iversen BF: Nontraumatic clavicular osteolysis in weight lifters. Am J Sports Med 20:463, 1992

21. Ogilivi-Harris DJ, Wiley AM: Arthroscopic surgery of the shoulder: a general appraisal. J Bone Joint Surg 68B:201, 1986

22. Small NC: Complications of arthroscopy of the knee and other joints. Arthroscopy 2:253, 1986

23. Wilkes J: Arthroscopy of the shoulder. p. 355. In Donatelli RA (ed): Physical Therapy of the Shoulder. 2nd Ed. Churchill Livingstone, New York, 1991

24. Zarin B, Boyle JJ: Shoulder arthroscopy and arthroscopic surgery. p. 79. In Rowe CR (ed): The Shoulder. Churchill Livingstone, New York, 1988

13

Glenohumeral Instability

EDWARD FEINBERG

The glenohumeral joint is the most mobile joint in the human body. To achieve such a large range of motion (ROM) at this joint, much stability is sacrificed. The shallow glenoid socket articulates with the large ball of the humeral head (Fig. 13-1). A loose joint capsule allows for this extreme mobility, but also creates a tendency for the humeral head to leave its centered glenoid contact. As a result, over 50 percent of all human dislocations occur at the glenohumeral joint,[1] and recurrent dislocations abound after the first event.[2-8] Glenohumeral instability is defined as a greater than normal tendency of the humeral head to leave its glenoid fossa.

The earliest known report of a shoulder dislocation was found in the Edwin Smith Papyrus, dated 3000–2500 BC.[9] Reduction techniques are depicted in Egyptian drawings from 1200 BC. By 400 BC, Hippocrates developed the first surgical techniques to stabilize recurrent dislocations. He endorsed burning of the anterior-inferior glenohumeral capsule with a "red hot poker" to produce postinjury scars that would stabilize the shoulder.[1] He carefully described procedures that would avoid damage to the major vessels and nerves. The ensuing scars would often reestablish stability at the cost of significant restriction in ROM. Since that time, over 100 surgical procedures have been developed to treat recurrent dislocating shoulders.

Our concern with glenohumeral instability is not limited to the subluxation or dislocation event. Risks of complications abound, including recurrence of the event, degenerative or traumatic joint changes, nerve injury, vascular injury, and fracture.

Proper management of instability must also consider the complications of the event.

DEGREE OF INSTABILITY
Dislocation

Dislocation is defined as the complete loss of articular contact between the humeral head and the glenoid socket (Table 13-1). When this occurs, the ligamentous and capsular nerve receptors are strongly stimulated causing reflex increases in muscle tensions that prevent spontaneous repositioning of the articular surfaces. First-time dislocations are usually traumatic, and resultant muscle spasms strongly hold the humeral head away from the glenoid surface. Careful leveraging procedures are usually necessary to replace the humeral head in its proper position, thus reducing the dislocation. Damage to the glenoid surface, glenoid labrum, glenohumeral ligaments, rotator cuff tendons, and/or the humeral head may result from dislocation. Resultant lesions are of diagnostic value and may indicate increasing risk of future events. Recurrent dislocations do not cause as massive a proprioceptive response and are generally easier to reduce. With each dislocation, the ligaments and muscles stretch and tear, further increasing the risk of future recurrence. Some individuals are able to voluntarily dislocate their shoulders by selectively contracting and relaxing particular muscles. This practice has been implicated in the development of involuntary, disabling instability, and should be strongly discouraged.

Subluxation

Subluxation of the glenohumeral joint is quite different from the chiropractic subluxation of the spine. Adjustable lesions in the extremities are called misalignments not subluxations.

331

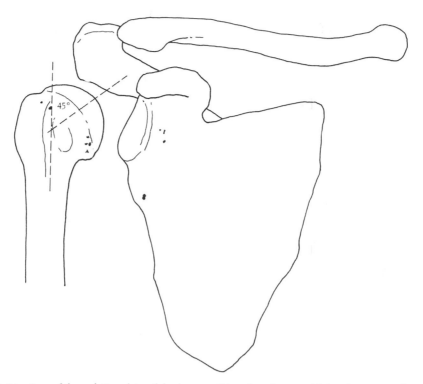

45°

Fig. 13-1. Anterior view of the relationship of the bones of the glenohumeral joint. (From Hertling and Kessler,[113] with permission.)

Subluxation occurs when the humeral head is partially displaced from the glenoid surface (Table 13-2). A sharp pain is experienced and the rotator cuff muscles contract forcefully to pull the humeral head back onto its glenoid throne. The sharp pain is often followed by weakness or paralysis that lasts for a few minutes. Called the "dead arm syndrome," this weakness or paralysis is considered a reflex response to the proprioceptive stimulus caused by a sudden stretch or injury of the glenohumeral muscles and ligaments.[3,10–12] Patients often report shoulder soreness that lasts for a few days, presumably caused by sprain and/or strain. Similar lesions of the glenoid surface, glenohumeral ligaments, rotator cuff tendons, and the humeral head may result from subluxation as with dislocation. These lesions further increase risk of both recurrent subluxations as well as dislocations. Glenohumeral subluxation is often misdiagnosed or complicated by other shoulder pain conditions. The significance of the glenohumeral subluxation has only been recognized in modern times. Some authors currently believe subluxation to be even more prevalent than dislocation as a cause of glenohumeral instability.

Many authors describe the severity of instability as a continuum from subluxation to dislocation.[4,13–18] Overuse syndromes that stretch and stress certain

Table 13-1. Primary Range of Motion Restrictions Associated with Glenohumeral Dislocation

Anterior dislocation
Internal rotation
Adduction
Abduction
Posterior dislocation
External rotation
Abduction

Table 13-2. Typical History of Glenohumeral Subluxation

Sudden sharp pain from stressful motion
The "dead arm syndrome"
Shoulder soreness for the next few days

shoulder soft tissues may represent early development in this continuum.[19] The degree or severity of instability is an important parameter in the classification and management of a patient.

DIRECTION OF INSTABILITY

Anterior Instability

Instability can occur in many different directions. Because the glenoid normally faces significantly anterior, its shape is unable to protect against anterior displacement. Anterior instability is the most common direction of shoulder instability, representing about 90 to 95 percent of cases studied.[8] Because it is so common, anterior instability has been most studied and is best understood. The ligaments and muscles that stabilize the anterior humerus are stressed by external rotation, abduction, and, to a lesser extent, extension. Throwing and swimming activities can cause external rotation overuse syndromes that may lead to anterior glenohumeral instability.

Traumatic anterior instability can develop from a direct blow to the shoulder or, more commonly, from a combination of rotation, extension, and abduction forces.[20] Anterior dislocations can be subcoracoid, subglenoid, subclavicular, or intrathoracic (Fig. 13-2). The subcoracoid dislocation is the most common ante-

rior glenohumeral dislocation. Usual causes involve some combination of abduction, extension, and external rotation forces. Each of the other anterior dislocations are quite rare and are usually associated with severe traumatic injury.[21] Such cases have a higher incidence of greater tuberosity avulsion, rotator cuff avulsion, and neurovascular injury. In the subglenoid dislocation, the humeral head is stuck inferior and anterior to the glenoid rim. The subclavicular dislocation presents with the humeral head medial to the position seen in the more common subcoracoid dislocation.[22–25] With the intrathoracic dislocation, the humeral head displaces anterior and medial between two adjacent ribs.[8] This inhibits normal respiratory function. The rare luxatio erecta is an anterior-inferior dislocation in which the arm is positioned vertically above the patient's head.[26]

Posterior Instability

Posterior instability is much rarer than anterior instability because the glenoid significantly resists posterior humeral motion. Reported rates of posterior instability range from 2 to 4 percent of all shoulders studied.[27] Some authors believe that the prevalence of posterior instability is higher than reported in these studies due to missed diagnoses. Over 60 percent of posterior dislocations are first mistaken for other conditions such as frozen shoulder.[21] The ligaments and muscles that resist posterior instability are stressed by flexion, adduction, and internal rotation or by direct anterior to posterior pressure to the forward flexed arm. Gymnastics, archery, butterfly swimming, rowing, boxing, and throwing sports can cause overuse syndromes that increase risks of posterior instability.[28]

Traumatic posterior directed forces on the forward flexed arm can cause posterior subluxation or dislocation. Motor vehicle accidents have reportedly caused posterior dislocation in this manner. Shoulder internal rotators (pectoralis major, latissimus dorsi, teres major, subscapularis) are far stronger than shoulder external rotators (infraspinatus, teres minor). Violent muscle contractions from electrical shock[29–31] or grand mal seizures[29,32–35] can also result in posterior dislocation. In such cases, the forceful internal rotation contractions vastly overpower the external rotation contractions.

The most common posterior dislocation is subacro-

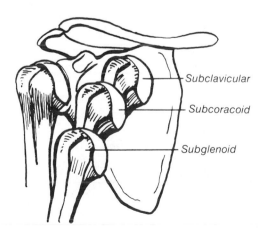

Fig. 13-2. Anterior subcoracoid, subglenoid, and subclavicular dislocations of the shoulder. (From Simon and Koenigsknecht,[95] with permission.)

Subclavicular

Subcoracoid

Subglenoid

mial, in which the humeral head is displaced directly posterior to the glenoid socket. In the subglenoid posterior dislocation, the humeral head is displaced posterior and inferior to the glenoid. The subspinous dislocation presents with the humeral head inferior to the scapular spine and further medial than the more common subacromial position.

Inferior Instability

Inferior instability occurs only with concurrent anterior or posterior instability. Incomplete surgical repair that does not address an inferior component of instability has been reported to result in unidirectional inferior instability. Such cases generally require further operative procedures.

Superior Instability

Superior instability occurs with neglected chronic rotator cuff tears, failed rotator cuff repairs, supraspinatus debridement, or acromioplasty.[27,36] Superior instability can cause impingement syndromes and degeneration of subacromial tissues. When postsurgical, this condition generally has a poor prognosis even to further surgical care unless supraspinatus repair and rehabilitation are possible.[36]

Superior dislocations can also occur from severe trauma. First reported in 1834, they usually result from extreme forward and upward force on the adducted arm. Fractures of the acromion, acromioclavicular joint, clavicle, coracoid, or humeral tuberosities can complicate a superior dislocation. The involved arm appears short and is adducted to the side. Neurovascular complications are common.[21]

Multidirectional Instability

Multidirectional instability is commonly congenital in origin, associated with ligamentous laxity or perilous bony presentations (see below). Symptoms are commonly bilateral and these patients usually respond best to conservative management. When surgery is necessary, the inferior capsule must be tightened to cause a positive result. Such patients have been classified by the term AMBRI (*a*traumatic, *m*ultidirectional instability with *b*ilateral symptoms that usually responds to rehabilitation and rarely requires an *i*nferior capsular shift).[21]

Any or all combinations of multidirectional instability can develop in a patient. It is vital to evaluate and diagnose all directions of instability for proper management.

ANATOMIC CONSIDERATIONS
Bony Attributes

In the ball and socket joint of the shoulder, the glenoid surface provides a very shallow socket. The glenoid contacts only 20 to 25 percent of the humeral head at any one time.[10] The percentage of articular contact varies among individuals and is believed to be associated with a risk of instability. This can be evaluated in the axillary radiograph by comparing the diameter of the glenoid to the diameter of the humeral head, called the glenohumeral contact head index. Cyprien et al.[37] demonstrated that patients with recurrent anterior dislocations had a significantly smaller contact index and a significantly smaller glenoid diameter than the general population.[37] These parameters were also smaller than the unaffected shoulder in the individual patients studied. Evaluation of glenoid diameter and contact index can identify patients at risk who engage in stressful activities such as competitive pitching, swimming, boxing, or gymnastics. One computed tomographic (CT) study of glenohumeral contact index did not support these radiographic findings.[38] Further studies are necessary to clarify contact index importance.

The relative position of the glenoid also appears to affect the risk of instability. Glenoid version is defined as the degree of anterior or posterior positioning of the articular surface. Some authors suggest that excessive retroversion predisposes to posterior instability.[15] They feel that glenoid version can be quantified on the axillary radiograph or with CT by measuring the angle between the spine of the scapula and the glenoid articular surface. Normal glenoid version is about 7 degrees resulting in a glenoid that faces about 45 degrees anterior during most shoulder function.[21] Significantly increased retroversion has been demonstrated in patients with clinically diagnosed posterior instability.[39,40] Some authors have successfully treated these patients with a wedge osteotomy to alter the glenoid version.[41] Increased anteversion has been observed in patients with recurrent anterior dislocations,[42] but the author is unaware of any surgical attempts at correction.

Scapulothoracic function also determines glenoid position and thus affects the risk of instability.[43,44] Scoliosis, thoracic hyperkyphosis, and scapulothoracic dysfunction can alter scapular position and motion. Altered glenoid position can affect shoulder stability by the same mechanism as variations in glenoid version. Restriction of scapular motion will functionally mimic glenoid retroversion and increase the risk of posterior instability. Scapular hypermobility will functionally

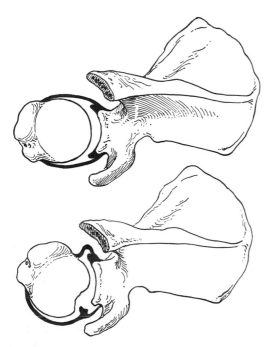

Fig. 13-3. Pathology of recurrent dislocation of the shoulder. *(Top)* Normal appearance. The labrum attaches to the margin of and deepens the glenoid. *(Bottom)* Pathologic appearance. A defect in the posterolateral aspect of the humeral head, avulsion of the labrum from the anterior lip of the glenoid, and stretching and separation of the capsule from the anterior neck of the glenoid. These factors contribute to but are not necessarily the primary causes of recurrent displacement. Not shown is the relaxed elongated subscapularis tendon, which lies anterior to and fuses with the anterior capsule. Its relative lengthening permits excessive external rotation of the humeral head, a necessary prerequisite to dislocation. (From Turek,[114] with permission.)

mimic glenoid anteversion and increase the risk of anterior instability. An altered scapular position also changes muscular length tension relationships and glenohumeral leverage systems, likely compounding instability risk.[43]

As the humeral head slips off the glenoid socket, it may be impaled on the glenoid rim causing a compression fracture. The fractured lesion is called the Hill-Sachs lesion (Fig. 13-3). The Hill-Sachs lesion can result from subluxation as well as dislocation. This lesion can result from instability in any direction and is often noted on routine radiographic studies. Specialized radiographic studies have been developed to provide greater sensitivity for this lesion.

Glenoid Labrum

Because of the shallow surface of the glenoid, the term "ball and saucer" can descriptively replace the term "ball and socket" for the glenohumeral joint. The glenoid saucer is deepened considerably by the glenoid labrum. Labrum size can vary widely. In most individuals, the glenoid labrum provides about 50 percent of the total socket depth.[45] The labrum is composed of both hyaline and fibrocartilage.[46] Being weaker than the bone, labrum injuries are commonly associated with shoulder instability.[3,10,19,47–50] Tears or degenerative changes in the labrum can significantly reduce the already shallow socket size. Most authorities agree that such lesions contribute to risk of future instability events.[51] A congenitally small glenoid labrum can be visualized by computed arthrotomography. A small labrum has also been reported to increase the risk of instability.[52]

In many individuals, the glenoid labrum can serve as an attachment, or partial attachment, for the glenohumeral ligaments, the glenohumeral capsule, and the long bicipital tendon. The glenohumeral capsule attaches to the labrum in 77 percent of patients studied.[49] Soft tissue attachments to the glenoid labrum result in less capsular laxity and greater stability. On the other hand, traumatic injury in such cases has a greater tendency to cause labral avulsion and further instability. Glenohumeral soft tissues sometimes attach further from the glenoid on the scapular neck causing increasing capsular laxity yet decreasing injurious risk to the labrum.

The glenoid labrum is analogous to the meniscus of the knee in both function and type of injury. Like the meniscus, loss of labral integrity can lead to increasing instability and degenerative changes.[53,54] It will be interesting to see whether research indicates an important proprioceptive role for the labrum as it has for the meniscus.[55] Labrum tear morphology is similar to that of meniscus tears. Possibilities include longitudinal or bucket-handle tears, radial tears, and radial tears with longitudinal components (flap tear). Various degrees of degenerative tears, fraying, and detachment are also possible.[54]

There are two common mechanisms of injury to the labrum. The first mechanism involves repetitive overhead activities such as throwing sports (particularly the deceleration phase), swimming, or weight training (bench or overhead press).[56,57] The second mechanism involves direct trauma such as dislocation, subluxation, fall, or the grounding of a bat or golf club. It is unclear whether the traumatic injuries are due to avulsions caused by violent biceps contractions or the mechanical entrapment of the humeral head against the glenoid rim.

Damage associated with overhead sports usually effects the upper labrum. The attachment of the long head of the biceps often includes the anterosuperior labrum and is proposed as the etiology of injury. In an attempt to slow the rapidly extending elbow during the deceleration phase of throwing, a strong eccentric biceps contraction may pull on the labral attachment.[56] These tears can cause mechanical interference to motion without causing instability. Patients presenting with labral tears and no instability are likely to respond well to surgical reattachment. Glenoid tears that present without instability are found mainly in the superior labrum. Superior labral tears can also be caused by a traumatic compression injury such as a fall on an outstretched arm.[54]

Damage to the inferior labrum is associated with dislocations and subluxations. These tears or detachments involve the attachments of the glenohumeral ligaments and are referred to as Bankart lesions[58] (Fig. 13-3). Pieces of the bony glenoid rim may also be avulsed. Functionally, this represents a loss of firm attachment for the anteroinferior glenohumeral ligament, which serves as the major passive restraint to anterior and inferior instability. In addition, loss of labral integrity can remove a mechanical buttress to ante-

rior translation. This factor plays an important role in therapeutic approach. If the labrum is resected, the symptoms can initially be relieved, creating an unstable shoulder likely to become symptomatic in the future. A conservative rehabilitation approach is usually the first therapy of choice.[12]

Passive Restraints: Glenohumeral Ligaments and Capsule

There are five ligaments that contribute to glenohumeral stability. These include the superior, middle, and inferior portions of the anterior glenohumeral ligaments, as well as the posteroinferior glenohumeral ligament and the coracohumeral ligament. All five ligaments contribute to all directions of glenohumeral stability.[59]

The glenohumeral ligaments are thickened folds of the glenohumeral capsule. The capsule is oriented with twisted fibers such that the anterior fibers run inferior and lateral. This orientation naturally restricts external rotation, a part of the capsular pattern. Anatomic variations in these ligaments can alter an individual's ability to remain stable with this motion. Failure of these ligaments when under stress can result in increasing laxity and instability.

The anterior glenohumeral ligaments provide primarily anterior stability to the glenohumeral joint. Fresh cadaver studies have demonstrated that the relative importance of the anterior glenohumeral ligaments will vary with arm position.[60] At 0 degrees abduction, the superior and middle glenohumeral ligaments restrain external rotation. At 45 degrees abduction, the middle and inferior glenohumeral ligaments restrain external rotation. At 90 degrees abduction, the inferior glenohumeral ligament restrains external rotation. The large inferior glenohumeral ligament usually attaches primarily to the labrum at its scapular side. This anterior ligament is considered the major passive stabilizer of anterior motion.[61] The middle glenohumeral ligament is often absent or anomalous in the recurrent dislocator.[62,63] Both the middle and inferior ligaments are often avulsed following traumatic anterior dislocation. A tight posterior capsule and ligament can increase stress to the anterior passive restraints, which may lead to anterior instability. This can develop following prolonged immobilization or excessive posterior capsular repair.

The posteroinferior glenohumeral ligament provides primarily posterior stability to the glenohumeral joint. Injury to this ligament is often associated with posterior dislocation. Tight anterior capsule and ligaments can increase stress to the posterior passive restraints leading to posterior instability. This can develop following prolonged immobilization or excessive anterior capsular repair.

The glenohumeral joint capsule provides similar stabilizing restraint as the glenohumeral ligaments. The anteroinferior capsule restrains anterior subluxation of the abducted humerus.[64] The inferior two-thirds of the anterior capsule limits abduction and external rotation.[65,66] The posterior capsule limits internal rotation.[65,67]

All of the passive restraining mechanisms come under stress only when the other restraining forces are overwhelmed.[21,68]

FUNCTIONAL CONSIDERATIONS

Finite Joint Volume: Adhesion/ Cohesion

The fluid mechanics of the glenohumeral joint also assist in providing joint stability. As a sealed structure, the glenohumeral joint is able to contain a limited or finite quantity of synovial fluid. Forces that attempt to increase this volume by subluxation or dislocation will be resisted by a vacuum of about 4 mmHg.[21] This vacuum is not strong enough to prevent dislocation or subluxation but it does contribute to stability. A loose or punctured glenohumeral capsule will not demonstrate these vacuum tendencies. Joint effusion or bleeding will also decrease these effects.

Probably more important fluidic forces at the glenohumeral joint are the intermolecular forces of adhesion and cohesion. These forces are best understood by trying to pull apart two pieces of wet glass. Intermolecular forces can hold those panes of glass very tightly. If increased fluid is placed between the panes of glass, the adhesion/cohesion forces diminish and the glass panes are easy to separate. Similarly, the fluid volume within the joint will determine the significance of these intermolecular actions. Increased fluid volumes from inflammation or hemorrhage will limit adhesive/cohesive forces.[21] Individual variations in the congruence of the humeral head and the glenoid socket may allow

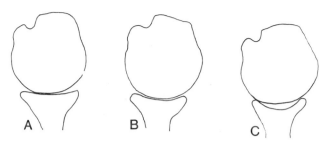

Fig. 13-4. Articular stability of the glenohumeral joint is enhanced or lessened according to the variation in articular congruence: **(A)** shallow glenoid surface; **(B)** conforming surfaces; and **(C)** excessively deepened glenoid surfaces. (Modified from Saha[70] as in Rockwood,[21] with permission.)

less contact of the articular surfaces, thus reducing adhesive/cohesive forces (Fig. 13-4).[21]

Glenohumeral adjustments cause a release of gas in the glenohumeral joint. Resultant increases in joint volume reduces adhesive/cohesive forces and allows larger ROM for about 20 minutes. Adjusting an unstable glenohumeral joint should be performed with great caution, limiting stressful motions or activities for at least the following 20 minutes.

Active Restraining Mechanisms

The muscles of the rotator cuff help hold the humeral head in the glenoid cavity. These include the supraspinatus, infraspinatus, teres minor, and subscapularis (Fig. 13-5). These are small muscles that all originate off the scapula and all insert on the humerus. Normally, the subscapularis inserts on the lesser tubercle; all others insert on the greater tubercle. In some individuals, anomalous attachments adversely affect joint stability.[69]

By reaching in front, behind, and on top of the humerus head, the rotator cuff muscles hold it in the glenoid socket (Fig. 13-6). In addition to their bony insertions, all of the rotator cuff muscles have fibers that blend with the joint capsule and control capsular tension. Many authors suggest that abnormal rotator cuff function is associated with glenohumeral instability.[5,21,49,61,69,70]

The subscapularis muscle has specific characteristics that likely contribute to joint stability. Positioned on the anterior aspect of the humerus, the subscapularis muscle acts as a physical barrier to control anterior translation of the humeral head. Contraction of the

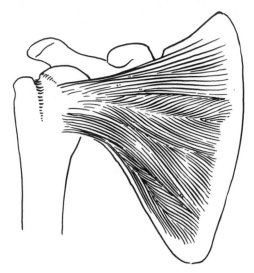

Fig. 13-5. The subscapularis muscle. (From Hollinshead,[115] with permission.)

subscapularis also prevents the excessive external rotation associated with anterior instability and ligament damage. This muscle has been observed to be lax and narrow, often with anomalous insertions in many patients who suffer recurrent anterior instability.[8,69] These studies also revealed post-traumatic subscapularis lesions on biopsies.[69] Cadaver and electromyographic studies have shown that the subscapularis prevents excessive external rotation only when the shoulder is at less than 90 degrees abduction,[21,49,61] thus limiting its clinical significance.

The teres minor and the infraspinatus likely contribute also to joint stability. Although these muscles cause external rotation at various degrees of abduction, cadaver and electromyographic studies show that they also limit excessive external rotation past 90 degrees abduction.[21,69,71] With the arm past 90 degrees abduction, these muscles cause posterior translation of the humeral head within the glenoid. This prevents unstable external rotation by reducing stress on the anterior glenohumeral capsule.[21,49] With this information, the clinician can use the historical details of injury or instability to help determine tissue specific lesions and rehabilitation plans.

The long head of the biceps can also play a significant role in the stabilization of the humeral head. The long tendon travels an intracapsular path over the humeral head to attach to the supraglenoid tubercle, and sometimes the labrum (Fig. 13-7). Tightening of this tendon will provide a force that will tether the humeral head into the glenoid socket. Analysis of the throwing mechanism in athletes with anterior shoulder instability reveals increased biceps activity during the acceleration phase presumably to reduce anterior humeral head translation.[72]

There is much controversy regarding the relative significance of the active and passive restraints of the shoulder. Patients with complete subscapularis rupture do not consistently present with shoulder instability.[73] On the other hand, subscapularis injury and tendinous laxity have been noted and repaired following recurrent anterior dislocation.[69] Electromyographic

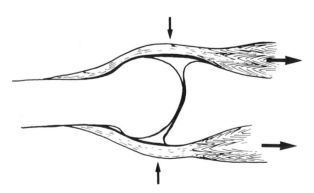

Fig. 13-6. Rotator cuff muscle action creates compressive and encircling shear forces to stabilize the humeral head on the glenoid fossa. (From Rowe,[116] with permission.)

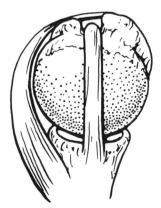

Fig. 13-7. Tension along the biceps tendon helps hold the humerus securely within the glenoid. (Modified from Petersson,[122] as in Rockwood,[21] with permission.)

analysis of patients with recurrent anterior instability has demonstrated lower than normal activity levels and activation rates of the subscapularis when placed in stressful positions.[74] Normal subscapularis function presumably prevents excessive humeral head motion in these positions and therefore probably contributes to stability.

Selective suprascapular nerve blocks can temporarily paralyze the supraspinatus and infraspinatus. Normal subjects given suprascapular nerve blocks do not demonstrate unstable glenohumeral kinematics.[57] On the other hand, posterior rotator cuff injury is common with anterior instability and rotator cuff strengthening exercise can reduce recurrent instability.[5–7,13,75] Furthermore, some patients with no ligament or capsular injury are able to voluntarily dislocate their shoulders by selectively contracting and relaxing particular shoulder muscles. This suggests that these muscles probably also contribute to glenohumeral stability.

Rockwood[21] summarized current understanding of the shoulder into a complex hierarchy of stabilizing factors. With minimal loads, such as gravity, ball and socket shape and size, finite joint volume, and adhesive/cohesive forces can maintain joint continuity. With larger loads, rotator cuff and biceps contraction maintain joint stability. Massive loads can overwhelm the active muscular restraints requiring the capsule, ligaments, and bony elements to provide stabilizing support.[21] Individual variation can increase or decrease the significance of each level of the hierarchy.

Circle Concept of Instability

Excessive translation in any one direction likely involves weakness, laxity, or damage to structures on multiple sides of the glenohumeral joint. This applies to both active and passive restraining structures. Some authors have called this the circle concept of instability and promote the need to stabilize all sides of the glenohumeral joint when any instability presents.[76] Rehabilitation of the active restraining structures requires strengthening of all of the rotator cuff muscles as well as the biceps. The specific muscular information presented above can be used to emphasize strengthening of particularly injured or weakened muscles in an individualized rehabilitation program.

Bilateral Instability

Many congenital factors determine relative glenohumeral stability in the population. These may include the following:

Variation of collagen makeup of ligaments
Variation of ligament size and position
Variation of ligament scapular/labral attachments
Variation of size, depth, and tilt of glenoid socket
Variation of labral thickness
Variation of rotator cuff attachments

Bilateral instability is found more often than would be randomly predicted. About 17 percent of unstable patients have bilateral symptoms.

Since a patient with a predilection for instability at one shoulder is likely to have similar influences at the other shoulder, evaluation for bilateral instability is prudent. This is particularly important for the patient with multidirectional instability, in whom congenital factors are of greater significance.

Congenital causes cannot be the only reason for the high incidence of bilateral instability. Other factors could include age, seizure, or tendency toward trauma.

Biokinetics

The glenohumeral joint normally functions as a true ball and socket joint. Throughout most motion, the center of rotation of the humeral head deviates very little from the center of the glenoid socket. This requires that the articular surfaces slide primarily with very little rolling motion. Motion in the coronal plane is called abduction. Throughout abduction, the center of rotation of the humeral head deviates only 6 mm in the normal shoulder. Most of the 6 mm excursion occurs at the extremes of abduction. The unstable shoulder demonstrates excessive excursion of the humeral head in abduction, measuring 10 mm or more.[77]

Motion in the horizontal plane also shows true ball and socket function. The center of rotation of the humeral head is precisely centered in the glenoid throughout the motions of horizontal abduction and horizontal adduction. If external rotation is added at the end of horizontal abduction, as in the cocking phase of the throwing activity, the humeral head deviates posteriorly 4 mm. In the normal shoulder, this posterior deviation will reduce stress to the anterior shoulder restraints. The patient with anterior instability does not exhibit this posterior humeral head deviation. In severe cases of instability, the humeral head may even deviate in an anterior direction when the cocking phase position is performed. In either case, the joint stabilizers are placed under greater stress and risk of injury than in the patient with normal joint biokinetics.[78]

The excessive and improper motion associated with glenohumeral instability can have multiple causes. Perhaps joint dysfunction in a specific direction limits articular sliding capability resulting in increased rolling motion. Thus greater excursion in specific directions would be noted. Evaluating excursions following specific shoulder adjustments may reveal therapeutic changes. Perhaps altered muscular tension permits inappropriate and excessive humeral head translation. Evaluating excursions following exercise and biofeedback programs may also reveal therapeutic changes. Perhaps passive restraints are weakened, thus permitting inappropriate and excessive excursion. Studies of excursion under anesthesia can produce meaningful results. It is possible that there may be multiple causes of the abnormal biokinetics associated with glenohumeral instability, suggesting that some techniques may be therapeutically useful for some patients and other techniques may be required for other patients. Clearly, further studies will help clarify instability mechanisms and help in the development of therapeutically useful treatment techniques.

Pitching and Instability

There are two phases during the throwing activity that risk glenohumeral instability. During the late cocking phase, the humeral head reaches the limits of horizontal abduction and external rotation. When approaching this phase, the normal athlete eccentrically contracts the pectoralis major, the latissimus dorsi, and the subscapularis to control the extreme of external rotation. The athlete with anterior instability demonstrates a decreased activity of all these muscles, thus allowing excessive external rotation and excessive stress to the passive shoulder restraints. Strengthening exercises and biofeedback programs can be used in a preventative program or in the treatment of anterior instability in the throwing athlete.[72,74]

One study suggests that the infraspinatus and teres minor are vital in the control of external rotation in the cocking phase of the throwing activity. In this position of abduction and rotation, these muscles pull the humeral head posterior to reduce stress on the passive restraints. Strengthening exercises and biofeedback therapy of these muscles can also be useful in prevention and treatment of anterior instability in the throwing athlete.[68]

The serratus anterior contracts from the end of the cocking phase, throughout the acceleration phase, and during the follow-through phase of the throwing activity. It actively protracts the scapula, thus allowing the glenoid to "catch up" to the progressive anterior displacement of the humeral head. This action limits anterior translation of the humeral head on the glenoid, thus reducing the risk of anterior instability. The athlete with anterior shoulder instability demonstrates decreased activity of the serratus anterior during these phases of throwing.[72] Again, appropriate strengthening exercise and biofeedback programs can be useful in prevention and treatment of instability disorders during throwing or pitching activities.[72]

The excessive internal rotation of the follow-through phase can cause a risk of posterior instability. The infraspinatus and teres minor act to control excessive internal rotation during this phase. The action of the serratus anterior also helps to control excessive glenohumeral internal rotation. Strengthening exercise and biofeedback programs can be useful for throwing athletes demonstrating tendencies toward posterior instability.

Contraction of the supraspinatus and the biceps brachii helps to hold the humeral head close to the glenoid cavity (see above). Throwing athletes with glenohumeral instability show increased activity of these muscles in the cocking and acceleration phases. This presumably helps compensate for the instability during stressful motions and positions. Strengthening exercises and biofeedback programs can be useful to help the unstable shoulder regain some stability during the throwing activity.[72]

CLASSIFICATION OF INSTABILITY

There are many different types of glenohumeral instability. Although there are similar attributes to all types, it is vital to classify specifically any individual patient's instability to safely and effectively develop a management plan. Parameters of instability include the following:

Degree of instability
Direction of instability
Recurrence of instability
Chronology of instability
Relationship to trauma
Neuromuscular or congenital factors

Degree of Instability

As previously stated, many authors describe the degree of instability as a continuum from subluxation to dislocation.[3,10,11,13,16–18] When dislocation is present, the first immediate objective of therapy is reduction of the dislocation. Once this is safely accomplished, treatment of subluxation and dislocation becomes very similar. In general, prognosis is better for the less severe subluxation.

Some authors have suggested that overuse syndromes are early precursors to subluxation and dislocation instabilities in the shoulder. Swimmer's shoulder and pitcher's shoulder are commonly considered presentations of impingement syndrome. Many of these patients may have unrecognized instability as a component of their condition. One study of patients with anterior instability revealed that 68 percent also had impingement signs.[19,79]

Direction of Instability

Glenohumeral instability can occur in any combination of directions previously discussed. It is important to evaluate all possible directions of instability to avoid the missed diagnosis of multidirectional instability. Anterior instability is the most common direction of instability due to the anatomic predispositions. Anterior dislocations can include the subcoracoid, subglenoid, subclavicular, intrathoracic, or the luxation erecta types.

Posterior instability is much rarer than anterior instability. Posterior dislocations can include the subacromial, subglenoid, or subspinous types. Inferior instability only occurs if other directions of instability are present. In the absence of severe trauma, superior instability only occurs following degenerative changes of the rotator cuff or acromioplasty.

Recurrence of Instability

Recurrence of dislocation or subluxation is a common complication of instability. The risk of recurrence is quite dependent on the patient's age. Patients less than 30 years of age have the highest risk of recurrence.[80] Some studies have found the incidence of recurrence to be 75 to 96 percent for this age group.[5,49,75,81–83] Specific rehabilitation protocols have, however, lowered this rate to 18 to 25 percent.[4–7,75] After each recurrent episode, the risk of future episodes increases.[2] For these reasons, it is important to classify a patient as first time or recurrent to better develop prognosis and management plans.

Chronology of Instability

Most cases of instability, whether first time or recurrent, are acute. These either reduce spontaneously or are quickly reduced in a therapeutic setting. An acute dislocation can be locked or fixed if the humeral head is impaled on the edge of the glenoid. Reduction is more difficult and if closed procedures are unsuccessful, open surgical procedures become necessary. In either case, the acute dislocation should be reduced as soon as possible. In a rare case, dislocation can remain unreduced for quite some time causing pathologic adaptation to the dislocated state. This has been reported following misdiagnoses. The posterior dislocation is not uncommonly mistaken for frozen shoulder. Patients regain some ROM but the condition usually degenerates and prosthesis is often necessary. Closed reduction may be successful up to 6 to 12 weeks following the injury but an earlier reduction has a consistently better prognosis.[8,18] Knowledge of chronicity is vital to correct management in these cases.

Relationship to Trauma

The presence or absence of trauma is another important factor when classifying shoulder instability. One study reports 96 percent of dislocations to be trauma related.[8] Most commonly, traumatic instability involves a specific injury or macrotrauma such as a blow to the shoulder, a fall on an outstretched arm, or a forced motion (i.e., a fall causing external rotation). When available, the details of the trauma provide clinically valuable information. In rare cases, traumatic instability can be caused by the forceful contractions of an epileptic seizure or an electrical shock. These dislocations are mostly posterior in direction.[3,11]

Microtrauma associated with repetitive activities can also cause instability. Repetitive motions such as swimming or pitching have been implicated.[11] The development of these overuse instabilities may involve ligamentous, labrum, or capsular damage in the absence of a macrotraumatic event.

Atraumatic instability causes fewer tissue lesions than traumatic instability. Atraumatic instability can present as subluxation or dislocation caused by merely placing the arm in a particular position. This condition can develop following long-standing traumatic instability or in a patient with ligamentous laxity.

Voluntary dislocations are a form of atraumatic instability. This type of patient intentionally dislocates a shoulder by contracting and relaxing individual glenohumeral muscles.[3,10,11] To the patient, this may seem a harmless party trick, but it can develop into a disabling instability with involuntary components. Voluntary dislocation is often associated with emotional disorders.[8,11]

Neuromuscular or Congenital Factors

Neuromuscular causes of instability include brachial plexus lesions resulting in paresis or paralysis of active stabilizers, cerebral palsy resulting in severely unbalanced muscle activity, seizures (as previously mentioned), or encephalitis. These conditions generally result in posterior instability.[35]

Congenital instability can be due to malformations of the humeral head or glenoid, such as excessive retroversion or anteversion.

COMPLICATIONS OF SHOULDER INSTABILITY

Complications of shoulder instability can include any of the following:

Joint lesions (labral fraying, Bankart, degenerative joint disease)
Bony lesions (Hill-Sachs, fracture)

Neurologic injury (usually axillary nerve)
Vascular injury (axillary artery, usually in elderly)
Recurrence

Either subluxations or dislocations can result in accelerated degenerative, arthritic changes in the glenohumeral joint. Both subluxations and dislocations can also cause specific lesions of the shoulder. The Hill-Sachs lesion is a compression fracture of the humeral head that results from smashing against the rim of the glenoid. Anterior instability results in posterior Hill-Sachs lesions. Posterior instability results in anterior Hill-Sachs lesions (Fig. 13-8). The Bankart lesion is a tear of the glenoid labrum from the glenoid, sometimes avulsing bone in the process (Fig. 13-9). Sclerosis often develops around the tear. These lesions can be seen on modified radiographic views or with other imaging methods. Either the Hill-Sachs lesion or the Bankart lesion can cause further destabilization of the shoulder, increasing risk of recurrence.

Dislocations can cause avulsion fractures of the greater tuberosity. These avulsions will not usually interfere with reduction. Postreduction radiographs can determine if further therapy is necessary. A greater tuberosity fracture requires no additional procedures if the postreduction space between the fracture segments is less than 0.5 cm.[6]

Dislocation can also result in nerve and/or vascular damage. The axillary nerve is most often affected yet any nerve of the brachial plexus can be involved. The

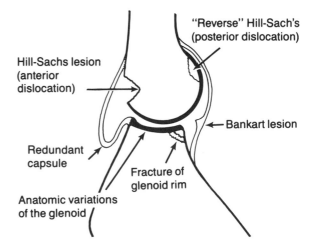

Fig. 13-8. Outline of the anatomic lesions producing instability of the shoulder. The muscular lesions are not shown. (From Rowe,[116] with permission.)

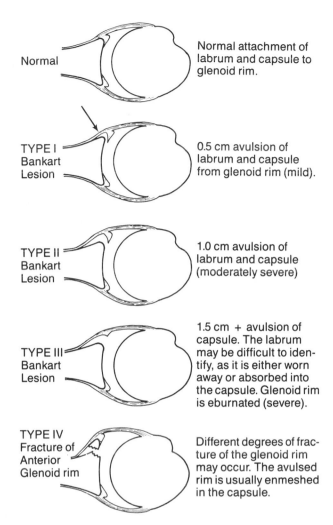

Normal — Normal attachment of labrum and capsule to glenoid rim.

TYPE I Bankart Lesion — 0.5 cm avulsion of labrum and capsule from glenoid rim (mild).

TYPE II Bankart Lesion — 1.0 cm avulsion of labrum and capsule (moderately severe)

TYPE III Bankart Lesion — 1.5 cm + avulsion of capsule. The labrum may be difficult to identify, as it is either worn away or absorbed into the capsule. Glenoid rim is eburnated (severe).

TYPE IV Fracture of Anterior Glenoid rim — Different degrees of fracture of the glenoid rim may occur. The avulsed rim is usually enmeshed in the capsule.

Fig. 13-9. Classification of the Bankart lesion (four types). (From Rowe,[116] with permission.)

axillary nerve originates from the posterior cord of the brachial plexus, crosses the anterior surface of the subscapularis tendon, and then travels posterior and around the inferior glenohumeral capsule. Its motor innervation includes the deltoid and teres minor. It supplies sensation to the lateral arm. Risk of axillary nerve damage is 5 to 30 percent for first-time dislocations.[84–86] Risk increases with age, duration of luxation, and degree of trauma.[84] Either dislocation or reduction may precipitate the injury. The musculocutaneous nerve is the second most common nerve injured. The musculocutaneous nerve innervates the biceps and is cutaneous to the lateral forearm. Minimal pre-reduction evaluation should include sensation to the lateral

arm and forearm if possible. Postreduction screen should also include isometric contraction of the deltoid and biceps. Screening tests can, however, be unreliable. Electromyographic evaluation is performed if recovery is delayed. Electromyography is accurate 3 to 4 weeks after the injury.[21]

Nerve injuries resulting from dislocations never exceed a second degree peripheral nerve lesion. Complete recovery is accomplished with only "watchful expectation."[21] Recovery is usually noted within 2 to 6 weeks with full electromyography demonstrated function at 3 to 5 months.[84,87] Interrupted galvanic stimulation is appropriate if no recovery is observed after 10 weeks to delay atrophy while nerve regeneration is accomplished. No cases of surgical necessity have been reported.

Vascular damage more commonly occurs in the elderly and is to be considered a medical emergency. Subluxation has no risk of neurovascular damage. Usually involving the axillary artery, these lesions have a 50 percent mortality rate with a high rate of morbidity in the survivors. Vascular injuries are usually seen with anterior-inferior dislocations. Signs and symptoms of vascular injury include pain, expanding hematoma, pulse deficit, peripheral cyanosis, peripheral coolness, pallor, neurologic dysfunction, and shock. Arteriograms confirm the diagnosis. Emergency surgery is necessary to save function, life, and limb.

Recurrence of dislocation or subluxation is a common complication of instability. Proper management of shoulder instability must minimize the risk of recurrence. Elderly patients require less attention to this complication.[80] Young adults require strict attention to avoid this complication. Management techniques include temporary immobilization, vigorous exercise, avoidance of stressful activities, and in some cases, surgical stabilization. Each occurrence of instability can further weaken active and passive restraints, thus increasing risk of additional incidents.[2]

DIAGNOSIS OF SHOULDER DISLOCATION

History

Glenohumeral dislocation usually presents with a history of predictable traumatic forces to the shoulder. A patient with anterior dislocation typically has a history of traumatic external rotation and abduction, traumatic

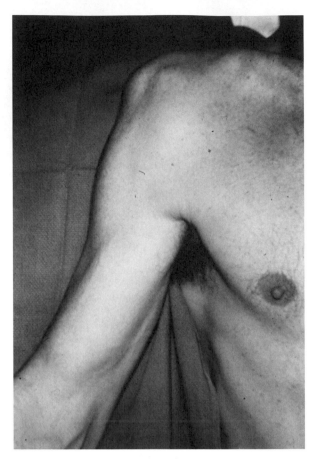

Fig. 13-10. An unreduced anterior dislocation of the right shoulder. Note that the arm is locked in external rotation. (From Rowe,[116] with permission.)

extension, or a forceful blow directly to the shoulder.[3,4,6,10,11,16] A patient with posterior dislocation typically has experienced an anterior to posterior force with the arm in flexion, adduction, and internal rotation. Examples could include a fall on an outstretched hand, a fall while holding a football, or a punch in boxing.[3,4,10,40,88,89] Forceful seizure contractions or electrical shock can also be the cause of posterior dislocation.

First-time dislocations usually require large traumatic forces. With a previous history of instability, minor traumatic force can result in dislocation. Patients who are voluntary dislocators also have increased risk of traumatic dislocation from minor traumatic incidents. First-time dislocations are very painful and disabling. Muscle spasms are quite prominent in first-time dislocation, and increase as time progresses after the traumatic event. Recurrent dislocations are typically less painful than first-time dislocations, and muscle spasms are less prominent.

When performing a history on a patient with glenohumeral dislocation, it is important to include questions of neurologic and vascular function. Neurovascular injury is a common complication of dislocation and should be identified early for proper management.

Physical Examination

Anterior Dislocation

Examination findings are usually reliable in a patient with frank anterior dislocation. Observation reveals the

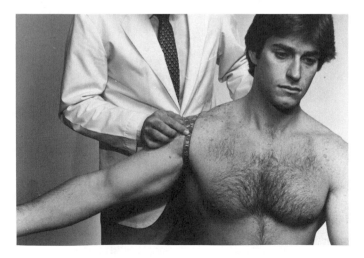

Fig. 13-11. Calloway's sign. (From Cipriano,[90] with permission.)

bulge of the humeral head anteriorly, which is palpably evident.[4] The acromion appears prominent and a posterior cavity is palpably present inferior to the acromion from where the humeral head was displaced[4] (Fig. 13-10). The deltoid is visibly and palpably flat. When an inferior component of displacement is present, the distance from the acromion to the lateral epicondyle is measurably greater than the uninvolved arm.[4] Calloway's sign is present because the circumference of the involved shoulder is larger than the uninvolved side[90] (Fig. 13-11).

The patient holds the arm in slight abduction and external rotation.[21] ROM is considerably restricted in internal rotation, adduction, or abduction.[3,4,6,21] This results in a positive Dugas test as the patient is unable to place his or her hand on the opposite shoulder[90,91] (Fig. 13-12). When first time and acute, a patient may allow no ROM at all due to the severity of the pain. Some authors claim that external rotation is also restricted in all patients with anterior dislocations.[6] ROM analysis is particularly helpful if observable and palpable findings are obscured by edema or in the obese. Neurovascular structures can be injured by dislocation and must be evaluated for proper management. In most cases, conservative management of neurologic injury is sufficient.[6,18] Vascular damage, although rare, is considered a medical emergency.

Posterior Dislocation

Posterior dislocations lack striking deformity and the arm is held adducted and internally rotated in the "sling position." They are quite rare and are often not considered in a patient with immobilizing shoulder pain. As a result, 50 percent of the posterior glenohumeral dislocations have delayed diagnoses, thus increasing the risk of degenerative change and the need for open reductions.[1] With posterior dislocation, observation reveals a prominent coracoid process and the anterior shoulder appears flattened relative to the uninvolved side.[4,41] This is best observed from behind and above the patient (Fig. 13-13). If a large hematoma or excessive edema is present these findings may be obscured.[88] The patient with posterior dislocation also

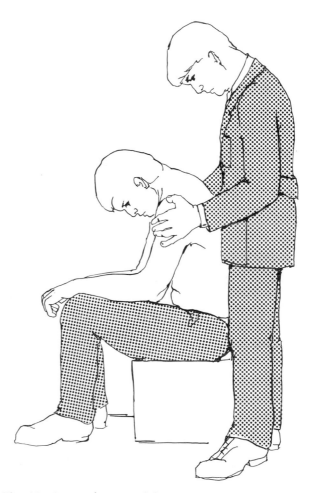

Fig. 13-13. Visualization of the anterior and posterior aspects of the shoulders can best be accomplished by having the patient sit on a low stool with the examiner standing behind him. Then the injured shoulder can easily be compared with the uninjured one. (From Rockwood,[123] with permission.)

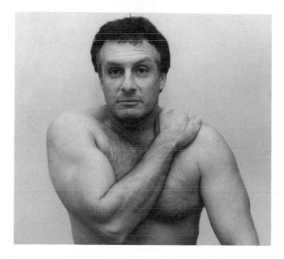

Fig. 13-12. Dugas test. (From Cipriano,[90] with permission.)

has a limited ROM. This patient is particularly unable to abduct or externally rotate.[3,4,48] Motion can be tested by having the patient fully supinate with the elbow extended. If posterior dislocation is present, the patient will be unable to reach the full palm up position as compared with the uninvolved side[3] (Fig. 13-14). A neurovascular examination should also be performed in posterior dislocations for reasons already stated.

Chronic posterior dislocation can develop due to the high incidence of misdiagnosis. One study found that it took an average of 8 months to diagnose posterior dislocation. Mistaken for frozen shoulder, aggressive physical therapy then deepens the bony degenerative lesions. Gradually, ROM increases slightly as the

bony lesions progress. This is a hazardous situation for the patient and the practitioner.

Inferior Dislocation

In the rare subglenoid dislocation, the arm is held internally rotated and abducted 30 degrees. The arm appears shortened in this position. In one reported case the involved acromion-olecranon distance was shortened by 1.5 inches as compared with the uninvolved side.[88]

Another type of rare inferior dislocation is the luxatio erecta in which the humerus is locked above the head at 110 to 160 degrees abduction. The humeral

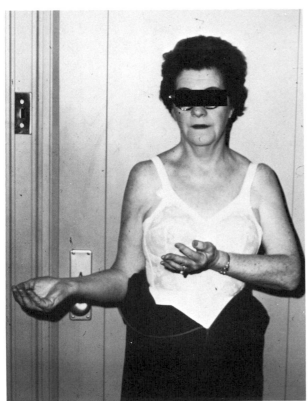
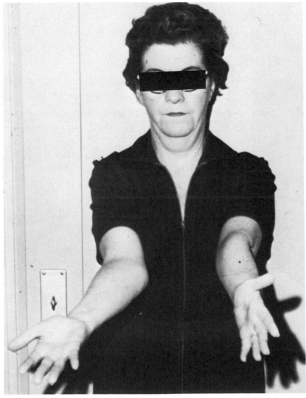

A   B

Fig. 13-14. The posterior dislocation of the patient's left shoulder had been unrecognized for 2 years, and treated for a "frozen" shoulder **(A)** The fixed internal rotation of the left shoulder is evident when the patient flexes the elbows to 90°. **(B)** With extension of the arms the patient is unable to turn her left palm up even though the arm is in complete supination (Rowe sign). (From Rowe,[117] with permission.)

head is palpable on the lateral chest wall. Pain is severe. Luxation erecta, usually due to a fall, is more common in the elderly.

Radiographic Evaluation

Anterior Dislocation

Any anterior posterior (AP) radiograph of the shoulder will clearly demonstrate a current anterior glenohumeral dislocation. Axillary and scapular radiographs also demonstrate anterior glenohumeral dislocation but these views are not necessary to make the diagnosis. The primary purpose of the AP radiograph is not to develop the diagnosis, but to investigate the presence of concurrent fracture. About 5 percent of gleno-

humeral dislocations are complicated by concurrent glenoid or humeral fracture.[81] Fractures are more common in the elderly and interposing bony fragments may prevent stable reduction. In such cases, surgical procedures may be necessary. Some fractures require no management beyond reduction. A greater tuberosity fracture requires no additional procedures if the postreduction space between the fracture segments is less than 0.5 cm.[82]

Posterior Dislocation

Posterior dislocations reveal only subtle changes on the AP films because the humeral head image overlaps the glenoid as in a normal projection. Axillary radiographs are capable of clearly demonstrating posterior

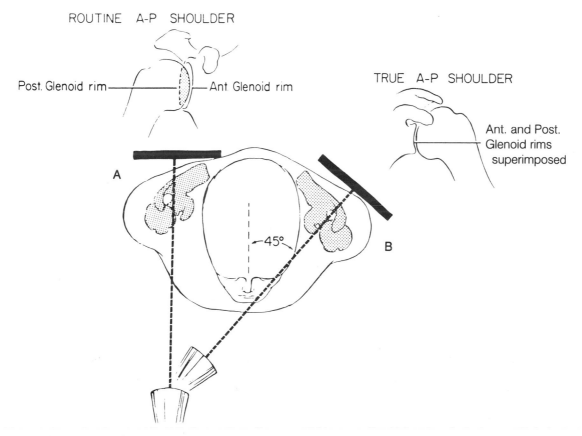

Fig. 13-15. Routine and true AP views of the shoulder. **(A)** Because the scapula sits at an angle in the chest wall, a routine AP view obtains an oblique silhouette of the joint. There should be an overlap of the humeral head with the glenoid. **(B)** 45° view minimizes the superimposition and allows a view of the glenoid margin and the joint space. (From Reid,[120] with permission.)

displacement. Some patients, however, are unable to abduct sufficiently for a true axillary film. The Velpeau axillary position is an option for these patients.[1] The Velpeau axillary radiograph is performed with the arm at the side. The central ray passes superior to inferior and slightly anterior to posterior through the shoulder allowing the clinician to visualize easily posterior dislocation.

Radiographs in the scapular plane demonstrate posterior dislocations conclusively with relative ease in several projections. In the scapulolateral procedure, the central ray passes medial to lateral along the scapula and through the glenoid as well as the humeral head. In the true AP shoulder, the central ray passes perpendicular to the scapula and through the glenohumeral joint space (Fig. 13-15). These views allow easier observation of any humeral displacement.[21]

MANAGEMENT OF ANTERIOR SHOULDER DISLOCATION

Reduction

A glenohumeral dislocation should be reduced as early as possible to minimize the risk of complications, such as degeneration or neurovascular insult.[6,18] Radiographic confirmation of the diagnosis may be reassuring to the clinician, but many authors suggest that the taking of radiograph is not necessary or desirable if it would delay reduction.[6,7] Aronen[6] states that any interposing tendons or bone fragments would simply prevent stable reduction. If proper reduction procedures are performed, there is no additional risk to such a patient.[6] Postreduction radiographs must always be evaluated to rule out glenoid or tubercle fracture.

Certain general procedures apply to all techniques of anterior glenohumeral reduction. All reductions should be performed with slow and gradual forces. Excessive speed or force is traumatic, and has been associated with iatrogenic fracture or neurovascular damage in multiple cases.[2,5,7] If gentle procedures are unsuccessful, the use of muscle relaxants or other sedatives is recommended to decrease muscle spasm thus allowing nontraumatic reduction. Gentle reduction is easiest immediately after the injury, when the least spasm is present. Spasm is typically less severe in the recurrent dislocation, and gentle reduction is generally easy to accomplish in such a patient.

The patient should be relaxed and as comfortable as possible during the reduction procedure. Slow, deep breathing exercises can help the patient relax and reduce muscle spasm.[92] The patient should also be comforted and encouraged throughout the procedure. This will help to minimize fear and its associated spasm. A relaxed, secure patient will permit a slow and gentle reduction even long after the injury.[3,9]

The following methods of glenohumeral reduction are discussed in some detail:

Kocher Method
Hippocratic method
Milch method
Scapular manipulation
Stimson method
Self-reduction

Kocher Method

The Kocher method of glenohumeral reduction begins with external rotation and inferior traction of the involved arm. External rotation reduces spasm and lifts the humeral head over the anterior lip of the glenoid.[4,7,8,92,93] In many cases, reduction will be accomplished once external rotation has occurred (see Fig. 6-35A–C).

During the procedure, the elbow is flexed 90 degrees to provide leverage for the maneuver. The flexed elbow also shortens the biceps to decrease bicipital muscle tension. When in spasm, the long head of the biceps holds the dislocated humeral head tightly against the scapula, preventing easy external rotation. Severe bicipital spasm may prevent a successful Kocher maneuver.[92,94] Attempting to forcefully overcome the biceps spasm can be quite hazardous. Iatrogenic nerve injuries, glenoid fractures, and humeral shaft fractures have been reported.[1,92,94]

Following external rotation, the elbow is adducted across the trunk. This sometimes provides the final leverage necessary for the humeral head to slip into the glenoid fossa. Internal rotation is then performed to reduce stress to the anterior glenohumeral capsule and the patient is immobilized in this position.[4,7,8,92]

Some modifications of the Kocher maneuver have involved external rotation while the arm is at 90 degrees abduction or 90 degrees flexion. No comparison studies regarding ease of reduction or incidence of complication have yet been reported.[95]

Hippocratic Method

Hippocrates described a technique of glenohumeral reduction that is used to this day. With the elbow extended, the arm is tractioned inferiorly while the trunk is stabilized.[4,6,7,96] Trunk stabilization is accomplished by placing a foot against the lateral ribs. A common mistake is to stabilize the trunk by placing the foot high in the axilla. This inappropriate foot placement compresses the axillary nerve and often results in nerve damage[4,96] (Fig. 13-16). An alternate method of stabilization uses an assistant to firmly hold the ribs.

Inferior traction gradually decreases muscle spasm to allow spontaneous reduction. Slight flexion or abduction can assist in reduction.[6,95] If reduction is not accomplished by 60 seconds of gradual traction, other methods should be applied.[95]

The main disadvantage of the Hippocratic method is the position of the elbow during the maneuver. The elbow is kept in full extension. This stretches the biceps and tightens its spastic hold on the scapula. For this reason, the Hippocratic maneuver is most successful with recurrent dislocations, when biceps spasm is minimal. Some variations of the Hippocratic method have kept the elbow bent to avoid tightening of the biceps (Fig. 13-17).

Milch Method

The Milch method is performed by gently and gradually moving the arm to full abduction and external rotation.[3,4,94] The elbow remains bent throughout the procedure to decrease biceps tension. The thumb of the doctor's uninvolved hand is used to stabilize the humeral head to prevent inferior slippage that may stress and injure the axillary nerve[3] (Fig. 13-18).

In the position of full abduction and external rota-

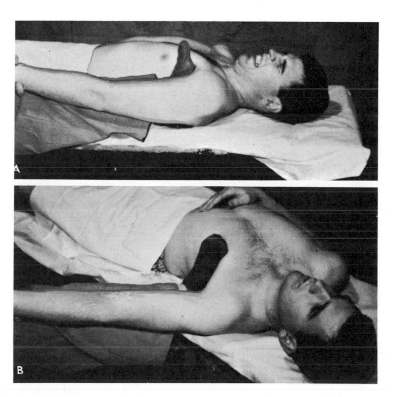

Fig. 13-16. (A) The improper method of reduction. Note the foot is directly in the axilla, impinging the brachial plexus against the dislocated humeral head while the arm is levered over the foot. This can cause serious damage to the brachial plexus and is quite painful. **(B)** The proper position is with the foot against the axillary wall for pressure while steady, even traction is made at about a 45 degree angle. (From O'Donoghue,[96] with permission.)

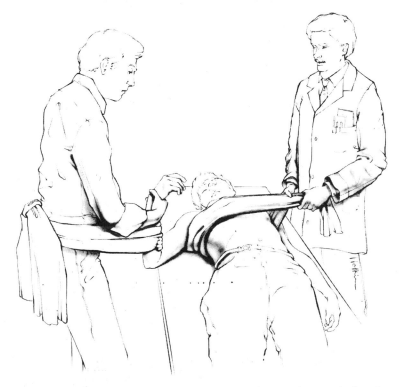

Fig. 13-17. This simple technique for reducing the dislocated shoulder applies gradual and steady traction along the axis of the dislocated limb. A bedsheet, wrapped around the supine patient's upper chest wall and over the unaffected shoulder, is either tied or held by an assistant, and acts as a fixed counterforce. A second bedsheet is placed around the patient's flexed forearm, just distal to the flexed elbow, and securely tied behind the physician's back. With the patient's forearm held in a neutral rotation and the hand in a vertical position the physician applies traction be leaning back. (Illustration by Bonnie Hofkin. From Respet,[118] with permission.)

tion, the long head of the biceps no longer holds the humeral head against the scapular fossa. Many cases will spontaneously reduce once this position is attained. In other cases, gentle superior pressure on the humeral head will complete the reduction. Superior traction from the shaft of the humerus has been associated with neurovascular damage and should be avoided.[3]

The Milch maneuver is a very safe method of glenohumeral reduction. It has been successful, without anesthesia, in many cases of spasmed, first-time dislocation. Early studies have found no fractures or nerve lesions attributable to the use of the Milch method.[3] A modification of the Milch method is performed in the prone position.[97]

Scapular Manipulation

Scapular manipulation is a recently developed technique of glenohumeral reduction, for dislocations that do not easily reduce. The patient is prone and 10 to 25 lb is used to traction the bent arm anteriorly. The doctor contacts and rotates the scapula so the lip of the glenoid no longer provides a barrier to the humeral head. Reduction spontaneously ensues.[3,98] The relative incidence of success or complication with this technique has yet to be studied (Fig. 13-19).

Stimson Method

The Stimson method of glenohumeral reduction was reported in 1900 and is used to this day.[99] The patient

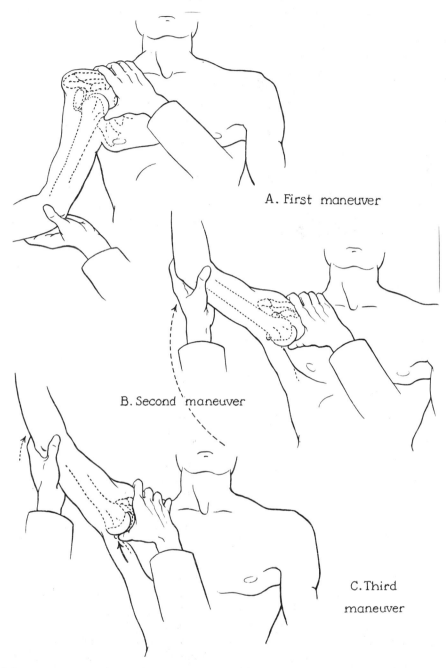

A. First maneuver

B. Second maneuver

C. Third maneuver

Fig. 13-18. **(A)** First maneuver: the patient supine; the surgeon's right hand is braced against the shoulder, while the thumb fixes the humeral head. **(B)** Second maneuver: the patient's dislocated arm is abducted in external rotation, the thumb pressure against the humeral head is still maintained. **(C)** Third maneuver: with the arm in the completely abducted position, the surgeon's thumb gently pushes the humeral head over the glenoid ridge into the fossa. (From Milch,[94] with permission.)

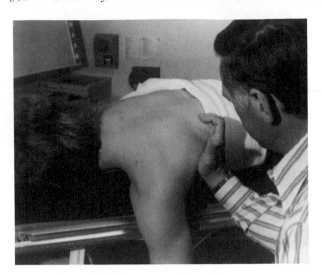

Fig. 13-19. Scapular manipulation involves pushing the inferior border of the scapula medially while the patient's arm is hanging. (From Rowe,[116] with permission.)

was originally placed in a lateral decubitus position. Modern modifications have successfully placed the patient in a prone position. A 10 lb weight is used to steadily traction the arm and reduce muscle spasm. Spontaneous reduction usually occurs within 6 minutes[4,7,8,96,99] (Fig. 13-20).

The disadvantage of the Stimson method is the position of the elbow during reduction. The elbow is kept in full extension, stretching the biceps and increasing its hold on the humeral head. Nevertheless, the Stimson method is usually a safe and effective reduction technique.

Self-Reduction

Patients who experience recurrent dislocations should be taught to safety perform reduction by themselves. This method is used to accomplish early reduction when professional assistance is not available. The patient sits on the ground or playing field with the leg bent on the involved site.[6] The patient then reaches around the knee and leans backward (Fig. 13-21). This reduces spasm and allows spontaneous reduction. This simple procedure is effective only for recurrent dislocations due to the generally lessened spasm and pain.

It is vital for these patients to understand that reduction is not synonymous with cure. Without rehabilitation, the risk of additional recurrence and any associated complications increases dramatically. Immobilization and rehabilitation are necessary to bring these risks down to acceptable levels.

Rehabilitation

After reduction is accomplished by any of the above methods, the patient experiences immediate relief and improved ROM.[7] At this time, radiographs are necessary to confirm reduction and assess for other injuries.[1] The patient should be iced, immobilized, and rehabilitated to reduce risk of recurrence.[1] Immobilization is usually performed by a sling and swathe that holds the arm in adduction and internal rotation (Fig. 13-22). This prevents the patient from abducting or externally rotating the arm, risking dislocation recurrence.

The period of immobilization for anterior dislocation is quite controversial. Anywhere from 3 to 9 weeks of immobilization is recommended by various authors.[2,50,81,83] It is believed by some that long periods of immobilization are required to heal the capsular ligament. Many patients, however, have difficulty complying with long periods of immobilization. It is also possible that long periods of immobilization cause weakening of the rotator cuff. One retrospective study showed that the rate of recurrence was unrelated to the period of immobilization.[50,81] They suggested that surgical stabilization may be appropriate for first-time dislocation in the high-risk age group—young adults.

Risk of recurrence, however, appears more related to the methods of rehabilitation than the period of immobilization. An aggressive rehabilitation exercise program can lower the recurrence rate from 75–96 percent to 18–25 percent.[5–7,13,75] The exercise program is designed to strengthen the stabilizing rotator cuff muscles. Isometric exercises are used first, even during the immobilization phase. As the patient is able, isotonic then isokinetic exercises are stressed. Most authors emphasize internal rotation exercise to control excessive external rotation postures.[2,3,5,6,83] The stabilizing effects of the external rotators, however, should not be forgotten. This rehabilitation program should be continued until the patient tests strong and apprehension free, at which time the patient may return to stressful sport activities.[5] Swimming is encouraged to develop neuromuscular balance in later stages of rehabilitation.[21]

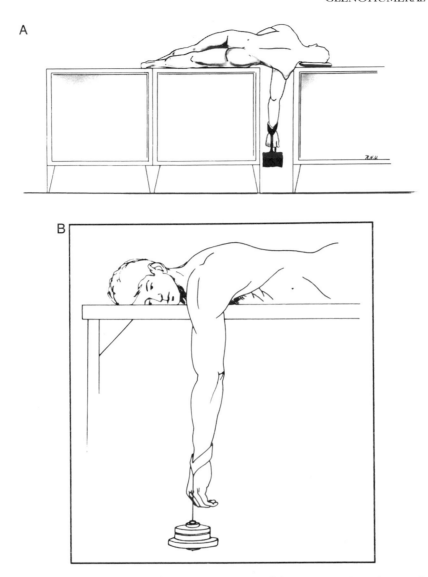

Fig. 13-20. Stimson Maneuver. **(A)** Lateral decubitis position. **(B)** Prone position. (Fig. **A** from Rowe,[7] with permission; Fig. **B** from Simon and Koenigsknecht,[95] with permission.)

Strengthening the pectoralis major and latissimus dorsi can also stabilize the shoulder by providing added eccentric control of external rotation. These muscles are strong internal rotators and may be important in shoulder stabilizers.[72] These exercises may not be appropriate in some pitchers with instability that already demonstrate internal rotation strength imbalances.

Strengthening of the serratus anterior can also provide added shoulder stability, especially in the athlete, by assisting the scapula in "keeping up" with the humeral head during high-speed, high-force activities.[72]

In addition to muscle strengthening procedures, neuromuscular pattern training can be beneficial. Fine wire biofeedback sensors can be placed on the muscles to train proper patterning during athletic or other activities. Although studies have yet to demonstrate consistent success with this approach, refinement of biofeedback techniques can provide invaluable adjuncts to rehabilitation.

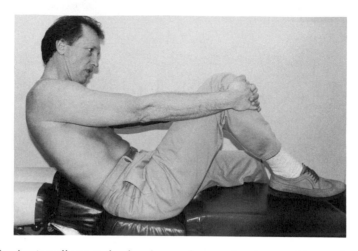

Fig. 13-21. Self-reduction allows early glenohumeral approximation resulting in fewer complications.

Because of the low risk of recurrence and the high risk of frozen shoulder, the elderly patient should be immobilized for only a short period. Some suggest only as long as pain persists.[80] Rehabilitation procedures are the same as above.

Elderly patients are at higher risk of vascular injury from dislocation. This is presumably due to the increased fragility of their vascular systems. All elderly dislocation patients should be given a complete vascular exam of the upper extremity.[80]

A sensible, progressive rehabilitation protocol can be summarized as follows:

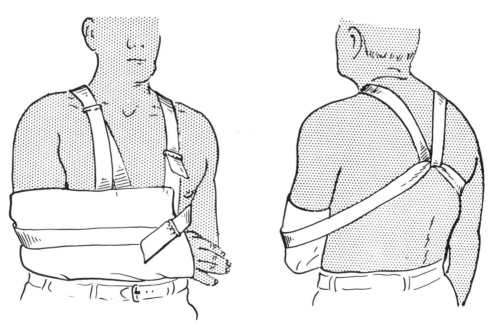

Fig. 13-22. Sling for an anterior dislocation. As long as the arm remains supported anterior to the coronal plane, the shoulder has not dislocated anteriorly. (From Rowe,[121] with permission.)

Short term immobilization (3 to 4 weeks)
Isometric rotator cuff exercises as soon as pain permits (emphasizing internal rotation in most cases)
Isotonic exercises used as immobilization is removed
Strengthening of the strong internal rotators, pectoralis major, and latissimus dorsi (not appropriate for some pitchers)
Strengthening of the biceps brachii and serratus anterior
Isokinetic exercise as increasing strength permits
Light swimming or other proprioceptive neuromuscular training
Continue above until patient is strong and apprehension free
Gradual return to stressful activities

Recurrent dislocations that cannot be controlled by conservative means require surgical stabilization. Arthroscopic procedures are less traumatic but some question the strength and durability of these less complete procedures. Surgical procedures have come a long way since Hippocrates and his red hot iron. They can provide necessary stability with minimal functional restriction in the patient who does not respond to conservative care.

MANAGEMENT OF POSTERIOR SHOULDER DISLOCATION

Reduction

Pain and spasm hold the humerus more tightly out of place when the patient dislocates in a posterior direction. Reduction is very difficult, even with muscle relaxants, tranquilizers, and/or intravenous narcotics. Closed reduction often requires general anesthesia. The procedure involves distracting the arm and gently lifting the humerus onto the glenoid. Internal rotation can help by loosening the joint capsule. External rotation should be avoided because it may deepen a humeral head compression fracture. An alternative procedure tractions the arm anteriorly from a flexed and adducted position.[21,29,31]

Early discovery of the posterior dislocation is paramount to proper management. Although quite painful, the rarity and lack of striking deformity result in typical delay in reduction. Chief complaints gradually subside although external rotation remains restricted with

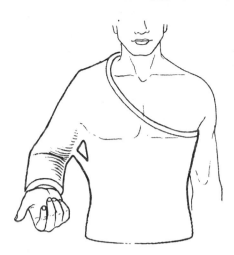

Fig. 13-23. A spica cast is often necessary to maintain a stable reduction following a posterior dislocation. (From De Palma,[119] with permission.)

pain. Years may pass before the diagnosis is ascertained.[21]

When closed reduction is not possible, one must consider the value of surgical intervention. It should be mentioned that some patients who remained dislocated gradually increased function and, years later, had minimal restriction or pain. An active patient has better prognosis. Some patients experienced progressive shoulder injury and required arthroplasty.

Rehabilitation

After reduction, the patient is immobilized with a sling and swathe for 3 weeks. Some patients must be placed in a spica cast, requiring some external rotation to maintain stable reduction (Fig. 13-23). This cast prevents internal rotation, which may destabilize the reduction. Rehabilitation involves rotator cuff strengthening. Excessive internal rotation exercises should be avoided. Swimming is encouraged to develop neuromuscular balance in later stages of rehabilitation.[21] Posterior dislocations less commonly recur than anterior dislocations due to the greater anatomic stability.

VOLUNTARY DISLOCATIONS

By relaxing and contracting selective muscles about the glenohumeral joint, some patients can voluntarily

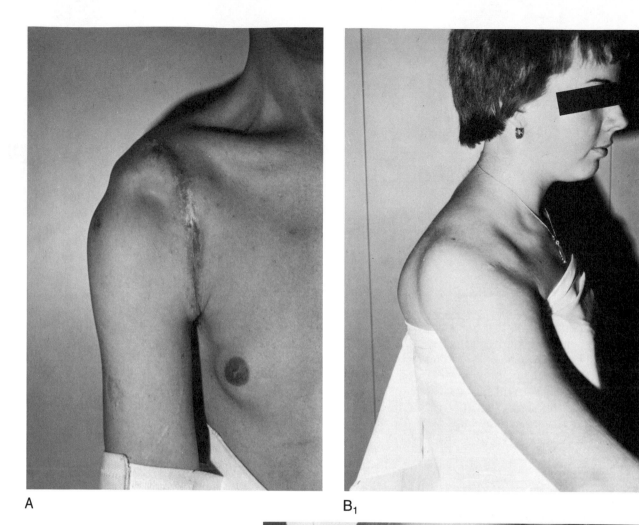

A

B₁

Fig. 13-24. Displacement of the humeral head can be accomplished with various positions of the arm or differing muscle combinations. **(A)** Inferior displacement is usually with the arm at side of body. (Patient's surgical repair had been unsuccessful.) **(B)** Posterior displacement (*1*) with the arm slightly flexed; (*2*) arm in forward flexion *(Figure continues.)*

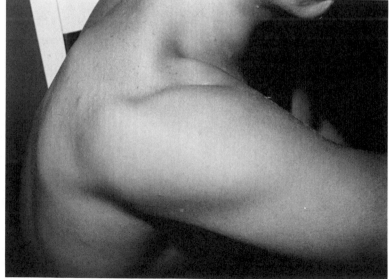

B₂

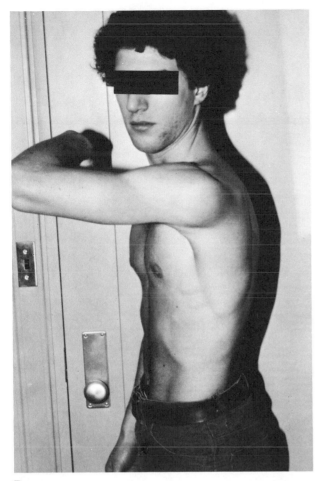

B₃

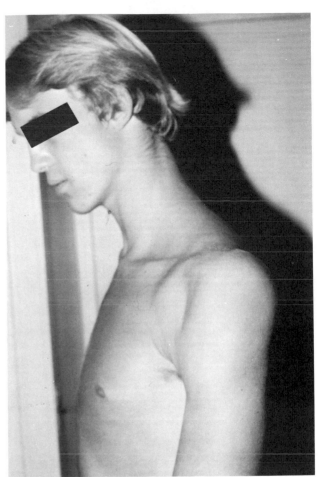

B₅

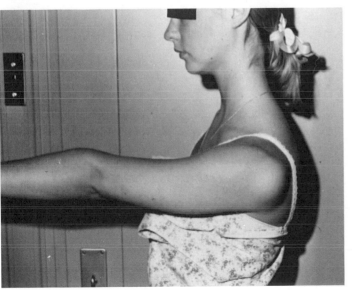

B₄

Fig. 13-24. *(continued). (3)* arm in forward flexion 90 degrees internal rotation; *(4)* arm in forward flexion 90 degrees and in neutral rotation; *(5)* with the arm in neutral at side of body. *(Figure continues.)*

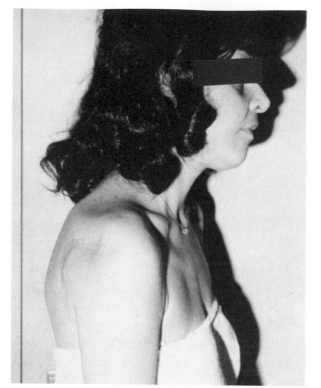

C₁

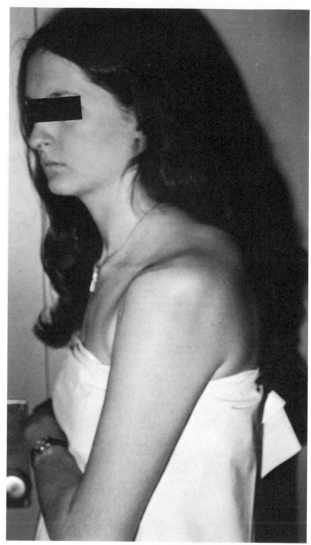

C₂

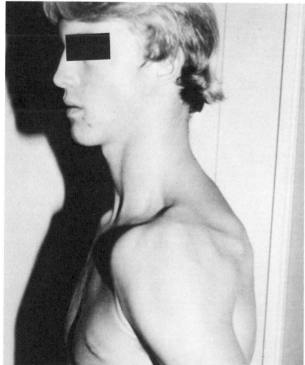

C₃

Fig. 13-24. *(continued).* **(C)** Anterior displacement (*1*) with arm in neutral position at side of body; (*2*) with arm in forward flexion and internal rotation; (*3*) with arm in backward extension. (From Rowe,[116] with permission.)

dislocate or subluxate their shoulders. It is believed that Houdini was able to voluntarily dislocate his shoulders to escape from strait jackets. This usually begins as a parlor trick by children. It may seem harmless to the patient, but it can progress into unstable and uncontrolled instability. Voluntary dislocation can be anterior, posterior, or inferior and can be performed in a variety of positions (Fig. 13-24). All patients with suspected instability should be questioned about voluntary dislocation during the history and subsequent examination.[21,100]

Rehabilitation procedures for voluntary dislocation are similar to rehabilitation programs for traumatic dislocation. Successful treatment of these patients requires high motivation on the patient's part. An uncooperative patient will not stabilize. Some uncooperative patients have benefited from psychiatric therapy. Motivated patients usually respond well to strengthening exercises that concentrate on the rotator cuff.[89,100] Electromyographic biofeedback therapy has provided a valuable adjunct to exercise therapy.[101] Rare, short-term immobilization may help the patient break the dislocation habit.

DIAGNOSIS OF SHOULDER SUBLUXATION

History

Subluxation of the glenohumeral joint occurs when hypermobility allows the humeral head to slip partially out of the glenoid. A sharp pain ensues followed by a strong muscle contraction that usually pulls the humerus back to the glenoid. After the subluxation, patients often experience the "dead arm syndrome," characterized by an inability to move the arm for a couple of minutes. Generally, the arm is sore and painful for the next few days. Most authors believe that the vast majority of subluxations occur in an anterior direction (Table 13-2). Subluxation may occur only once, or may become disabling with recurrence preventing the patient from placing the arm in certain positions without devastating effects.[3,10,11,13,14,102] Subluxations, previously thought to be very rare, may be even more common than dislocations.[13] The forces that cause anterior instability or posterior instability are the same as those for dislocation or subluxation.

Some authors believe that overuse syndromes, such as "swimmer's shoulder" or "pitcher's shoulder," often also present with demonstrable instability. They feel that excessive mobility may allow the humerus to slide superiorly and impinge the rotator cuff, biceps tendon, or bursa against the acromion. These patients will not necessarily present with a subluxation history. Physical stress tests are required to reveal the presence of instability. These patients do respond better to therapy if rehabilitation for instability is considered.

EXAMINATION

There are no observable findings in a patient with subluxation, or risk of recurrent dislocation. The patient who suffers from subluxation will typically not present with the joint displaced. In these cases, the clinician must stress the supporting structures of the shoulder to determine the presence of instability. Other secondary findings may also be present.

Physical Examination

Anterior Instability

Posterior rotator cuff tenderness and hypermobility in external rotation are common physical findings in patients with anterior instability.[3,10,11,103] Passive motion in external rotation is best tested with the patient supine and the arm at 90 degrees abduction. Hypermobility alone may be normal for any individual patient. Some authors suggest that capsular laxity or "normal" hypermobility may predispose to instability.[3,10] Hypermobility in passive external rotation may be masked by a restricting muscle tension if the patient feels the shoulder begin to subluxate.

Anterior instability is tested by providing a force that attempts to push the humeral head anteriorly out of its socket. Positive signs include pain, clicking, or a sense of apprehension that a subluxation or dislocation will occur. The clicking sounds are presumably due to labral tears. The mechanism of labral clicking is believed to be the same as the McMurray test in the knee.[48] Sometimes patients with instability will strongly contract muscles to prevent a risky position required by a particular test. Although not as meaningful in diagnosis, this response is also considered a positive test.

A number of tests may be used to evaluate anterior instability. The force is applied from a variety of arm positions to demonstrate varying degrees or regions of instability. Descriptions of these tests are presented below.

Anterior Shoulder Drawer Test

The patient is seated or supine with the shoulder relaxed. The scapula is stabilized with one hand while the other hand maneuvers the humerus. First the humerus is gently pushed medially to center it in the glenoid. From this neutral position, the humerus is pushed forward to evaluate the amount of anterior translation present. The normal shoulder allows only slight anterior translation with a firm end-feel[21,40] (Fig. 13-25).

This test can be performed from various arm positions to demonstrate differing degrees or regions of instability. With the arm at the side, very little anterior translation is normally allowed. At 80 to 120 degrees abduction, slightly more anterior translation is present. Adding external rotation up to 30 degrees will tighten the capsular ligaments further limiting translation. This position better tests the passive glenohumeral restraints. Forward flexion up to 20 degrees normally loosens the capsule and allows slightly more anterior displacement. This variety of arm position provides varying degrees of sensitivity to the anterior shoulder drawer test. It also allows the clinician to evaluate pa-

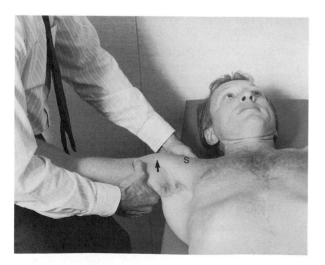

Fig. 13-25. Anterior shoulder drawer test. *S,* stabilize.

tients whose arm positions are limited for other reasons.[14,21,40,104]

Positive findings of the anterior shoulder drawer test include excessive anterior motion, pain, apprehension of impending dislocation, and/or a clicking sound. Hypermobility may be confirmed with a radiograph while the arm is stressed during the test.[14] The clicking sounds can be indications of a labral tear or a Bankart lesion. Excessive motion without other positive findings may simply indicate the presence of ligamentous laxity without pathologic instability. Evaluation of an asymptomatic shoulder, as well as other joints, can be informative in such cases.

Apprehension Test

The apprehension test is the most common method of evaluation for anterior instability.[3,10–12,14,16,17,21,40,82,103,104] To perform this test, the patient is seated or supine with the arm relaxed. The patient's arm is then placed in 90 degrees of abduction and full external rotation. The clinician then pushes the humeral head from posterior to anterior. In a positive test, the patient will feel apprehension as the humerus begins to slip toward an impending luxation. This test should be performed slowly to avoid iatrogenic dislocation.[40] Pain or a clicking sound is also considered a positive test. Some patients may contract muscles to prevent the horizontal abduction that occurs from the clinician's pressure. Such a response is also considered a positive test. Neurologic symptoms may be present (see Fig. 6-29A–D).

This test can also be performed in varying degrees of abduction, indicating involvement of different rotator cuff muscles.[10,14] At 0 degrees or 45 degrees, the subscapularis is likely involved. At 90 degrees or 135 degrees, the infraspinatus, teres minor, and glenohumeral ligaments are more likely involved.[49]

Relocation Test

The relocation test is used to confirm the apprehension test as positive for anterior instability. From a supine position, the patient is stressed at 90 degrees abduction and full external rotation, just like the apprehension test. The humeral head is then pushed from anterior to posterior to reverse abnormal biomechanics and prevent apprehension. If a patient with a positive apprehension test is relieved with a relocation test,

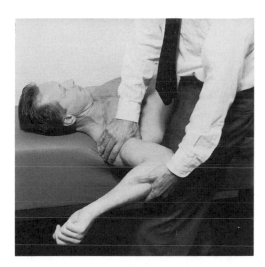

Fig. 13-26. Relocation test.

there is confirmation that instability is present. These patients will often also allow greater external rotation when the humerus is stabilized within the glenoid in this manner[40,104,105] (Fig. 13-26).

Release Test

Following a relocation test, the stabilizing AP pressure may be suddenly released. The humeral head is suddenly pushed forward in the unstable abduction and external rotation position. The positive sign of dramatically increased pain is again confirmation of anterior instability.[40]

Augmentation Test

Following a release test, the humerus is again pulled anterior to augment these painful and apprehensive responses. This again may confirm anterior instability.[40] This test is only necessary in confusing cases.

Clunk Test

The patient is supine with the arm at full abduction. The clinician stands at the head of the table. One hand is placed behind the humeral head, the other hand holds the humerus near the elbow. The clinician then pushes the humeral head anteriorly while externally rotating the humerus at the elbow. Positive findings include a clunk, click, or grinding sound, which is indicative of labral or Bankart lesions. Circular motions at the humerus may help reveal a positive finding. Following the test, the arm can be moved through horizontal abduction to relocate the humerus. An additional click or clunk is also confirmation of a positive finding[104] (Fig. 13-27).

Anterior Instability Test

The patient is seated while the clinician stands behind the patient on the involved side. The clinician's hand is placed on the shoulder so that the index finger contacts the anterior humeral head and the middle finger contacts the coracoid process. The thumb contacts the posterior humeral head. The clinician's other hand grasps the forearm to position the arm at 90 degrees

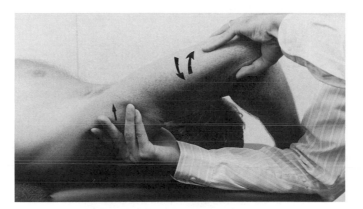

Fig. 13-27. Clunk test.

abduction and full external rotation. This movement should be performed carefully to avoid injury.

Normally, the index finger will remain in the same transverse plane as the coracoid process because the humerus remains centered in the glenoid. Anterior movement of the index finger indicates excessive anterior translation of the humeral head and is a positive finding of instability. Returning the arm to the neutral position will allow the humeral head and index finger to glide back to the starting position.[104]

Protzman Test

The patient is seated with the clinician standing on the involved side. The patient's arm is passively abducted to 90 degrees and supported against the clinician's side to allow relaxation of all shoulder muscles. The clinician's anterior fingers gently contact the anterior humeral head deep in the patient's axilla. The clinician's other hand contacts the posterior humeral head and pushes in an anterior, inferior direction. Humeral head movement greater than 25 percent of the humeral head diameter is indicative of instability. Apprehension may also be present in the unstable patient[104] (Fig. 13-28).

Posterior Instability

Posterior subluxations are far more common than posterior dislocations.[40] Posterior subluxations present with similar symptoms as anterior subluxations. Most patients complain of pain when the arm is flexed, ad-ducted, and internally rotated with an axial loading force. Such situations can include boxing, the push-up, or the bench press.

Posterior instability is tested by providing a force that attempts to push the humeral head posteriorly out of its socket. Positive signs include pain, clicking, or a sense of apprehension that a subluxation or dislocation will occur. The force is applied from a variety of arm positions to demonstrate varying degrees or regions of instability. Descriptions of these tests are presented below.

Posterior Shoulder Drawer Test

This test is analogous to the anterior shoulder drawer test in many ways. The goal of the posterior shoulder drawer test is to determine the amount of posterior translation available at the glenohumeral joint. Hypermobility, apprehension, pain, and clicking are all positive signs of instability. Hypermobility alone, without pain or other symptoms, may only suggest ligamentous laxity without pathologic instability. Evaluation of the uninvolved shoulder, as well as other joints, can clarify the clinical presentation.

The posterior shoulder drawer test can be performed in different positions, allowing differing degrees of stress and apprehension. When performed in the seated position, risk of iatrogenic dislocation is minimal and the patient is less likely to prevent meaningful findings with protective muscle contractions.[21]

To perform this test, the patient is seated with the

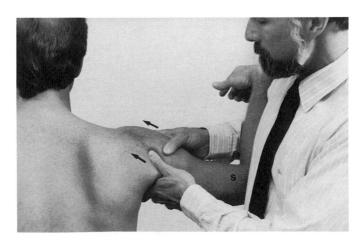

Fig. 13-28. Protzman test. *S,* stabilize.

arm at the side and the shoulder muscles relaxed. The scapula is stabilized with one hand while the other hand maneuvers the humerus. First the humerus is gently pushed medially to center it in the glenoid. From this neutral position, the humerus is pushed backward to evaluate the amount of posterior translation present. Normal posterior translation is up to one-half the diameter of the humeral head. Excessive translation, apprehension, clicking, or pain is indicative of posterior instability.[21]

A very sensitive posterior drawer test can be performed in the supine position. The patient's arm is positioned more precariously. False negatives due to protective muscle contraction are more common because of increased risk of iatrogenic dislocation. This test does allow more sensitivity with the patient who is able to relax during the maneuver. The patient's arm is held passively at 80 degrees to 120 degrees abduction and 20 degrees to 30 degrees horizontal flexion. The clinician supports the arm in this position by grasping the forearm with the elbow bent. The clinician's other hand grasps the scapula with the index and middle fingers. The patient's arm is horizontally flexed an additional 40 to 50 degrees while the arm is internally rotated. The clinician's thumb simultaneously slips off the coracoid to push the humeral head posteriorly. Both the thumb and index finger can then evaluate the amount of posterior translation produced. Apprehension and hypermobility are both positive signs of this test.[104]

Posterior Apprehension Test

The patient lies supine with the arm internally rotated and flexed to 90 degrees. One hand contacts the elbow and axially loads the humerus by pushing in a posterior direction. The other hand palpates the scapula and posterior humeral head to evaluate posterior displacement. Posterior translation greater than 50 percent of the diameter of the humeral head is excessive. Excess motion, apprehension, muscular resistance to motion, and pain are all positive signs of instability. The test may be accompanied by a clicking sound. In rare cases, the humerus may lock posteriorly as a result of this test. If this occurs, the arm is gently moved through horizontal abduction to reduce the subluxation or dislocation[27,41,104] (see Fig. 6-31).

This test is also performed with the arm at 90 degrees abduction to evaluate hypermobility in alternate positions.

Norwood Stress Test

The patient lies supine with the clinician standing superior to the patient facing caudad. The patient's arm is held passively at 90 degrees abduction with the elbow flexed to 90 degrees. The clinician supports the arm by holding the forearm near the elbow. The clinician's other hand palpates the lateral scapula and glenohumeral joint. To perform the test, the clinician brings the arm through horizontal flexion followed by about 20 degrees of internal rotation. The clinician palpates for posterior slipping of the humeral head. A posterior axial load at the elbow can make the test more sensitive. Caution is prudent, however, because iatrogenic subluxation or dislocation can occur without apprehension. Clicking may be noted as the arm is brought back through horizontal extension[104] (see Fig. 6-25A&B).

Jerk Test

The patient is seated with the arm flexed 90 degrees and internally rotated. The clinician grasps the elbow and axially loads the joint by pushing in a posterior direction while stabilizing the scapula with the other hand. The arm is then moved across the body through horizontal flexion. A sudden jerk is produced in the unstable patient when the humeral head slips off the posterior lip of the glenoid. The jerk or snapping motion is the positive sign. A second jerk may be observed on returning the arm to the original position[21] (see Fig. 6-26A&B).

Push/Pull Test

The patient lies supine with the humeral head positioned just off the edge of the table. The arm is positioned at 90 degrees abduction and 30 degrees horizontal flexion. The clinician grasps the patient's wrist with one hand and gently pulls anteriorly while the other hand contacts the proximal humerus and pushes posteriorly. This simultaneous stress causes posterior glenohumeral translation. A positive sign of hypermobility is a posterior translation greater than 50 percent of the diameter of the humeral head. Apprehension may also be present[21,104] (Fig. 13-29).

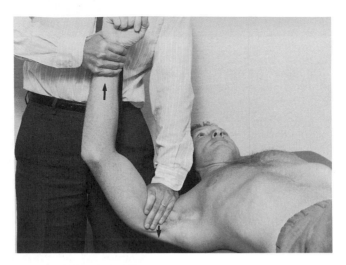

Fig. 13-29. Push/pull test.

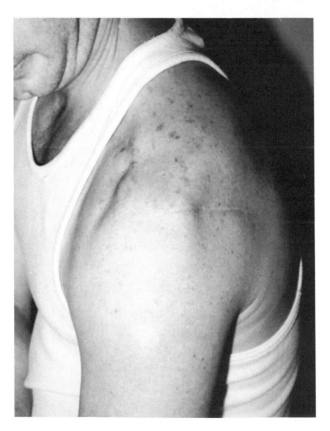

Fig. 13-30. Positive sulcus test. This patient had a posterior repair for glenohumeral instability. However, he continues to have inferior instability and demonstrates the sulcus (or hollow) just inferior to the anterior acromion during this sulcus test. A capsular shift is indicated. (From Rockwood,[21] with permission.)

Inferior Instability

Inferior instability is usually detected only in the presence of anterior and/or posterior instability.[10,11,14] Inferior instability should always be tested as an evaluation of multidirectional instability. Tests for inferior instability include the Sulcus test and Feagen test.

Sulcus Test

The patient is seated with the arm relaxed at the side. The clinician grasps and stabilizes the distal forearm at 90 degrees flexion. The other hand contacts the

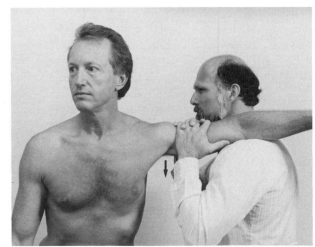

Fig. 13-31. Feagen test.

proximal forearm and pushes the humerus distally. A positive sign is the presence of a sulcus inferior to the acromion[10,11,14,21,104] (Fig. 13-30 and see Fig. 6-20C). Apprehension may also be present.

Feagen Test

The Feagen test is simply a sulcus test performed with the patient's arm positioned at 90 degrees abduction. The arm is stabilized on the clinician's shoulder. A positive sign is the presence of a sulcus inferior to the acromion[104] (Fig. 13-31). Apprehension may also be present.

Radiographic Evaluation for Shoulder Instability

The diagnosis of subluxation is often quite subtle. The subluxation rarely occurs in the doctor's office so the doctor must stress the joint to determine presence or absence of instability. These stresses can be applied under anesthesia for greater confirmation and displacement may be radiographically verified.[11] Since the mobility of the glenohumeral joint varies among individuals, the presence of hypermobility can be misleading.[10,106] Comparison with an unaffected shoulder is often helpful. Radiographic studies may show subtle post-traumatic degenerative changes if Bankart lesions are present.[10,11,13,16,47,48] Hill-Sachs compression frac-

tures may also be present. Because the diagnosis is sometimes obscure, it is important in these patients to rule out other shoulder conditions such as impingement syndrome, arthritis, frozen shoulder, strain, etc. It is also important to remember that simultaneous presentations of multiple conditions is possible. Especially noted are instability and impingement syndromes.

Routine radiographic views do not always demonstrate the subtle changes found in patients with glenohumeral instability. A variety of special views are more effective in such instances.

The Stryker (notch) view provides the best view of the Hill-Sachs defect.[10,13,21,107] This is an AP radiograph in which the arm is flexed slightly more than 90 degrees with the patient's hand on top of the head. The central beam is angled slightly cephalad. In this position, the defect is viewed longitudinally to reveal mild bony changes (Fig. 13-32).

A variety of modified axillary views are taken to provide an unobstructed image of the glenoid. These include the West Point prone axillary,[10,11,13,16,21,47,107] Ciullo supine axillary,[13] and Hermodsson axillary.[13] In these views, the central ray is angled to avoid coracoid or humeral head projection within the glenoid. A clear view of the glenoid allows the clinician to see the subtle calcific and degenerative changes associated with the Bankart lesion. The modified Didee is not an axillary film, but involves an oblique position that also

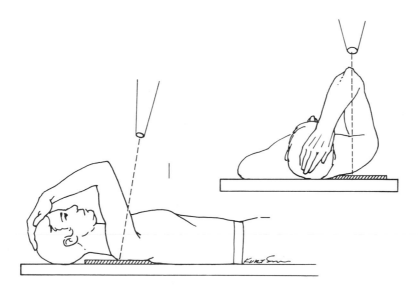

Fig. 13-32. Stryker radiograph procedure.

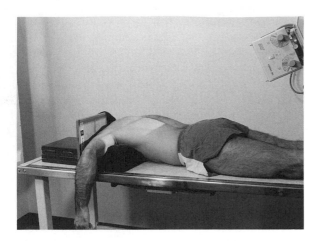

Fig. 13-33. West Point modified axillary radiograph procedure.

provides an unobstructed glenoid image.[13,107] The West Point prone axillary is the most common of the above views used for this purpose (Fig. 13-33).

Special Studies for Shoulder Instability

A variety of special imaging studies have been used to demonstrate lesions that are not visible on x-rays. These include single and double contrast arthrography,[10,11] CT[10,18] and axillary and AP arthrotomography.[11,48,108,109] In addition to the previously mentioned radiographic signs, these studies reveal labral fraying, tears, and degenerative attrition.[11] Capsular bodies may also be visualized.[110] Because it is a more comfortable procedure with low radiation exposure and a high degree of detail, the double contrast computed arthrotomography is considered by some the adjunctive study of choice for shoulder instability.[11]

Until recently, magnetic resonance imaging (MRI) has not been considered consistently sensitive at demonstrating labral lesions. One recent study using modern equipment compared imaging techniques. In the 25 patient sample, MRI showed better diagnostic results than other methods.[110a]

MANAGEMENT OF SHOULDER SUBLUXATION

Rehabilitation: Active Restraints

It is important to recognize that subluxation and dislocation are simply different degrees of the same biome-chanical problem, shoulder instability. All the management principles of shoulder subluxation also apply to the patient who is at risk of recurrent dislocation or subluxation. These procedures may be preventative for patients in high-risk groups.

Patients who suffer from shoulder subluxation should avoid activities and positions that risk recurrence until glenohumeral stability returns. Anterior subluxation patients should avoid abduction and external rotation postures, as seen in swimming activities and the cocking phase of throwing. Posterior instability patients should avoid adduction, flexion, and internal rotation, as seen in the bench press or punching activities. Immobilization is typically not necessary for those patients who are willing to restrict their activities.

Exercise programs are used to increase the strength and performance of the active restraining muscles about the glenohumeral joint. All of the rotator cuff muscles are strengthened for this purpose. Initial programs involve isometric workouts from safe and comfortable positions. The patient with anterior instability performs early isometrics from an adducted, internally rotated position. The patient with posterior instability performs early isometrics from an arm neutral or 30 degrees abducted position. Progression to resisted isotonic or isokinetic exercise is preferred when safe. The anterior subluxation patient should also exercise the pectoralis major, latissimus dorsi, biceps, and serratus anterior to help further prevent anterior displacement. These strengthening procedures continue until the patient presents as strong and apprehension free. One study demonstrated a 63 percent success rate using conservative care as described above for the treatment of posterior subluxation.[111] It is interesting that the likelihood of success was unrelated to the severity of the patients' symptoms.[111]

In addition to increasing muscle strength, a proper neuromuscular response is necessary to increase glenohumeral instability. A strong rotator cuff is not advantageous if it does not spontaneously contract in vital positions. Swimming has been recommended during late stages of rehabilitation to develop a spontaneous neuromuscular response. Other complex movement exercises have been developed to improve proper neuromuscular balance. These usually utilize **S** shaped or **C** shaped movements with little or no resistance. They should be performed in comfort to be effective. These can even be performed while the patient balances on a wobble board to help develop complex habit patterns. Advancements in biofeedback training may also prove valuable in promoting a stable neuromuscular response to the proprioceptive stimuli of risky shoulder positions.

ADJUSTING PROCEDURES AND INSTABILITY

Adjustive maneuvers to the unstable shoulder can be beneficial if used with forethought and care. The center of rotation of the humeral head moves very little in the normal glenohumeral joint. Normal arthrokinetic motion is mostly sliding with very little rolling thus providing for an unmoving center of rotation. The patient with anterior instability presents with a humerus center that shifts anterior when horizontally abducting. Passive stretching or manipulative forces in this position may help the humeral head stay centered in the glenoid. As stability increases, external rotation can be added prior to administering the therapeutic force. Mechanisms of benefit may include the normalization of arthrokinetic or a proprioceptive training of the active muscle restraints. No studies have investigated the use of adjustive procedures in the treatment of shoulder instability but the author believes such adjustments have their place within a comprehensive program of rehabilitation.

Adjustive procedures in the unstable shoulder can be quite dangerous if performed indiscriminantly without regard to specifically diagnosed pathophysiology. Simply put, forces should never be applied in a direction that could further displace an unstable humerus. It is contraindicated for a patient with anterior instability to receive adjustments that force the humerus anteriorly. It is similarly contraindicated for a patient with posterior instability to receive adjustments that force the humerus posteriorly. It is further contraindicated for a patient with anterior instability to receive adjustments that force the humerus into external rotation, thus mimicking an apprehension test. These forces risk capsular sprain, dislocation, subluxation, labral tears, Hill-Sachs lesions, Bankart lesions, and recurrent instabilities. Some patients present with multidirectional instability thus rendering all glenohumeral adjustments inappropriate and dangerous.[112]

Rehabilitation of the shoulder girdle is very important to the conservative care of the unstable shoulder. The shoulder acts not as an individual unit, but as part of a kinetic chain. If the scapular movement is excessive or restricted, stress at the glenohumeral joint is altered risking recurrent instabilities. Restricted scapulothoracic motion increases risk of posterior instability from punching activities and anterior instability from the follow-through phase of the throwing activity. Excessive scapulothoracic motion increases risk of anterior activity from the cocking phase of the throwing act. Shoulder girdle therapy can include adjustive procedures to the cervical, thoracic, costovertebral, sternoclavicular, acromioclavicular, and scapulothoracic regions. Exercise programs can include serratus anterior, trapezius, levator scapula, and rhomboids. Details of shoulder girdle rehabilitation are not the purpose of this chapter.

If a 3 to 6 month trial period of conservative care does not result in improved stability, or if episodes of recurrence increase in frequency or severity, it is time to consider surgical stabilization. Surgical stabilization is the only way to strengthen the passive restraining effects of the capsule and ligaments. Arthroscopic procedures are sometimes used, but the relative stability of these procedures remains controversial. Other surgical procedures have demonstrated stabilizing effects although sometimes at the risk of diminished ROM. Surgical stabilization is not highly successful for all types of instability.[40] Competent consultation is prudent during this phase of clinical management.

REFERENCES

1. Bloom MH, Obata WG: Diagnosis of posterior dislocation of the shoulder with use of Velpeau axillary and angle-up roentgenographic views. J Bone Joint Surg 49A:943, 1967
2. Simonet WT, Cofield RH: Prognosis in anterior shoulder dislocation. Am J Sports Med 12:19, 1982
3. Zarins B, Rowe CR: Current concepts in the diagnosis and treatment of shoulder instability in athletes. Med Sci Sports Exerc 16:444, 1984
4. Henry JH: How I manage dislocated shoulders. Phys Sports Med 12:65, 1984
5. Aronen JG, Rehan K: Decreasing the incidence of recurrence of first time anterior shoulder dislocations with rehabilitation. Am J Sports Med 12:283, 1984
6. Aronen JG: Anterior shoulder dislocations in sports. Sports Med 3:224, 1986
7. Rowe CR: Acute and recurrent anterior dislocations of the shoulder. Orthop Clin North Am 11:253, 1980

8. Post M: The Shoulder—Surgical and Non-surgical management. Lea & Febiger, Philadelphia, 1978
9. Zimmerman LM, Veith I: Great Ideas in the History of Surgery: Clavicle, Shoulder, Shoulder Amputations. Williams & Wilkins, Baltimore, 1961
10. Norris TR: Diagnostic techniques for shoulder instability. p. 239. In Stauffer ES (ed): AAOS Instructional Course Lectures. Vol 34. CV Mosby, St. Louis, 1985
11. Cofield RH, Irving JF: Evaluation and classification of shoulder instability. Clin Orthop 223:32, 1987
12. Rowe CR, Zarins B: Recurrent transient subluxation of the shoulder. J Bone Joint Surg 63A:863, 1981
13. Strauss MB, Wrobel LJ, Neff RS, Cady GW: The shrugged-off shoulder: a comparison of patients with recurrent shoulder subluxations and dislocations. Phys Sports Med 11:85, 1983
14. Gerber C, Reingold G: Clinical assessment of instability of the shoulder. J Bone Joint Surg 66B:551, 1984
15. Samilson RL: Congenital and developmental anomalies of the shoulder girdle. Orthop Clin North Am 11:219, 1980
16. Hastings DE, Coughlin LP: Recurrent subluxation of the glenohumeral joint. Am J Sports Med 9:352, 1981
17. Martin, Blazine E, Satzman JS: Recurrent anterior subluxation of the shoulder in athletics—a distinct entity. J Bone Joint Surg 51A:1037, 1969
18. Danzig L, Resnick D, Greenway G: Evaluation of unstable shoulders by computed tomography. Am J Sports Med 10:138, 1982
19. Garth WP, Allman FW, Armstrong WS: Occult anterior subluxations of the shoulder in noncontact sports. Am J Sports Med 15:579, 1987
20. O'Brien SJ, Warren RF, Schwartz E: Anterior shoulder instability. Orthop Clin North Am 18:395, 1987
21. Rockwood CA, Matsen FA: The Shoulder. WB Saunders, Philadelphia, 1990
22. Glessner JR: Intrathoracic dislocation of the humeral head. J Bone Joint Surg 42A:428, 1961
23. Moseley HF: The basic lesions of recurrent anterior dislocations. Surg Clin North Am 43:1631, 1963
24. Patel MR, Pardee ML, Singerman RC: Intrathoracic dislocation of the head of the humerus. J Bone Joint Surg 45A:1712, 1963
25. Saxena K, Stavas J: Inferior glenohumeral dislocation. Ann Energ Med 12:718, 1983
26. Moseley HF: Shoulder Lesions. Williams & Wilkins, Baltimore, 1969
27. Schwartz E, Russell WF, O'Brien SJ, Fronek J: Posterior shoulder instability. Orthop Clin North Am 18:409, 1987
28. Norris TR: Recurrent posterior shoulder dislocations. Hosp Med 26:45, 1990
29. Hawkins RJ, Neer CS II, Pianta RM, Mendoza FX: Locked

posterior dislocation of the shoulder. J Bone Joint Surg 69A:9, 1987
30. O'Flanagan PH: Fracture due to shock from domestic electric supply. Injury 6:244, 1975
31. Taylor RG, Wright PR: Posterior dislocations on the shoulder: report of six cases. J Bone Joint Surg 34B:624, 1952
32. Demos TC: Radiologic case study. Orthopedics 3:887, 1980
33. Din KM, Meggit BF: Bilateral four-part fractures with posterior dislocation of the shoulder. J Bone Joint Surg 65B:176, 1983
34. Lindholm TS, Elmstedt E: Bilateral posterior dislocation of the shoulder combined with fracture of the proximal humerus. Acta Orthop Scand 51:485, 1980
35. Shaw JL: Bilateral posterior fracture-dislocation of the shoulder and other trauma caused by convulsive seizures. J Bone Joint Surg 34A:584, 1952
36. Wiley AM: Superior humeral dislocation: a complication following decompression and debridement for rotator cuff tears. Clin Orthop 263:135, 1991
37. Cyprien JM, Vasey HM, Burdet A et al: Humeral retrotorsion and glenohumeral relationship in the normal shoulder and in recurrent anterior dislocation (scapulometry). Clin Orthop 175:8, 1983
38. Randelli M, Gambrioli PL: Glenohumeral osteometry by computed tomography in normal and unstable shoulders. Clin Orthop 208:151, 1986
39. Brewer BJ, Wubben RC, Carrerra GF: Excessive retroversion of the glenoid cavity. J Bone Joint Surg 68A:724, 1986
40. Hurley JA, Anderson TE, Dear W et al: Posterior shoulder instability: surgical versus conservative results with evaluation of glenoid version. Am J Sports Med 20:396, 1992
41. Norwood LA, Terry GC: Shoulder posterior subluxation. Am J Sports Med 12:25, 1984
42. Saha AK: Anterior recurrent dislocation of the shoulder. Acta Orthop Scand 42:491, 1967
43. Gould JA, Davies GJ: Orthopedic and sports physical therapy. CV Mosby, St. Louis, 1985
44. Hertling D, Kessler RM: Management of Common Musculoskeletal Disorders. Harper & Row, New York, 1983
45. Howell SM, Galinat BJ: The glenoid-labral socket: a constrained articular surface. Clin Orthop 243:122, 1989
46. Andrews JA, Carson WG, Ortega K: Arthroscopy of the shoulder: technique and normal anatomy. Am J Sports Med 12:1, 1984
47. Rokous JR, Feagin JA, Abbott HG: Modified axillary roentgenogram. Clin Orthop 82:84, 1972
48. Pappas AM, Goss TP, Kleinman PK: Symptomatic shoul-

der instability due to lesions of the glenoid labrum. Am J Sports Med 11:279, 1983

49. McGlynn FJ, Caspari RB: Arthroscopic findings in the subluxating shoulder. Clin Orthop 183:173, 1984

50. Hovelius L, Eriksson K, Fredin H et al: Recurrences after initial dislocation of the shoulder. J Bone Joint Surg 65A:343, 1983

51. Howell SM, Kraft TA: The role of the supraspinatus and infraspinatus muscles in glenohumeral kinematics of anterior shoulder instability. Clin Orthop 263:128, 1991

52. Rafil M, Firooznia H: Variations of normal glenoid labrum. AJR 152:201, 1989

53. Levy IM, Tojrxilli PA, Warren RF: The effect of medial meniscectomy on the anterior/posterior motion of the knee. J Bone Joint Surg 64A:883, 1982

54. Andrews JR, Kupferman SP, Killman CJ: Labral tears in throwing and racquet sports. Clin Sports Med 10:901, 1991

55. Cerulli G, Ceccarini A, Alberti PF et al: Mechanoreceptors of some anatomical structures of the human knee. p. 50. In Muller W, Hackenbruch W (eds): Surgery and Arthroscopy of the Knee. Springer-Verlag, Berlin, 1988

56. Andrews JR, Angelo BL: Shoulder arthroscopy for the throwing athlete. Tech Orthop 3:75, 1988

57. McMaster WC: Anterior glenoid labrum damage: a painful lesion in swimmers. Am J Sports Med 14:383, 1986

58. Bankart ASB: The pathology and treatment of recurrent dislocation of the shoulder. Br J Surg 26:23, 1938

59. Schwartz RR, O'Brien SJ, Warren RF, Torzilli PA: Capsular restraints to anterior-posterior motion in the shoulder. Paper presented at the 4th open meeting of the American Shoulder and Elbow Surgeons, Atlanta, 1988

60. O'Connell PW, Nuber GW, Mileski RA, Lautenschlager E: The contribution of the glenohumeral ligaments to anterior stability of the shoulder joint. Am J Sports Med 18:579, 1990

61. Turkel SJ, Panio MW, Marshall FL, Girgis FG: Stabilizing mechanisms preventing anterior dislocation of the glenohumeral joint. J Bone Joint Surg 63A:1208, 1981

62. Moseley HF, Overgaard B: The anterior capsular mechanism in recurrent anterior dislocation of the shoulder. J Bone Joint Surg 44B:913, 1962

63. Ferrari DA: Capsular ligaments of the shoulder, anatomical and functional study of the anterior superior capsule. Am J Sports Med 18:20, 1990

64. Ovensen J, Nielsen S: Stability of the shoulder joint: cadaver study of stabilizing structures. Acta Orthop Scand 56:149, 1985

65. Ovensen J, Nielsen S: Anterior and posterior shoulder instability. A cadaver study. Acta Orthop Scand 57:324, 1986

66. Ovensen J, Sojbjerg JO: Lesions in different types of

anterior glenohumeral joint dislocations. An experimental study. Arch Orthop Trauma Surg 105:216, 1986

67. Ovensen J, Sojbjerg JO: Posterior shoulder dislocation. Muscle and capsular lesions in cadaver experiments. Acta Orthop Scand 57:535, 1986

68. Cain PR, Mutschler TA, Fu FH, Lee SK: Anterior stability of the glenohumeral joint: a dynamic model. Am J Sports Med 15:144, 1987

69. Symeonides PP: The significance of the subscapularis muscle in the pathogenesis of recurrent anterior dislocation of the shoulder. J Bone Joint Surg 54B:476, 1972

70. Saha AK: Dynamic stability of the glenohumeral joint. Acta Orthop Scand 42:491, 1971

71. Jobe F, Tibone J, Perry J: An EMG analysis of the shoulder in throwing or pitching. Am J Sports Med 11:3, 1983

72. Blousman R, Jobe F, Tibone J et al: Dynamic electromyographic analysis of the throwing shoulder with glenohumeral instability (anterior) in the athlete. J Bone Joint Surg 70A:220, 1988

73. Gerber C, Krushell RJ: Isolated rupture of the tendon of the subscapularis muscle. J Bone Joint Surg 73B:389, 1991

74. Brostrom LA, Kronberg M, Nemeth G: Muscle activity during shoulder dislocation. Acta Orthop Scand 60:639, 1989

75. Yoneda B, Welsh DL, MacIntosh DC: Conservative treatment of shoulder dislocation in young males. J Bone Joint Surg 64B:254, 1982

76. Silliman JF, Hawkins RJ: Current concepts and recent advances in the athlete's shoulder. Clin Sports Med 10:693, 1991

77. Poppen NK, Walker PS: Normal and abnormal motion of the shoulder. J Bone Joint Surg 58A:195, 1976

78. Howell SM, Galinat BJ, Renzi AJ, Marone PJ: Normal and abnormal mechanics of the glenohumeral joint in the horizontal plane. J Bone Joint Surg 70A:227, 1988

79. Warner JP, Micheli J, Arslanian LE et al: Patterns of flexibility, laxity, and strength in normal shoulders and shoulders with instability and impingement syndrome. Am J Sports Med 18:336, 1990

80. Wenner SM: Anterior dislocation of the shoulder in patients of 50 years of age. Orthopedics 3:1155, 1985

81. Henry JH, Genung JA: Natural history of the glenohumeral dislocation. Am J Sports Med 10:135, 1982

82. McLaughlin HL: Preoperative and postoperative care of shoulder injuries. Clin Orthop 38:58, 1965

83. Donatelli R. Physical Therapy of the Shoulders. Churchill Livingstone, New York, 1987

84. Blom S, Dahlback LO: Nerve injuries in dislocations of the shoulder joint and fractures of the neck of the humerus. Acta Chir Scand 136:461, 1970

85. Gugenheim S, Sanders RJ: Axillary artery rupture caused by shoulder dislocation. Surgery 95:55, 1984
86. Leffert RD, Seddon H: Infraclavicular brachial plexus injuries. J Bone Joint Surg 47B:9, 1965
87. Brown JT: Nerve injuries complicating dislocation of the shoulder. J Bone Joint Surg 34B:526, 1952
88. Nobel W: Posterior traumatic dislocation of the shoulder. J Bone Joint Surg 44A:523, 1962
89. May VR: Posterior dislocation of the shoulder: habitual, traumatic, and obstetrical. Orthop Clin North Am 11:271, 1980
90. Cipriano J: Photographic Manual of Regional Orthopedic and Neurologic Tests. Williams & Wilkins, Baltimore, 1991
91. Degowin EL, Degowin RL: Bedside diagnostic examination. Macmillan, New York, 1981
92. Horaguchi T: Case studies: painless reduction of dislocation and fracture of the shoulder joint utilizing normal respiration. Orthop Sport Phys Ther 6:296, 1985
93. Riebel GD, McCabe JB: Anterior shoulder dislocation: a review of reduction techniques. Am J Emerg Med 9:180, 1991
94. Milch H: Treatment of dislocation of the shoulder. Surgery 3:732, 1938
95. Simon RR, Koenigsknecht SJ: Emergency Orthopedics: The Extremities. Appleton-Century-Crofts, East Norwalk, CT, 1987
96. O'Donoghue DH: Treatment of Injuries to Athletes. 3rd Ed. WB Saunders, Philadelphia, 1984
97. Lacey T, Crawford H: Reduction of anterior dislocations of the shoulder by means of the Milch abduction technique. J Bone Joint Surg 34A:108, 1952
98. Bosely RC, Miles JS: Scapular manipulation for the reduction of anterior-inferior shoulder dislocations. Orthop Trans 3:270, 1980
99. Stimson LA: An easy method of reducing dislocations of the shoulder and hip. Med Rec 57:356, 1900
100. Rowe CR, Pierce DS, Clark JG: Voluntary dislocation of the shoulder. J Bone Joint Surg 55A:445, 1973
101. Beall MS, Diefenbach G, Allen A: Electromyographic biofeedback in the treatment of voluntary posterior instability of the shoulder. Am J Sports Med 15:175, 1987
102. Morton KS: The unstable shoulder: recurring subluxation. J Bone Joint Surg 59B:508, 1977
103. Protzman RR: Anterior instability of the shoulder. J Bone Joint Surg 62A:909, 1980
104. Magee DJ: Orthopedic Physical Assessment. WB Saunders, Philadelphia, 1992
105. Hammer WI: Functional Soft Tissue Examination and Treatment by Manual Methods: The Extremities. Aspen, Rockville, MD, 1991
106. Alder H, Lohmann B: The stability of the shoulder joint in stress radiography. Arch Orthop Trauma Surg 103:83, 1984
107. Pavlov J, Warren RF, Weiss CB et al: The roentgenographic evaluation of anterior shoulder instability. Clin Orthop 194:153, 1985
108. McGlynn FJ, El-Khoury G, Albright JP: Arthrotomography of the shoulder. J Bone Joint Surg 64A:506, 1982
109. Braunstein EM, O'Connor G: Double-contrast arthrotomography of the shoulder. J Bone Joint Surg 64A:192, 1982
110. Singson RD, Feldman F, Bigliani LU, Rosenberg ZS: Recurrent shoulder dislocation after surgical repair: double contrast CT arthrography. Radiology 164:425, 1987
110a.Janke AH, Petersen SA, Neuman C et al: A prospective comparison of computerized arthrotomography and magnetic resonance imaging of the glenohumeral joint. Am J Sports Med 20:695, 1992
111. Fronek J, Warren RF, Bowen M: Posterior subluxation of the glenohumeral joint. J Bone Joint Surg 71A:205, 1989
112. Feinberg EF: A clinical approach to anterior glenohumeral instability. Chirop Tech 1:113, 1989
113. Hertling D, Kessler RM: Management of Common Musculoskeletal Disorders: Physical Therapy Principles and Methods. 2nd Ed. JB Lippincott, Philadelphia, 1990
114. Turek SL: Orthopaedics: Principles and Their Application. JB Lippincott, Philadelphia, 1984
115. Hollinshead WH, Roose C: Textbook of Anatomy. 4th Ed. Harper & Row, Hagerstown, MD, 1974
116. Rowe CR: The Shoulder. Churchill Livingstone, New York, 1988
117. Rowe CR: Chronic unreduced dislocations of the shoulder. J Bone Joint Surg 64A:494, 1982
118. Respet RB: A practical technique for reducing shoulder dislocations. J Musculoskel Med 1:29, 1988
119. DePalma AF: The Management of Fractures and Dislocations An Atlas. 2nd Ed. WB Saunders, Philadelphia, 1982
120. Reid DC: Sports Injury Assessment and Rehabilitation. Churchill Livingstone, New York, 1991
121. Rowe CR, Marble AC: Shoulder girdle injuries. p. 254. In Cave EF (ed): Fractures and Other Injuries. Yearbook Medical Publishers, Chicago, 1958
122. Petersson CJ: Degeneration of the glenohumeral joint: an anatomical study. Acta Orthop Scand 54:277, 1983
123. Rockwood CA, Green DP, Bucholz RW (eds): Rockwood and Green's Fractures in Adults. 3rd Ed. JB Lippincott, Philadelphia, 1991

14

Impingement Syndrome, Tendinopathies, and Degenerative Joint Disease

THOMAS A. SOUZA

Tendon involvement about the shoulder is a common source of pain and dysfunction. Disagreement still exists regarding whether a tendinitis or bursitis is due to a primary cause or secondary involvement due to impingement. This has led to confusion regarding the terminology and distinction among the various etiologies and added a complexity to decision making with regard to further evaluation and treatment approaches. Although impingement is likely a common thread that connects may of these causes it is still difficult to determine the relative importance of each and to distinguish between which are cause and which are result. It is important to recognize that a tendinopathy more often represents a process rather than an acute cause-and-effect result. Although attention to the acute, symptomatic phase is of immediate concern, prevention of progression is the primary goal. The progressive nature of a tendinopathy is not restricted to the tendon itself but requires adaptive movement modification or compensation that often impacts many other peripheral structures such as the scapula, forearm, and trunk. Following is a discussion of the impingement syndrome and tendinopathies in general. Although not all cases of tendinopathies are due to impingement the general principles of evaluation and management apply.

The impingement syndrome was first emphasized by Neer[1] as representing a frictional irritation due to overhead activities of the structures that pass through the subacromial outlet. McMaster[2] also recognized the connection with the overhead position in sports, specifically with swimming. Although commonly referred to as swimmer's shoulder, impingement is not limited to the swimmer and McMaster recommended that injuries should be diagnosed on an anatomic basis only. Although originally conceived as a mechanical process, much doubt has arisen as to the true etiology of the majority of cases. Adding to the difficulty in differentiation is that, traditionally, anterior shoulder pain was a hallmark of impingement; however, overlay of involved structures makes distinction difficult. Finally, impingement may be primarily due to instability or due to a tendinopathy that secondarily creates this entity. Many feel that the process is accumulative and potentially degenerative, and therefore early recognition, prevention, and treatment are important. Neer[3] identifies several stages of involvement based on age and pathologic changes; however, his observations may represent more a complicated form of impingement.

FUNCTIONAL ANATOMY
Tendons

Tendons are relatively avascular structures made up primarily of three components:

Collagen: Collagen is responsible for the tensile force capabilities of the tendon. Synthesized by fibroblasts, collagen accounts for 70 percent of the tendon's dry weight.[4] The collagen is so strong it has a breaking point close to that of steel. However, strong collagen is not flexible, allowing elongation of only 4 percent before failure.[5]

Elastin: Elastin is the flexibility component of the tendon. Rich in glycine and proline, the content of hydroxyproline or lysine is low. Amazingly, elastin will elongate up to 70 percent of its length without failure. Breakage occurs at 150 percent of its length.[6] Very little elastin is found in healed tissue, which indicates a loss of flexibility after injury.

Ground Substance: The ground substance is a gel-like material that adds to the structure, aids in nutrition, and plays a role in the regulation of fibril formation.

Woo et al.[7] in studies of tendon insertion have demonstrated four zones (Fig. 14-1). They found that in the first zone, which is the tendon itself, there is no nerve supply and that the blood supply comes entirely from the bone. The second zone is uncalcified fibrocartilage followed by calcified fibrocartilage and finally bone. No vessels cross the middle fibrocartilage zones. The fibrocartilaginous zone protects the collagen fibers from sharp angulation and potentially protects the tendon from excessive rubbing against the humeral head.

Four Zones Within 1 mm

Zone 1
Tendon itself; Type 1 collagen
Vascular supply runs parallel
No nerve supply

Zone 2
Fibrocartilage
Large chondrocytes in single rows

Zone 3
Mineralized fibrocartilage
Enclosed in lacunae but biochemically active

Zone 4
Bone
Type 1 collagen fibrils embeded in bony matrix

Fig. 14-1. Histology of tendon insertion.

Another interesting finding is that the insertions of the rotator cuff interlace with the adjoining tendons. This interdigitation occurs between the supraspinatus and subscapularis, and is even more evident between the supraspinatus and infraspinatus. This observation was first made by Codman[8] and confirmed by Clark.[9]

Although it may be common for tendon avulsion to occur in other joints of the body, it is not as likely to occur with the rotator cuff. Instead, the more common occurrence is a distal midsubstance tear. Schneider[10] demonstrated that the structure of the attachment site varies depending on how a muscle is stressed. Continuous use of the forearm in supination as opposed to pronation would change the structure of the biceps insertion over time.

Tendons elongate in a phased reaction to stress. At rest, tendons have a more wavy appearance due in part to the crimpled collagen fibers. The straightening of this configuration accounts for the first 2 percent of lengthening. The next 2 percent of lengthening is through collagen deformation allowing tendon lengthening linearly. If this 4 percent stretch is not exceeded, the tendon will return to its baseline length. Exceeding this length up to 8 percent, the collagen fiber crosslinks begins to fail on a microscopic level.[5]

Nerve supply is via the organs of Golgi and lamellated corpuscles.[11] This largely afferent supply is located at the musculotendinous junction and essentially serves the function of monitoring muscle tension. They lie in series with the extrafusal fibers and will decrease muscular tension when excessive loads are encountered.

The blood supply to the rotator cuff tendons is from both the osteotendinous junction and the muscular branches of arteries. It was previously believed that this led to an area of avascularity for the supraspinatus, the superior portion of the infraspinatus, and the biceps. Currently, this concept has been challenged by several studies discussed below. Avascularity does seem to increase with age beginning as early as 20 years of age.[12]

It is important to understand that the healing process is relatively slow with tendons due to the slow rate of collagen metabolism and vascular supply. During the first few days following injury the fibroblasts lay down the ground substance and tropocollagen. This is a vulnerable phase where no cross-links between the tropocollagen molecules exist. They may be broken down by enzymes associated with the inflammatory process. The cross-links do develop between days 6 and 14. The collagenous tissue organizes over the next 2 weeks. Fibers initially form in disarray and are gradually aligned to tensile loads applied to the tendon. The musculotendinous junction is where a tendon elongates due to an increased population of collagen-producing cells. Growth capacity decreases as one reaches the insertion point.

A delicate balance exists. Although initially the fibers are weaker, excessive immobilization in an attempt to allow proper organization results in the opposite intention. As much as 20 to 40 percent of the ground substances is lost if immobilized for too long.[4] Add to that the decrease in elastin content of the newly formed tissue and a dangerous situation exists. Passive mobilization has been recommended soon after tendon injury to accelerate repair. This probably occurs through alignment of the collagen fibers increasing tensile strength.

The production of new collagen can be affected by many factors. A decrease in protein, inadequate nerve or vascular supply, corticosteroids, aging, some inborn errors, and hereditary tendencies can decrease collagen production. Estrogen, testosterone, and insulin increase collagen production.

The Subacromial Space

The subacromial space or arch (Fig. 14-2) is formed by the acromion and coracoacromial ligament anterosuperior and the superior aspect of the humeral head inferiorly. The contents consist of the tendons of the rotator cuff and biceps sharing space with the subacromial bursa. The size of this space is functionally variable. Forward flexion combined with internal rotation significantly compresses the contents of the subacromial region by the greater tuberosity and decreases the subcoracoid space. Abduction above 80 to 90 degrees without concomitant external rotation will also lead to impingement (Fig. 14-3). Repeated compression with shearing or eccentric loading will lead to irritation. Abduction greater than about 120 degrees clears the greater tuberosity from the arch.

Although most theories are based on acromial abnormalities, Gerber et al.[13] using computed tomography (CT) scans evaluated the distance between the coracoid and humerus in normal individuals to determine

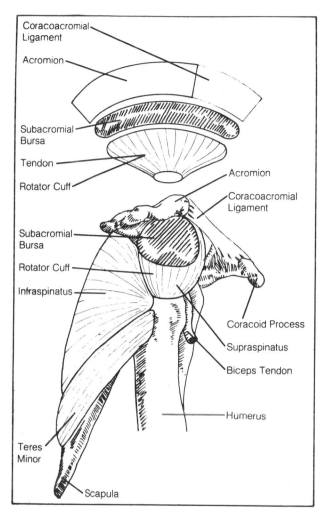

Fig. 14-2. The subacromial outlet or space. (From Brunet et al,[99] with permission.)

if this relationship was a factor in impingement. They found with forward flexion and internal rotation that the coracohumeral distance was decreased to an average of 6.7 mm. This must accommodate 2 to 3 mm of humeral articular cartilage, 1 to 2 mm of joint capsule, and 2 to 4 mm of the subscapularis muscle leaving enough room for glide; this is a difficult task.

The supraspinatus has a unique vascular supply. Lindblom[14] and Codman[8] were the first to recognize a critical zone that lies slightly proximal to the supraspinatus insertion point. Moseley and Goldie[15] concluded from their studies on cadavers that the area described as the critical zone is more likely a zone of anastomo-

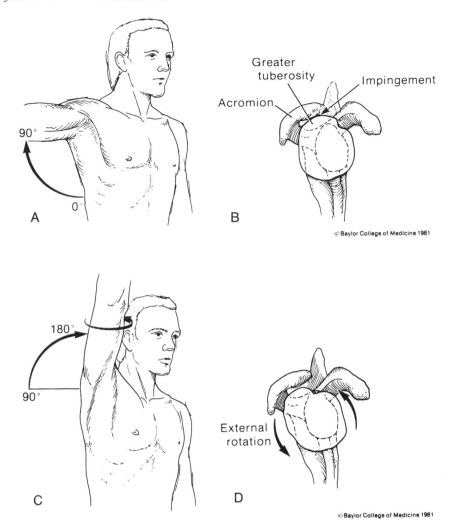

Fig. 14-3. (A & B) Abduction external rotation of the shoulder joint and the relationship of the greater tuberosity of the humeral head to the acromion, 0 to 90 degrees abduction. **(C & D)** Abduction external rotation of the shoulder joint and the relationship of the greater tuberosity of the humeral head to the acromion, 90 to 180 degrees abduction. (From Tullos and Bennett,[100] with permission.)

ses between the vessels supplying the bone and tendon. They felt that this zone was not less vascular and that the morphology did not significantly change with age. Iannotti et al.[16] have confirmed this observation using laser Doppler studies. Adequate blood flow in the area of the critical zone was noted. Rathburn and Macnab[17] felt that this zone was compromised with the arm in a neutral dependent position due to the compression of the humeral head against the tendons. This observation was further confirmed by other au-

thors who found the vessels to be filled with abduction.[17] With the arm at rest a zone of avascularity extended from 1 cm proximal to the point of insertion. Compounding this positional tendency toward avascularity, the blood supply to the supraspinatus does not enter at intervals along the course of the tendon as occurs with most other tendons. Instead the vessels run longitudinally along the course fiber, which predisposes them to structural or functional constriction due to humeral head compression or long axis distraction of the arm, respectively.[5] Sigholm et al.[18] have demonstrated significant subacromial pressure increases with active flexion. However, given that most usage of the shoulder is intermittent, it is unlikely to be the single cause. Rathbun and Macnab[17] also noted that the avascular zone preceded degenerative changes and so is not the result of degeneration.

The infraspinatus may also have an area of avascularity near its humeral insertion. The intracapsular portion of the biceps also demonstrates an area of avascularity when stretched over the humeral head.[7]

IMPINGEMENT THEORIES

An evolution of understanding occurred regarding impingement. The first clarification of possible cause began with Neer.[1] He advocated the mechanical theory, which placed emphasis on the anterior acromion. As a result of this theory, he developed a surgical procedure, the acromioplasty, to eliminate the offending structure. Initially, the reported success was quite high, indirectly supporting Neer's theory.[1] However, a much higher rate of failure, particularly in the athlete, has led to a reassessment of this single etiology theory.

Focus shifted to the concept of secondary impingement (impingement due to a separate but inter-related etiology). Jobe and Kvitne[19] recognized impingement in young throwers with associated instability. They proposed the concept that instability allowed migration of the humeral head, in particular anterior and superior, resulting in secondary impingement.

Similar concepts have arisen with other authors. Nirschl,[20] a major opponent to the primary concept of Neer, feels that the major initiator of rotator cuff tendinitis (a major source of impingement signs) is eccentric overload due to repetitive microtrauma in overhead activities. This leads to a reactive inflammatory process that, if not resolved, leads to progressive degenerative changes (Fig. 14-4).

The findings of Ozaki et al.[21] fail to support the Neer concept of rotator cuff injury due to acromial impingement. The presence of normal acromial architecture with rotator cuff tears was demonstrated by Ozaki et al. They made the observation that most rotator cuff tears occurred on the articular side of the tendon. Ozaki et al. did find a correlation between the degree of acromial changes and the severity of the tear. Full

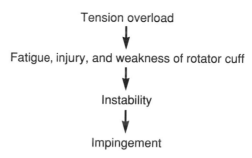

Fig. 14-4. Nirschl concept of impingement.

ruptures were more common with abnormal acromial changes. They concluded that the process of degeneration is intrinsic and age related. Full ruptures were then due to a weakened tendon subjected to trauma.

The theories of causation are still abundant and represent a current controversy in sports medicine (Table 14-1). It seems likely that elements of each theory contribute in varying degrees based on individual anatomy and activity. These theories can generally be categorized into structural and functional. There often is overlap among these causes. Additionally, it must be remembered that impingement can coexist with other pathologies that may contribute to the progression of changes (secondary impingement).

Structural causes include

1. An abnormally shaped acromion, unfused acromial apophysis (before age 21), infraacromial traction spurs, and acromioclavicular arthritis
2. Vascularity of the supraspinatus and other rotator cuff musculature
3. Laxity of the capsule
4. Decrease in the subacromial space due to inflammation of the tendons or bursa

Table 14-1. Possible Factors Involved with Impingement

Structural	Functional
Acromial shape and acromioclavicular degeneration	Imbalance between internal rotators/adductors and external rotators/abductors
Vascularity of the rotator cuff	Dysfunction of scapular stabilizers
Capsular laxity	Tight posterior capsule
Decrease in outlet due to inflammation	Overhead positions
Or a combination of the above	

5. Subcoracoid impingement due to pathology of the long head of the biceps or the subscapularis muscle

Functional possibilities include the following:

1. An imbalance between the external rotators/abductors and internal rotators/adductors
2. Dysfunction of the scapular movers, particularly the serratus anterior
3. Lack of coordination between deltoid and rotator cuff (especially supraspinatus)
4. A tight posterior capsule
5. Overhead activities, particularly with internal rotation and also with factors increasing resistance to arm movement in this position (e.g., swim paddles)

Structural Theories

Acromion Shape

An os acromiale has been identified by several authors[22–25] as a possible cause of impingement. Liberson[22] found an os acromiale to be, when present, bilateral 62 percent of the time. In a review of 1,000 radiographs the os acromiale was found in only 2.7 percent of individuals. It was most visible on an axillary view. The size of the unfused acromion can be quite large with direct impingement possible from the unfused segment or by bony or soft tissue overgrowth at the

unfused site. Fusion usually occurs by age 22. Failure to fuse usually occurs at the mesoacromion or meta-acromion.

Bigliani et al.[26] recognized a variation in the slope and shape of the acromion in the normal population. They classified these according to increase in slope with type III being the most likely contributor to impingement due to its hooked appearance (Fig. 14-5). More specifically, it appears that a hooked acromion may be a predisposition to full-thickness rotator cuff tears. Bigliani et al.[25] found that 70 percent of 50 patients with full-thickness tears had a hooked acromion. This observation led to the common practice of acromioplasty for the treatment of impingement syndrome. This past common procedure did help some individuals, but not all, illustrating again that there is no single cause for impingement.

Avascularity

In the past, it was believed that the supraspinatus had a zone of hypovascularity a few centimeters from its insertion into the greater tuberosity.[8] It was felt that this was the weak link in the structure of the supraspinatus. Although some authors subscribe to the critical zone concept, others do not. Several factors contribute to potential for this area to become a factor with tendon degeneration or rupture. The first involves the variation in blood supply to the tendon as described

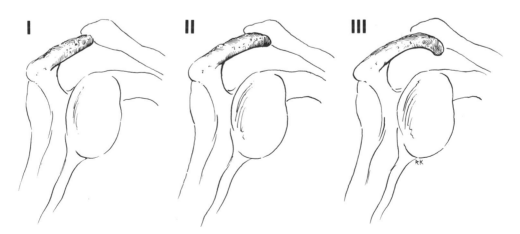

Fig. 14-5. The three types of acromion morphology defined by Bigliani and Morrison. Type I, with its flat surface, provided the least compromise of the supraspinatus outlet, whereas type III's sudden discontinuity or hook was associated with the highest rate of rotator cuff pathology in a series of cadaver dissections. (From Jobe,[101] with permission.)

above. Secondly, the orientation of the blood supply is such that as the tendon is pulled or compressed the vasculature is stretched or compressed, and thereby functionally constricted. This postural component has been demonstrated by several authors. The blood supply to most tendons is at right angles to the tendon. However, with the supraspinatus the blood supply runs parallel to the fibers of the tendon. As the tendon is tractioned so is the blood supply.[7]

Theoretically, the critical zone is not able to repair itself properly following damage leading to a process of continued degeneration. This is especially true if the underlying damage is unrecognized clinically and the individual is allowed to use the muscle. For example, weightlifters often describe a "burn" at the end of an exercise set that indicates a maximum workout. Unfortunately, a burn may be a subtle sign of damage and may be misinterpreted by the athlete. The difference is usually identifiable by the indoctrinated weightlifter.

The critical zone is specifically the area that is compressed under the coracoacromial ligament. A process of degeneration, with or without calcification, is possible. If calcium deposition is present there is a risk of irritation and possible rupture into the overlying subacromial bursa.

Cuillo[27] disagrees with the avascular concept and proposes that the area of supposed avascularity is a protective mechanism that evolved to prevent repeated hemorrhage and repair in an area that is inherently susceptible to trauma. The more current research suggests that this is unlikely.

Capsular Laxity

Capsular laxity may be present due to trauma (acute/macro or chronic/micro) or genetically determined. When present, the rotator cuff muscles, in concert with the deltoid, have difficulty supplementing the intended function of the capsule. Migration of the humeral head anterosuperior can then create impingement. This may in part be due to excessive deltoid contraction or mistiming of the deltoid with the supraspinatus allowing a vertical line of pull into the subacromial space.

Jobe and Kvitne[19] feel that many sports activities lead to repetitive microtrauma to the glenohumeral ligaments. Although gross tears may not be present, the ligaments are attenuated to such a degree as to provide less support requiring more cooperation from the rotator cuff muscles. Fatigue of the rotator cuff might then lead to secondary impingement. This theory bridges the gap between structural and functional theories and primary and secondary impingement.

Narrowing Due to Inflammation

A vicious cycle develops when tendon or bursal inflammation is present. Whether due to impingement or other causes of tendinitis, swelling of an involved tendon or the subacromial bursa narrows the available space for the other occupying structures within the subacromial outlet. This leads to irritation of the normal structures, which in turn diminishes the available space. It becomes painfully obvious that if any degree of structural or functional instability is added to this scenario the result is predictable.

Subcoracoid Impingement

As early as 1901, Goldthwait[28] mentioned two possible sites of impingement: subacromial and subcoracoid. Although impingement can be due to trauma with resultant coracoid fracture, the most common causes cited are a subscapularis tear or dislocation of the tendon of the long head of the biceps medially.[29] In addition, displacement of the humeral head anteromedial toward the coracoid process can occur concomitantly. Therefore, Patte[30] believes that laxity of the anterior capsule or ligaments due to various causes can also result in subcoracoid impingement. The position accentuating impingement is forward flexion with internal rotation (Fig. 14-6).

Functional

The most common observation of muscular imbalance in individuals with impingement is between the external rotators/abductors and the internal rotators/adductors. Inherent and sometimes acquired imbalance exists allowing migration of the humeral head. The infraspinatus and teres minor both act as external rotators; however, in the higher positions of arm elevation they have a depressing effect on the humeral head providing stability. Weakness or dysfunction may then allow impingement.

Kibler and Chandler[31] suggest that impingement can also occur without proper synchrony between the hu-

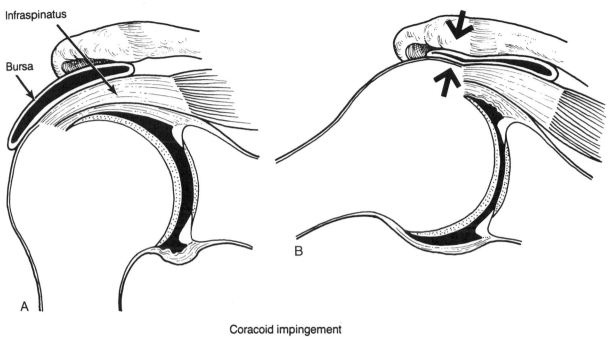

Fig. 14-6. (A–C) Subcoracoid impingement. (From Rowe,[95] with permission.)

merus and scapula. Without the humeral head being supported by a stable glenoid platform, movement is restricted and impingement is likely. They noted the need for balanced muscular positioning of the scapula with particular emphasis placed on the role of the serratus anterior.

Andrews et al.[32] and others[33] feel that the biceps tendon plays a role in the development of the impingement syndrome. The biceps may contribute to stabilization of the humeral head preventing superior migration. Electromyographic studies have suggested a role due to increased activity in the cocking phase of throwing.[34] Also there is an increase in activity when instability is present.[35] Two potential injuries may be involved. An eccentric load injury due to repetitive motions is suggested. Also Superior Labrum Anterior to Posterior (SLAP) lesions are common with throwing athletes and may correlate with instability and impingement.

Pappas et al.[36] and others have observed a decrease in passive/active internal rotation and horizontal adduction in throwing athletes with impingement. Probably a secondary reaction to repetitive microtrauma, posterior contracture can result in superior translation of the humeral head during forward flexion. Harryman et al.[37] demonstrated that tightening the posterior capsule in cadaver specimens increased anterior translation of the shoulder, particularly with forward flexion or horizontal adduction.

Relationship to Sports

Many sports require an overhead positioning. The determination of whether impingement occurs or not is apparently dependent on several factors:

1. Is there underlying instability (structural or functional)?
2. Is the position of abduction or elevation coupled with internal rotation?
3. Is there an increase in resistance added to the impingement position?

The most common sport in which the answers to all three questions would be yes is swimming. In the catch phase as the hand enters the water, the arm is in an unstable position acting against the resistance of the water. Then it progresses into an impingement position with internal rotation with even more resistance provided.

HISTORY AND EXAMINATION FOR IMPINGEMENT

History

The categorization of the typical impingement patient has changed since the suggestion of age-related factors by Neer.[3] He felt that as a degenerative process, severity and symptomatology would be progressive, which led to the four stages of impingement (Table 14-2).

Jobe and Kvitne[19] have combined the structural and functional theories into a composite patient not necessarily related to age but based primarily on whether instability is present. This categorization includes

Group I—Athletes with pure impingement (Fig. 14-7)
Group II—Athletes with TUBS (*t*raumatic instability, *u*nilateral in nature, with a *b*ankart lesion that usually responds to *s*urgery) and secondary impingement (Fig. 14-8)
Group III—Athletes with AMBRI (*a*traumatic, *m*ultidirectional, *b*ilateral, and usually responding to *r*ehabilitation) and secondary impingement (Fig. 14-9)
Group IV—Athletes with pure anterior instability (Fig. 14-10)

Although it might seem that a consistent patient presentation would be found and agreed upon, there is a marked discrepancy in the descriptions of presentation with regard to signs and symptoms.

Matsen and Arntz[38] feel that most patients will not present in an acute stage but after failure of the symptoms to resolve. In this scenario the patient would present with pain and weakness felt with activities of daily living. Penny and Welsh[39] describe two types of patients with supraspinatus involvement. The first involves a patient with sharp catching pain relieved by full overhead elevation. The second (found more commonly in swimmers) is the overuse patient who does not complain of catching pain but a deep ache with activity.

Palpation

Matsen and Arntz[38] do not feel that tenderness is a primary finding with impingement. Most authors disagree.[3,4,26,30] Perhaps the distinction is based on the criteria and definition of the term impingement. Matsen and Arntz[38] feel it is important to separate the signs of

Table 14-2. Neer's Classification of Impingement

Stage	Typical Patient
Stage I	**History**
	Patient usually younger than 25 with a report of repetitive overhead activity initiating symptoms; dull ache after activity that progresses to pain during activity
	Clinical Findings
	Tenderness at supraspinatus insertion and anterior acromion
	A painful arc between 60° and 120°; increased with resistance 90°
	A positive impingement sign (injection)
	Muscle testing may reveal weakness due to pain
	Radiographs are typically normal
	Treatment
	Usually resolve with activity modification and a rehabilitation program
Stage II	**History**
	Found more typically in athletes aged 25–40 years
	(Hawkins et al.[47] feel that age is secondary; duration of signs and symptoms is a better indicator)
	Severity of symptoms worse than stage I progressing to pain with activity and night pain
	Simple overhead movement painful
	Clinical Findings
	Same as Stage I plus:
	—More soft tissue crepitus and/or a catching sensation at 100 degrees abduction
	—Some restrictions in passive ROM due to fibrosis
	—Radiographic changes may be evident in the later stages including
	a. Cystic changes at the greater tuberosity
	b. Osteophytes on the acromial undersurface
	c. Degenerative acromioclavicular joint changes
	Treatment
	No longer reversible with activity change and rest; cautious rehabilitation over a prolonged period may be effective
Stage III	**History**
	Found more typically in patients 40 years and older
	History of chronic tendinitis; prolonged periods of pain/stiffness
	Often unable to perform athletic activities
	Clinical Findings
	Same as Stage II plus:
	—More limitation in active and passive ROM
	—Biceps tendon and acromioclavicular joint have more positive findings
	—Infraspinatus atrophy due to disuse
	—X-ray findings as stage II plus possible superior migration of humeral head due to rotator cuff tear
	Treatment
	Typically surgical following a failed conservative approach

subacromial impingement from signs of tightness or tendon involvement. They believe that subacromial crepitus is the major indication of impingement whereas limited movement indicates tightness, and pain, weakness, or atrophy indicates tendon involvement. Although it is true that each of these entities can exist separately, it is more likely that all are found with the impingement patient.

Tenderness is usually found in relationship to the irritated structure. Therefore, anterior tenderness between the coracoid and acromion is common with impingement.[26] Cuillo[27] feels that the most common site of tenderness is over the coracoacromial ligament.

Tenderness at the biceps tendon (compare bilaterally) and the supraspinatus insertion are often found. Palpation of the biceps is assisted by internal rotation of the arm from neutral to 10 degrees. The supraspinatus insertion is slightly more accessible with the arm in extension (the arm behind the back). Palpation anterior and inferior to the acromioclavicular joint will usually be tender. The bursa is best palpated with the patient prone. The examiner passively stretches the arm into extension while palpating anterior to the acromioclavicular joint. Tenderness found on extension eliminated with flexion is indicative of bursal irritation.

Orthopaedic Testing

Due to the recent suggestion that impingement is often secondary to instability,[8] it is extremely important to evaluate the athlete for instability, general impingement signs, and specific muscular function.

Instability

The standard approach to evaluating instability (see Figs. 6-20A–D and 6-32) is the load and shift maneuver by Hawkins et al.[40] This procedure can be applied in various patient positions: standing (bent forward 45 degrees), seated, and supine.

In the standing and seated approaches the patient's arm is relaxed while the examiner stabilizes the scapula with one hand. Grabbing the proximal humerus between the thumb and fingers the shoulder is pushed anteriorly, to test anterior instability, posterior for posterior instability, and finally inferiorly, which tests for coupled or global instability.

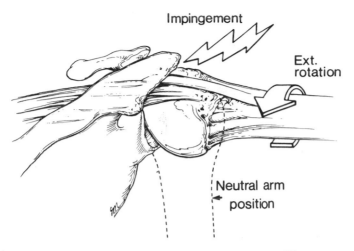

Fig. 14-7. Group 1: impingement. (From Jobe and Bradley,[102] with permission.)

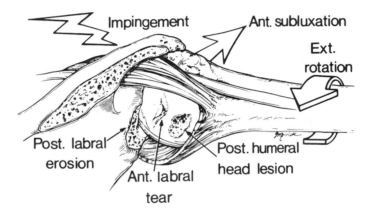

Fig. 14-8. Group 2: anterior instability due to chronic microtrauma. (From Jobe and Bradley,[102] with permission.)

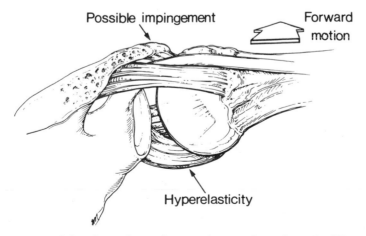

Fig. 14-9. Group 3: instability due to hyperelasticity. (From Jobe and Bradley,[102] with permission.)

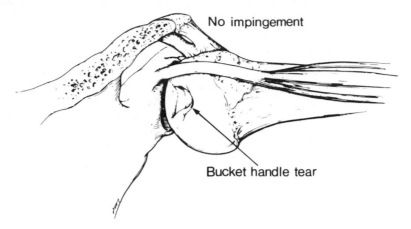

No impingement

Bucket handle tear

Fig. 14-10. Group 4: instability due to a single episode of traumatic subluxation. (From Jobe and Bradley,[102] with permission.)

The standard apprehension sign is a test for anterior instability usually performed standing or seated. The patient's arm is placed in abduction of 90 degrees. While pressing anteriorly on the proximal humerus the arm is brought back into horizontal extension and external rotation. Further testing at 120 degrees is also recommended. Either a sense of discomfort, pain, or the arm feeling like it might "go out" is indicative of a positive test. A functional addition that helps identify functional instability is to have the patient mimic the throwing act starting with the cocking phase. The examiner resists the movement at the forearm or elbow through an isotonic contraction. This functional apprehension test is suggested by Kulund[41] as an alternative with equivocal findings.

The supine test involves grasping the patient's hand between the examiner's arm and side. The arm is then positioned in 80 to 120 degrees abduction, forward flexed 0 to 20 degrees, and externally rotated 30 degrees. The examiner palpates the coracoid process and humeral head as the pressure is exerted anteriorly to test anterior stability. Posterior testing involves flexing the elbow 120 degrees, abducting the shoulder 80 to 120 degrees while forward flexing to 20 to 30 degrees. With the examiner's thumb palpating lateral to the coracoid and the scapula stabilized, a posterior directed force is applied to the shoulder.

The relocation test is used to further qualify a positive apprehension sign.[42] The supine patient is placed in the apprehension position of abduction and external rotation, but the humeral head is pushed poste-

riorly rather than anteriorly. Relief of the sensation of pain and/or apprehension is indicative of a positive test further confirming instability.

Silliman and Hawkins[43] recommend an additional test they call the release test. After a positive relocation test, the arm is suddenly released while the shoulder is maintained in the apprehension position. A sudden increase in pain is suggestive of instability.

Uhthoff and Sarkar[44] suggest that to distinguish between anterior shoulder pain due entirely to instability as opposed to impingement, the examiner should use the relocation test. If the pain is relieved by the relocation test, instability is probably the primary cause. Unfortunately, if both coexist, this finding would be less clear.

Labrum tears are often associated with instability. Clinical testing is rather indirect, consisting of the clunk test and the Kocher maneuver. The clunk test is an extension of the supine apprehension test. Added is a rotational component in an effort to elicit grinding or a clunk. The Kocher maneuver, originally developed for replacing a dislocation, may through a distractive force elicit the clunk response described above.

General Impingement Tests (Fig. 14-11)

Neer developed one of the first tests for impingement.[1] He found that with passive forward flexion with the arm supinated, end-range pain would be present with impingement, particularly with anterior involvement. Penny and Welsh[39] suggest that if internal rotation re-

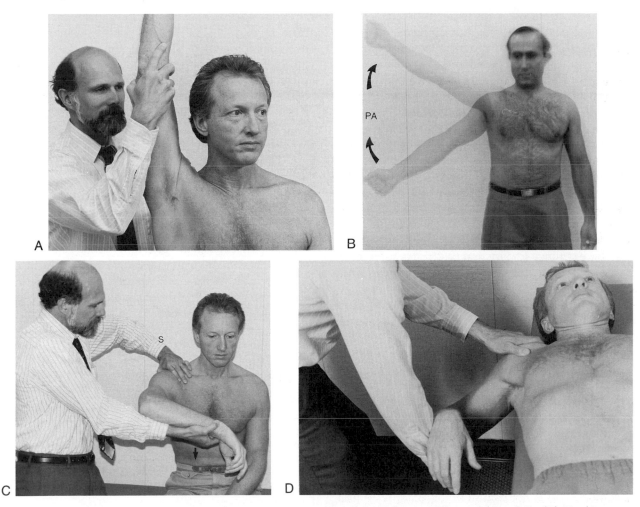

Fig. 14-11. Impingement testing. **(A)** Neer's test with passive forward flexion, **(B)** painful arc *(PA)* , **(C)** Hawkins-Kennedy's test with abduction/internal rotation, and **(D)** the locking maneuver. *S,* stabilize.

lieves the positive finding of painful catching a differentiation between supraspinatus and biceps involvement may be indicated. They believe that the biceps is cleared from the coracoacromial arch with internal rotation. Neer also developed the impingement test involving injection of 10 ml of 1 percent lidocaine into the subacromial space. Relief of pain is suggestive of impingement. However, one study demonstrated equal success with gluteal injections raising the question of specificity of involved structures versus systemic effects.[1]

Cyriax[45] recognized the entity we know as the painful arc. He observed that while abducting the arm an arc of discomfort or pain would be felt between about 70 and 110 degrees with little or no pain before and little pain after this range. He theorized that subacromial structures were mechanically compressed during this range. If the patient could actively move beyond this range or the examiner could assist the patient passively, clearance of the greater tuberosity would allow more subacromial space relieving compression. Kessel and Watson[46] attempted to differentiate various types of painful arcs. They felt that adding external rotation to the painful range indicated subscapularis involvement or possibly supraspinatus and/or infraspinatus involvement when the pain was increased. Tenderness was more evident over the lesser tuberosity. When adding internal rotation, the supraspinatus or infraspinatus was more likely the source of involvement if the pain was increased. Tenderness is more over the greater tuberosity. Finally, they suggest a superior type where pain continues from 60 to 180 degrees unaffected by rotation. This usually indicates acromioclavicular involvement or degenerative lesions of the supraspinatus, subscapularis, or biceps. This last group was less amenable to treatment.

Hawkins and Kennedy[47] developed a test that takes advantage of the maximum compression position (forward flexion with internal rotation). The examiner passively positions the patient's arm into forward flexion of 90 degrees. Supporting the patient's elbow with one arm, the examiner imparts internal rotation by pressing down on the forearm toward the ground while preventing scapular movement with the other hand. This may be repeated with varying degrees of horizontal adduction. An increase or reproduction of anterior pain is suggestive of impingement. Adding resisted internal rotation with this same position may increase the patient's pain response.

A similar concept, applied in a slightly different manner, is the locking maneuver.[48] The supine patient relaxes the arm and allows the examiner to passively extend the arm off the table with the elbow bent. Then the arm is passively abducted until resistance or pain is felt. Normally, the arm can be abducted to just shy of 90 degrees with a detectable blockage to further movement. This is not painful in the uninvolved individual. With impingement, pain is felt.

Specific Muscle Testing

Given that tendon involvement can either be primary or secondary to impingement it would seem clear that an attempt at specific identification should be made. In addition, an attempt at evaluating muscular dysfunction should be made. It would be advantageous to distinguish between tendon and muscle involvement for treatment purposes, but this is probably not feasible. It has been suggested that tendon involvement will be more evident on stretch testing while muscle involvement is revealed with contraction testing. If this distinction is unequivocal, then treatment can be more specifically applied. It would seem prudent to also check for reactive trigger point involvement.

The distinction between tendon and muscle involvement might better be applied using the current concepts of impingement causation. The anterior tendons, the biceps and supraspinatus, are the victims of impingement, while muscular involvement would not necessarily be primary. In addition, muscular dysfunction would more likely be found in the external rotators, teres minor and infraspinatus, and the scapular stabilizing musculature.

Supraspinatus

Palpation of the insertion of the supraspinatus is best performed with the patient's hand behind the back or with the arm passively extended by the examiner (see Fig. 6-7). This brings the insertion point more forward from the acromion making approximation of the insertion point more likely.[49] An attempt at abduction against the resistance of the examiner can be requested from this position of stretch to determine involvement that may be undetected by traditional testing. Palpation for trigger point involvement is best performed with the patient lying prone. This position will relax the overlying trapezius making identification of the supraspinatus more likely.[50]

Contraction of the supraspinatus is performed with the empty can test (Fig. 14-12).[51] The patient abducts the internally rotated arm to about 90 degrees. The arm is brought forward of the coronal plane by 30 degrees. The thumb will be pointing toward the floor if internal rotation is complete. Lack of full internal

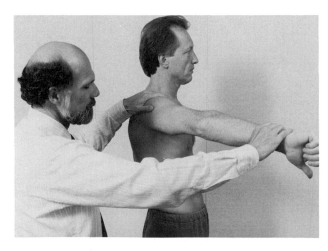

Fig. 14-12. Supraspinatus empty can test.

rotation capabilities in this position might represent posterior capsular tightness that may also contribute to impingement. If the patient can actively accomplish this position against gravity, the examiner can then introduce resistance to fully evaluate involvement.

Biceps

Although the biceps tendon is not a rotator cuff muscle, its relationship to the coracoacromial arch, glenoid labrum, and rotator cuff muscles warrants an evaluation in all cases of impingement (see Figs. 6-8C and 6-43). The biceps has often been accused of being the primary source of discomfort with anterior shoulder pain. In addition to bicipital tendinitis, dislocation or subluxation of the tendon and detachment of the superior labrum have been proposed.

Standard orthopaedic muscle testing of the biceps by resisted flexion at the elbow is relatively useless. Even patients with a rupture of the long head maintain substantial strength. An alternative muscle testing position is the Speed's test,[52,53] which attempts to reproduce the position of impingement with contraction of the biceps. The patient holds the arm at 90 degrees forward flexion with the forearm supinated, elbow extended. The examiner attempts downward pressure at the forearm as the patient resists. This is repeated several times. An increase in anterior shoulder pain is suggestive of bicipital involvement.

Yergason's test[54] is sometimes helpful. With the elbow flexed and pronated, arm at the side, the patient attempts flexion with supination against the resistance of the examiner testing both functions of the biceps. This does not cause any significant movement to occur between the bicipital groove and tendon rendering this test relatively insensitive. In fact, Post[55] found that only 50 percent of patients with primary bicipital involvement had a positive test.

Several tests have been devised to test subluxation of the biceps tendon medially. This is, in fact, a rare occurrence and when it does occur is not due to rupture of the transverse ligament but damage to either the glenohumeral ligament or the subscapularis muscle. Snapping of the tendon seems to be most common when returning the arm from abduction to the side. The Gilcrest sign and Abbott-Saunders tests[56] reproduce this movement with and without weight, respectively.

The Ludington's test[57] is also a relatively useless means of trying to determine rupture of the long head of the biceps although it may increase tenderness with bicipital tendinitis. If rupture has occurred visualization and palpation are usually all that is necessary. The Ludington's test involves the patient placing the hands behind the neck and contracting the biceps while the examiner palpates. Lack of palpation of the tendon is supposed to indicate rupture. This author has found it difficult to palpate the tendon in heavily muscled individuals with this position, and interpretation of the results is impossible in these cases.

Infraspinatus/Teres Minor

In later stages of impingement observation for atrophy of the infraspinatus should be included (see Figs. 6-8A and 6-40). Palpation of the combined insertions of the infraspinatus/teres minor is facilitated by forward flexion to 90 degrees, horizontal adduction plus external rotation. The insertion point is at the posterior aspect of the greater tuberosity. Testing for strength is usually performed with the elbow bent 90 degrees. The patient attempts external rotation against the resistance of the examiner at a neutral arm-by-the-side position, and at 90 degrees abduction. The main trigger point for the infraspinatus is in the belly of the muscle in the center of the scapula. The teres minor trigger point is on the lateral border of the scapula at the posterior aspect of the shoulder.

Subscapularis

Although the subscapularis is not commonly involved in impingement syndromes, it is possible to strain the muscle or cause a tendinitis especially in throwing sports. Palpation of the insertion onto the lesser tuberosity is more discernible with the patient seated with the arm relaxed at the side. Slight external rotation will bring the lesser tuberosity more anterior and accessible to palpation (see Figs. 6-41 and 6-42).

To search for trigger points, the patient lies supine. The examiner drags the abducted arm away from the side in order to expose the scapula away from the chest wall. A pincer action is used to reach the lateral border of the scapula where some trigger points may be found.

Scapular Movement

An examination for scapular stabilization and a search for interference with normal scapular movement should always be included when examining the athlete (see Figs. 6-9, 6-46, 6-47, and 6-48). Observation for winging of the scapular should be performed first in a neutral standing position. Kibler and Chandler[58] describe a test referred to as the lateral scapular slide. The test involves measuring the distance from the spinous processes to the medial border of the scapula. An increased distance compared with the opposite side may indicate a lack of stabilization. They found that the more symptomatic throwers had increased distances with the lateral scapular slide test.

Functional approaches to evaluate scapular stabilization involve muscle testing while screening for scapular movement. Initial observation includes an evaluation of a normal scapulohumeral ratio. Through the first 30 degrees the scapula moves as it stabilizes itself. Beyond this range the ratio is approximately 2 to 1. The serratus anterior may be tested by having the patient flex to 90 degrees with the elbow extended palm down. The examiner pushes downward at the forearm with one hand while palpating the medial border of the scapula with the other noting any movement. The scapula should remain stabilized with this challenge. Movement indicates need for stabilization exercises.

Rhomboid testing can be performed with the athlete seated and the hand placed on the hip, elbow flexed 90 degrees. The examiner pushes the elbow forward against the resistance of the patient while noting any movement of the medial scapula during contraction.

Finally, traditional testing for winging with contraction can be used. This includes a push-up against the wall, with and without resistance. Note that winging may be indicative of several disorders including scoliosis, neurologic, and/or muscular weakness.

Tightness of the medial scapular musculature can be palpated in several positions. With the relaxed patient prone or side-lying the examiner pushes the shoulder posteriorly, which wings-out the medial border of the scapula allowing palpation. Trigger points along the medial border are common, particularly at the superior medial border at the attachment site of the levator scapula. With this same position general movement can be evaluated by circumducting the scapula over the posterior thorax. Crepitus or grinding warrants a

further evaluation historically for a prior history of rib fracture or irritating crepitus during functional movements. Pitchers may be plagued by an inflamed bursa at the inferior medial border of the scapula.[59]

Tightness of the posterior capsule should be evaluated through passive horizontal adduction (Fig. 14-13). Adding internal rotation places more stress to the posterior capsule and the posterior shoulder muscles. It is important to determine where pain or stretching is produced. Anterior produced pain is more indicative of a compressive effect on anterior structures such as the bursa or anterior acromioclavicular joint.

Chiropractically it is important to evaluate for cervical and thoracic vertebral subluxation or rib subluxation, which may mechanically or neurologically interfere with normal scapular movement. Many of the midthoracic muscles have attachment sites in the cervical region suggesting a potential mechanical etiology when both neck and shoulder pain are found together. Maigne[60] suggests two possible causes of constant pain medial to the scapula that may interfere with normal scapular movement. The first is an anomalous branch of the posterior primary rami (PPR) of T2. The medial branch of the PPR courses down the entire extent of the medial border of the scapula and ascends back up

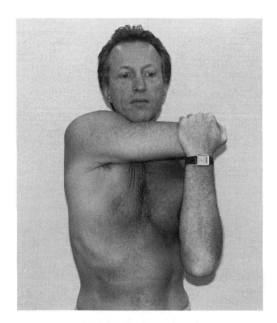

Fig. 14-13. Passive horizontal adduction for stretching posterior capsule and musculature.

as far as the acromion. Irritation can be due to vertebral misalignment. Adjustment of the T2-T3 area can eliminate discomfort caused through this mechanism.

Maigne[60] also describes the "doorbell sign," which is used to implicate the cervical region as the source of midthoracic pain. Given that the midthoracic musculature is primarily innervated by the cervical region, Maigne devised a test where pressure is applied to the transverse processes of the mid to lower cervical vertebrae for 10 to 20 seconds in an attempt to reproduce a midthoracic complaint. Treatment is then to adjust the involved cervical component.

Most rib subluxations are affected to some degree through adjustment of their associated vertebrae. In other instances, the rib itself may need adjustment. To determine the need for adjustment, palpate with pressure along the course of the rib to the rib angle if possible. Adding rotational trunk movements may add overpressure to the area revealing a lack of normal springy motion. Most rib adjusting is similar to thoracic adjusting but with a more lateral contact. Caution should be used in thin and older patients.

Bursal Tests

The subacromial bursa is one of the three major structures possibly impinged (Fig. 14-6). When chronic adhesions develop, significant crepitus is often palpable on movement of the arm. Direct palpation of the bursa is not always distinct; however, two tests have been devised to assist in approximation of their location, and more importantly to provide relief of tenderness when the bursa slides under the acromial hood.

The first palpation is done with the patient prone and the arm relaxed. The examiner takes the arm and passively extends it while palpating anterior to the acromion. If tenderness is present with the arm in extension but disappears with the arm in flexion, the bursa is likely the cause. This is due to the sliding of the bursa underneath the arch with flexion making palpation less sensitive.

Dawbarn's test is similar, but it attempts to reproduce the same mechanism with the arm moving through abduction. The examiner passively abducts the arm while palpating anterolateral to the acromion. If tenderness is evident with the arm by the side, but reduces with abduction, the bursa is the suspected cause based on the assumption of retraction.

Radiographic Evaluation

It is generally agreed that the use of radiographs to determine or diagnose impingement syndrome is useless. Until the later stages of the Neer classification, or when the athlete is in the senior age group, radiographic changes are rare. The finding of calcification may be incidental since this finding does not correlate with symptomatology. When radiographs are taken the following should be evaluated:[61]

1. Hooked acromion
2. An unfused acromial apophysis before age 21
3. Subacromial sclerosis ("sourcil" or "eyebrow" sign) or traction spurs
4. Acromioclavicular arthritis
5. Superior migration of the humeral head (suggestive of rotator cuff rupture)

The most revealing view is the supraspinatus outlet view. The outlet view is taken by positioning for a true lateral scapular view and then angling the tube between 10 and 40 degrees (Fig. 14-14).[62] In a search for a bipartite acromion, the axillary view is indicated.

Special imaging can be useful in distinguishing between inflammatory changes versus ruptures and tears. Magnetic resonance imaging (MRI) is probably most

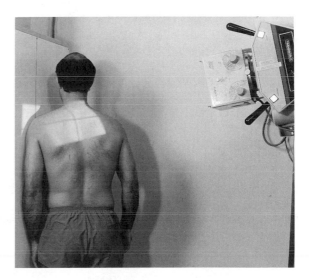

Fig. 14-14. Outlet view with tube angled between 10 and 40 degrees.

valuable in evaluation of inflammatory lesions (see Ch. 11). Complete tears can be detected with ultrasonography (see Ch. 10). Partial tears can also be appreciated, but with less sensitivity. The advantages of ultrasonography and MRI are the avoidance of ionizing radiation and the lack of invasiveness. Full-thickness tears are evident on CT–arthrography, but this represents an invasive and not necessarily superior means of evaluation.

Treatment

Treatment for impingement is best approached from several standpoints:

1. Evidence of instability and its grading. Matsen's and Thomas' acronyms are helpful[63] in this approach:

    *TUBS: T*raumatic instability, *u*nilateral in nature, with a *b*ankart lesion that usually responds to *s*urgery

    *AMBRI: A*traumatic, *m*ultidirectional, *b*ilateral, and usually responding to *r*ehabilitation

    Combining this distinction with the groupings of Jobe et al.[8] helps clarify the relation between instability and impingement and their effects on treatment and rehabilitation outcome.

    Group I: Athletes with pure impingement. No instability is evident in this group.

    Group II: Athletes with TUBS and secondary impingement. These athletes have labral damage and thinning of the cuff, which leads to primary instability with secondary impingement.

    Group III: Athletes with AMBRI and secondary impingement. These athletes have hyperelastic ligaments and capsule. Athletes with Ehlers-Danlos syndrome probably fit this category. No traumatic lesions are initially evident.

    Group IV: Athletes with pure anterior instability. The instability is usually due to a single traumatic lesion evident with most patients exhibiting anterior labral damage.

2. Evidence of muscular dysfunction based on range of motion (ROM) findings and orthopaedic evaluation
3. Degenerative changes evident
4. Acuteness of problem
5. Prior treatment outcomes
6. Age and activity level of patient

Conservative care seems appropriate in most cases with the possible exception of the group II athlete. However, given the low rate of success with surgical decompression in elite athletes, conservative care is worth an attempt. Even Neer[3] suggests conservative care initially to prevent progression through his conceptual stages.

Conservative care means different things to different health care providers. To an orthopaedic surgeon, a steroid injection is conservative, while to a chiropractor it would be considered conservative yet unnecessarily invasive due to a documented potential for tendon degenerative changes and other complications.[64,65]

The two issues in the care of impingement are treatment of acute versus chronic problems, and treatment that is specific to involved structures. Leadbetter[66] suggests a distinction of the type of tendon involvement based on a physiologic/histologic categorization. Under this classification tendinosis represents a degenerative, noninflammatory, and possibly asymptomatic involvement of a tendon, whereas tendinitis represents an inflammatory, symptomatic entity that may overlap with tendinosis (Table 14-3). The clinical point to this distinction is that addressing tendinitis as a self-resolving inflammatory process without considering underlying, possibly asymptomatic, degeneration ignores important considerations when devising rehabilitation approaches and return-to-play decisions. Curwin and

Table 14-3. Distinction Between Tendinitis and Tendinosis

Term	Pathophysiology	Clinical Signs	Treatment Approach
Tendinitis	Vascular disruption with inflammatory repair process	Inflammatory signs of swelling/ tenderness	Initially, decrease inflammation then assist healing
Tendinosis	Degeneration of tendon due to factors such as aging, avascularity, repetitive microtrauma. Changes include collagen degeneration, hypocellularity, and possible necrosis	May be asymptomatic. Palpable nodule in tendon	Avoid positions of irritation such as overhead positions or positions to compromise vascularity

Table 14-4. Staging of Tendinitis and Overuse Syndrome

Grade	Symptoms	Treatment
I	Pain only after activity Does not interfere with performance Often generalized tenderness Disappears before next exercise session	Modification of activity Assessment of training pattern Possibly NSAIDs
II	Minimal pain with activity Does not interfere with intensity or distance Usually localized tenderness	Modification of activity Physical therapy; NSAIDs; consider orthotics
III	Pain interferes with activity Usually disappears between sessions Definite local tenderness	Significant modification of activity Assess training schedule Physical therapy; NSAIDs[a]; consider orthotics
IV	Pain does not disappear between activity sessions Seriously interferes with intensity of training Significant local sign of pain, tenderness, crepitus, swelling	Usually need to temporarily discontinue aggravating motion Design alternate program May require splinting Physical therapy and NSAIDs
V	Pain interferes with sport and activities of daily living Symptoms often chronic or recurrent Signs of tissue changes and altered associated muscle function	Prolonged rest from activity NSAIDs plus other medical therapies[b] Consider splint or cast Physical therapy May require surgery

[a] In some circumstances, injection of steroids into the tendon sheath may be considered, along with other medications such as heparin.
[b] Occasionally, systemic steroids are used with appropriate reference to the benefit/risk ratio.
(From Reid,[67] with permission.)

Stanish[5] have staged tendon involvement based on functional criteria. Reid[67] has added treatment approaches based on these stages (Table 14-4).

Acute Impingement

Treatment of the acute presentation of an impingement patient is similar to that of most acute scenarios. The major goals are the reduction of pain and inflammation. Pain can be reduced through aspirin or nonsteroidal anti-inflammatory drugs (NSAIDs), cryotherapy (cold pack or ice massage), transcutaneous electrical nerve stimulation (TENS) or other neural stimulators. Also restriction of activity without immobilization is usually possible and desirable.

The Subacute Phase

In the subacute phase, ultrasound might be used at low frequency. At this stage, cross-friction massage might be effective in the treatment of the supraspinatus or biceps if involved.

Cross-friction massage is applied slightly distal or proximal to the site of maximum tenderness. The application involves a 7 to 9 minute treatment time divided into 2 minute reassessment periods. Application is skin to skin and does not involve the use of lotions.

Pressure is directed at right angles to the fibers being treated. Initially the doctor applies the maximum amount of bearable pressure as directed by the patient. After 2 minutes, without releasing the pressure, the patient is asked if tenderness is still present. If it is not or a sense of improvement is perceived, more pressure is added. This process is repeated for a total time of 7 to 9 minutes and followed by ice. After treatment the patient should attempt ROM to determine any immediate effects. Treatment is directed at the involved structures evident on examination. Common areas include the supraspinatus and biceps tendons, and the coracoacromial ligament. Specific directions for patient positioning and angle of application are demonstrated in Chapter 18.

In an attempt to decrease pressure and maintain normal accessory movement, the doctor may impart an inferior mobilization technique to the prone or supine patient. The patient's arm is stabilized between the doctor's knee. The doctor grasps the humeral head and directs an inferior oscillation or thrust inferiorly.

To maintain flexibility in a subacute stage lightweight Codman pendulum exercises are used. These are first performed without weight and then with a light weight added if the nonweighted version is performed pain-free. Patterns begin in a straight flexion/

extension plane progressing to circumduction maneuvers. Progression can then add outlining numbers or letters in the air requiring some mild acceleration and deceleration function of the muscles.

Muscle energy techniques or post–isometric techniques can be helpful in relaxing any spasmed musculature or simply reflexly inhibit pain through contraction. In-office and home prescription is recommended. These post–isometric techniques usually involve a concentric contraction of the involved muscle in a stretched position. The contraction is submaximal, approximately 25 to 50 percent for 8 to 10 seconds, followed by a stretch into an increased range. This then becomes the new starting position for the next stretch. Most self-stretches can be facilitated by a contraction against a supporting structure or gravity followed by further stretch. Particular attention must be paid to the posterior capsule, which has been implicated as a cause of superior migration of the humeral head resulting in impingement. Cross-body (horizontal adduction) stretching should be a daily routine unless anterior structures are irritated. Modification with external rotation added may help.

Rehabilitation

It is likely that the long-term goals of a treatment program for impingement could, in general, be applied to most shoulder problems with some modification. In other words, the mainstay of rehabilitation is

1. Balancing the ratio of strength between the internal rotators/adductors and the external rotators/abductors
2. Stabilize the glenohumeral joint directly through training that is specific to the rotator cuff
3. Stabilize the glenohumeral joint indirectly through stabilization and freedom of movement of the scapulothoracic joint
4. Stretch the posterior capsule
5. Slow retraining and modification of sporting activity to reduce further irritation

Specific approaches are presented in Chapter 20.

Rehabilitation usually involves a sequence of isometric contraction to tone or facilitate the muscles followed by isotonic contractions either performed with weights or elastic tubing. Both isometrics and elastic tubing should be initially performed at a submaximal level with the arm at the side to avoid recruitment and impingement. All exercises should progress away from the waist avoiding the 90 degree impingement position of abduction.

Isometrics can be performed several ways. First, through squeezing a tennis ball in various positions of elevation/abduction, the shoulder muscles are functionally facilitated (Fig. 14-15). Second, isometrics performed against the well-arm hand or against a wall can be used as pre-isotonic stabilizing exercises. Shoulder shrugs held for 3 to 5 seconds are also beneficial.

Eccentric training is advocated by Curwin and Stanish.[5] They feel that eccentric training is important for the treatment and prevention of tendon overload. The program is phased to assure a safe progression. The program sequence is

1. Static stretching for 15 to 30 seconds repeated 3 to 5 times.
2. Next, eccentric exercise is begun with gravity or light weight. For the first 2 days they are performed slowly. During days 3 to 5 they are performed at moderate speed. On days 6 and 7 the exercises are performed quickly. Three sets of 10 are performed.
3. After the eccentric phase, a repeat of the static stretching phase is performed as in 1.
4. Follow with 5 to 10 minutes of icing.

Although most exercise programs caution about pain experienced during the exercise, Curwin and Stanish feel that there should be some pain during the last set of 10 repetitions. If not, the resistance is increased slightly. Pain felt during either of the first two sets indicates too much resistance.

Isotonic exercise can be accomplished first with elastic tubing. Several approaches have been developed. A sequence of beginning with slow mid-range followed by fast mid-range exercises can be used for facilitation. Strength can be addressed next with full-range contractions held isometrically at the end and slowly guided through the eccentric phase. The final phase involves endurance. Fast full-range exercises are used. This provides an excellent primary approach to shoulder stabilization (see Ch. 20).

Electromyographic analysis of common shoulder exercises has demonstrated a core group that involves both weight resistance and body resistance (Ch. 20).

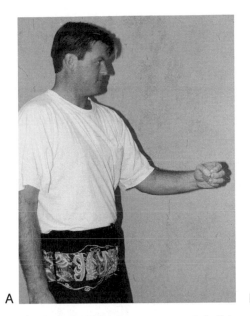
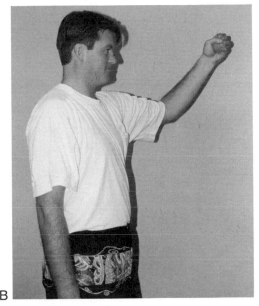

Fig. 14-15. (A & B) Squeezing a tennis ball in various positions for an isometric total arm contraction.

This group of exercises should function to strengthen all the supportive rotator cuff and scapular musculature. Figure 14-16 demonstrates some core exercises. Flexion is effective in stimulating most of the rotator group and the deltoids, as is scaption (abduction 30 degrees forward). Internal and external rotation should be performed without accompanying abduction or adduction.

More advanced prone exercises (against gravity) are demonstrated in Figure 14-17. Prone horizontal extension is effective for the whole rotator cuff group with specific emphasis on the supraspinatus and posterior deltoid. Prone external rotation is effective in stimulating the infraspinatus and teres minor. Prone extension is effective for the teres minor and infraspinatus.

If available, isokinetic training should include high-speed training between 180 and 300 degrees per second to more functionally stimulate the speed of most sports activities.

A summary of the above general approach to treatment and rehabilitation is given in Table 14-5. Following are some specific suggestions for specific sports.

Specific Sports Suggestions

Although many sports can be directly associated with impingement through repetitive positioning or sec-ondarily through the development of instability, some sports are more commonly involved. A brief description of specific recommendations is given for some of these sports.

Swimming is probably the most common sport with regard to impingement. Modifications of the basic stroke patterns can have major impact on future occurrence. The first is the use of body roll. Using body roll instead of arm lift prevents the early fatigue of the external rotators and serratus anterior.

Avoidance of the use of hand paddles is requisite. While attempting to strengthen the larger muscles, the increased resistance provided by the paddles can be detrimental to the cuff musculature.[68]

Based on recent electromyographic analysis of the shoulder with swimming,[69,70] several recommendations have been made regarding emphasis on specific rehabilitation:

1. Endurance training of the subscapularis and serratus anterior should be used.
2. Focus should be on concentric contractions of the posterior scapular musculature (performed mainly prone, against gravity).
3. Flexibility exercises should be stressed, but not overstressed (in particular with the young swim-

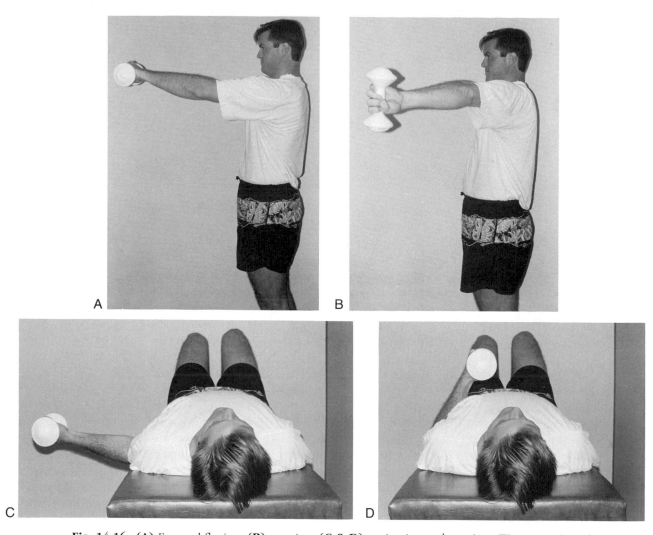

Fig. 14-16. (A) Forward flexion, **(B)** scaption, **(C & D)** supine internal rotation. *(Figure continues.)*

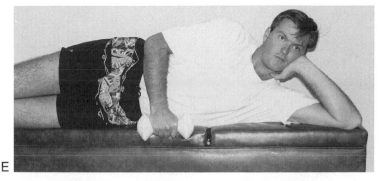

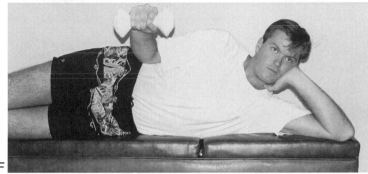

Fig. 14-16. *(continued).* **(E & F)** side-lying external rotation.

mer).[71] Ciullo and Guise[72] demonstrated in one study that the incidence of impingement symptoms dropped from 90 percent to approximately 14 percent with adolescent swimmers using a stretching program. Results in Master's swimmers were less dramatic.

With tennis it is important to avoid the 90 degree position in the serve. Raising the arm to a higher level around 135 degrees will allow the humeral head to clear the subacromial space. Other recommendations include

1. Use a midsize racquet with an open-throat leather grip; the racket should be strung between 62 and 67 lb with nylon.
2. For novices a larger racquet with a large "sweet spot" strung between 72 and 80 lb with nylon is recommended.
3. Proper grip size is important. Nirschl[73] suggests measuring along the radial side of the ring finger

from the tip to the palmar crease to determine proper grip handle size.
4. Do not play on wet courts.
5. Train the trunk and lower extremity musculature, which will decrease the stress to the shoulder.

Weightlifting requires specific attention to position.[74] Positions that either cause impingement at the 90 degree abducted or 90 degree horizontally adducted position should be avoided. In addition, when instability coexists with impingement, all straining positions should be avoided or modified. Some suggestions include

1. All elevation maneuvers with internal rotation should be restricted to below 90 degrees abduction
2. Front raises for the deltoids should be initially avoided
3. If anterior instability is present:
   a. Avoid dumbbell flys

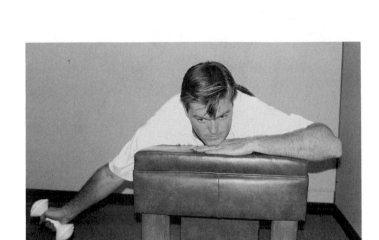

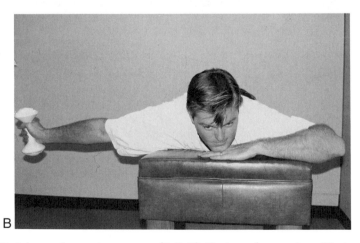

Fig. 14-17. Advanced exercises prone. **(A & B)** Horizontal extension. *(Figure continues.)*

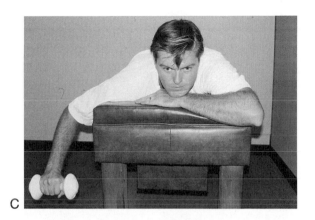

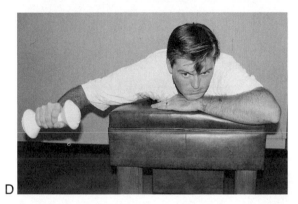

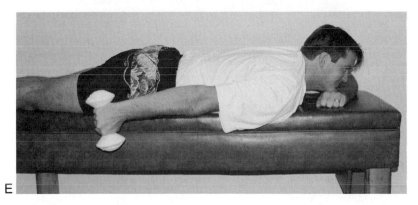

Fig. 14-17. *(continued).* **(C & D)** prone external rotation, **(E)** extension with external rotation.

Table 14-5. General Treatment Protocol to Impingement Syndrome and Rotator Cuff Tendinitis

Acute Phase

No sport activity involving upper extremity for 2 to 6 weeks
Ice and TENS or possibly microamperage stimulation for pain relief
Isometrics involving squeezing a tennis ball throughout diagonal patterns
Isometric contractions performed at the side against opposite hand
Codman/pendulum exercises (if performed pain-free)
Maintain aerobic capacity with lower body exercise such as bicycling
Manipulation of cervical/thoracic or rib subluxations

Sub-Acute Phase

Continue ice and TENS or microamperage stimulation if necessary
Cross-friction massage of involved tendons or over coracoacromial ligament (3 times/week for 2 to 4 weeks)
Continue isometrics and progress to first phase of elastic tubing exercise
Stretching with focus on posterior capsule
Inferior mobilization or manipulation if indicated
Manipulation of cervical/thoracic or rib subluxations

Return to Sport

Progress through elastic tubing program with emphasis on eccentric phase
Flexibility should be emphasized with focus on pectoral and posterior capsular stretching
Use a core exercise program (see Ch. 20) including
  1. Scaption
  2. Flexion
  3. Horizontal abduction with external rotation
  4. The press-up
  5. Bent-over rowing
  6. Push-up with a plus
PNF diagonal patterns progressing to resisted simulated sport patterns
Exercise program may progress using DAPRE or PRE approaches; for rotator cuff exercise limit weight to 5 to 10 lb
After progression through exercise program for several weeks progress to:
  1. Isokinetics at high speed (if available)
  2. Plyometrics using push-ups or medicine ball toss
  3. Proprioceptive training using Apley's or diagonal patterns with light free-weights or tubing
Educate patient regarding offending positions of individual sport and suggest modifications
Return to sport is gradual with icing after activity
Emphasis should be placed on off-season conditioning to prevent recurrence

Abbreviations: TENS, transcutaneous electrical nerve stimulation; PNF, proprioceptive neuromuscular facilitation; DAPRE, daily adjustable progressive resistance exercise; PRE, progressive resistance exercise.

  b. Avoid wide-grip bench and standing barbell/dumbbell maneuvers
  c. Substitute narrow-grip bench presses

BICIPITAL TENDON DISORDERS

The tendon of the long head of the biceps may be involved in a variety of disorders. Primary involvement apparently is rare, but secondary involvement is very common. Primary disorders include direct trauma and damage due to excessive contractile force. Discussed above is the common secondary involvement with impingement.

The unique features of the tendon of the long head of the biceps that predisposes it to involvement are

1. Sliding of the bicipital groove on the tendon as the arm is elevated
2. Anomalies of the bicipital groove due to congenital factors or acquired exostosis
3. Angulation over the head of the humerus
4. Potential impingement with the supraspinatus under the coracoacromial arch (the tendon runs directly under the supraspinatus critical zone)
5. Potential avascularity due to arm position
6. Increased demand when there is damage to the capsule or rotator cuff

The biceps can be affected in several ways including tendinitis/tenosynovitis, subluxation/dislocation, and avulsion of the superior glenoid labrum.

It appears that bicipital groove anomalies and impingement are the most common cause in the younger athlete, whereas in the older athlete degenerative changes are the most common predisposition.

Tendinitis/Tenosynovitis

Tendinitis is believed by most authors to be secondary to the impingement process discussed in detail above. There is disagreement regarding whether the tendon sheath is involved initially. Slatis and Aalto[75] distinguish this secondary involvement from a more primary involvement that they call attrition tendinitis. Due primarily to an acquired stenosis of the groove, processes such as reactive bone formation and adhesion development damage the tendon as the anomalous tunnel runs over the tendon with arm elevation. Examples of these anomalies include supratubercular ridges[76] (Fig. 14-18), medial wall spurs (reactive to either traction exostosis or bicipital tendon pressure), and spurs on the floor of the bicipital groove.

Inflammation of the synovium and tendon degeneration are common reactions. Paavolainen et al.[77] feel that attrition tendinitis is the most painful type of tendinitis. They also believe that it is the most common precursor to rupture.

Evaluation by radiographs can include bicipital groove views. The first is described by Cone et al.[78] and involves directing the central beam horizontally with a medial tilt of 15 degrees. The patient is supine with the cassette placed above the shoulder. The arm is externally rotated. The second view is taken with the standing patient supporting the cassette on the forearm. The central ray is directed straight down the groove with the patient positioned under the tube with the forearm flat on the table supporting the shoulder (Fig. 14-19). Indirect views are the outlet view mentioned above used to evaluate subacromial spurring.

Treatment is similar to the approaches described above. Additionally, counterforce bracing has been advocated for bicipital tendinitis. The theory is that by displacing the force distally, the tendon is not placed under as much tension or at the same location. The counterforce brace is a band of material similar to the tennis-elbow brace, which encircles the arm high up on the arm just below the humeral tuberosities.

Additionally, tenosynovitis can be a feature of adhesive capsulitis, septic arthritis of the shoulder, rheumatoid arthritis, rheumatoid variants, and crystalline arthritis.[79] Tuberculosis and syphilis can also lead to eventual rupture.

Subluxation/Dislocation

One of the more controversial topics regarding the biceps is subluxation and dislocation out of the bicipital groove. In the past it was assumed based on gross visualization of cadavers that the transverse ligament was the primary restraint to dislocation. Meyer[80] and Codman[8] commented on the tendency for the cuff and capsule to be torn in cases of dislocation. Recently, it has been demonstrated by observation and selective dissection that the thickened area of capsule over the superior sulcus is the primary restraint.[80] This area is formed by the coracohumeral ligament and the edges of the supraspinatus and subscapularis tendons. The primary restraint below the tuberosity is the tendinous extension of the pectoralis major (sternal division) referred to as the falciform ligament.[79]

Dislocation/subluxation of the tendon of the long head of the biceps is primarily due to the chronic de-

generative changes that result from chronic impingement. Other contributing factors include

1. Direct blows to the shoulder (either to the biceps or capsular/cuff damage from a blow in the apprehension position)
2. Falls on an outstretched arm leading to capsular/cuff damage
3. Overexertion/contraction with
   a. Weightlifting
   b. A checked swing in baseball
   c. Quarterback passing
   d. Various support positions in gymnastics

In the past it was believed that the tendon displaced medially over the lesser tuberosity and over the subscapularis. The findings of Petersson[85] and DePalma[81] have disputed this concept. When dislocation occurs the tendon slides under the subscapularis.

Patient presentation usually includes a complaint of anterior shoulder pain and snapping when the arm is used in the overhead position. Locking can occasionally occur. There are several tests (described previously) that can be used to elicit this snapping sensation, including Yergason's, Ludington, Abbott-Saunders, and Gilcrest sign tests. Kulund[41] suggests that migrating tenderness with positional changes is an important clue with all bicipital disorders. He feels that tenderness moves with the position of the bicipital groove so that internal rotation causes medial migration; external rotation causes lateral migration of tenderness.

Cowper[82] was apparently the first person to document repositioning of the tendon almost 300 years ago in 1694. Currently, chiropractors and osteopaths use a relocation maneuver that anecdotally seems to produce results. The arm of the relaxed supine patient is extended toward the floor. The examiner pulls laterally at the superior bicipital groove while circumducting the arm into external rotation abduction completing the maneuver with the arm across the chest and down to the side in internal rotation (Fig. 14-20). Variations of this maneuver are common. In reoccurring episodes that initially respond to this maneuver, 1 to 2 weeks of splinting can allow sufficient healing to occur.

Medically, surgical reattachment is recommended in the professional athlete if conservative treatment fails to effect full recovery.

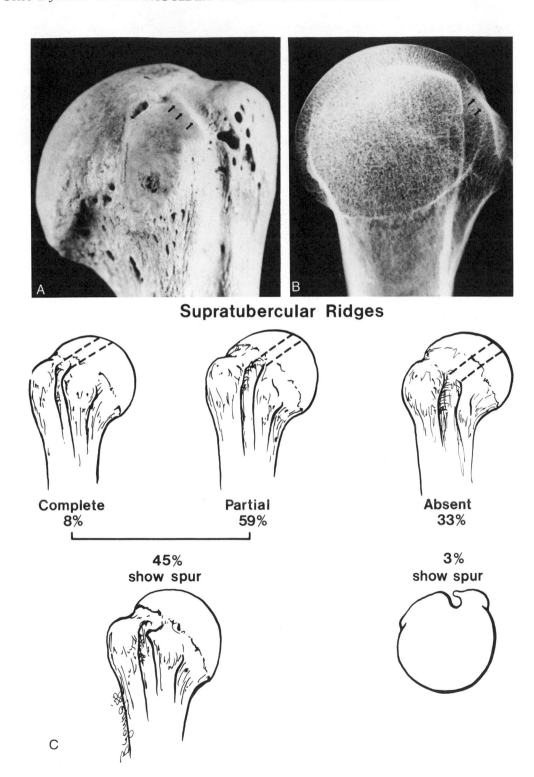

Supratubercular Ridges

Complete
8%

Partial
59%

Absent
33%

45%
show spur

3%
show spur

C

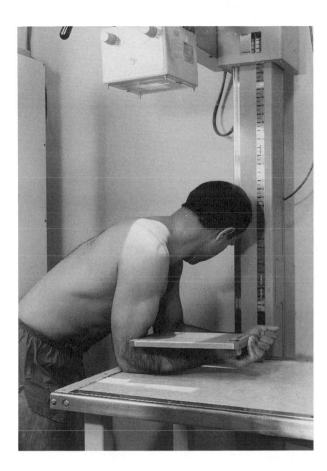

Fig. 14-19. Bicipital groove view.

Ruptures of the Biceps

Ruptures of the tendon of the long head of the biceps is usually an extension of the attrition process described above where chronic degeneration occurs or in the older athlete where aging-degeneration is present. At the time of injury a pop may be heard. On examination, the muscle belly of the long head is displaced distally leaving an obvious proximal gap. Injury is most common with underhand maneuvers such as softball pitching, weightlifting, and gymnastic maneuvers.

Treatment is palliative for the nonathlete. Serious athletes will often require surgical repair. Rupture of the tendon of the long head of the biceps results in a decrease of elbow flexion strength by 20 percent.[25] The effects on glenohumeral stability have not been studied. However, given the apparent increased requirements for bicipital participation with throwers who have unstable shoulders, it seems likely that the effects would be more apparent with sports requiring the throwing action.[35] In this author's experience most individuals not involved in competitive sports show

Fig. 14-18. **(A)** Externally rotated view of a cadaveric specimen showing the supratubercular ridge *(black arrows).* **(B)** Internally rotated radiograph showing the prominent supratubercular ridge *(small black arrows).* **(C)** The presence of the supratubercular ridge (seen extending from the lesser tuberosity, altering the angle of the biceps tendon) and narrowing of the groove, both partial and complete in the specimens of Hitchcock and Bechtol are shown. Medial wall spurs are much more common in specimens with supratubercular ridges. (Figs. **A & B** from Cone et al.,[104] as adapted in Burkhead,[79] with permission.) (Fig. **C** from Hitchcock and Bechtol,[105] as adapted in Burkhead,[79] with permission.)

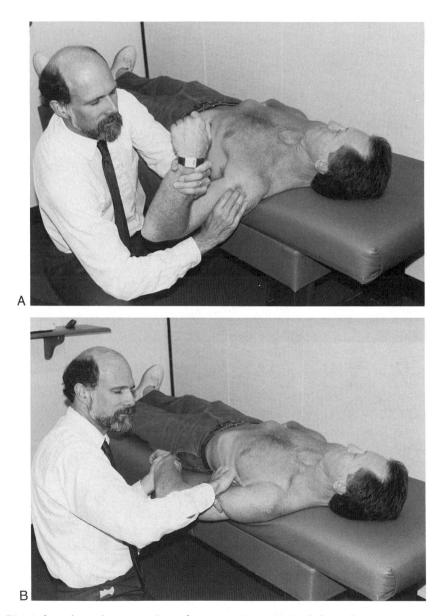

Fig. 14-20. Bicipital tendon adjustment. Lateral pressure is maintained throughout the maneuver. **(A)** Arm is brought into external rotation/abduction and then **(B)** circled around into internal rotation/extension.

no objective loss of elbow flexion on manual muscle testing and rarely complain of weakness.

Avulsion Injuries

As mentioned above, the biceps has been implicated as a cause of glenoid labrum tears contributing to instability. Andrews et al.[32] have noted that during a forceful eccentric contraction in an attempt to decelerate the elbow, the biceps may tear the glenolabral attachment. This is most common in the follow-through phase of throwing sports. Treatment is usually surgical resection and reattachment of the biceps tendon.

RUPTURES OF THE ROTATOR CUFF

The terms rupture and tear are often used synonymously with regard to the rotator cuff. Ruptures represent full substance or complete tears when they extend the entire thickness of the tendon allowing communication between the glenohumeral joint space and the subacromial/subdeltoid bursal area. The size of these complete tears varies considerably, ranging from small to large defects. Partial-thickness or incomplete tears also exist either as superficial, deep, or intrasubstance lesions (Fig. 14-21).

Generally, the two major (often overlapping) causes of tendon rupture/tear are trauma and degeneration. Trauma can further be divided into macro (single-event trauma) and micro (repetitive trauma). Single-event trauma requires a massive force that exceeds the tensile strength of the tendon. In the majority of these scenarios a greater tuberosity avulsion is more likely due to the lower tensile strength of bone as compared with tendon. When a single event does cause a complete rupture, underlying chronic degeneration predisposed the occurrence. This would be more common in the older athlete.

As discussed earlier, degenerative changes occur as the athlete ages due to structural changes that involve fascicular splitting and thinning. The interfascicular tissue may increase while the tendon becomes hypocellular. Theoretically, these changes are due to the hypovascularity that may exist in several of the tendons. Augmentation of this proposed hypovascular tendency can occur through position either involving compression or stretch or a combination of both.

It has been demonstrated that vascular supply is minimal on the articular side of the tendon.[83] Articular-sided tears constitute the majority of partial-thickness tears. It is possible that this represents an inability to heal appropriately due to the relative hypovascularity. However, it has also been demonstrated that some tendons derive the majority of their nutrition from diffusion of tissue fluids, not from perfusion. The vascularity of the bursal side of the tendon is more abundant.

Complete tears often occur between the tendon fibers and Sharpey's fibers. In the supraspinatus tendon, this occurs in the interval between the subscapularis and supraspinatus tendons.[1] Complete tears often present with a concomitant subacromial bursitis.[84]

Patients with cuff tears are likely to be symptomatic, but this is not always true. Pettersson[85] performed arthrography on 71 asymptomatic patients and found 13 with positive findings for partial- and full-thickness tears. When symptomatic, patients will present with the same signs and symptoms as the impingement patient. Full tears due to trauma can exhibit more dramatic losses in strength and severity of symptoms. The Codman drop-arm maneuver may reveal inability to lower the arm when a full rupture of the supraspinatus is present. Gerber and Krushell[86] describe the "lift-off" test to determine rupture of the subscapularis. With the back of the hand of the involved side placed on the lower back, the patient is asked to lift the hand away and is unable to do so with a tear of the subscapularis. The patients examined by Gerber and Krushell did not present with complaints of instability in the presence of a subscapularis rupture.

Lyons and Tomlinson[87] have reported on the sensitivity and specificity of palpation for full tears. They report a 91 percent sensitivity and a 75 percent specificity using palpation alone. Palpation is performed with the elbow flexed to 90 degrees. Palpation of the humeral head is performed with internal and external rotation followed by hyperextension. The authors claim that an anterior supraspinatus tear may be felt in external rotation, with internal rotation a posterior tear may be felt, and with hyperextension a tear in the infraspinatus is palpable. Unfortunately, no more localizing information or diagrams were included.

Treatment of rotator cuff tears is variable. The first

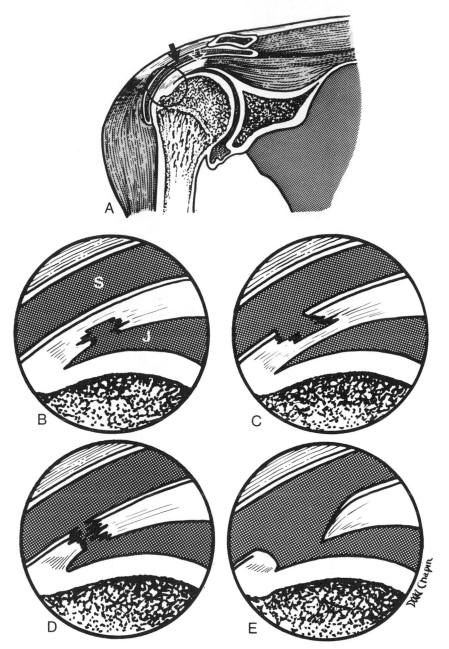

Fig. 14-21. Rotator cuff tears. **(A)** Diagram showing the intact tendons of the rotator cuff *(open arrow)* separating the shoulder joint from the subacromial-subdeltoid bursa *(arrow)*. The circle indicates the critical area of the cuff, through which most tears occur. This is the area shown in parts **B–E**. **(B)** A partial tear of the inferior aspect of the rotator cuff is shown. This tear would be demonstrated by shoulder arthrography. *J*, joint; *S*, subacromial-subdeltoid bursa. **(C)** A partial tear of the superior aspect of the rotator cuff is shown. This tear would be demonstrable on bursography but not on arthrography. **(D)** A complete tear of the cuff, with the irregular margins typical of an acute tear, is shown. A shoulder arthrogram would show filling of the subacromial-subdeltoid bursa. **(E)** Chronic complete rotator cuff tear. The smoothly tapered margins are characteristic. (From Weismann,[103] with permission.)

Table 14-6. Indications for Surgical Repair of Rotator Cuff Tear

A patient younger than 60 years of age with the following:
Demonstration of a full-thickness tear with an imaging modality such as magnetic resonance imaging, arthrography, or sonography
Failure of a nonoperative treatment program for no less than 6 weeks and up to 1 year
Need for patient to use the involved arm in overhead activities
Willingness of patient to accept a trade-off of reduction in pain for decreased strength and some loss of active abduction

distinction is between surgical and nonsurgical treatment. Samilson and Binder[88] offer some criteria for this decision as illustrated in Table 14-6. Although Takagishi[89] demonstrated a 44 percent success rate with nonoperative repair and Samilson and Binder[88] demonstrated a 59 percent success, there appears to be no confirmation of the extent of the tears. It is suggested that most were partial-thickness tears. Conservative treatment often involved corticosteroid injections, which carries with it some inherent risk of further damage.

Conservative care is recommended following the same approach as discussed with a tendinitis. A 1 week period of immobilization may be necessary prior to initiating any rehabilitation. Rehabilitation should involve neutral, mild isometrics prior to progressing to isotonic maneuvers. If the patient does not respond to a conservative approach over several months, surgery may be needed.

Surgical repair is beyond the scope and intention of this text. In summary, these approaches usually involve combinations of acromioplasty and various approaches to primary tendon repair. Tendon repair can be tendon-to-tendon, tendon-to-bone, or further mobilization or advancement of major tendon flaps.[90] Review of the success of these various approaches varies considerably due to the techniques used and the criteria for success. Cofield[91] summarizes some of these results and averaged them indicating that pain relief ranged from 71 to 100 percent, averaging 87 percent. Patient satisfaction ranged between 72 and 82 percent, averaging 77 percent.

RUPTURE OF THE PECTORALIS MAJOR

Rupture of the pectoralis major is usually at or near the insertion to the humerus. The most common mechanism is overcontraction in a position of stretch as occurs with the bench press. Another mechanism is a fall with the arm flexed and horizontally abducted catching all the weight of the body on one arm. The patient presentation includes a history of a ripping sensation at the time of injury followed by pain and swelling in the anterior shoulder. Over time ecchymosis usually is evident indicating the severity of damage. Palpation of the defect is not always obvious, but having the athlete contract the pectorals by pushing the palms together usually makes it more palpably evident. If treated conservatively, full ruptures will heal, but with a loss of strength.[92] For full return to strength, surgery is recommended.[93]

CALCIFYING TENDINITIS

For many years it was an accepted belief that calcification of the tendons about the shoulder represented a progressive degenerative disorder.[6] The assumption was also that radiographic demonstration confirmed tendon involvement as the source of the patient's problem (Fig. 14-22). Recently, some important arthroscopic discoveries and empirical observations have clarified the entity known as calcific tendinitis.[94]

The major clinical radiologic clue was observed by Rowe[95] who found that calcification did not occur before the age of 30 and not after the age of 60. This questioned the past belief of a progressively degenerative process. Many of the patients were inadvertently found to have calcification that did not correlate to symptomatology.

Arthroscopically it became evident that there were two forms of calcification process. The first is referred to as reactive, and the second dystrophic. With reactive calcification, surrounding bony structures are normal and reflect no degenerative process. Hydroxyapatite crystals are deposited. The dystrophic type demonstrated a stippled calcification process associated with irregularity of the greater tuberosity and other glenohumeral degenerative signs.

In the initial formative stages the deposits have a chalklike appearance. Radiographically these dense homogenous deposits are usually well defined. Clinically, symptoms may be created by impingement due to increase in tendon size by this process. These deposits may remain unchanged for months or years.

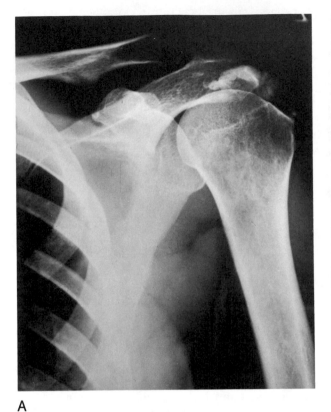

A

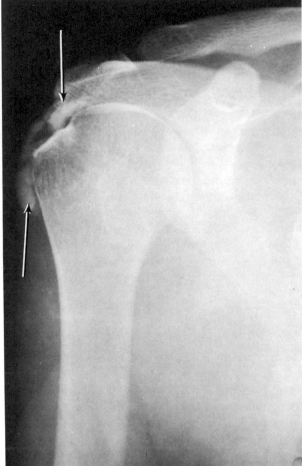

B

C

Fig. 14-22. (A) The most common site of calcific deposits in the shoulder is the supraspinatus tendon. The deposit may be a single foci, or **(B)** multiple foci deposits. **(C)** Occasionally, a deposit may occur in the subscapularis tendon. (From Rowe,[95] with permission.)

At some time there is a trigger for a reabsorptive process that is accompanied by increased vascularity to the region. This increase in vascularity causes swelling in the region of deposit and often initiates a very painful, apparently acute reaction. Therefore, the more acute presentation is more likely due to the reabsorption process and not the initial calcification process. Arthroscopically, the calcification becomes less chalky and more creamy in consistency and is gradually reabsorbed over time.

These new discoveries should alert the surgeon to avoid the unnecessary surgical attempts at correction. It is within the natural course of the process to self-resolve. Even the use of corticosteroids might be questioned. In the acute resorptive phase, pain medication is usually necessary.

DEGENERATIVE JOINT DISEASE

Although the nonathletic population will usually not demonstrate degenerative findings in the glenohumeral joint until at least the fifth and sixth decades, degenerative findings and symptoms may be evident in the athletic population at a much earlier age. There are several suggestions as to why this may occur. Primarily, instability seems to be the unifying concept. Instability may accelerate changes directly or indirectly.

Directly, it appears that instability allows abnormal wear on the glenoid. Neer[96] noted that the average age of the athletic individual with severe changes was 37. This arthritis of dislocation was further confirmed by a review by Brems[97] of 500 patients with degenerative disease of the shoulder. Interestingly 103 patients had a prior history of instability and 97 of these patients had surgery for their instability. So it appears that in addition to instability itself being a cause, the treatment may be a factor. Theoretically, it is suggested that one major reason may be when multidirectional instability is not recognized with the attempted surgery allowing subluxation into areas not stabilized.[98] In addition, the placement of screws and other apparatus may be associated with early degenerative changes.

Patient Presentation

As mentioned, the average age of the athlete with degeneration is 37 years old. They will probably have a history of active involvement in sports such as golf, swimming, or tennis. The complaints will usually be one of a deep poorly localized pain with associated stiffness. The stiffness is often the capsular pattern of external rotation and abduction restricted most followed by internal rotation. Overhead activity is very limited. Associated with the stiffness is weakness on external rotation and atrophy of the external rotators in long-standing cases.

Radiographically, it is important to include an axillary view such as the West Point view or similar positioning. It has been observed by Brems[97] that there is often a posterior displacement of the humeral head seen on the axillary view. Degeneration changes on the posterior glenoid rim are also apparent. These may be missed on routine views. It is interesting to note that this observation of posterior displacement with the associated limitations in external rotation and abduction resemble both the patient with undetected posterior dislocation and the patient with frozen shoulder (adhesive capsulitis).

Treatment

Treatment is very similar to the treatment of frozen shoulder (see Ch. 16). Pain is usually alleviated by over-the-counter medications with appropriate physical therapy and stretching. Most beneficial is ultrasound, which may be used prior to in-office stretching. Stretching should focus on the anterior capsule in most cases. Tightness in the anterior capsule will allow excessive translation posteriorly of the humeral head.[37] Stretching in-office can include rhythmic stabilization and other reflex approaches. A mild to moderate contraction is held isometrically for 8 to 10 seconds followed by a stretch into a new position.

Recalcitrant cases may need operative repair and occasionally joint replacement. With operative repair it is crucial to recognize the patient with multidirectional instability in an attempt to avoid accelerating the already existing degeneration with an inadequate stabilization.

REFERENCES

1. Neer CS II: Anterior acromioplasty for the chronic impingement syndrome in the shoulder: a preliminary report. J Bone Joint Surg 54A:41, 1972
2. McMaster WC: Painful shoulder in swimmers: a diagnostic challenge. Phys Sports Med 14:108, 1986

3. Neer CS II: Impingement lesions. Clin Orthop 173:70, 1983
4. O'Brien M: Functional anatomy and physiology of tendons. Clin Sports Med 11:505, 1992
5. Curwin S, Stanish WD: Tendinitis: Its Etiology and Treatment. Collamore Press, Lexington, MA, 1984
6. Borynsenko M, Beringer T: Functional Histology. p. 105. Little, Brown, Boston, 1989
7. Woo S, Maynard J, Butler et al: Ligament, tendon, and joint capsule insertions to bone. p. 133. In Woo S, Buckwalter JA (eds): Injury and Repair of the Musculoskeletal Soft Tissue. American Academy of Orthopaedic Surgeons, Park Ridge, IL, 1988
8. Codman EA: The Shoulder. Rupture of the Supraspinatus Tendon and Other Lesions in or about the Subacromial Bursa. Thomas Todd, Boston, 1934
9. Clark JC: Fibrous anatomy of the rotator cuff. Abstract presented at the meeting of the American Academy of Orthopaedic Surgeons, 1988
10. Schneider H: Zur Struktur der Schnenansatzzonen. Z Anat Entwickl Gesch 119:431, 1980
11. Stillwell TL Jr: The innervation of tendons and aponeurisms. Am J Anat 100:289, 1957
12. Ling SC, Chen SF, Wan RX: A study of the vascular supply of the supraspinatus tendon. Surg Radiol Anat 12:161, 1990
13. Gerber C, Terner F, Ganz R: The role of the coracoid process in the chronic impingement syndrome. J Bone Joint Surg 67B:703, 1985
14. Lindblom K: On pathogenesis of ruptures of the tendon aponeurosis of the shoulder joint. Acta Radiol 20:563, 1939
15. Moseley HF, Goldie I: The arterial pattern of the rotator cuff of the shoulder. J Bone Joint Surg 45B:780, 1963
16. Iannotti JP, Swiontkowski M, Esterhafi J, Boulas HJ: Intraoperative assessment of rotator cuff vascularity using laser Doppler flowmetry. Abstract presented at the meeting of the American Academy of Orthopaedic Surgeons, Las Vegas, 1989
17. Rathburn JB, Macnab I: The microvascular pattern of the rotator cuff. J Bone Joint Surg 52B:540, 1970
18. Sigholm G, Styf J, Kormer L, Herberts P: Pressure recording in the subacromial bursa. J Orthop Res 6:123, 1988
19. Jobe FW, Kvitne RS: Shoulder pain in the overhand or throwing athlete: the relationship of anterior instability and rotator cuff impingement. Orthop Rev 18:963, 1989
20. Nirschl RP: Rotator cuff tendinitis: basic concepts of pathoetiology. p. 439. AAOS Instr. Course Lect, 1989
21. Ozaki J, Fujimoto S, Nakagawa Y et al: Tears of the rotator cuff of the shoulder associated with pathological changes in the acromion: a study of cadavers. J Bone Joint Surg 70A:1224, 1988
22. Liberson F: Os acromiale—a contested anomaly. J Bone Joint Surg 19:683, 1937
23. Norris TR, Fischer J, Bigliani LU et al: The unfused acromial ephiphysis and its relationship to impingement syndromes. Orthop Trans 7:505, 1983
24. Mudge MK, Wood VE, Frykman GK: Rotator cuff tears associated with os acromiale. J Bone Joint Surg 66A:427, 1984
25. Bigliani LU, Norris TR, Fischer J et al: The relationship between the unfused acromial epiphysis and subacromial impingement lesions. Orthop Trans 7:138, 1983
26. Bigliani LU, Morrison DS, April EW: The morphology of the acromion and its relationship to rotator cuff tears. Orthop Trans 10:216, 1986
27. Cuillo J: Swimmer's shoulder. Clin Sports Med 5:115, 1984
28. Goldthwait JE: An anatomic and mechanical study of the shoulder joint. Am J Orthop Surg 6:579, 1909
29. Patte D, Goutallier D, Bernageau J: Desinsertions traumatiques de sous-scapulaire avec ou sans subluxations du long biceps. Deuxieme congres de la Societe Europeene pour la chirugie de l'epaule et du coude, Berne, Switzerland, October 16, 1988
30. Patte D: The subcoracoid impingement. Clin Orthop Relat Res 254:55, 1990
31. Kibler WB, Chandler TJ: Functional scapular instability in throwing athletes. Presented at the meeting of the American Orthopaedic Society for Sports Medicine, Traverse City, MI, June 19–22, 1989
32. Andrews JR, Broussard TS, Carson WG: Arthroscopy of the shoulder in the management of partial tears of the rotator cuff: a preliminary report. Arthroscopy 1:117, 1985
33. Rodosky MW, Rudert MJ, Harner CD et al: S.L.A.P. lesions of the shoulder (lesions of the superior labrum anterior to posterior). Presented at the 8th Annual Meeting of the Arthroscopy Association of North America, Seattle, WA, April 13–16, 1989
34. Jobe FW, Moynes DR, Tibone JE, Perry J: An EMG analysis of the shoulder in pitching: a second report. Am J Sports Med 12:218, 1984
35. Glousman R, Jobe FW, Tibone JE et al: Dynamic electromyographic analysis of the throwing shoulder with glenohumeral instability. J Bone Joint Surg 70A:220, 1988
36. Pappas A, Zwacke R, McCarthy C: Rehabilitation of the pitching shoulder. Am J Sports Med 13:223, 1985
37. Harryman DT, Sidles JA, Clark JM et al: Translation of the humeral head on the glenoid with passive glenohumeral motion. J Bone Joint Surg 72A:1334, 1990
38. Matsen FA, Arntz CT: Subacromial impingement. In Rockwood CA, Matsen FA (eds): The Shoulder. Vol. 1. WB Saunders, Philadelphia, 1990
39. Penny JN, Welsh RP: Shoulder impingement syndromes

in athletes and their surgical management. Am J Sports Med 9:11, 1981

40. Hawkins RJ, Abrams JS, Schutte JP: Multidirectional instability of the shoulder: an approach to diagnosis. Orthop Trans 11:246, 1987

41. Kulind DN: The Injured Athlete. JB Lippincott, Philadelphia, 1982

42. Jobe FW, Tibone JE, Jobe CM et al: The shoulder in sports. p. 961. In Rockwood CA, Matsen FA (eds): The Shoulder. Vol. 1. WB Saunders, Philadelphia, 1990

43. Silliman JF, Hawkins RJ: Current concepts and recent advances in the athlete's shoulder. Clin Sports Med 10:693, 1991

44. Uhthoff HK, Sarkar K: Classification and definition of tendinopathies. Clin Sports Med 10:707, 1991

45. Cyriax J: Textbook of orthopaedic medicine. Vol. l. Diagnosis of soft tissue lesions. 8th Ed. Balliere-Tindall, London, 1982

46. Kessel L, Watson M: The painful arc syndrome: clinical classification as a guide to management. J Bone Joint Surg 59B:2,166, 1977

47. Hawkins RJ, Kennedy JC: Impingement syndrome in athletes. Am J Sports Med 8:151, 1980

48. Corrigan B, Maitland GD: Practical orthopaedic medicine. Butterworths, London, 1983

49. Jackson D, Einhorn A: Rehabilitation of the shoulder. p. 103. In Jackson DW (ed): Shoulder Surgery in the Athlete. Aspen, Rockville, MD, 1985

50. Travell J, Simons DG: Myofascial dysfunction: The trigger point manual. Williams & Wilkins, Baltimore, 1983

51. Jobe FW, Jobe CM: Painful athletic injuries of the shoulder. Clin Orthop 173:117, 1983

52. Gilcrest EL, Albi P: Unusual lesions of muscles and tendons of the shoulder girdle and upper arm. Surg Gynecol Obstet 69:903, 1939

53. Crenshaw AH, Kilgore WE: Surgical treatment of bicipital tenosynovitis. J Bone Joint Surg 48A:1496, 1966

54. Yergason RM: Rupture of the biceps. J Bone Joint Surg 13:160, 1931

55. Post M: Primary tendinitis of the long head of the biceps. Paper presented at the Closed Meeting of the Society of American Shoulder and Elbow Surgeons, Orlando, FL, 1987

56. Abbott LC, Saunders LB de CM: Acute traumatic dislocation of tendon of the long head of the biceps brachii. Report of 6 cases with operative findings. Surgery 6:817, 1939

57. Ludington NA: Bicipital tendinitis. Am J Surg 77:358, 1923

58. Kibler WB, Chandler TJ: Functional scapular instability in throwing athletes. Paper presented at the 15th Annual Meeting of the American Orthopaedic Society of Sports Medicine, Traverse City, MI, June 19–22, 1989

59. Sisto DJ, Jobe FW: The operative treatment of scapulothoracic bursitis in professional pitchers. Am J Sports Med 14:192, 1986

60. Maigne R: Orthopaedic Medicine: A New Approach to Vertebral Manipulation. Charles C Thomas, Springfield, IL, 1972

61. Hardy DC, Vogler JB III, White RH: The shoulder impingement syndrome: prevalence of radiographic findings and correlation with response to therapy. AJR 147:557, 1987

62. Neer CS II, Poppen NK: Supraspinatus outlet. Paper presented at the 3rd Open Meeting of the Society of American Shoulder and Elbow Surgeons, San Francisco, 1987

63. Matsen FA, Thomas SC: Glenohumeral instability. In Evarts CM (ed): Surgery of the Musculoskeletal System. 2nd Ed. Churchill Livingstone, New York, 1989

64. McWhorter JW, Francis RS, Heckmann RA: Influence of local steroid injections on traumatized tendon properties: a biomechanical and histological study. Am J Sports Med 19:435, 1991

65. McFarland R, Dugdale TW, Gerbino P, Nielsen R: Neurovascular complications resulting from corticosteroid injections. Phys Sports Med 18:89, 1990

66. Leadbetter WB: Cell-matrix response in tendon injury. Clin Sports Med 11:533, 1992

67. Reid DC: Sports Injury Assessment and Rehabilitation. Churchill Livingstone, New York, 1990

68. McMaster WC: Painful shoulder in swimmers: a diagnostic challenge. Am J Sports Med 14:108, 1986

69. Pink M, Perry J, Browne A et al: The normal shoulder during freestyle swimming: an electromyographic and cinematographic analysis of twelve muscles. Am J Sports Med 19:569, 1991

70. Scovazzo ML, Browne A, Pink M et al: The painful shoulder during freestyle swimming: an electromyographic cinematographic analysis of twelve muscles. Am J Sports Med 19:577, 1991

71. Greipp JF: Swimmer's shoulder: the influence of flexibility and weight training. Phys Sports Med 13:92, 1985

72. Ciullo JV, Guise ER: Adolescent swimmer's shoulder. Orthop Trans 7:171, 1983

73. Nirschl RP: Prevention and treatment of elbow and shoulder injuries in the tennis player. Clin Sports Med 7:289, 1988

74. Reider B: Strength training. p. 19. In Reider B (ed): The School-Age Athlete. WB Saunders, Philadelphia, 1990

75. Slatis P, Aalto K: Medial dislocation of the tendon of the long head of the biceps. Acta Orthop Scand 50:73, 1979

76. Hitchcock HH, Bechtol CO: Painful shoulder: observations on the role of the tendon of the long head of the biceps brachii in its causation. J Bone Joint Surg 30A:263, 1948

77. Paavolainen P, Slatis P, Alto K: Surgical pathology in

chronic shoulder pain. p. 313. In Bateman JE, Welsh RP (eds): Surgery of the Shoulder. BC Decker, Philadelphia, 1984

78. Cone RO, Danzig L, Reznick D, Goldman AB: The bicipital groove: radiographic, anatomic, and pathologic study. AJR 41:781, 1983

79. Burkhead WZ: The biceps tendon. In Rockwood CA, Matsen FA (eds): The Shoulder. WB Saunders, Philadelphia, 1990

80. Meyer AW: Spontaneous dislocation of the long head of the biceps brachii. Arch Surg 13:109, 1926

81. DePalma AF: Surgery of the Shoulder. JB Lippincott, Philadelphia, 1983

82. Cowper W: Myotomia Reformata. London, 1694

83. Uhthoff HK, Lohr J, Hammond I et al: Aetiologie und pathogenese von rupturen der rotatoremmanschette. In Helbig B, Blauth W (eds): Schulterschmerzen und Rupturen der Rotatoremmanschette. Springer-Verlag, Heidelberg, 1980

84. Uhthoff HK, Sakar H, Hammond DI: The subacromial bursa: a clinico-pathological study. p. 121. In Bateman JE, Welsh RP (eds): Surgery of the Shoulder. BC Decker, Philadelphia, 1984

85. Pettersson G: Rupture of the tendon aponeurosis of the shoulder joint in anterior inferior dislocation. Acta Chir Scand, suppl. 77:1, 1942

86. Gerber C, Krushell RJ: Isolated rupture of the tendon of the subscapularis muscle: clinical features in 16 cases. J Bone Joint Surg 73B:389, 1991

87. Lyons AR, Tomlinson JE: Clinical diagnosis of tears of the rotator cuff. J Bone Joint Surg 74B:414, 1992

88. Samilson RL, Binder WF: Symptomatic full-thickness tears of the rotator cuff: an analysis of 292 shoulders in 276 patients. Orthop Clin North Am 6:449, 1975

89. Takagishi N: Conservative treatment of the ruptures of the rotator cuff. J Jpn Orthop Assoc 52:781, 1978

90. Matsen FA, Arntz CT: Rotator cuff tendon failure. In Rockwood CA, Matsen FA (eds): The Shoulder. WB Saunders, Philadelphia, 1990

91. Cofield RH: Current concepts review rotator cuff disease of the shoulder. J Bone Joint Surg 67A:974, 1985

92. Gudmundsson B: A case of agenesis and a case of rupture of the pectoralis major muscle. Acta Orthop Scand 44:213, 1973

93. Berson B: Surgical repair of the pectoralis major rupture in an athlete. Am J Sports Med 7:348, 1979

94. Uhthoff HK, Sarkar K: Calcifying tendinitis: its pathogenic mechanism and a rationale for its treatment. Int Orthop 2:187, 1978

95. Rowe CR: Tendinitis, bursitis, impingement, "snapping" scapula, and calcific tendinitis. p. 105. In Rowe CR (ed): The Shoulder. Churchill Livingstone, New York, 1988

96. Neer CS, Watson KC, Stanton FJ: Recent experiences in total shoulder replacement. J Bone Joint Surg 64A:319, 1982

97. Brems JJ: Arthritis of recurrent dislocations. Presented at the annual meeting of the New York Orthopaedic Hospital Alumni Meeting, New York, 1984

98. Brems JJ: Degenerative joint disease in the shoulder. p. 237. In Hershman JA, Hershman EB (eds): The Upper Extremity in Sports Medicine. CV Mosby, St. Louis, 1990

99. Brunet ME, Haddad RJ, Porche EB: Rotator cuff impingement syndrome in sports. Phys Sports Med 10:86, 1982

100. Tullos HS, Bennett JB: The shoulder in sports. p. 110. In Scott WN, Nisonson B, Nicholas J (eds): Principles of Sports Medicine. Williams & Wilkins, Baltimore, 1984

101. Jobe C: Gross anatomy of the shoulder. In Rockwood CA, Matsen FA (eds): The Shoulder. WB Saunders, Philadelphia, 1990

102. Jobe FW, Bradley JP: The diagnosis and non-operative treatment of shoulder injuries in athletes. Clin Sports Med 8:430, 1989

103. Weismann S: Orthopedic Radiology. WB Saunders, Philadelphia, 1986

104. Cone RO, Danzig L, Resnick D, Goldman AB: The bicipital groove: radiographic, anatomic, and pathologic study. Am J Roentgenol 41:781, 1983

105. Hitchcock HH, Bechtol CO: Painful shoulder: observations on the role of the tendon of the long head of the biceps brachii in its causation. J Bone Joint Surg 30A:263, 1948

15

Sternoclavicular, Acromioclavicular, and Scapular Disorders

THOMAS A. SOUZA

The shoulder is a complex of joints and requires cooperation as a kinesiologic linkage for efficient movement. Dysfunction of any of the joints will have some degree of effect on the others. Movement among the joints of the shoulder complex is dependent on a balance between timing and function.

Dvir and Berme[1] describe a sequence of joining and uncoupling between the joints of the shoulder complex to allow function while maintaining stability through four phases of elevation. Phase 1 is the setting phase representing scapular stabilization. Then as the conoid ligament becomes taut there is a uniting of the previously independent units of the clavicle and scapula. This claviscapular linkage then rotates around an imaginary axis that extends from the sternoclavicular joint through a point at the medial spine of the scapula during phase 2. Phase 2 ends with tightening of the costoclavicular ligament. At this point the clavicle begins to rotate and the scapula follows. During phase 3 the scapula rotates about an axis extending through the acromioclavicular joint. This provides a stable yet moving platform for the humeral head. When the trapezoid ligament becomes taut phase 4 begins as the claviscapular linkage is re-established until further movement is structurally limited.

STERNOCLAVICULAR JOINT

Compared to the acromioclavicular and glenohumeral joints, the sternoclavicular joint is injured less often.[2]

This seems unusual when considering the bony anatomy and function of the joint. The sternoclavicular joint is one of the most mobile joints in the body due mainly to its inherent incongruency. It moves with most movements of the shoulder. However, it is supported by a very strong capsule. Additionally, when considering the mechanism of injury necessary to damage the sternoclavicular joint, it becomes apparent that the location of the joint is somewhat positionally protected so that direct trauma would require large forces, and indirect trauma requires unusual positioning of the shoulder. Also indirect forces are more likely to cause damage to the clavicle rather than the joint due to leverage and the ligamentous protection at the joint. Sports that might involve a side-lying position with compression such as wrestling or a pile-up in football are more likely to damage the sternoclavicular joint indirectly than direct blows or falls.[3]

Functional Anatomy

The medial end of the clavicle articulates with the sternum in a most incongruent manner (Fig. 15-1). Less than half of the articular surface is in contact with the sternum.[4] The shape of the medial clavicle is rather bulbous with a concave morphology anterior to posterior and convex vertically. Acting as mainly a saddle joint, the clavicle is capable of most movements. Limitation of these movements is mainly ligamentous.

There are several ligaments that contribute in varying degrees to the stability of the sternoclavicular joint.

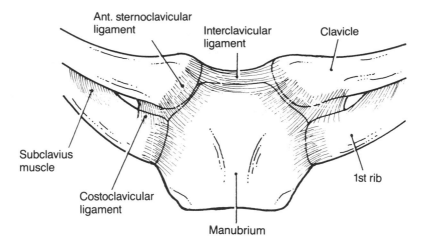

Fig. 15-1. Anatomy of the sternoclavicular joint. (From Rowe,[9] with permission.)

The extra-articular costoclavicular or rhomboid ligament is composed of two divisions with an intervening bursa. Analogous to the coracoclavicular, the costoclavicular ligaments have an anterior section and posterior section that are oriented in an oblique fashion crossing each other to provide support during rotation and elevation. The anterior section is oriented in a superolateral direction off of the first rib to the clavicle. The posterior section is lateral to the anterior and is directed superomedial. The anterior fibers prevent excessive superior or lateral displacement. The posterior fibers restrict excessive inferior and medial displacement.[5]

A dissecting intra-articular ligament divides the sternoclavicular joint connecting the junction of the first rib and sternum to the superior aspect of the medial clavicle, creating in essence two separate spaces. Apparently, the intra-articular disc ligament acts as a "checkrein" to medial displacement of the clavicle, in particular with elevation of the medial clavicle (as may occur in downward displacement of the arm).

The interclavicular ligament connects the two medial clavicle ends with the sternum and capsule. It acts to help support the suspensory role of the capsular ligaments thereby assisting in what Bearn[5] calls "shoulder poise." Shoulder poise describes the nonmuscular suspension of the arm at the clavicle. Grant[4] feels the interclavicular ligament may be homologous to the wishbone in birds. The interclavicular function can be indirectly appreciated by a palpable tautness felt on lowering of the arm and with a decrease in elevation illustrating its suspensory function.

Although the interclavicular ligament aids in suspending the shoulder, the main element is tension in the capsular ligaments. Thickenings of the joint capsule on the superior, anterior, and posterior aspects represent strong resistance to upward displacement of the medial clavicle. These capsular ligaments resist forces at the clavicle created by forceful downward movement of the shoulder. Bearn,[5] in his historical evaluation of the hierarchy of ligamentous support at the sternoclavicular joint, demonstrated through selective cutting that the capsular ligaments were necessary for the maintenance of "shoulder poise." In other words, elimination of the support from the intra-articular, costoclavicular, and interclavicular ligaments had no effect on poise. Only after division of the capsular ligaments was there a displacement of the outer clavicle downward. It must be noted that downward displacement may also occur with trapezius paralysis. Theoretically, this would be due to stretching of the capsular ligaments.

Movement at the sternoclavicular joint is described in relation to movements of the clavicle (Fig. 15-2). With full elevation of the arm there is a range of 30 to 35 degrees of upward movement combined with approximately 45 to 50 degrees of rotation about its long axis. With adduction and extension the clavicle has a combined range of about 35 degrees.[6]

Accessory movement is palpable due to the superfi-

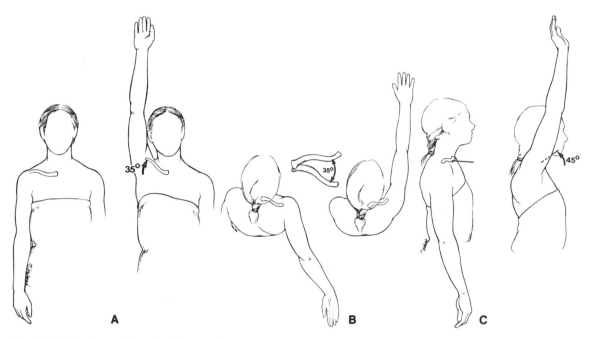

Fig. 15-2. Motions of the clavicle and the sternoclavicular joint. **(A)** With full overhead elevation the clavicle elevates 35 degrees. **(B)** With adduction and extension, the clavicle displaces anteriorly and posteriorly 35 degrees. **(C)** The clavicle rotates on its long axis 45 degrees, as the arm is elevated to the full overhead position. (From Rockwood and Green,[58] with permission.)

cial nature of the sternoclavicular joint location. Inferior glide is necessary for arm elevation. Anterior glide is necessary for shoulder (scapular) retraction; protraction requires posterior glide. Rotation is also a requisite accessory movement with humeral elevation.

Injuries of the Sternoclavicular Joint

Due to the stability provided by the capsular ligaments, it is unlikely for subluxation or dislocation to occur without outside force application. There are those individuals, however, with enough ligament laxity or those with previous trauma (leaving the ligaments attenuated but not torn) who may have spontaneous subluxation or dislocation. Usually this is not a painful process.[7]

The most common cause of dislocation/subluxation is an indirect force applied to the lateral aspect of the shoulder anteriorly or posteriorly. Both Mehta et al.[3] and Heinig[8] found in their small sample groups a vast majority of cases due to indirect force at the shoulder. The mechanism is simple to understand. With the per-

son lying on the uninvolved side, a force is applied to the lateral shoulder with either the arm in extension or in flexion (scapula protracted). In the extended (retracted) position the distal clavicle is directed posteriorly causing the more common anterior displacement of the medial clavicle (Fig. 15-3A). With the scapula protracted the distal aspect of the clavicle is forced forward driving the medial clavicle posteriorly (Fig. 15-3B). The most common sports scenario would be a pile-up in football on a player lying on his side. Falling on an outstretched hand with the arm abducted can also provide a similar mechanism.

Direct force application is more likely to cause the less common posterior dislocation. In sports, either a kick to the medial clavicle or perhaps a player landing on the clavicle of a supine player will drive the clavicle posteriorly behind the sternum. Due to the proximity of the trachea, aorta, and other vessels, this injury is life-threatening (Fig. 15-4). Jockeys have described this injury as "a brush with death."[9]

A review of dislocations by Omer[10] suggests that approximately 80 percent of injuries were due to either

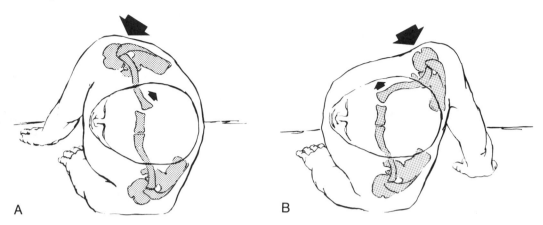

Fig. 15-3. Mechanisms that produce anterior or posterior dislocations of the sternoclavicular joint. **(A)** If the patient is lying on the ground and a compression force is applied to the posterior lateral aspect of the shoulder, the medial end of the clavicle will be displaced posteriorly. **(B)** When the lateral compression force is directed from the anterior position, the medial end of the clavicle is dislocated anteriorly. (From Rockwood and Green,[58] with permission.)

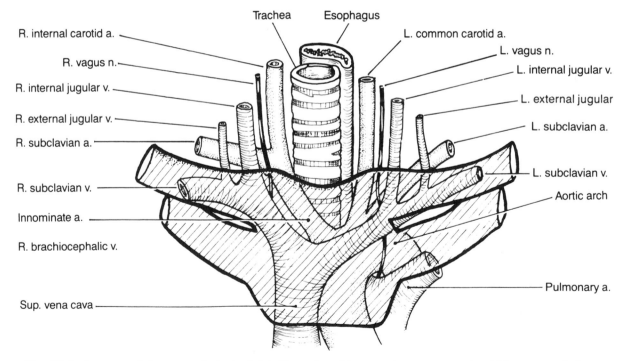

Fig. 15-4. Anatomy of the sternoclavicular joint. The vulnerable posterior structures should be constantly kept in mind. (From Rowe,[9] with permission.)

motor vehicle accidents or sports injuries. The motor vehicle accidents caused slightly more injuries. The incidence is so low that some orthopaedists may never see a sternoclavicular dislocation.[11]

As with all joint/ligament injuries, there is a gradation of severity. Mild strains may present with mild to moderate pain increasing with upper extremity elevation. Swelling and tenderness may be present. Moderate sprains involving partial tearing of the ligaments will present with similar signs and symptoms with the addition of either visual static subluxation or palpable subluxation upon movement. It is important to note that the differences between second and third degree sprains may represent perhaps attenuation to the point of nonfunctioning of the ligaments without total rupture.

Third degree sprains represent rupture, in most cases with an obvious deformity. Pain is severe and increased by any movement of the arm or lateral compression of the shoulders bilaterally (pressing them together). The patient position will usually include a forward looking shoulder usually supported across the trunk. Lying back, the shoulder does not reach the table and pain is increased. Due to sternocleidomastoid spasm the head may be tilted toward and rotated away from the dislocated side.[7]

Differentiating between anterior and posterior dislocations may academically appear obvious; however, the signs and symptoms may be similar and the mechanism of injury may not be readily apparent. Some differentiating signs may include a more prominent medial clavicle with anterior dislocation. Posterior dislocation is usually much more painful with accompanying signs of vessel, nerve, esophageal, or tracheal compression. Therefore, the patient with a posterior dislocation may have difficulty breathing or swallowing with a sensation of choking possible. Venous congestion signs or decreased circulation to the ipsilateral upper extremity may be evident. A pneumothorax may complicate the presentation.

Rockwood[7] notes that several patients who presented clinically with an anterior dislocation were later found to have posterior dislocation on radiograph. This observation conflicts with the older concept that clinical evaluation was more accurate than radiographic evaluation. This view was in part held because of the difficulty interpreting standard or oblique views. Due to the overlap of the sternoclavicular joint on oblique views and the inability to obtain a true 90 degree tangential view, confusion was common. Many specialized views have been recommended by a host of authors. The two views that are recommended by Rockwood and others include the Hobbs' and serendipity views.

The Hobbs'[12] projection view is almost a lateral view from a superior-inferior perspective (Fig. 15-5). The patient sits or stands at the table bucky and leans forward over the cassette, which rests on the table top. Leaning on the elbows the patient rests the anterior rib cage on the edge of the cassette positioning the neck to be parallel with the film. The beam is directed through the cervical spine and sternoclavicular joints.

The serendipity view by Rockwood[13] involves the patient lying supine on the table with an 11 × 14 cassette placed under them (Fig. 15-6). The beam is directed through the superior sternum at an angle of 40 degrees from the vertical at a distance of 60 inches with adults or 45 inches with children. The technique

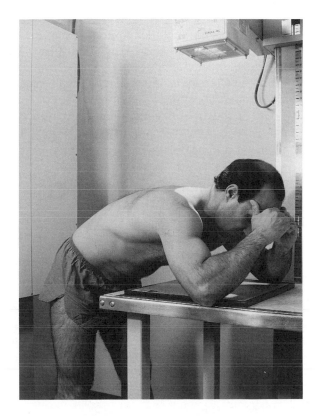

Fig. 15-5. The Hobb's projection view.

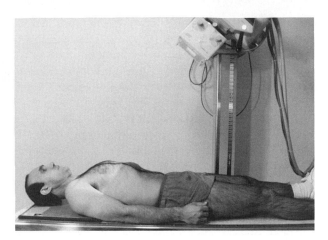

Fig. 15-6. The serendipity view.

should be similar to a posterior to anterior chest view. Both sternoclavicular joints must be included to gain a comparative perspective. A clavicle that appears to ride high on the medial end represents an anterior dislocation. An inferior positioning indicates a posterior dislocation.

Advanced imaging includes tomograms and computed tomography (CT) scans. They both provide a better evaluation for distinguishing fractures from dislocations, but CT scans are superior.[7] The CT scan can clearly illustrate, for example, compression of vascular and other structures from a posterior dislocation. It is important that both sternoclavicular joints be included for comparative purposes.

Treatment of Sternoclavicular Injuries

Mild strains of the sternoclavicular joint are managed with the standard approach for all strains: ice, rest, and support for a few days in a sling. Second degree sprains, by some definitions, may be subluxated. The reduction can be accomplished by drawing the shoulders back whether anterior or posteriorly subluxated. There are many different suggestions for bracing ranging from a soft figure-eight with a shoulder splint to a hard figure-eight splint. The intent of the shoulder support or splint is to reduce the traction stress on the sternoclavicular ligaments. If not reducible, it is probably better to splint without reduction. Surgical pinning with moderate sprains carries with it serious complications.[9] If pain is persistent, a torn articular disc or ligament may be demonstrated on surgical exploration.

A dilemma exists for the closed reduction of anterior sternoclavicular dislocations. Although it may be possible to reduce without anesthesia, they rarely stay reduced. This is apparently acceptable. Long-term subluxation or recurrent dislocation can be treated with Steinmann pins or Kirschner's wires, but there have been reports of migration of these stabilizing apparatus. Rockwood[7] and others feel that it is best left untreated or surgically approached with medial resection of the clavicle.

Chronic Sternoclavicular Disorders

When a patient presents with a long-standing sternoclavicular complaint it usually will be of pain or crepitus. Swelling may be present and necessitates a long list of differentials. One of the first considerations is the possibility of an unreduced dislocation. In an older individual, the possibility of osteoarthritis or other arthritides should be considered (Table 15-1). Ankylosing spondylitis is a specific condition that has been noted to create marked radiographic changes at the sternoclavicular and acromioclavicular joints and present with glenohumeral restriction patterns. However, the correlation between radiographic changes and clinical presentation seems to be poor.[14]

There are several unusual disorders. Sonozaki et al.[15] reported a number of cases in Japan that involved sternoclavicular hyperostosis. This peculiar disorder affects either sex usually between the ages of 30 and 50 years. The process involves an ossification of the ligaments about the sternoclavicular joint later to involve the bone. Sonozaki et al. found varying degrees of involvement ranging from mild cases of ligamentous involvement to a full bony block between the rib, clavicle, and sternum. The more severe stages may significantly impair motion at the glenohumeral joint as reported by Dohler.[16]

Another condition is referred to as condensing osteitis of the medial clavicle.[17] Apparently more common in women over the age of 40, the patient will usually have a tender swollen joint and a history of chronic overuse. Radiography may reveal sclerosis of the inferior medial border of the clavicle. Bone scans may show an increase in uptake. CT scans are reported as

Table 15-1. Differential Diagnosis of Chronic Sternoclavicular Disorders

Disorder	Findings
Sternoclavicular hyperostosis	Age 30–50 Ossification of ligaments and possibly bone Radiograph diagnosis
Osteitis of medial clavicle	More common in women over 40 Tender swollen joint; history of overuse Radiograph may show sclerosis if inferior/medial clavicle Bone scan may show increased uptake Computed tomography scan is best imaging tool
Friedreich's disease	Aseptic necrosis of the medial clavicle
Postmenopausal arthritis	Involves dominant arm sternoclavicular joint Probably represents acceleration of normal degeneration Involved sternoclavicular joint is enlarged Radiograph demonstrates degenerative arthritis with possible enlargement or subluxation
Hypermobile sternoclavicular joint	Patient complains of constant clicking or snapping at sternoclavicular joint Possible history of past sternoclavicular injury or repetitive activity More common with specific maneuvers such as retracting or protracting shoulders Popping at sternoclavicular should be reproducible Adjusting the sternoclavicular joint may bring relief temporarily Modification of activity to avoid extreme protraction/retraction of shoulders
Tietze syndrome	Patient usually female; middle-aged History may be unremarkable or report of overuse from pushing or coughing Pain is over costochondral junction and in intercostal space of upper ribs usually Treatment may include a trial of "drop-table" adjusting with a broad contact over area If conservative care fails, cortisone injection usually effective
Arthropathies	Literally any arthropathy can affect the sternoclavicular joint Usually a comprehensive history coupled with lab and radiograph reveal the cause

the best imaging tool to visualize this idiopathic process. Differentiation will need to be made between other arthropathies, Tietze syndrome, Paget's disease, sternoclavicular hyperostosis, Friedreich's disease (aseptic necrosis of the medial end of the clavicle), and postmenopausal arthritis.

Postmenopausal arthritis involves the dominant arm sternoclavicular joint and probably represents an acceleration of a normal degenerative process.[18] The patient may present with a lump over the involved sterno-

clavicular joint. Radiographic findings are those of degenerative arthritis with possible sclerosis, enlargement, and possible subluxation.

Patients with hypermobile sternoclavicular joints often present with a complaint of audibly irritating, yet painless, clicking or crepitus. It is often found that this occurs with any extreme of motion such as full horizontal adduction, horizontal abduction, or elevation. Add to these movements an extension or weight to the long lever of the arm such as a ball, bat, racquet, or weight apparatus, and the problem is naturally magnified. In particular with weightlifting, it must be assumed that either through chronic attenuation the capsular ligaments have become stretched enough not to support the sternoclavicular joint, or that repetitive microtrauma has resulted in degenerative changes with the intra-articular disc or ligament perhaps being torn. Modification includes avoiding end range on the descent of a bench press or the fully open position of a fly maneuver.

Chiropractic management may include adjusting the sternoclavicular joint. Immobilization for a few days may aid in resolving the complaint, but aggravating maneuvers must be religiously avoided.

Static palpation can be misleading. Asymmetry is not uncommon. Hypomobile sternoclavicular joints are best palpated with passive and active movement of the involved side shoulder. Restrictions can affect glenohumeral movement indirectly. Adjustment for the sternoclavicular joint is described in detail in Chapter 19.

Fractures of the Proximal and Distal Clavicle

Although fractures may or may not be within the scope of the chiropractor, depending on the state practiced in, it is important to understand that although anecdotally benign, fractures of the clavicle may present with serious complications. Fragments can injure the lung apices, subclavian vessels, or brachial plexus with accompanying related signs and symptoms.

Fractures of either end of the clavicle are most likely due to a fall on an outstretched arm. Other possibilities include the same mechanisms for sternoclavicular dislocation with direct and indirect forces possible. The signs and symptoms are typical of most long bone fractures such as an audible snap or pop at the time of injury accompanied by pain and possibly crepitus on

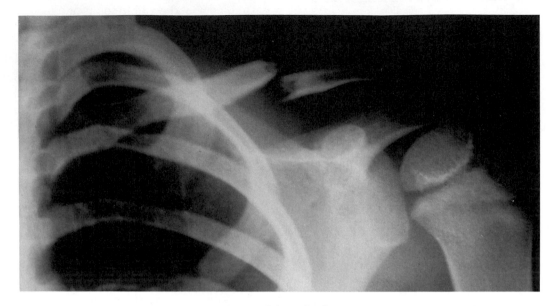

Fig. 15-7. Midclavicular fracture.

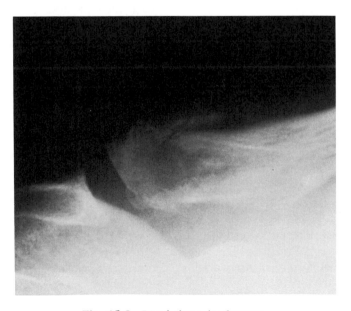

Fig. 15-8. Distal clavicular fracture.

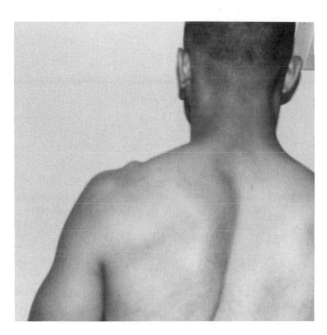

Fig. 15-9. Bump deformity from a third degree acromioclavicular separation.

movement. Swelling, tenderness, and deformity will usually be obvious. Identification is easily made radiographically (Fig. 15-7). Fractures of the distal end of the clavicle are possible with a fall on the tip of the shoulder and should be considered in all cases clinically resembling acromioclavicular separation (Fig. 15-8).

On-the-field management of a suspected fracture would be dependent on whether an open wound was present. Sterile protection should be provided to an open wound with no attempt at reduction. Even reduction of nonpenetrating fractures on-the-field may involve risk due to the inability to determine where fragments are positioned.

Reduction after radiographic clarification is usually the same as for the dislocation of the sternoclavicular joint with retraction of the shoulders posteriorly. A figure-eight brace is worn for about 6 weeks at which time callus formation should be readily apparent on radiography. Return to sports must involve proper rehabilitation prior to return to full activity.

When fractures are unstable it is important to remember that, like second and third degree acromi-

oclavicular separations, the residual problem is primarily cosmetic and not functional. A general rule is not to expect perfect congruent union (avoid criticizing the lack of acumen of the treating orthopaedist) but expect full function. The same complications of migration of wires or pins are still possible with an attempt at surgical fixation.

ACROMIOCLAVICULAR JOINT

Acromioclavicular injuries are extremely common in sports. If the athlete falls directly on the tip of the shoulder acromioclavicular damage is likely. Given the superficial and peripheral location of the acromioclavicular joint, the deformity from a second or third degree separation is usually quite evident (Fig. 15-9). It was recognized as early as the time of Hippocrates[19] several hundred years BC. He, in fact, advised physicians on the importance of differentiating between a glenohumeral dislocation and acromioclavicular separation, warning that disastrous results would occur if the acromioclavicular separation was treated with the then standard relocation techniques for dislocation at the glenohumeral joint.

Functional Anatomy of the Acromioclavicular Joint

The acromioclavicular joint is a diarthrodial joint. The acromial and clavicular ends change from hyaline to fibrocartilage at different rates. The acromial end reaches later maturity at age 23 or 24. The clavicle reaches maturity at about age 17.[20] A disc or meniscus exists between these two bones that may be complete or partial. Marked degeneration occurs in the disc leaving it functionally useless by age 40.[21-23] Osteoarthritic changes on the undersurface may predispose an individual to impingement of the underlying tendons and bursa. Like the sternoclavicular joint there are many variations to the slope and angle of the acromioclavicular articulation (Fig. 15-10). The slope of the acromion and angulation of the acromioclavicular joint may be important factors with regard to impingement and separation of the joint. DePalma[24] and Moseley[25] have classified these variations in slope and angulation into different types. The three general possibilities include a vertical articulation, one where the clavicle overrides the acromion at varying degrees, and an underriding clavicle. Statistically, the most common is the overrid-

ing type representing about half of the articulations. Moseley[25] found that from experience (and from visual understanding of the injury mechanism), the vertical and underriding types were more prone to injury. The vertical type would be less stable osseously and the underriding type would be more prone to compressive injury.

Ligamentous support of the acromioclavicular joint is provided by a relatively thin capsule with some reinforcement from the acromioclavicular ligaments. The superior and inferior portions are not as well developed as the anterior and posterior components. This reinforcement anteriorly and posteriorly prevents horizontal movement. The true support, however, is provided by the coracoclavicular ligaments, which prevent excessive movements of the clavicle on the acromion (Fig. 15-11). There are two components: the more medial cone-shaped conoid ligament and the more lateral trapezoid ligament. Both arising from the coracoid process and inserting on the undersurface of the clavicle, the conoid attaches to the conoid tubercle with the trapezoid attaching just anterior and lateral to this point with an occasional intervening bursa. The two divisions of the coracoclavicular ligament function to prevent vertical movement.[26] The sternoclavicular ligaments help maintain the distal elevation of the clavicle while the coracoclavicular ligaments prevent excessive elevation. The trapezoid aids in rotation of the clavicle during elevation.

Although a ligamentous connection exists between the coracoid process and acromion, the coracoacromial ligament represents more a source of irritation than support of any kind. It is the primary culprit in impingement syndrome of the glenohumeral joint.

It is important to note the muscular support provided by the deltoid and upper trapezius muscles, which find attachment at the site of the acromioclavicular joint. Consideration of this factor is important in devising a rehabilitation program for moderate to severe sprains/separations.

Movement at the acromioclavicular joint was first discussed by Codman,[27] who noted very little movement, yet in many directions. This was contradicted by the work of Inman et al.[28] who suggested as much as 20 degrees of movement occurring mainly in the first and last degrees of abduction. This conclusion was reached following a set of interesting experiments where a coracoclavicular pin was inserted to observe

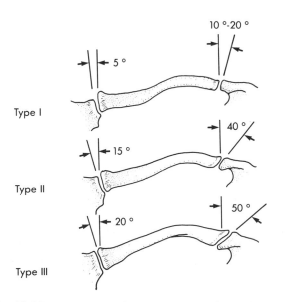

Fig. 15-10. Variations in the acromioclavicular and sternoclavicular articulations. (From Hurley,[59] with permission.)

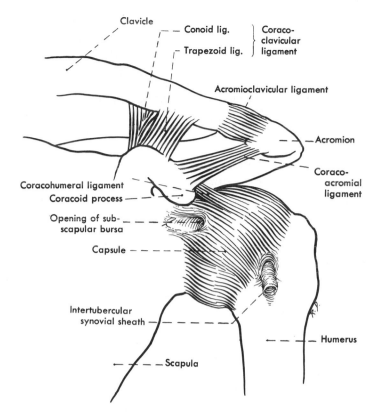

Fig. 15-11. Ligaments of the acromioclavicular and glenohumeral articulations. (From Hollinshead and Jenkins,[57] with permission.)

movement and note the consequent restrictions. Their observations indicated that abduction (or overhead elevation) was limited to 110 degrees. This led to the assumption that the corrective coracoclavicular pins would be detrimental to full function of the shoulder.

More recently, it has been reported by numerous authors that when an arthrodesis at the acromioclavicular joint (imposed surgically or acquired) or between the coracoid and clavicle was present, minimal dysfunction at the end range of elevation resulted. Examples include the coracoclavicular screw technique of Kennedy and Cameron and Kennedy,[30] which demonstrated that limitation was based on how far down the pin or screw was depressed. In other words, the more inferior the clavicle was depressed the more restriction occurred. Rockwood and Young[31] noted that with acquired arthrodesis of the coracoid and clavicle following acromioclavicular surgery, no restriction to full elevation was evident. It would be interesting to note

in a retrospective study the effects of a fixation over time in an athletic individual. In other words, full function in a nonstressful situation may be different than chronic overload in an overhead position such as occurs in many sports.

Separate pins placed in the acromion and clavicle in close proximity to the joint were used to observe movement. The degree of pin movement remained within 5 to 7 degrees at the joint whether passive or active movements were used.[13] This further illustrates the observation that the clavicle and scapula rotate together (synchronous scapuloclavicular rotation). Therefore, although there is a fair amount of rotation about the long axis of the clavicle, movement specific to the joint is limited due to the combined movement of both bones. This explanation serves well to explain Caldwell's observation[32] in 1943 that patients retained almost full range of motion (ROM) following arthrodesis of the acromioclavicular joint.

Mechanism of Injury

The acromion and distal clavicle can be chronically irritated through repetitive compression as occurs in weightlifting. Traction injury can occur from the pull of the deltoid or trapezius muscle from repetitive maneuvers or a fall on the tip of the shoulder. Other disorders are insidious or reveal a past history of damage with chronic complaints.

For the stabilizing ligaments of the acromion and clavicle to be injured or disrupted, the acromion must be forced inferior on the clavicle. This mechanism is the most common cause usually due to a fall on the tip of the shoulder with the arm in adduction. Other mechanisms are a fall on the hand or elbow of an outstretched arm and a hit to the posterior shoulder with the arm in an outstretched position. This latter mechanism can drive the clavicle away from the acromion with injury more specific to the acromioclavicular joint. The coracoclavicular ligaments are not at risk due to the approximation rather than stretch of these ligaments. The author has seen a second degree tear imposed by a palm-hit to the bottom of the clavicle.

There is a sequence of stress acceptance with either mechanism. First the sternoclavicular ligaments tense to prevent upward displacement of the clavicle. This resistance is quite strong resulting in stress distribution to the clavicle itself or the acromioclavicular/coracoclavicular ligaments. Therefore, either a fracture or varying degrees of tearing of the ligaments may occur. Further disruption can involve tearing of the muscular support including the deltoid and upper trapezius.

The sequence of tearing has led to a grading process of separation (Fig. 15-12).[33] There is some discrepancy in this classification, but, generally it is accepted that a type I separation involves minimal tearing of the acromioclavicular ligament with no laxity. Type II involves complete disruption of the acromioclavicular ligament with accompanying upward movement of the clavicle. Type III tears represent a three ligament disruption involving the acromioclavicular, conoid, and trapezoid ligaments. The deltoid and trapezius muscle are often detached from their clavicular attachment. An extended classification was developed by Rockwood.[34] A type IV is similar to type III with the addition of posterior translation of the clavicle into or through the upper trapezius. A type V injury is a more severe type III injury with severe dislocation of the acromion (as much as 100 to 300 percent greater than the comparative normal). The type VI injury is again similar to the type III; however, the clavicle is displaced inferior to the acromion or coracoid process. The mechanism of injury for the type VI injury is probably a direct blow to the superior distal clavicle while the arm is abducted and the scapula retracted.

When instability is present a deformity exists at the acromioclavicular joint (Fig. 15-9). Visually this would appear to be due to upward displacement of the clavicle. It is true that some minor displacement is probably caused by the trapezius muscle; however, the majority of the deformity is caused by the downward sagging of the unsupported upper extremity.[31] This is clearly evident on radiographs demonstrating a second or third degree sprain where the involved clavicle is es-

Fig. 15-12. Schematic drawings of the classification of ligamentous injuries to the acromioclavicular joint. **(A)** In the type I injury a mild force applied to the point of the shoulder does not disrupt either the acromioclavicular or the coracoclavicular ligaments. **(B)** A moderate to heavy force applied to the point of the shoulder will disrupt the acromioclavicular ligaments, but the coracoclavicular ligaments remain intact. **(C)** When a severe force is applied to the point of the shoulder both the acromioclavicular and the coracoclavicular ligaments are disrupted. **(D)** In a type IV injury not only are the ligaments disrupted but the distal end of the clavicle is also displaced posteriorly into or through the trapezius muscle. **(E)** A violent force applied to the point of the shoulder not only ruptures the acromioclavicular and coracoclavicular ligaments, but also disrupts the muscle attachments and creates a major separation between the clavicle and the acromion. **(F)** This is an inferior dislocation of the distal clavicle in which the clavicle is inferior to the coracoid process and posterior to the biceps and coracobrachialis tendons. The acromioclavicular and coracoclavicular ligaments are also disrupted. (From Rockwood and Green,[61] with permission.)

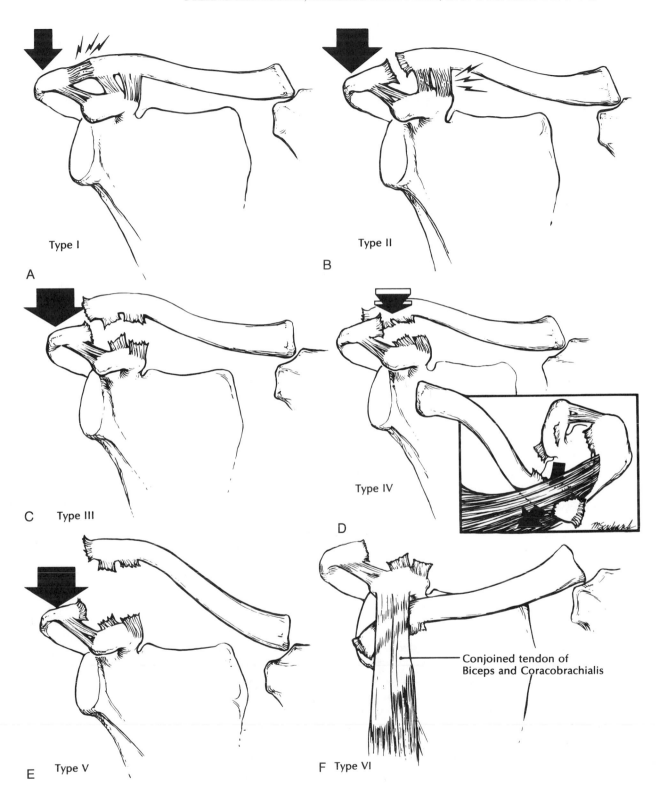

Type I

A

Type II

B

Type III

C

Type IV

D

Type V

E

Type VI

F

Conjoined tendon of
Biceps and Coracobrachialis

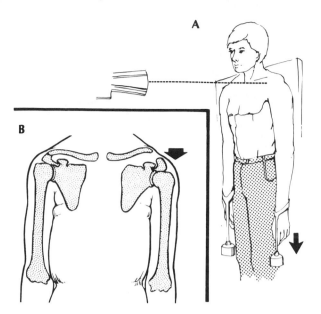

Fig. 15-13. Technique of obtaining stress radiographic views of the acromioclavicular joint. **(A)** Anteroposterior radiographs are made of both acromioclavicular joints with 10 to 15 lb of weight hanging from the wrists. **(B)** The distance between the superior aspect of the coracoid and the undersurface of the clavicle is measured to determine whether the coracoclavicular ligaments have been disrupted. One large horizontal 14 × 17 inch x-ray cassette can be used in small patients to visualize both shoulders on the same film. In large patients it is better to use two horizontal smaller cassettes and take two separate radiographs for the measurements. (From Rockwood and Green,[61] with permission.)

sentially in line with the opposite clavicle (no upward displacement). However, the upper extremity "sags" below the contralateral normal side (Fig. 15-13).

Testing of the Acromioclavicular Joint

In acute injuries it is often possible to deduce from the injury mechanism and patient appearance that the acromioclavicular joint is injured. However, occasionally there is a questionable or unclear mechanism and the pain is less localized. In these situations and with patients presenting with chronic complaints, provocative maneuvers are helpful. It is necessary to test the acromioclavicular joint for pain reproduction with positions that maximally compress the joint (the close-

packed position). For the acromioclavicular joint, the extremes of elevation and horizontal adduction maximally compress the joint. This may be accomplished actively or passively. Due to pain constraints, the passive testing approach seems easiest. Classically, passive movement of the arm into full abduction will not give a painful arc of discomfort in the range of 70 to 110 degrees with acromioclavicular joint involvement, but after this "impingement" range. Active and passive horizontal adduction also provides a clear reproduction of the patient's complaint toward end range (Fig. 15-14A). A squeeze test will locally compress the joint, but the examiner must be careful to use a broad palm contact to eliminate "palpation" tenderness as opposed to compression pain (Fig. 15-14B). Finally, upward compression using the flexed elbow as the support and directing an axial force upward through the shoulder may elicit pain (Fig. 15-14C). However, this maneuver may impinge other structures and is not specific.

Radiographic examination of the acromioclavicular joint is specific and separate from evaluation of the glenohumeral joint. To achieve a quality film the acromioclavicular joint requires about half of the intensity used on a glenohumeral technique. Also there must be a 10 to 15 degrees cephalad tilt of the tube,[35] otherwise there is superimposition of the acromioclavicular joint over the spine of the scapula making detection of small fractures difficult (Fig. 15-15).

Radiographic evaluation is often necessary to determine the degree of acromioclavicular separation. Differentiating between a type II and type III injury is often difficult on clinical evaluation. Weighted and nonweighted bilateral views are taken (Fig. 15-16). Most patient's shoulders will fit on a 14 × 17 cassette; however, larger individuals may require two 10 × 12 cassettes. The importance of strapping the weights to the wrist as opposed to having the patient grip the weights cannot be overemphasized.[31] A simple self-test will demonstrate that while gripping tightly with the hand, muscles in the shoulder contract, possibly decreasing the amount of measurable instability on the radiograph. A separation visible on the nonweighted view would represent a third degree tear.

Although the coracoclavicular distance can be measured to determine the amount of separation, many factors can distort this measurement. For example, the distance of the patient to the cassette and the distance

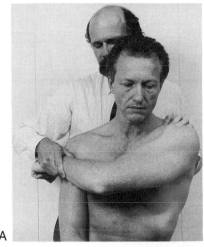

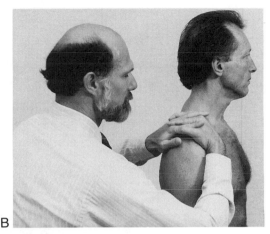

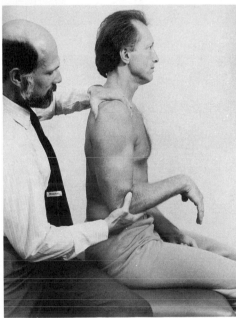

Fig. 15-14. Acromioclavicular joint testing. **(A)** Horizontal adduction; **(B)** compression; and **(C)** Shultz test.

from the tube can alter the measurement. Normally, the coracoclavicular distance is between 1.1 cm and 1.3 cm (Fig. 15-17).[26,36] More importantly, however, is the comparison with the opposite (assumed well) shoulder. Bearden et al.[26] indicate that a difference of 40 to 50 percent indicates complete dislocation (separation). However, Rockwood and Young[31] suggest that as little as 25 percent difference may indicate complete disruption of the coracoclavicular ligaments.[31]

Treatment of Acromioclavicular Separations

There is little disagreement as to the treatment of first and second degree strains of the acromioclavicular joint (Table 15-2). Conservative care consisting of rest, ice, and splinting is considered standard. Often return to sports activity is within days to a week with the application of protective padding and/or taping. Rehabilita-

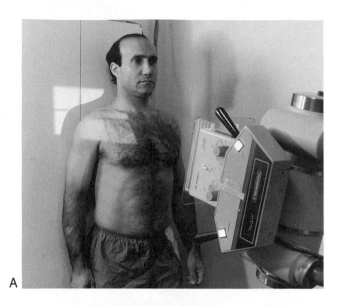

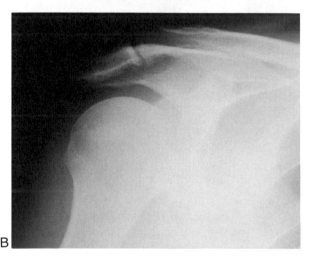

Fig. 15-15. (A) 10 degree tilt view of acromioclavicular joint; **(B)** spur formation at acromioclavicular joint.

tion of second degree sprains involves mainly a focus on the deltoid and trapezius muscles.

Specifically, type I sprains are rehabilitated when any swelling has dissipated and ROM is near maximum. For a period of 4 to 6 weeks it is ill-advised to perform any overhead activities or horizontal flexion exercises. Specifically bar dips, bench presses (especially with a wide grip), or moderate to heavy dead lifts should be avoided for at least 2 to 3 weeks. All of these exercises will potentially aggravate any residual inflammation.

Type II sprains require a period of immobilization. Usually a Kinney-Howard type of sling is preferred (Fig. 15-18).[37] It offers the advantage of addressing both the concern of support of the upper extremity as well as compression of the distal clavicle. These actions are provided by stabilizing the clavicle with the dependency of the ipsilateral arm. Modification of the brace allows stabilization against the contralateral chest to avoid sliding off the shoulder. Rehabilitation is begun with isometrics while wearing the brace followed by

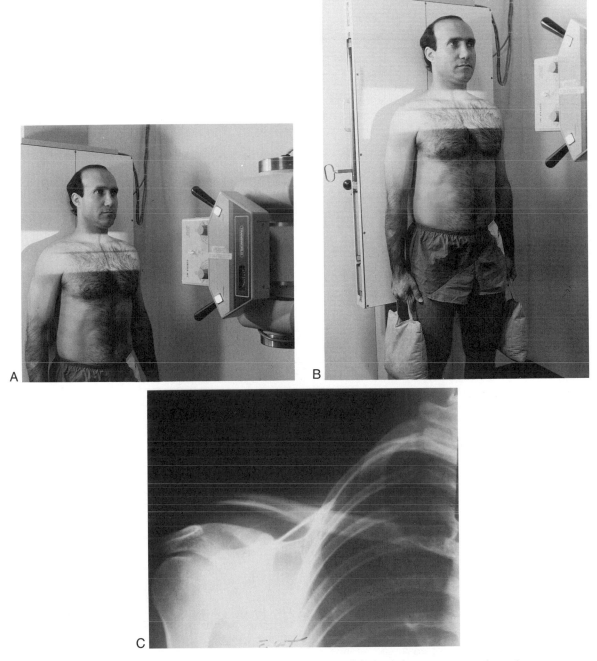

Fig. 15-16. **(A)** Nonweighted view setup; **(B)** weighted setup; **(C)** third degree acromioclavicular separation.

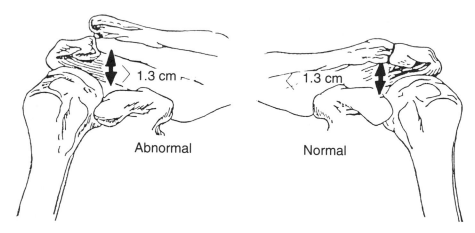

Fig. 15-17. One hundred percent displacement or more than 1.3 cm between the coracoid silhouette and the distal clavicle usually indicates a third degree acromioclavicular joint sprain. (From Reid,[60] with permission.)

elastic tubing or free weight exercises after 1 to 2 weeks. The focus of the exercises is to restore stability of the glenohumeral and acromioclavicular joints while avoiding end-range elevation and horizontal adduction. Specifically for the acromioclavicular joint, deltoid and trapezius exercises involving forward flexion and shoulder shrugs are incorporated. Return to sports is often possible within 2 to 3 weeks depending on the athlete, specific sport involved, and rehabilitation adherence. The previously mentioned caution with bar dips, bench presses, and heavy dead lifts should be in effect for at least 6 weeks. Residual pain and crepitus is not uncommon with type II separations. Relief can be achieved in some cases with mobilization or manipulation (see Ch. 19).

Treatment of third degree tears is more controversial, but the trend is toward a more conservative approach. Focus in the acute stage is the prevention of pain. The strapping method used by Hippocrates is still used by some. Galen in the second century found it to be very painful and removed it when treating his own acromioclavicular separation.[19] Taping or tight strapping causes compression of an already irritated joint and often results in excruciating pain. The author finds that a figure-eight clavicular brace worn with a Kinney-Howard sling is effective, usually worn for a

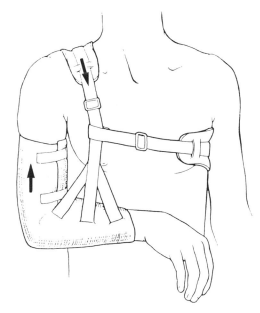

Fig. 15-18. Severe second and third degrees injuries can be treated by a modified Kinney-Howard shoulder harness. The strap that runs over the top of the shoulder and under the elbow is tightened sufficiently to reduce the clavicle to the acromion. A halter strap around the trunk keeps the pad from slipping off the shoulder. (From Reid,[60] with permission.)

Table 15-2. Treatment of Acromioclavicular Joint Injury

Acromioclavicular separations
  Type I—sprain (first degree separation)
    Ice and analgesics for pain control
    Rehabilitative exercises may begin quickly because acromioclavicular joint is stable
    Protective doughnut pad should be worn during contract sport participation
  Type II—partial subluxation (second degree separation—torn acromioclavicular ligament)
    Ice and analgesics
    Immobilization with Kinney-Howard sling with following recommendations:

1. Two slings are used so that the athlete may shower with support
2. Changing slings should be done only with the elbow supported
3. Tightening of the sling should also be done with elbow support
4. Sling is worn for 2–6 weeks depending on extent of injury

  Isometrics may be performed while in the sling using the opposite hand (elevation of the arm or shoulder is avoided)
  After sling, rehabilitation of shoulder muscles with emphasis on:

1. Deltoid with shrugs and raises (limited to below 90 degrees initially)
2. Trapezius with shrugs and front rows
3. Biceps
4. Pectorals with light weights and avoiding extremes of horizontal adduction initially

  Return to sport requires protective pad sewn or taped in place
  Type III—total separation (third degree separation—torn acromioclavicular and coracoclavicular ligaments)
    Ice, analgesics for pain
    Options suggested by various authors:

1. Immobilization for 4–6 weeks in a Kinney-Howard sling with above rehabilitation (author's choice)
2. No immobilization with use of progressive exercises and sports participation with protection in 2–4 weeks
3. Surgical repair which includes the following options:

    a. Stabilize clavicle to coracoid with a screw
    b. Resection of lateral clavicle
    c. Transarticular acromioclavicular fixation with pins
    d. Use of coracoacromial ligament as substitute acromioclavicular ligament

Osteolysis of the Distal Clavicle
  Suggested options include
    Athlete retires from competitive weightlifting
    Modification of weightlifting activities including

1. Substitute bench press with incline or decline press, or cross-cable exercises
2. Modify bench press using close grip instead of wide grip; reduce weight used
3. Eliminate dips and substitute with above pectoral exercises and triceps extensions

    Surgery—usually resection of lateral/distal clavicle

Shoulder Pointer and Acromial Apophysitis
  Ice and analgesics
  Avoid overhead activities for several weeks, in particular, with weights
  Protect with acromial (doughnut) pad

week or two. Slippage can be prevented by a modification that stabilizes the brace against the opposite thorax.

When the athlete is ready to return to play it is advisable to protect the acromioclavicular joint with padding taped on or worn under other protective padding. Figure 15-19 demonstrates a taping approach that has two purposes: (1) stabilization of a protective pad, and (2) some mild support. Three anchor strips are used: one on the arm, another on the chest, and a third over the shoulder binding down part of the foam pad. Next a weave pattern begins with cross strips applied to the shoulder and down the arm. These are followed by a basket weave following the pattern of the shoulder and chest anchors. This can then be stabilized with a figure-eight shoulder spica using 3 inch elastic taping. This approach is probably most helpful in athletes who may be involved in contact or collision sports who do not wear protective padding as part of the regular equipment.

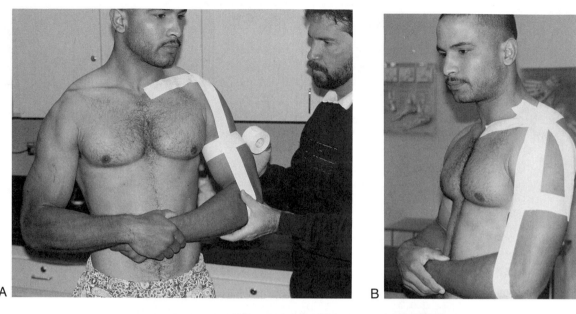

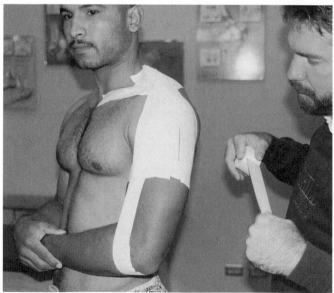

Fig. 15-19. (A–I) Protective taping for acromioclavicular injury. *(Figure continues.)*

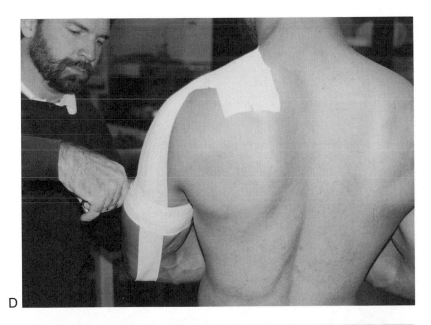

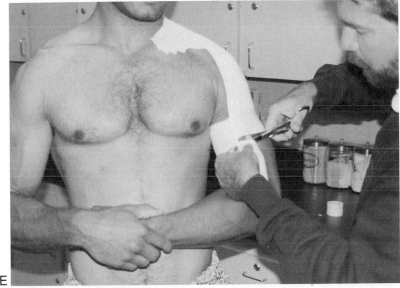

Fig. 15-19. *(Figure continues.)*

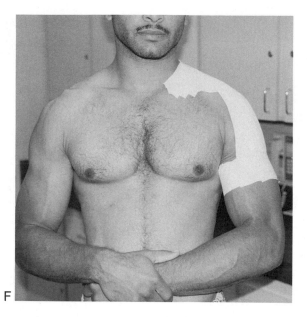

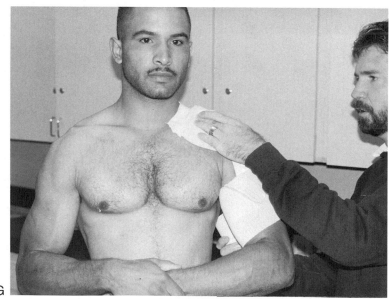

Fig. 15-19. *(Figure continues.)*

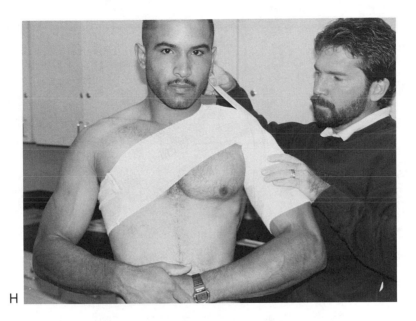

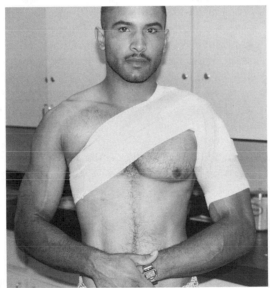

Fig. 15-19. *(Figure continues.)*

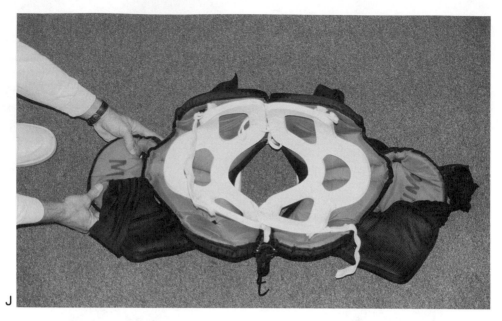

Fig. 15-19. *(continued).* **(J)** Protective shoulder padding for football with acromioclavicular with protection *(white insert).*

In a study by Glick et al.[38] that followed the status of 35 unreduced acromioclavicular separations over time, it was found that the vast majority were able to return to full sports activity very quickly when properly rehabilitated without immobilization after injury. Most of those who were not able to return for weeks had associated injuries that complicated return. Some of the patients included professional football quarterbacks, a javelin thrower, and a tennis instructor. Nineteen of the 35 patients were football players. Eighty percent of the throwers had no effect on their activity. It is important to note that conservative nonsurgical care resulted in a comparatively earlier return to sports activity with comparable long-term follow-up. The trade-off for the athlete in most cases is a residual bump deformity with conservative care or a scar with surgery.

Although the trend has switched back and forth between conservative and surgical management of type III separations, currently the tendency is shifting back to a conservative trend advocated in the 1940s. Others have found conservative treatment effective in the treatment of type III separations.[39–41] More recently Tibone et al.[42] have demonstrated in a follow-up of 20 male patients with type III acromioclavicular tears, no significant strength deficit as a result of conservative management. These patients were examined with a Cybex II dynamometer in all movements at 60 and 120 degrees/s comparing the injured to the uninjured side. The average follow-up was 4.5 years. Their recommendation is that most type III separations be treated conservatively. They do note that subjective complaints are fairly common, yet functional capacity is maintained.

There are a number of surgical procedures that have developed over the years starting in 1861 with Samuel Cooper who performed the first repair with a single silver wire.[43] Currently, surgical treatment usually involves distal clavicular resection. Although the results are excellent, this approach should be reserved for those with unsuccessful attempts at conservative management.

OSTEOLYSIS OF THE DISTAL CLAVICLE

A sequela that may occur several months following severe injury to the acromioclavicular joint is osteolysis of the lateral end of the clavicle. Injury may be due to subluxations, dislocations, or fractures. Pain is usually diffuse and aggravated by compressive positions of the acromioclavicular joint. Radiography will reveal lateral clavicular subchondral defects, cystic changes, and a gap of translucency at the joint. Treatment involves rest from aggravating positions, especially sports if possible for a prolonged period of time until symptoms are eliminated. Recurrence with activity requires cautious rehabilitation. Failure of conservative care requires resection of the distal clavicle, which is usually quite effective.

A newly recognized entity is "weightlifter's shoulder" or nontraumatic osteolysis of the distal clavicle (Fig. 15-20). Cahil[44] first described this condition in 1982 with athletes. Scavenius et al.[45,46] have specifically found a subgroup with the weightlifter using heavy weights as the prime candidate. Scavenius et al. found the prevalence to be about 27 percent.

The typical presentation is a serious amateur weightlifter who reports diffuse shoulder pain in particular abducting beyond 90 degrees. Aggravating maneuvers include the bench press, the clean and jerk, and the dip among others. Palpation reveals point tenderness over the acromioclavicular joint with increases in pain with compressive end-range positions such as horizontal adduction and full abduction.

Radiographically, the same findings are present as

are found in traumatic osteolysis. These again include loss of subchondral detail, cystic changes, and a gap of radiolucency at the acromioclavicular joint.

Treatment may follow one of three paths. The first is complete abstinence for 4 to 6 months. During this time degeneration may decrease with an increase in repair, but the widened acromioclavicular gap apparently is permanent. Another approach is initial rest followed by modification and substitution exercises with weightlifting. Narrow grip bench presses should replace wide grip presses or substitution with cable crossovers, or decline or incline presses is acceptable. Dips should be avoided. Symptoms should resolve with this program. If unsuccessful, resection of the distal clavicle is suggested.[47]

SHOULDER POINTER

A common diagnostic difficulty is discriminating between a first degree acromioclavicular sprain and a contusion about the acromioclavicular joint. The mechanism is similar, but the consequence may be different. Commonly referred to as a "shoulder pointer," a contusion to the deltoid or the trapezius muscle produces local pain on top of the shoulder, yet not specifically at the acromioclavicular joint. Avulsion of some trapezius fibers may occur at the insertion on the posterior aspect of the clavicle. This injury is rather common in sports such as rugby where protective padding is not worn over the shoulders.[48]

Ice and padding are usually sufficient to allow quick return to play. Restriction of exercises involving the deltoid or upper trapezius should be in effect for several days to a week. Since most pointers occur with players without equipment, padding in the shape of a doughnut is usually sewn into the jersey or taped onto the shoulder.

ACROMION APOPHYSITIS

An apophysitis can develop in the adolescent at the lateral acromion due to repeated traction by the deltoid attachment. A single traumatic event is not reported. Because the apophysis closes between the ages of 16 and 19 years, athletes below this age presenting with nontraumatic acromial pain are most suspect. Ra-

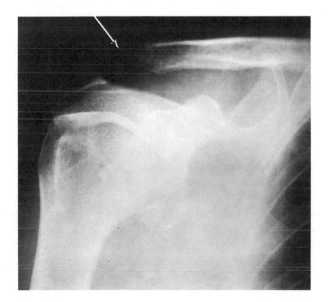

Fig. 15-20. A 25-year old man with osteolysis of distal end of clavicle from weightlifting. (From Rowe,[9] with permission.)

diographs may not be valuable; however, if the athlete is a weightlifter, exclusion of the possibility of osteolysis of the lateral clavicle may need to be made. Diagnosis is usually one of exclusion based on the nontraumatic onset and fairly quick resolution with rest and ice.

CORACOID DISORDERS

Although rare, it is possible to injure the coracoid process through two mechanisms. The first is direct trauma as occurs with target or game shooting. Recoil of the butt of the gun can result in a bruise or bursitis. The second mechanism is excessive pull of the pectoralis minor or short head of the biceps during the acceleration phase of tennis or throwing, which may avulse part of the coracoid. Radiographic evaluation is important; however, reference to the appearance of secondary ossification centers should be made in young athletes to avoid confusion with a true avulsion. Treatment initially involves rest and immobilization. Internal fixation is reserved for unresolved healing or symptoms.[49]

SCAPULOCOSTAL (LEVATOR SCAPULA) SYNDROME

Acute or chronic strain of the levator scapula can cause pain at the superior medial border of the scapula associated at times with neck and shoulder pain. Referred to as levator scapulae syndrome by Estwanik,[50] superior scapula syndrome by Moseley,[51] and scapulocostal syndrome by Shull,[52] it is found in sports. It has been reported to occur in wrestling, weightlifting, sailing, swimming, gymnastics, boxing, karate, and golf. The function of the levator scapula is to act as a checkrein to forward neck flexion when acting bilaterally. When acting unilaterally the function is to lift the superior medial border of the scapula, which results in depression of the glenoid and lowering of the connected humeral head. Tightening of the muscle over time or through protective splinting can restrict elevation of the lateral border by the upper trapezius. Slumped postures and carrying heavy objects can chronically stretch the muscle/tendon leading to chronic irritation. Attachment to the transverse process of the upper four cervical vertebrae may lead to cervical pain.

Evaluation is performed with the patient prone, leaning onto the elbows. By bearing the upper body weight onto the elbows, the superior medial border of the scapula is lifted away from the thorax making palpation more possible. Extreme tenderness with reproduction of the patient's associated complaints is a true positive. Caution should be used in overdiagnosing this disorder given that this is usually a tender area to palpate. Palpation of the opposite side for comparison is essential.

Treatment involves adherence to a stretching, and eventually strengthening, program. Stretching involves grasping under a chair to fix the shoulder while using the opposite hand (or examiner with spray and stretch maneuvers) to stretch the head away from the side of involvement. This procedure, in office and prescribed at home, should be frequently applied until pain relief is accomplished. Assisting with this process is upper cervical adjusting. The long-term goal is to prevent recurrence with ergonomic correction of occupational and sports postures plus a stretching/strengthening program to correct postural abnormalities.

SNAPPING SCAPULA SYNDROME

An interesting phenomenon recognized as early as the 1930s by Codman[53] is the "snapping scapula" syndrome. Patients report a snap or thud sensation especially on raising the arm. Rowe[54] considers two general classifications of etiology: mechanical and dysfunctional.

Mechanical causes are due to processes on the undersurface of the scapula such as an osteochondroma, bursitis, or fibrous scar tissue. Adventitial bursa or irritation of a medial scapular bursa do develop as a reactionary process to repetitive irritation on the undersurface of the scapula. This is seen most commonly in throwing sports during the follow-through phase. Fibrous scar tissue can develop secondary to repeated trauma in contact sports as reported by Rowe.[54] Additionally, any disruption of the normal contour or positioning of the ribs such as subluxation, fracture, or arthritic irregularities can produce this presentation. These irregularities can be primary to the development of adventitial bursitis or fibrous tissue. Some of the mechanical processes can be visible directly or indirectly on an oblique or profile view of the scapula.

Chiropractic treatment of associated vertebral subluxations, mechanically and through elimination of an irritative focus, may neurologically assist in proper scapulothoracic movement.

Other mechanical causes include a Luschka's tubercle, which represents a bony extension of the superior medial border of the scapula and Sprengel's deformity with an associated omovertebral bone.

Removal of an osteochondroma or arthritic spur will be beneficial. Subluxations can be adjusted and bursitis relieved by rest, injection, or surgery.[55]

A snapping scapula due to muscular dysfunction is yet another example of the varied disorders resulting from imbalance in a finely tuned shoulder mechanism. Rowe[54] theorizes that the patient will have a tendency, either protective or emotional, to contract the scapulothoracic musculature at the initiation of elevation. He uses the analogy of a car, instructing the patient to take the foot off the brake before accelerating. Both premature contraction or overtightening of the musculature have the effect of grinding the scapula against the thorax with the potential of initiating a bursal or degenerative reaction.

Ironically, these patients will most likely irritate this process and augment this tendency with strengthening exercises if the underlying dysfunction is not recognized. Insistence on leaving shoulder muscle contraction out of elevation is the only conservative solution. This involves practicing over time (first without resistance and then with), to lift the arm while palpating the shoulder musculature with the other hand. Although muscles need to contract to elevate the shoulder, if the patient can concentrate on staying as "relaxed" as possible during the movement, the more likely premature scapulothoracic contraction will be diminished. Surgical attempts at correction should be reserved for mechanical blockage processes only.

INTERSCAPULAR PAIN

Limitation of throwing or swimming activities may be due to persistent pain between the scapula. Overuse injuries to the rhomboids, middle trapezius, levator scapula, and the serratus posterior superior are not uncommon, particularly during the follow-through and deceleration phases of the throwing act. Underlying complicating factors may include hyperkyphosis or scoliosis.

A search for specific muscle involvement should in-

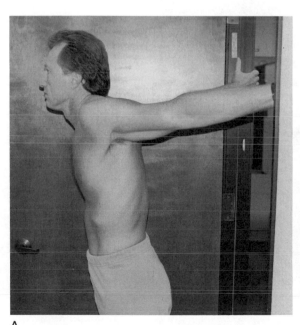
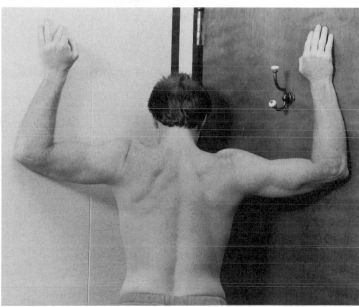

A B

Fig. 15-21. Pectoral stretching. **(A)** In the doorway; **(B)** in the corner.

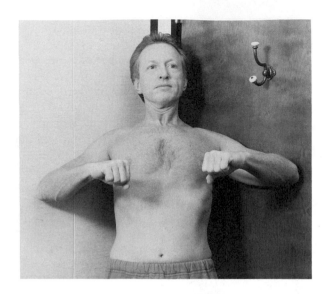

Fig. 15-22. Middle trapezius and rhomboid corner exercise.

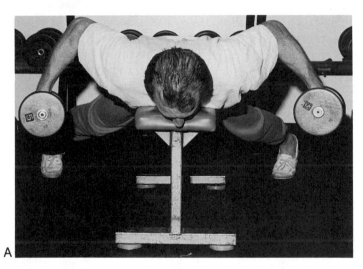

A

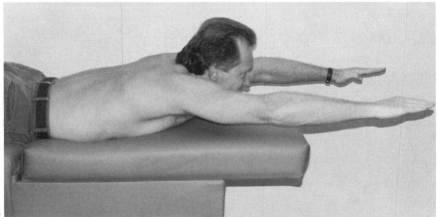

B

Fig. 15-23. (A) Reverse flys for midscapular muscles. **(B)** Airplane exercise for trapezius and erector spinae muscles.

436

clude contraction of the muscle, stretch of the muscle, and a search for trigger points. Although the referral pattern for the rhomboids, middle trapezius, and serratus remain relatively local to the muscle, the referral zone for the serratus posterior superior may cause posterior shoulder pain that extends down to the hand in an ulnar-like distribution. Treatment is similar for all trigger points as described in Chapter 18.

In addition to attention to individual muscles, a general program of pectoral stretching and midscapular strengthening should be included. Corner or doorway stretches for the pectoral muscles should be performed first, followed by corner scapular exercises (Fig. 15-21). Stretches can be localized to different portions of the pectorals through elevation of the arms. Stretches should be static and held for at least 10 seconds, repeated several times. For scapular muscle strengthening the patient steps back into a corner (preferably in a shower) and takes one step forward. Leaning back onto the forearms with the shoulders abducted just shy of 90 degrees (Fig. 15-22), the patient attempts contraction of the muscles between the scapula. The added resistance of partial body weight by this position makes it more effective. The incorrect result is a chicken or bird appearance during the exercise. The patient must understand that only slight forward and upward protrusion of the chest will result from a focused, properly executed exercise. Held for 3 to 5 seconds the patient slowly releases back into the corner. Repetitions should initially be kept low, and within 2 weeks should be increased to 25 to 35 repetitions 2 to 3 times per day. An alternative is to perform light weight reverse flys in the prone position and "airplane" isometrics (Fig. 15-23).

As mentioned, thoracic vertebra and rib subluxations may be a source of mechanical blockage and irritation. Appropriate adjusting techniques can be found in various texts. In addition, Maigne[56] suggests that an anomalous branch of the posterior primary rami of T2 may be the source of medial scapular pain. The branch descends down along the medial border of the scapula and then ascends back and across the scapular spine. He recommends manipulation of the T2 area to relieve pain from this source.

Maigne[56] also refers to a cervical source of midscapular pain and has devised a test referred to as the "doorbell" sign. By pressing on the transverse process of the lower cervical vertebra for 10 to 20 seconds, pain can be reproduced in the midscapular region usually around T7. This is an indication to adjust the corresponding cervical vertebra in an attempt to relieve the thoracic pain.

SCAPULAR FRACTURES

Fractures of the body of the scapula are relatively rare. The mechanism must involve a direct blow of considerable magnitude. Displacement of fragments are usually minimal due to the surrounding muscle support; therefore, treatment is usually nonoperative with rest, and supportive immobilization unless associated fractures are involved.

REFERENCES

1. Dvir Z, Berme N: The shoulder complex in elevation of the arm: a mechanism approach. J Biomech 11:219, 1978
2. Cave EF: Fractures and Other Injuries. Year Book Medical Publishers, Chicago, 1958
3. Mehta JC, Sachdev A, Collins JJ: Retrosternal dislocation of the clavicle. Injury 5:79, 1973
4. Grant JCB: Method of Anatomy. 7th Ed. Williams & Wilkins, Baltimore, 1965
5. Bearn JG: Direct observations on the function of the capsule of the sternoclavicular joint in clavicle support. J Anat 101:159, 1967
6. Lucas DB: Biomechanics of the shoulder joint. Arch Surg 107:425, 1973
7. Rockwood CA: Disorders of the sternoclavicular joint. p. 477. In Rockwood CA, Matsen FA (eds): The Shoulder. WB Saunders, Philadelphia, 1990
8. Heinig CF: Retrosternal dislocation of the clavicle: early recognition, x-ray diagnosis, and management. J Bone Joint Surg 50A:830, 1968
9. Rowe CR: Acromioclavicular and sternoclavicular joints. p. 293. In Rowe CR (ed): The Shoulder. Churchill Livingstone, New York, 1988
10. Omer GE: Osteotomy of the clavicle in surgical reduction of anterior sternoclavicular dislocation. J Trauma 7:584, 1967
11. Salvatore JE: Sternoclavicular joint dislocation. Clin Orthop 58:51, 1968
12. Hobbs DW: Sternoclavicular joint: a new axial radiographic view. Radiology 90:801, 1968
13. Rockwood CA, Green DP, Bucholz RW (eds): Rockwood and Green's Fractures in Adults. 3rd Ed. JB Lippincott, Philadelphia, 1991

14. Emery RJ, Ho EK, Leong JC: The shoulder girdle in ankylosing spondylitis. J Bone Joint Surg 73A:1526, 1991

15. Sonozaki H, Azuma A, Okai K et al: Clinical features of 22 cases with inter-sterno-costo-clavicular ossification. Arch Orthop Trauma Surg 95:13, 1979

16. Dohler JR: Ankylosing hyperostosis of the sternoclavicular joint. J Disch Med Wochenschr 112:304, 1987

17. Brower AC, Sweet DE, Keats TE: Condensing osteitis of the clavicle: a new entity. AJR 121:17, 1974

18. Sadr B, Swann M: Spontaneous dislocation of the sternoclavicular joint. Acta Orthop Scand 50:269, 1979

19. Adams FL: The genuine works of Hippocrates. Vol. 1 and 2. William Wood, New York, 1886

20. Tyurina TV: Age-related characteristics of the human acromioclavicular joint. Arkh Anat Gistol Embriol 89:75, 1985

21. DePalma AF, Callery G, Bennett GA: Variational anatomy and degenerative lesions of the shoulder joint. AAOS Instructional Course Lectures 6:255, 1949

22. Petersson CJ: Degeneration of the acromioclavicular joint: a morphological study. Acta Orthop Scand 54:904, 1983

23. Salter EG, Shelley BS, Nasca R: A morphological study of the acromioclavicular joint in humans, abstracted. Anat Rec 211:353, 1985

24. DePalma AF: Surgery of the Shoulder. 2nd Ed. JB Lippincott, Philadelphia, 1973

25. Moseley HF: Athletic injuries to the shoulder region. Am J Surg 98:401, 1959

26. Bearden JM, Hughston JC, Whatley GS: Acromioclavicular dislocation: method of treatment. J Sports Med 1:5, 1973

27. Codman EA: Rupture of the supraspinatus tendon and other lesions in or about the subacromial bursa. In Codman EA (ed): The Shoulder. Thomas Todd & Co, Boston, 1934

28. Inman VT, Saunders JB, Abbott LC: Observations on the function of the shoulder joint. J Bone Joint Surg 26:1, 1944

29. Kennedy JC, Cameron H: Complete dislocation of the acromioclavicular joint. J Bone Joint Surg 36B:202, 1954

30. Kennedy JC: Complete dislocation of the acromioclavicular joint 14 years later. J Trauma 8:311, 1968

31. Rockwood CA, Young DC: Disorders of the acromioclavicular joint. p. 413. In Rockwood CA, Matsen FA (eds): The Shoulder. WB Saunders, Philadelphia, 1990

32. Caldwell GD: Treatment of complete permanent acromioclavicular dislocation by surgical arthrodesis. J Bone Joint Surg 25:368, 1943

33. Tossy JD, Mead NC, Sigmond HM: Acromioclavicular separations: useful and practical classification for treatment. Clin Orthop 28:111, 1963

34. Rockwood CA: Injuries to the acromioclavicular joint. p. 860. In Rockwood CA, Green DP, Bucholz RW (eds): Rockwood and Green's Fractures in Adults. 3rd Ed. JB Lippincott, Philadelphia, 1991

35. Zanca P: Shoulder pain: Involvement of the acromioclavicular joint: analysis of 1,000 cases. AJR 112:493, 1971

36. Bosworth BM: Complete acromioclavicular dislocation. N Engl J Med 241:221, 1949

37. Allman FL Jr: Fractures and ligamentous injuries of the clavicle and its articulation. J Bone Joint Surg 49A:774, 1967

38. Glick JM, Milburn LJ, Haggerty JF, Nishimoto D: Dislocated acromioclavicular joint: follow-up study of 35 unreduced acromioclavicular dislocations. Am J Sports Med 5:264, 1977

39. Bjerneld H, Hovelius L, Thorling J: Acromio-clavicular separations treated conservatively: a 5-year follow-up study. Acta Orthop Scand 54:743, 1983

40. Dias JJ, Steingold RA, Richardson RA et al: The conservative treatment of acromioclavicular dislocation: review after five years. J Bone Joint Surg 69B:719, 1987

41. Schwarz N, Leixnering M: Results of nonreduced acromioclavicular Tossy III separations. Unfallchirurg 89:248, 1986

42. Tibone J, Sellers R, Tonino P: Strength testing after third-degree acromioclavicular dislocations. Am J Sports Med 20:328, 1992

43. Cadenat FM: The treatment of dislocations and fractures of the outer end of the clavicle. Int Cli 1:145, 1917

44. Cahil BR: Osteolysis of the distal part of the clavicle in male athletes. J Bone Joint Surg 64A:1053, 1982

45. Scavenius M, Iversen BF: Nontraumatic clavicular osteolysis in weight lifters. Am J Sports Med 20:463, 1992

46. Scavenius M, Iversen BF, Sturup J: Resection of the lateral end of the clavicle following osteolysis, with special emphasis on non-traumatic osteolysis of the acromial end of the clavicle in athletes. Injury 18:261, 1987

47. Reider B: Strength training. p. 19. In Reider B (ed): Sports Medicine: The School-Age Athlete. WB Saunders, Philadelphia, 1991

48. Mitchell LJ, Riseborough EM: The incidence of injuries in rugby football. Am J Sports Med 2:93, 1974

49. Benton J, Nelson C: Avulsion of the coracoid process in an athlete: report of a case. J Bone Joint Surg 53A:356, 1971

50. Estwanik JJ: Levator scapulae syndrome. Phys Sports Med 17:57, 1989

51. Moseley HF: Shoulder Lesions. p. 74. Charles C Thomas, Springfield, IL, 1945

52. Shull JR: Scapulocostal syndrome: clinical aspects. South Med J 62:956, 1969

53. Codman EA: The Shoulder. Kreiger, Melbourne, FL, 1984

54. Rowe CR: Tendinitis, bursitis, impingement, "snapping" scapula, and calcific tendinitis. p. 105. In Rowe CR (ed): The Shoulder. Churchill Livingstone, New York, 1988

55. Sisto DJ, Jobe FW: The operative treatment of scapulothoracic bursitis in professional pitchers. Am J Sports Med 14:192, 1986

56. Maigne R: Orthopaedic Medicine: A New Approach to Vertebral Manipulation. Charles C Thomas, Springfield, IL, 1972

57. Hollinshead WH, Jenkins DB: Functional Anatomy of the Limbs and Back. 5th ed. WB Saunders, Philadelphia, 1991

58. Rockwood CA. Injuries to the sternoclavicular joint. p. 1257. In Rockwood CA, Green DP, Bucholz RW (eds): Rockwood and Green's Fractures in Adults. 3rd Ed. JB Lippincott, Philadelphia, 1991

59. Hurley JA: Anatomy of the shoulder. p. 23. In Nicholas JA, Hershman EB (eds): The Upper Extremity in Sports Medicine. CV Mosby, St. Louis, 1990

60. Reid D: Sports Injury Assessment and Rehabilitation. Churchill Livingstone, New York, 1991

61. Rockwood CA, Williams GR, Young DC: Injuries to the acromioclavicular. p. 1192. In Rockwood CA, Green DP, Bucholz RW (eds): Rockwood and Green's Fractures in Adults. 3rd Ed. JB Lippincott, Philadelphia, 1991

16

Frozen Shoulder

THOMAS A. SOUZA

DEFINITION AND THEORIES OF CAUSATION

Frozen shoulder remains an enigma. It is rarely found in individuals before the age of 40; rarely after 60.[1] This distribution seriously questions the past assumption that frozen shoulder is a progressive degenerative process. In relation to sports activity, the clinician would most likely encounter this entity in the senior athlete. Incidence in the athlete as compared with the average individual has not been documented. If a younger athlete presented with the typical restriction findings of limited external rotation and abduction, other causes should be investigated (Table 16-1). Topping this list of differentials would be an undiagnosed posterior shoulder dislocation. Many go undetected.[2] The intent of the physician in the older population of athletes is to return them to activity as quickly as possible, realizing that even shortening of this condition still leaves a natural course of several months to a year. Additionally, too aggressive a treatment in the early phases may lead to a protracted recovery, sometimes with permanent residuals.[2,3]

It becomes obvious with even a cursory review of the literature that the term frozen shoulder is, and has been, used to describe a multitude of disorders that present with some restriction of shoulder movement. Much of the confusion arises from the many historical descriptions of etiology and clinical presentations. This is in part due to a now recognized sequence of progression that mimics other conditions based on the phase at which the condition is clinically seen. Adding to the confusion, frozen shoulder often coexists with other conditions. Terms that are often used synonymously with frozen shoulder are adhesive capsulitis,

capsulitis, and periarthritis. Often throughout the text and in references to various authors these terms will be used interchangeably; however, frozen shoulder or adhesive capsulitis are the preferred terms. Periarthritis covers a large group of disorders including tendinitis and tears of the rotator cuff, calcifying tendinitis, and bursitis. Therefore, this is not an acceptable classification.

Presently, it is suggested that the diagnosis of frozen shoulder be one of exclusion (i.e., other conditions should be ruled out before identifying the condition as frozen shoulder). The conditions regarded as subgroups under the term periarthritis should be eliminated before the term frozen shoulder is applied. Therefore, the term frozen shoulder should be reserved for limitation of specific active and passive ranges of motion (ROM) that is due to no known underlying disorder. If an underlying disorder is found and frozen shoulder is present, a qualification as secondary frozen shoulder should be given.

Although some of the pathologic changes seen with frozen shoulder have been discovered, the cause of these changes is still a mystery. Relationship to specific diseases such as diabetes,[4,5] hyperthyroidism,[6,7] and certain psychiatric conditions[8–10] has suggested a metabolic cause. Others have recognized an obvious connection to disuse.[1] Still others have suggested either an autoimmune etiology[11] or a consequence of reflex triggering of sympathetic reactions.[12] All of these theories, to some degree, have been recognized as related, yet no one single cause has been discovered.

Table 16-2 lists some of the many authors and theories that deal with frozen shoulder. A quick survey indicates that literally any soft tissue structure in the shoulder area has been implicated. Lippman[13] and Pasteur[14]

Table 16-1. Differential Diagnosis of Restricted Abduction/External Rotation

Condition	Diagnosis
Frozen shoulder	Limitation in active and passive motion preceded by an immobilization phase and pain phase
Posterior dislocation	History of trauma, usually a fall on outstretched hand or adducted arm; radiographic confirmation
Glenohumeral osteoarthritis	Past history of shoulder surgery and radiographic documentation
Reflex sympathetic dystrophy	Similar to frozen shoulder presentation plus sympathetic signs and symptoms included swelling of the arm/hand and skin changes

both believed that the primary pathology was in the biceps tendon. Lippman believed that the syndrome gradually resolved as fibrosis progressed and tethering occurred in the bicipital groove. DePalma[15] felt that bicipital tendinitis was a predisposing factor. He recommended that in refractory cases, the tendon be detached and moved to the coracoid process. Simmonds[16] believed that the primary pathology was in the supraspinatus tendon. He felt that the degree of revascularization would determine the final outcome. Codman[17] felt that the subacromial bursa was at fault. Withers[18] theorized that, analogous to the peritoneum, the bursa is rarely the original site of pathology, but

Table 16-2. Conflicting Theories Regarding Frozen Shoulder

Author	Suspected Structure or Theory
Lipman[13] and Pasteur[14]	Biceps tendon pathology is primary cause
DePalma[15]	Muscular inactivity is main cause; biceps tendinitis predisposes to frozen shoulder
Simmonds[16]	Supraspinatus pathology is primary cause
Codman[17]	Subacromial bursitis is primary cause
Withers[18]	Bursa is not primary, however, highly pain sensitive
Reeves[19]	Adhesive capsulitis is attempt to heal small cuff tears
Kopell and Thompson[20]	Supracapsular nerve entrapment leading to muscular dysfunction
Neviaser[22]	Adhesions in the capsule are primary pathology
Travell and Simons[12]	Trigger points primarily in the subscapularis muscle
Macnab[11]	An autoimmune mechanism leading to diffuse capsulitis

being pain sensitive, alerts the patient to an underlying pathology.

Reeves[19] came to the conclusion that adhesive capsulitis was an attempt to heal small and medium-sized cuff tears. By obtaining bilateral arthrograms on patients in the recovery phase of frozen shoulder, Reeves observed that only 4 out of 49 involved shoulders had rotator cuff tears while in the opposite shoulders a defect was found in 23.

Kopell and Thompson[20] were convinced that the suprascapular nerve could be entrapped causing local discomfort and lead to muscular dysfunction. Their solution to this problem was to release the nerve from the superior transverse scapular ligament. A similar functional entrapment has been suggested as a cause of impingement due to dysfunction of the infraspinatus compromising stability.

The variety of theories regarding causation is due to theoretical or surgical observations of the process at varying stages and perhaps processes initiated by different stimuli. Failure to recognize the natural course of the disorder might cause clinicians to feel that their procedure was successful when in fact it reflected the natural self-resolution of the painful aspect of this condition. Agreement to date is that the capsule is primarily involved with secondary involvement of many of the previously suggested primary causes.[21]

PATHOLOGIC CHANGES

As the term frozen shoulder implies, there is a marked reduction of active and passive range of motion in the shoulder. The characteristic loss usually follows a pattern with most of the restriction found with external rotation and abduction. The most accepted explanation of this gross loss of movement has been an adhesive process in or about the capsule. Neviaser[22] felt that adhesions developed within the capsule, particularly in the larger inferior recess, preventing downward movement of the humerus upon elevation. Interestingly, signs of a reparative inflammatory process were visible in the subsynovial layer only but not in the synovial layer itself.[23] Lundberg[24] also failed to notice significant changes in the synovial layer. Lundberg did find increased fibroblastic collagen formation, loss of hyaluronic acid, and increased sulfated GAGs. McLaughlin[25] found that the capsular folds and pouches were adherent in a small minority of his cases at operative release. He also noted involvement of the rotator cuff muscle bellies with sparing of the biceps tendon sheath and relative sparing of the subacromial bursa. There is agreement, however, that the restriction is due to a tightened inflexible capsule. Bland et al.[26] hypothesize that fibrosis without adhesions may in fact be due to impaired circulation, perhaps autonomic in origin. Travell and Simons[12] also feel that a reflex autonomic reaction may be the underlying cause due to subscapularis trigger points.

Recently, Nobuhara et al.[27] and Uhthoff and Sarkar[28] described fibrosis of the coracohumeral ligament. Nobuhara et al.[27] feel that this is the reason for limited external rotation seen in patients with frozen shoulder. Limitation does not occur in flexion due to the relaxed coracohumeral ligament in this position. They also felt that subacromial bursal adhesions would possibly limit abduction. In the later stages they felt that the tendons of the pectoralis major, latissimus dorsi, and teres major were affected.

According to Fareed and Gallivan,[29] the initial area of adhesion development is in a triangular area of synovial tissue that lies between and in contact with the subscapularis and biceps tendons. This allows a bridging fibrosis to surrounding rotator cuff muscles and the glenoid.

HISTORY

Historical clues to the suggestion of a connection between idiopathic loss of range of motion and frozen shoulder include the following:

1. A sequence of painful restriction followed by a gradual shift to stiffness with less pain. This sequence requires time to recognize and in the early stages is very difficult to distinguish from other conditions.
2. A history of disuse following shoulder injury or immobilization. Patients first presenting with early signs and symptoms will intuitively immobilize the arm. Bulgen et al.[3] found that up to 50 percent of patients were never instructed to maintain ROM when presenting to their primary care physician. On the other hand, Bateman[30] argues against the disuse theory due to the fact that frozen shoulder does not develop in those with paralysis and degen-

erative tendinitis of the rotator cuff. Perhaps disuse or immobilization must be coupled with an inherent tendency in some individuals.

3. Being a woman between the ages of 40 and 70. Although males are also affected, the female incidence is higher. Note that the process is not degenerative or would be found in the higher age groups. This resembles a similar poorly understood process referred to as calcifying tendinitis.
4. A history of diabetes. Diabetics have an incidence of between 10 to 20 percent compared to a normal population incidence of 2 to 5 percent. Bilateral involvement is common, being between 42 and 77 percent. Patients with chronic diabetes, in particular insulin dependent for more than 10 years, or those with other advanced signs are more likely to develop frozen shoulder.[4,5]
5. A history of hyperthyroidism. Here the frozen shoulder seems to resolve with treatment of the underlying condition.
6. A history of cardiopulmonary involvement. Patients who have emphysema or chronic bronchitis may be more prone.[31] Post myocardial infarction patients often develop frozen shoulder[32] (due to immobilization or reflex autonomic changes?). Earlier ambulatory requirements for post myocardial infarction patients seem to have reduced the incidence.

It has also been suggested that there might be a psychiatric personality type associated with frozen shoulder. The inability to adapt to life's situations or the type of patients who fail to take responsibility for their own care are potentially predisposed. However, studies have failed to agree on this personality type.[33] Therefore, categorization based on a patient with past psychiatric problems may not be an accurate assumption.

CLINICAL PRESENTATION

The patient with frozen shoulder may present at any stage of the process. Each stage has distinct signs and symptoms that are easier to recognize the longer the patient has the disorder. The first phase is a painful one with only the suggestion of progressive stiffness. This phase blends with the second phase where stiffness predominates. The acute painful phase is variable, lasting between 2 and 9 months[34] or longer if too aggressive therapy is applied.

If patients present to the clinician in the second phase after having been diagnosed and treated in the early phase, they may report as Rowe[2] states a "guilt complex" from being told they are not working hard enough in their program to maintain mobility. Yet, to the patient's dismay, the harder they work the worse the stiffness and pain become. This puritanical condemnation is a misunderstanding of the natural course of this disorder and has led to many frustrating encounters for patients simply wanting assurance that the condition will get better.

In the initial stages inflammation is present causing often an acute presentation that may mimic rotator cuff involvement. Although it would be expected that contraction of the muscles would be painless, and so help differentiate cuff involvement from frozen shoulder, up to 40 percent of patients reported pain on resisted movement.[28]

The pain is often difficult for the patient to localize. The beginnings of movement restriction may have begun. Again, the restriction is usually in both active and passive ROM. The patient often reports an impairment of a normal daily activity such as combing the hair, fastening a bra strap, putting on a coat, etc. The pain most often interrupts sleep and sleeping on the affected side is impossible.

The second stage is usually weeks to months later when the stiffness may be advancing as the primary complaint. In this phase the primary restriction pattern is external rotation, abduction, followed by internal rotation. There are, of course atypical presentations where this sequence may not be true. It is more likely in this phase to find restrictions in active and passive ranges of motion with little pain on resisted movement if kept within the restricted range. The entity of frozen shoulder is now more obvious during the second stage. The length of this phase is between 4 and 12 months.[35]

The final thawing phase represents a release of some of the restrictions in ROM; however, many people feel less restricted while objective measurement shows only minor improvements.[28]

The total course of the disorder has been reported to self-resolve in 18 to 24 months.[35,36] However, several studies, in particular Reeves,[19] have demonstrated patients being symptomatic as long as 5 to 10 years post onset. It appears that the length of the painful phase correlates with the length of the recovery time.

DIAGNOSIS

The diagnostic criteria for frozen shoulder are varied depending on the author reviewed. Literally any intrinsic and many extrinsic shoulder disorders may present as a painful stiff shoulder. An attempt at consensus seems to indicate, in general, the observations of Cyriax,[37] which require an examination that rules out other causes of limitation through an extensive comparison of restriction patterns in both active and passive patterns. Cyriax[38] describes the capsular pattern as a position that indicates arthritis, undifferentiated. The pattern involves a sequence of restriction starting with abduction being the most limited, followed by abduction, and then internal rotation. There are some variations to this pattern, but this is the most typical.

Many orthopaedic testing maneuvers are not even attainable by the patient with frozen shoulder, often limiting the clinical evaluation to the restricted ranges. Within the restricted ranges it is important to determine degrees of restriction, whether they occur passively, actively, or both. Resisted attempts should also be made in the pain-free ranges. Although not a hallmark of frozen shoulder, resisted movements may be painful in as many as 40 percent of individuals and do not necessarily rule out frozen shoulder if typical restriction patterns are found. Measurement of passive ranges should follow the recommendations of the American Academy of Shoulder and Elbow Surgeons as outlined below:

1. Measurement of passive and active external rotation performed at the side and at 90 degrees of abduction
2. Measurement of active internal rotation by measurement of the highest spinal level the patient can reach with the hand behind the back
3. Measurement of passive internal rotation with the arm at 90 degrees and the scapula stabilized
4. Recording of the patient's reported restrictions in a number of activities of daily living

Given that the glenohumeral area is restricted with frozen shoulder, it is important to evaluate the contribution of the scapula to abduction. Patients with frozen shoulder will often initiate abduction with hiking of the shoulder through use of the upper trapezius or through trunk leaning placing the arm in a position of relative abduction.

The cervical region should be evaluated for several reasons. The first is to differentiate between cervical etiologies of shoulder pain, both radicular and referred. The second reason is that due to the painful nature of frozen shoulder and the altered biomechanics (in particular, related to the scapulae), associated musculature may be involved. Extension of the thoracic spine may also be used by the patient to substitute for loss of shoulder motion.

A general orthopaedic screen should involve cervical compression, distraction, and shoulder depression tests. Included would be thoracic outlet screening tests, and a full sensory, motor, and reflex evaluation of the upper extremity. Although frozen shoulder may mimic a C6 nerve root problem, the pain is usually more diffuse, not isolated to the specific dermatome.

Although attempts have been made to correlate laboratory findings such as HLA-B27 and an increased erythrocyte sedimentation rate, these initially promising theories have been discounted.[39,40]

TREATMENT

Decision making in the treatment of frozen shoulder is directed by several motivations. These include the desire to relieve pain in the acute primary stage, to see a successful long-term outcome with resolution of both pain and stiffness, and to possibly shorten the potential protracted 2 to 5 year recovery.

Ethically, it would appear that all should be the goals of the treating physician, but controversy blurs these good intentions. It is apparent that several forms of treatment have actually worsened the condition (sometimes causing permanent damage). Additionally, not any single form of treatment seems consistently effective. The questions that arise are: When to apply different forms of treatment? How much treatment is necessary; how much is too much?

In the past, the goal of therapy was to prevent the shoulder from "freezing up." It became apparent to many clinicians that this often made the condition worse. This approach was applied during the early

stages when apparently the inflammatory process may be aggravated. Rowe,[2] Grey,[35] DePalma,[15] and Post[41] independently tested the "wait and see" attitude only addressing the pain complaint with analgesics. They all felt that the patient was much better off than those enduring painful forced physical therapy. Yet again, full or close to full resolution took 2 years or more. This resolution often meant that the patient felt a return to acceptable, functional range of motion, but compared to the well-arm did not have full range.

Determining the effectiveness of different treatment approaches for frozen shoulder has been difficult due to the varying criteria for making a diagnosis (Table 16-3). The studies that have been done agree that exercise is the common ingredient in successful treatment programs. It seems likely from the studies of Bulgen et al.[3] and others that corticosteroid injections, mobilization, and ultrasound do not significantly alter the course of the disorder. In a study by Hazelman,[42] 28 percent of the patients treated had an exacerbation with physiotherapy treatment.

The hallmark of treatment for any phase of frozen shoulder is the maintenance and restoration of ROM. The techniques used to accomplish this goal are variable, depending on phase presentation. A generalized treatment protocol is summarized in Table 16-4.

In the acute phase, no more than passive Codman or pendulum exercise should be permitted (Fig. 16-1). This allows a passive ranging without potential exacerbation from muscle contraction. The patient uses the body to range the passive dependent arm. Initially gravity is sufficient followed by the use of small weights when symptomatology permits. An attempt at active treatment with aggressive mobilization or manipulation is contraindicated in the acute stage. Actively performed Codman or pendulum exercise should be reserved for patients in whom pain is not of an acute nature and passive ranging has been performed pain free.

Treatment using transcutaneous electrical nerve stimulation (TENS) is reported to be effective in the alleviation of pain with frozen shoulder (Fig. 16-2).[43] Recommended acupuncture points used for pad placement include LI 14, LI 15, LI 16, and TW 14. Other points that have been recommended include the distal points ST 38 and UB 57 or LI 15, SI 10, GB 34, and LI 11 (see Ch. 18 for specific locations).[44]

Table 16-3. Review of Various Treatment Approaches for Frozen Shoulder

Author	Findings
Hazelman[42]	No difference in patients treated with either local corticosteroid injections, physical therapy using pendulum/pulley exercises with short-wave diathermy, or manipulation under anesthesia
Hamer & Kirk[61]	No distinct advantage with treatment using ultrasound or ice; both seemed effective in decreasing pain (acute stage)
Dacre et al.[63]	Local steroid injection, physical therapy with passive mobilization, or a combination of both were effective in decreasing pain and increasing shoulder ROM
Lee et al.[62]	No significant difference in patients treated with local cortisone and exercise or infrared therapy and exercise; they concluded that patients who exercised improved more than patients using analgesics alone
Liang & Liang[64]	Active exercise was beneficial when combined either with intra-articular injection plus heat, heat alone, or injection alone; concluded exercise was only useful treatment
Bulgen et al.[3]	No significant differences in long-term follow-up with patients treated with intra-articular steroids, passive mobilization (Maitland-type), ice, or no treatment
Biswas et al.[68]	Exercise is most important treatment; patients treated with combinations of active and passive exercise coupled with intra-articular cortisone, short-wave diathermy, and aspirin benefited
Rizk et al.[46]	Combination of TENS with prolonged pulley traction was more effective than heat modalities and exercise
Pothmann et al.[65]	Acupuncture treatment of stomach 38 is effective
Nicholson[69]	Patients performing mobilizations and active exercises were compared to patients performing active exercise alone; passive abduction was significantly better with the mobilizing group
Leclaire & Bourgouin[71]	Magnetic field therapy was found not to be effective in the treatment of frozen shoulder
Roy & Oldham[70]	Significant pain relief and moderate ROM increase with patients treated with intraarticular and bursal injections weekly for maximum of three injections (prednisolone)
Andren & Lundberg[51] Hsu & Chan[52]	Distension arthrography effective
Helbig et al.[66] Connolly et al.[67]	Manipulation under anesthesia effective

Table 16-4. Treatment of Frozen Shoulder

Stage I—Painful
  Attention is given to pain relief with emphasis on maintaining ROM
  Aggressive mobilization/manipulation is contraindicated in this stage
  TENS and analgesics for pain relief
  Passive Codman/pendulum exercises
  Grade I–III mobilization for pain
  Adjustment of involved cervical or thoracic vertebrae
  Stretching of upper trapezius and levator scapula
  Sleep with involved arm up and supported by a pillow to prevent internal rotation

Stage II—Stiffening
  Emphasis is placed on increasing ROM through the use of:
    Rhythmic stabilization and other PNF approaches
    Passive stretching with gravity and hot pack for up to 60 minutes
    Spray and stretch (particularly the subscapularis)
    Continuation of Codman/pendulum exercises at home with weight
    Wall walking
    Self-mobilization with emphasis on inferior glide
    Overhead pulley with TENS (use with caution)
  (In-office stretching should be preceded by ultrasound or short-wave diathermy if not contraindicated)
    Isometric exercises (squeezing ball or using opposite arm resistance) are used to prevent atrophy and maintain "tone"
  Grade IV mobilization to increase ROM

Stage III—Thawing
  Continuation of stiffening program plus:
    Elastic tubing program if tolerated
    Pool exercises

In the second stage, ROM may be increased through the use of a variation of proprioceptive neuromuscular facilitation (PNF). This variation is of a simple technique referred to as *hold-relax*. Hold-relax is a technique that takes advantage of reflex inhibition induced through a contraction of either the agonist or antagonist in a stretched position. The variation is referred to as *rhythmic stabilization* and requires that the patient be challenged to reciprocally contract first one group (agonist or antagonist) than the other rhythmically with contraction against the doctor's resistance (Fig. 16-3).[45] The contraction is minimal, between 20 and 25 percent, and held for 8 to 10 seconds with no rest period between reciprocal activation. This is repeated several times before an attempt at accessing more range. Fairly remarkable gains can often be demonstrated within several minutes. However, like all viscoelastic structures, the soft tissues of the shoulder will attempt to return to their initial contracted state causing some loss of improvement. Even this transitory im-

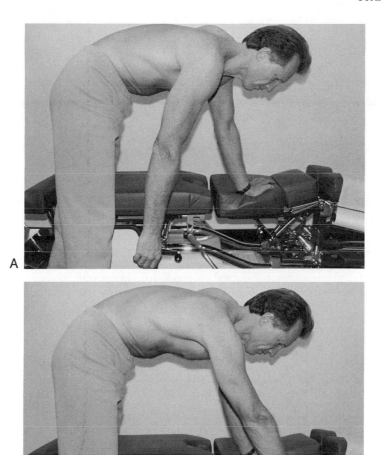

Fig. 16-1. (A & B) Pendulum exercises.

provement reflects the contractile tissue component of a primarily capsular problem. Repeating the procedure 3 to 4 times a week will probably realize the best results.

Addressing the concern of loss due to viscoelastic "memory," Rizk et al.[46] and Sapega et al.[47] have designed a protocol where soft tissue structures can be lengthened without overstrain. The following approach is a modification using minimal load to induce stretching while heating the area being stretched. Before relieving the load, the tissue is cooled. The prescription is

1. Warm the shoulder with a most heat pack for 10 to 15 minutes.
2. Lie in a supine position with the arm abducted and externally rotated as far as tolerable (discomfort is acceptable but not pain). First the patient attempts gravity-induced stretch with the moist heat pack applied to the anterior shoulder (Fig. 16-4). This should be maintained for 45 minutes to 1 hour (change heat packs every 10 to 15 minutes to retain the effect).
3. During the last 10 to 15 minutes, ice is substituted for heat prior to release of the stretch position.

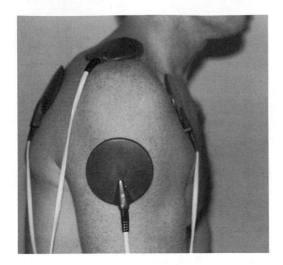

Fig. 16-2. Placement of pads for transcutaneous electrical nerve stimulation treatment of shoulder.

The procedure should be repeated daily for 1 week (5 to 6 days). If the patient is able to perform this pain free, 1 to 2 lb weights can be strapped to the wrist to add an increased load and stretch. Again, pain is the restrictor to continuation.

In the second and final stages, Travell and Simmons[12] recommend treatment primarily of subscapularis trigger points (Fig. 16-5). They contend that active trigger points cause a reflex tightening of the subscapularis, an internal rotator. Attempts by the patient to externally rotate are then resisted by this pseudocontracture of the subscapularis. The subscapularis has several trigger points. The most palpable is in the lateral superior border in the axillary region. To access the lateral trigger point the patient is placed in a supine position. By abducting the arm (as far as possible) and tractioning laterally, palpation through the teres major and latissimus will usually reveal a tender area with associated firm bands of muscle fibers between the serratus anterior and subscapularis (Fig. 16-6).

The options for treatment of trigger points are usu-

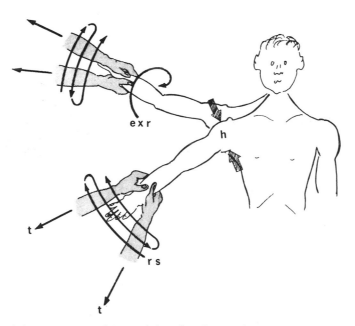

Fig. 16-3. Rhythmic stabilization manipulation of the glenohumeral joint. While the patient applies isometric contraction of the glenohumeral joint to "prevent motion," the therapist attempts to move the arm in abduction external rotation, then reverses to adduction internal rotation. Traction *(t)* is constantly applied. Motion by the therapist is smooth and gradually increasing then decreasing in force and amplitude, with the patient resisting it with equal force. After one cycle at a specific range of abduction, the arm is passively abducted and externally rotated to a further point, and the cycle is repeated. The author performs this technique with the patient's elbow bent. (From Caillett,[45] with permission.)

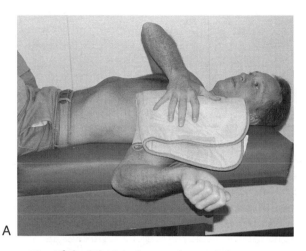
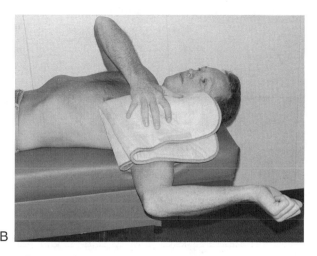

Fig. 16-4. (A) Moist heat pack stretch for increasing range of motion, beginning position. **(B)** Advanced position.

ally ischemic pressure, stretch and spray, and injection (needling). Stretch and spray is a technique whereby the muscle in question is passively stretched. A vapocoolant spray is applied while the stretch is maintained in an attempt to take advantage of a reflex relaxation. The primary caution is not to overcool the skin. To avoid this, the following suggestions are made:

Do not spray at right angles to the skin.
Spray in one direction only using ¼ inch strips.
Hold the bottle about 14 to 18 inches away from the target area.
Use only a few passes being cautious not to frost the skin.

Use fluoromethane not ethylchloride (ethylchloride is colder and may overcool the skin).

The procedure is a sequential approach that can be repeated several times. It consists of the following steps:

Stretch specifically in a manner to effectively stretch the involved muscle (ice may be substituted for spray).

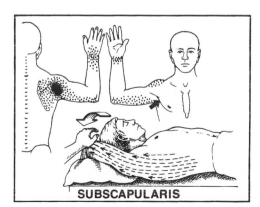

Fig. 16-5. Subscapularis trigger point *(arrow)*. Pain pattern is indicated by dots. (From Basmajian and Kirby,[72] with permission.)

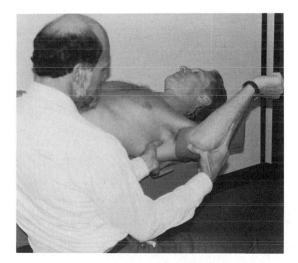

Fig. 16-6. Position to access the subscapularis trigger point. Drag the arm away to expose the ventral surface of the scapula.

Spray parallel to the muscle fibers including both the trigger point and reference zone while maintaining stretch.

Rewarm the area with a moist pack for 20 to 30 seconds.

Follow with a full range active movement by the patient incorporating the involved muscle pattern.

Various stretching procedures, both office and home, have been suggested for increasing ROM. They fall under two categories: stretching of the muscles and articular accessory-movement "stretching." Each attempts to address different aspects of the frozen shoulder. Theoretically, passive stretching of soft tissue without restoration of joint play movement will not demonstrate significant gains in active movement. The most common recommendation is to establish inferior glide of the humerus due to the relationship with abduction and the blockage to downward movement of the humerus by obliteration of the inferior recess.

A summary of glide and stretch maneuvers is illustrated in Figure 16-7. The essence of these maneuvers is to impart a patient or examiner downward glide to the humerus during passive elevation maneuvers. Given that forward flexion is not usually as restricted as abduction, it is often recommended to begin accessing this movement first, while gradually "sneaking up" on abduction over time.

Doorway or overhead pulley stretches are often incorporated with acceptable success. Murray[48] has noted some cautions and limitations of this application.

These include (1) the scapula is not stabilized allowing excessive abduction and rotation; (2) there is no extrinsic force to assure the accessory motion of humeral head depression with abduction; and (3) the patient has a tendency to use the spine through extension, to increase the ROM.

Another home prescription often used is wall walking. Patients are instructed to place their fingers on the wall and walk up the wall to increase abduction. There are many problems with this simple instruction that may render this technique useless or even aggravating. It is extremely important that the patient understand that the movement comes from the wrist and hand and not from the shoulder. The involved shoulder must be totally relaxed to allow stretching. This may be accomplished by monitoring the patient to assure proper technique. A helpful addition is to have the patient place the hand of the well arm on the involved shoulder to detect any unnecessary contractions or scapular contribution.

The wall walk is often given to the patient to begin in abduction. Given that the most restricted range is abduction and one of the least is forward flexion, the patient is instructed in forward flexion wall walking first (Fig. 16-8). Sneaking up on abduction, using progressive yet slight angle changes in relationship to the wall, will gradually access the abduction plane and allow safe, less aggravating movement.

Sleep is usually impossible on the involved side; therefore, it is imperative that with the involved shoulder up, excess internal rotation be prevented. This is

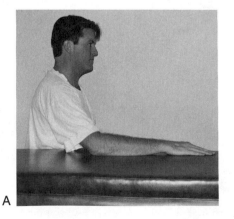
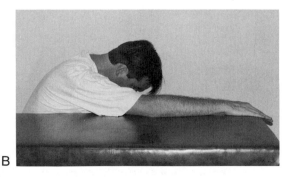

Fig. 16-7. (A & B) Flexion stretch. Patient presses lightly against the table for 8 to 10 seconds followed by a cautious attempt at increased range. *(Figure continues.)*

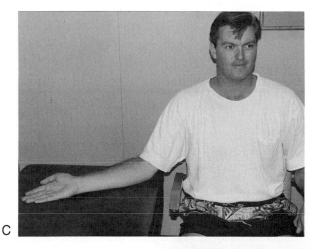
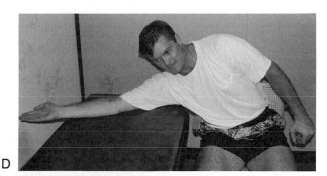
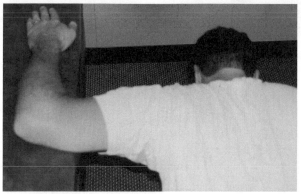

Fig. 16-7. *(continued).* The same procedure is used for the following stretches. **(C & D)** Abduction stretch. **(E)** External rotation stretch.

accomplished by placing a pillow between the involved forearm and the bed as illustrated in Figure 16-9. This prevents a relatively long period of adaptation to a shortened position, perhaps decreasing the degree of contracture.

Murray[48] notes that patients with frozen shoulder have a tendency to overuse the upper trapezius and levator scapula in compensating for the loss of glenohumeral motion. As part of a comprehensive treatment program it is often necessary to address this overuse with office and home stretching. Lateral traction stretching with the shoulder depressed is effective in stretching the upper trapezius while adding flexion addresses the levator scapula.

The cervical spine must be evaluated and treated in most cases of frozen shoulder due to the effects on attaching muscles and their effect on vertebral move-

ment. Lundberg[24] and other researchers[25,49] feel that there may be a relationship between intervertebral disc disorders of the cervical spine and frozen shoulder.

Less Conservative Forms of Treatment

Injections

Steroids with local anesthetic have been recommended in the treatment of frozen shoulder. Injection sites have included subacromial, capsular, and the area of the biceps. Studies have not indicated any significant advantage over other forms of treatment.[50] Travell and Simons[12] suggest that instead of injecting 0.5 percent procaine into the referral zone of the deltoid and glenohumeral areas (common areas of complaint), that

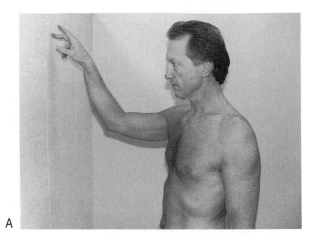
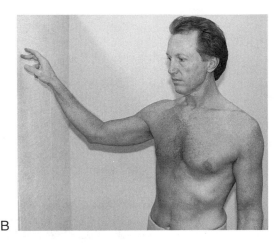
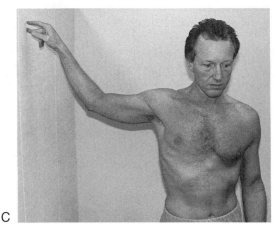

Fig. 16-8. (A) Wall walking beginning in flexion. **(B)** Wall walking progressing to abduction. **(C)** Wall walking in abduction.

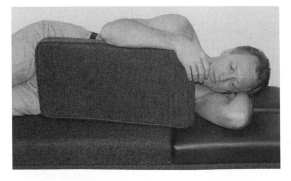

Fig. 16-9. Position of support for sleep to prevent excessive internal rotation and subsequent contracture.

sites in the primary muscles such as the subscapularis should be considered first.

Distension Arthrography

It has been found that arthrography, initially used for diagnostic purposes, may create a therapeutic result. Apparently, the distension that occurs with fluid pressure developed during arthrography is enough to rupture adhesions in some individuals providing temporary and sometimes permanent relief.[51,52] The technique involves serial injections to gradually increase intra-articular pressure. Capsular tears occur in the area of the biceps tendon or subscapularis bursa. Patients with mild to moderately restricted ROM have the most chance of success using this technique. Pain relief may be abrupt or over several hours. ROM may not increase with the reduction in pain.

Manipulation Under Anesthesia or Open Surgery

Many surgeries had been advocated in the past based on the theory of the individual practitioner. Today, manipulation under anesthesia is still recommended in refractory cases. Cautions exist due to the tendency to tear more than adhesions. Tearing of the capsule, in particular the inferior capsule, is common. In addition, the long head of the biceps and the subscapularis tendon are often torn.[25,53] Possible but uncommon complications include recurrent hemorrhagic effusion, hematoma, shoulder dislocation, and humeral fracture.[54,55]

Open surgery has been suggested in refractory cases and with secondary frozen shoulder associated with fracture or postsurgery. Release of the coracohumeral ligament has been suggested to increase external rotation restriction.[56] McLaughlin[25] recommends a combination of manipulation and release of the subscapularis, excising the intra-articular section of the biceps, and surgically releasing adhesions if necessary. Arthroscopic treatment for frozen shoulder is not considered a standard option at this time.

Other Approaches

Although a plethora of other approaches have been advocated, none seem to be beneficial in the long-term outcome. Some of the other approaches include stellate ganglion block,[57] radiotherapy,[58] and oral corticosteroids.[11]

REFLEX SYMPATHETIC DYSTROPHY AND SHOULDER-ARM-HAND SYNDROME

Dysfunction of the sympathetic nervous system may result in a group of disorders referred to as reflex sympathetic dystrophy syndrome.[59,60] Major and minor classifications are used. Major disorders include causalgia, phantom limb pain, and central pain of the thalamus and related neural tracts. The minor classification includes the shoulder-hand syndrome. The terminology is often used interchangeably, which makes distinction difficult. It is convenient to consider the shoulder-hand syndrome as a reflex sympathetic dystrophy syndrome variant. Common historical and clinical ties to the shoulder-hand syndrome include

1. Usually a sequence of pain (with or without trauma) followed by immobilization or disuse, which seems to initiate a sympathetic vasomotor response
2. Dysfunction or failure of the venous and lymphatic circulation pumps to eliminate fluid buildup in the arm and hand
3. The development of a stiff painful shoulder
4. Metacarpophalangeal movement restriction due to edema and contracted ligaments
5. Wrist in flexed position with "intrinsic minus" appearance (extension of phalanges with flexion of metacarpophalanges)
6. Variable sympathetic vasomotor involvement

When there is sympathetic involvement additional signs may include

1. Trophic skin changes
2. Osteoporosis (Sudeck's atrophy)
3. Swelling of the shoulder-arm-hand
4. When exposed to fluctuations in ambient temperature, such as taking a bath, there is an exaggerated erythema alternating with pallor, associated with sweating disturbances
5. History of myocardial infarction, pulmonary disorder, stroke, or trauma is not uncommon; however, many cases are without known cause
6. Vast majority of cases after age 40

Apparently reflex sympathetic dystrophy syndrome or the shoulder-arm-hand syndrome begins with an initiating event that leads to a painful stiff shoulder. The lack of shoulder elevation plus sympathetic involvement leads to edema and further disuse of the entire limb. Resolution is not unlike frozen shoulder in that there is often a protracted course lasting months to years. Usually the syndrome is unilateral. It is bilateral in 20 to 35 percent of cases.

Treatment is difficult, but retaining use of the arm is imperative including mild exercise and stretching. Calliett[45] describes various techniques to decrease hand and arm swelling. Through the use of elevation and compression from twine at the fingers or elastic wrap at the forearm swelling may be reduced. Caution must be used when applying hot or cold. A mild cool pack at approximately 70°F is appropriate. The mainstay of many medical practitioner's treatment are stellate ganglion blocks.

Other suggested forms of treatment include

1. Sympathetic blocks—usually 5 to 7 stellate ganglion blocks (1 block every 1 to 3 days)
2. Sympathectomy in recalcitrant cases
3. TENS over the vascular supply but not the neural supply (to a maximum of on 1 hour, off 1 hour during waking hours)
4. Nonsteroidal anti-inflammatory drugs and beta-blockers
5. Splinting—standard splint modified with support on opposite shoulder. (Do not allow wrist to be in a position of ulnar deviation or palmar flexion or edema will develop.) Splinting should not be worn for extended periods of time without intermittent mild exercise
6. Elevation with exercise to remove edema
7. Intermittent compression through the use of an air-splint with the arm elevated to an angle of 40 to 45 degrees

REFERENCES

1. Bruckner FE, Nye CJS: A prospective study of adhesive capsulitis of the shoulder in a high-risk population. Q J Med 198:191, 1981
2. Rowe CR: The Shoulder. New York, Churchill Livingstone, 1988
3. Bulgen DY, Binder AI, Hazelman BL et al: Frozen shoulder: prospective clinical study with an evaluation of three treatment regimens. Ann Rheum Dis 43:353, 1984
4. Bridgman JF: Periarthritis of the shoulder and diabetes mellitus. Ann Rheum Dis 31:69, 1972
5. Fisher L, Kurtz A, Shipley M: Relationship of cheiroarthropathy and frozen shoulder in patients with insulin dependent diabetes mellitus. Br J Rheumatol 25:141, 1986
6. Wohlgathan JR: Frozen shoulder in hyperthyroidism. Arthritis Rheum 30:936, 1987
7. Oldham BE: Periarthritis of the shoulder associated with thyrotoxicosis. NZ Med J 29:766, 1959
8. Coventry MB: Problem of the painful shoulder. JAMA 151:177, 1953
9. Oestericher W, Van Dam G: Social psychological researchers into brachialgia and periarthritis. Arthritis Rheum 6:670, 1964
10. Tyber MA: Treatment of the painful shoulder syndrome with amitriptyline and lithium carbonate. Can Med Assoc J 111:137, 1974
11. Macnab I: The painful shoulder due to rotator cuff tendinitis. Br Med J 54:367, 1971
12. Travell JG, Simons DG: Myofascial Pain and Dysfunction: The Trigger Point Manual. Williams & Wilkins, Baltimore, 1983
13. Lippman RK: Frozen shoulder: bicipital tenosynovitis. Arch Surg 47:283, 1943
14. Pasteur F: Les aglies de L'epaule et la physiotherapie. J Radiol Electro 16:419, 1932
15. DePalma AF: Loss of scapulohumeral motion (frozen shoulder). Ann Surg 135:193, 1952
16. Simmonds FA: Shoulder pain with particular reference to the frozen shoulder. J Bone Joint Surg 31:834, 1949
17. Codman EA: The Shoulder. Thomas Dodd, Boston, 1934
18. Withers RJW: The painful shoulder: review of one hundred personal cases with remarks on the pathology. J Bone Joint Surg 31:414, 1949
19. Reeves B: The natural history of the frozen shoulder syndrome. Scand J Rheumatol 4:193, 1975
20. Kopell HP, Thompson WAL: Pain and the frozen shoulder. Surg Gynecol Obstet 109:92, 1959
21. Murnaghan JP: Frozen shoulder. p. 837. In Rockwood CA, Matsen FA (eds): The Shoulder. Vol. 1. WB Saunders, Philadelphia, 1990
22. Neviaser JS: Adhesive capsulitis of the shoulder. J Bone Joint Surg 27:211, 1945
23. Neviaser JS: Arthrography of the Shoulder, Charles C Thomas, Springfield, IL, 1975
24. Lundberg BJ: The frozen shoulder. Acta Orthop Scand, suppl. 119:1, 1969
25. McLaughlin HL: The frozen shoulder. Clin Orthop 20:126, 1961
26. Bland JH, Merti JA, Boushey DR: The painful shoulder. Semin Arthritis Rheum 7, 1977
27. Nobuhara K, Sugiyama D, Ikeda H, Makiura M: Contracture of the shoulder. Clin Orthop 254:105, 1990
28. Uhthoff HK, Sarkar K: An algorithm for shoulder pain caused by soft tissue disorders. Clin Orthop 254:121, 1990
29. Fareed DO, Gallivan WR: Office management of frozen shoulder syndrome: treatment with hydraulic distension under local anesthesia. Clin Orthop Relat Res 242:177, 1989
30. Bateman J: The Shoulder and Neck. WB Saunders, Philadelphia, 1978
31. Saha ND: Painful shoulder in patients with chronic bronchitis and emphysema. Am Rev Respir Dis 94:455, 1966
32. Askey JM: The syndrome of painful disability of the shoulder and hand complicating coronary occlusion. Am Heart J 22:1, 1961

33. Wright V, Haq AM: Periarthritis of the shoulder I: aetiological considerations with particular reference to personality factors. Ann Rheum Dis 35:213, 1976

34. Quin EH: Frozen shoulder: Evaluation of treatment with hydroxycortisone injections and exercises. Ann Phys Med 8:22, 1965

35. Grey RG: The natural history of idiopathic frozen shoulder. J Bone Joint Surg 60:554, 1978

36. Haggart GE, Digman RJ, Sullivan TS: Management of the frozen shoulder. JAMA 161:1219, 1956

37. Cyriax J: The shoulder. Br J Hosp Med 19:185, 1975

38. Cyriax J: Textbook of Orthopaedic Medicine. Balliere Tindall, London, 1975

39. Kessel L: Clinical Disorders of the Shoulder. Churchill Livingstone, Edinburgh, 1982

40. Rizk TE, Pinals RS: Histocompatibility type and racial incidence in frozen shoulder. Arch Phys Med Rehabil 65:33, 1984

41. Post M: The Shoulder. Lea & Febiger, Philadelphia, 1978

42. Hazelman BL: The painful stiff shoulder. Rheumatol Rehabil 11:413, 1972

43. Mannheimer J, Lampre G: Clinical Transcutaneous Electrical Nerve Stimulation. FA Davis, Philadelphia, 1984

44. The Academy of Traditional Chinese Medicine: An Outline of Chinese Acupuncutre. Foreign Languages Press, Peking, 1975

45. Calliett R: Shoulder Pain. 2nd Ed. FA Davis, Philadelphia, 1981

46. Rizk TE, Christopher RP, Pinals RS et al: Adhesive capsulitis (frozen shoulder): a new approach to its management. Arch Phys Med Rehabil 64:29, 1983

47. Sapega AA, Quedenfeld TC, Moyer RA et al: Biophysical factors in range of motion exercise. Phys Sports Med 93:57, 1981

48. Murray W: The chronic frozen shoulder. Phys Ther Rev 40:866, 1960

49. Kamieth H: Radiology of the cervical spine in shoulder periarthritis. Z Orthop 100:162, 1965

50. Loyd JA, Loyd HM: Adhesive capsulitis of the shoulder: arthrographic diagnosis and treatment. South Med J 76:879, 1983

51. Andren L, Lundberg DJ: Treatment of rigid shoulders by joint distension during arthrography. Acta Orthop Scand 36:45, 1965

52. Hsu SY, Chan KH: Arthroscopic distension in the management of frozen shoulder. Int Orthop 15:79, 1991

53. Reeves B: Arthrographic changes in frozen and post-traumatic stiff shoulders. Proc R Soc Med 59:827, 1966

54. Haines JF, Hargadon EJ: Manipulation as the primary treatment of frozen shoulder. J R Coll Surg Edinburgh 27:271, 1982

55. Quigley TB: Indications for manipulation and corticosteroids in the treatment of stiff shoulders. Surg Clin North Am 43:1715, 1969

56. Leffert RD: The frozen shoulder. Inst Course Lect 34:199, 1985

57. Wiley AM: Arthroscopic examination of the shoulder. p. 113. In Bayley J, Kessel L (eds): Shoulder Surgery. Springer-Verlag, Berlin-Heidelberg, 1982

58. Ziberberg CH, Leveille-Nizerolle M: La radiographic anti-inflammatoire dans 200 cas de periarthite scapulo-humerale. Sem Hop 52:909, 1976

59. Steinbrocker O: The shoulder-hand syndrome: associated painful homolateral disability of the shoulder and hand with swelling and atrophy of the hand. Am J Med 3:402, 1947

60. Kozin F, McCarty DJ, Sims J, Genant H: The reflex sympathetic dystrophy syndrome. I & II. Am J Med 60:321, 1976

61. Hamer J, Kirk JA: Physiotherapy and the frozen shoulder: a comparative trial of ice and ultrasonic therapy. NZ Med J 83:191, 1976

62. Lee M, Haq AM, Wright V et al: Periarthritis of the shoulder: a controlled trial of physiotherapy. Physiotherapy 59:312, 1972

63. Dacre JE, Beeney N, Scott DL: Injections and physiotherapy for the painful stiff shoulder. Ann Rheum Dis 48:322, 1989

64. Liang H, Lien I: Comparative study in the management of frozen shoulder. J Formosan Med Assoc 72:243, 1973

65. Pothmann R, Weigel A, Stux G: Frozen shoulder: differential acupuncutre therapy with point ST-38. Am J Acupunct 8:65, 1980

66. Helbig B, Wagner P, Dohler R: Mobilization of frozen shoulder under general anesthesia. Acta Belgian Belg 49:267, 1983

67. Connolly J, Regan E, Evan OB: Management of the painful, stiff shoulder. Clin Orthop 84:97, 1972

68. Biswas AK, Star BN, Gupta CR: Treatment of periarthritis shoulder. J Indian Med Assoc 72:276, 1979

69. Nicholson GG: The effects of passive joint mobilization on pain and hypomobility associated with adhesive capsulitis of the shoulder. Orthop Sport Phys Ther 6:238, 1985

70. Roy S, Oldham R: Management of painful shoulder. Lancet 1:1322, 1976

71. Leclaire R, Bourgouin J: Electromagnetic treatment of shoulder periarthritis: a randomized controlled trial of the efficiency and tolerance of magnetotherapy. Arch Phys Med Rehab 72:284, 1991

72. Basmajian JV, Kirby RL: Medical Rehabilitation. Williams & Wilkins, Baltimore, 1984

17

Cervicogenic and Other Extrinsic Causes of Shoulder Pain

THOMAS A. SOUZA

To the medical practitioner, the term cervicogenic, used in reference to the cause of shoulder pain, is a euphemism for radicular pain due to nerve root, spinal cord, or brachial plexus involvement. Common examples in sports include the "burner" or "stinger" and the "burning hands" syndrome found with traumatic injury to the brachial plexus and/or cervical spine. With the exception of osteoarthritic causes of referral pain to the shoulder, most physicians would not recognize other cervical connections. The chiropractor and osteopath recognize an entity of referred pain that involves the segmentally related soft tissue and bony structures. In addition to this neurologic relationship, mechanical dysfunction can result in altered functional capabilities of muscles and their bony attachments. Although this chapter is limited specifically to cervicogenic causes, thoracic and lumbar spinal involvement can also, from a mechanical perspective, alter function of the shoulder through kinesiologic linkage.

THEORIES OF REFERRED PAIN

In an attempt to explain unusual presentations, not typically radicular, several investigators have theorized the possibility of referral from soft tissue and bony structures that are segmentally related. Two distinct approaches have been used in this research. The first involves the use of irritating substances in a group of "normal" individuals. This was first performed by Inman and Saunders[1] in 1944. Feinstein et al.[2] performed similar investigations in 1954. Secondly, Bogduk and Marsland[3] and others[4,5] attempted relief of symptomatic patients with injections of the medial branch of the posterior primary rami with a more specific theory of facet etiology.

Inman and Saunders[1] injected a variety of substances into a variety of tissues to determine the effects. There were several consistent findings, which are listed below:

1. Radiation of pain with associated soreness and tenderness over bony prominences was found to occur with injection of the periosteum, ligamentous, and tendinous attachment sites. This radiation was often latent occurring minutes to hours after the injection. Compared to other tissues stimulated, the periosteum and ligaments were most sensitive.
2. The stimulus was difficult to locate, and more difficult the deeper the irritation.
3. Referral zones were consistent and were charted.
4. Autonomic signs and symptoms often accompanied the stimulation (not uncommon with painful scenarios).

Feinstein et al.[2] were able to confirm the findings of Inman and Saunders[1] but in addition were able to answer questions regarding the relationship of referred pain to the sympathetic and peripheral nervous sys-

457

tems. The patterns of referral are illustrated in Figure 17-1. The following are some other important findings:

1. By performing a sympathetic block the authors found that the pain was not relieved but in fact intensified.
2. Referral pain was similar in location when segmentally related musculature was stimulated.
3. Even after a block of the brachial plexus, pain could still be produced by irritating injection.
4. Hypoalgesia of the skin over the referred areas with deep tenderness and muscle spasm were noted consistently.

The interpretation of these findings indicate that the referral of pain must occur at the spinal cord level or above. Given that anesthetically eliminating the sympathetic and peripheral nervous systems did not prevent the production of pain and that segmentally related musculature produces similar referral pain suggest that referred pain is a function of spinal cord integration and/or cortical misinterpretation.

In addition to the segmental relationship theory, there is the Korr[6] theory of facilitation that would explain why referral pain may be a self-sustaining entity.[6] At the spinal cord level there may be overflow of stimulation. According to the Korr model, when sufficient aberrant sensory stimulation is received, there may be stimulation of both motor and sympathetic efferents, via interneurons, leading to a new source of aberrant sensory stimulation (a vicious cycle) (Fig. 17-2).

Bogduk and Marsland[3] contended that the source of referral pain from the neck is more likely from the facet (zygapophysial) joints. Noting that cervical pain had been treated successfully with denervation of the facet joints, they set out to treat patients with neck pain and associated complaints such as headaches and shoulder pain.

The facet joints are innervated by the medial branch of the posterior primary rami. Bogduk and Marsland[3] performed medial branch blocks on patients to determine specificity of relief in relation to their complaints. They obtained relief in consistent patterns as indicated in Figure 17-3. Shoulder pain was relieved with facet injection at C5 to C6.

It is extremely important to note that the segmentally referred pain zones of Feinstein et al.[2] (scleratogenous?) do not correlate with the relief patterns of Bogduk and Marsland.[3] Feinstein et al.[2] injected multiple structures; Bogduk and Marsland[3] just intra-articular. Marks,[7] who performed intra-articular injections in the lumbar region similar to Feinstein et al.,[2] noted that no distinct segmental or scleratogenous pattern could be recognized in the vast majority of his patients.

Trigger Points

An additional, possibly overlapping concept with the above observations is that of Travell and Simons[8]: trigger point referral. Trigger point referral from muscles inserting at the humerus has been discussed in previous chapters. Trigger point referral from cervicogenic muscles is worth consideration when both neck and shoulder pain coexist. Travell and Simons postulate that due to a myriad of mechanical, environmental, and emotional traumas, areas of localized hypersensitivity develop in muscles. With a continuation of sensitivity these points may become "active" referring to areas that are primarily myotogenous. Examples of potential referrals to the shoulder are illustrated in Chapter 18.

The T4 Syndrome

An entirely empirical entity tagged the T4 syndrome is based on the observation that patients may have a diffuse arm pain, numbness, or paresthesias (nondermatologic).[9] The symptoms usually begin distally moving proximally, and are reproducible by examiner applied movement to the midthoracic area. Relief of symptoms may occur following manipulation of this area. The sympathetic supply to the upper extremity has been found to range from T1 to as far down as T7. Theoretically, from probably a reflex mechanism, the nerve cell bodies are affected by manipulation of the corresponding vertebral level. If true, a similar mechanism could be part of the cause of some "frozen shoulder" cases.

APPROACH TO THE PATIENT WITH CERVICOGENIC INVOLVEMENT

In assessing a patient with possible cervicogenic contribution to the shoulder complaint, it is important to consider both direct (radicular) and indirect (re-

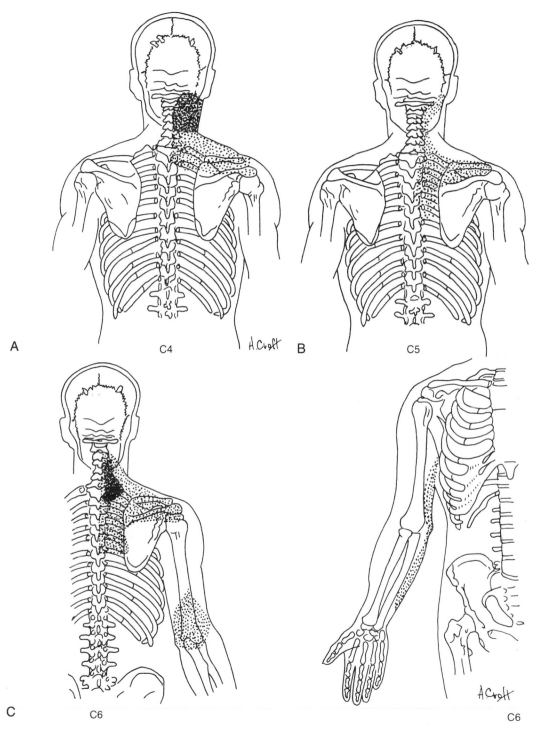

A   C4   H.Croft   B   C5

C   C6   A.Croft   C6

Fig. 17-1. (A–G) Referred patterns of Feinstein (From Foreman and Croft,[71] with permission.) *(Figure continues.)*

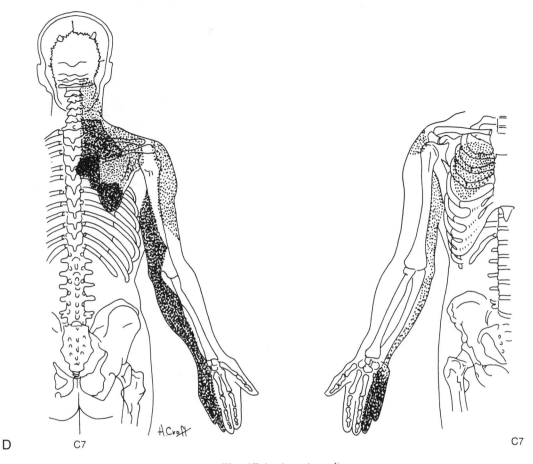

D   C7   C7

Fig. 17-1. *(continued).*

ferred) neural involvement. The evaluation of each overlaps to some degree.

Standard testing of the cervical spine includes both an orthopaedic examination that attempts to reproduce neurologic signs or symptoms and a direct neurologic examination. The general findings indicating radicular involvement include

Reproduction or relief of the patient's radicular complaint with orthopaedic testing, particularly in a specific dermatome
Detection of a nerve root involvement due to:
    a. Loss of muscle strength related to a segmental level
    b. Objectifiable numbness or pain with pinwheel

and similar evaluations that are limited to specific dermatomes
c. Deep tendon reflex changes

Examination distinctions that indicate referred etiology include

Reproduction of a patient's "radicular" complaint with orthopaedic testing that is not limited to a specific dermatome
Production of local discomfort in the neck without reproduction of the "radicular" complaint
Lack of evidence for nerve root involvement even though the patient's complaint is "radicular":
    a. No distinctive loss of muscle strength although

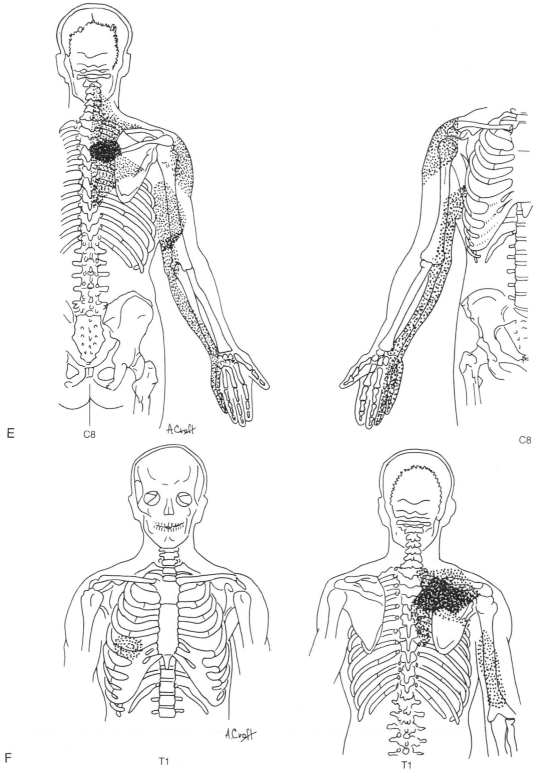

E   C8   A.Croft   C8

F   T1   A.Croft   T1

Fig. 17-1. *(continued).*

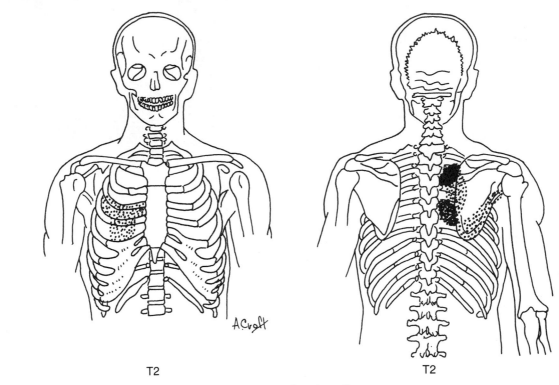

G   T2   T2

Fig. 17-1. *(continued)*.

a sense of weakness or general gripdynamometer evaluation is positive
b. Subjective numbness present but not objectifiable, or not within a dermatome
c. Deep tendon reflexes normal

A quick review of a cervical spine examination should help illustrate the distinctions listed above. Initial orthopaedic testing without prior radiographs or other imaging should be reserved for scenarios where traumatic cervical injury is not reported.

Standard evaluation begins with range of motion (ROM) testing first performed actively then passively. Restrictions may be due to several possibilities:

1. Soft tissue restrictions including spasmed or contracted muscles, or capsular and ligamentous adhesions.
2. Bony restrictions due to fracture/dislocation or osteoarthritic spurring.
3. Neural involvement causing protective recruitment due to pain or instability (overlap with soft tissue

category), or weakness with inability to perform movement.
4. Psychological—willingness to perform the movement.

The distinction between muscular restriction and osseous may be exposed by asking the patient to perform mild isometric contractions of the agonist or antagonist in a stretched position for 8 to 10 seconds. If then more range is accessed, more attempts should be made until a firm end-feel is perceived. This scenario would be reflective of a contractile involvement. Inability to attain more range with this procedure does not rule out muscular involvement, particularly with the protective splinting of a painful condition. However, the ability to access significantly more motion rules out a primarily bony cause.

Finding evidence of osteoarthritic involvement on radiographs does not confirm a cause of a patient's restrictions. Often the range can be increased by muscular relaxation, ligamentous stretching, or in the case of instability, strengthening of cervical musculature.

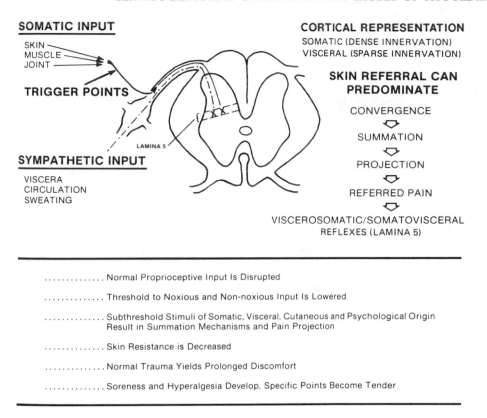

SOMATIC INPUT
SKIN
MUSCLE
JOINT

TRIGGER POINTS

LAMINA 5

SYMPATHETIC INPUT

VISCERA
CIRCULATION
SWEATING

CORTICAL REPRESENTATION
SOMATIC (DENSE INNERVATION)
VISCERAL (SPARSE INNERVATION)

SKIN REFERRAL CAN PREDOMINATE

CONVERGENCE
⇩
SUMMATION
⇩
PROJECTION
⇩
REFERRED PAIN
⇩
VISCEROSOMATIC/SOMATOVISCERAL
REFLEXES (LAMINA 5)

. . . . Normal Proprioceptive Input Is Disrupted

. . . . Threshold to Noxious and Non-noxious Input Is Lowered

. . . . Subthreshold Stimuli of Somatic, Visceral, Cutaneous and Psychological Origin
Result in Summation Mechanisms and Pain Projection

. . . . Skin Resistance is Decreased

. . . . Normal Trauma Yields Prolonged Discomfort

. . . . Soreness and Hyperalgesia Develop, Specific Points Become Tender

Fig. 17-2. Facilitated segment. Disruption of normal excitation threshold of a vertebral segment by abnormal physiologic input and the resultant objective and subjective changes theorized to occur. (From Mannheimer and Lampre,[72] with permission.)

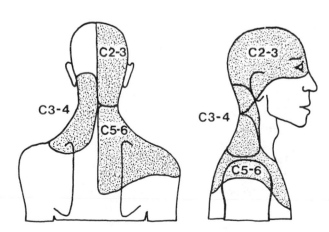

Fig. 17-3. Pain relief patterns from facet injection. (From Bogduk and Marsland,[3] with permission.)

Degenerative changes are less likely a direct stimulus for pain as they are for altered biomechanics leading to local or referred soft tissue pain.

Protective splinting can, in part, be gravity stimulated. An elimination of gravity-induced spasm may occur when the patient is supine. Further distinction can be made with passive testing in the relaxed supine position.

Testing for Nerve Root or Spinal Related Etiology

Standard approaches include cervical compression, distraction, and shoulder depression. Cervical compression is an attempt to compress nerve roots in their foramina reproducing a radicular complaint (Fig. 17-4). However, these same maneuvers may compress the facet capsules or other soft tissue structures producing either a local or nondermatologic radiation response. The patient is first tested in neutral, then with

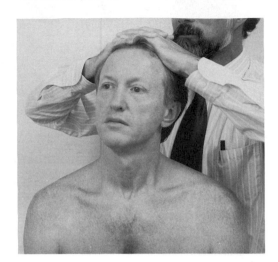

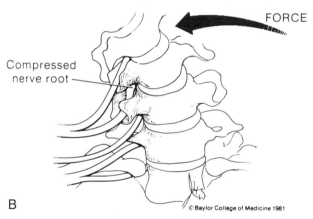

Fig. 17-4. **(A)** Cervical compression testing. **(B)** Mechanism with coupled right lateral bending and compression. (Fig. **B** from Tullos and Bennett,[73] with permission.)

rotation added, followed by rotation coupled with extension and finally flexion. Spurling's test is a variation that involves adding a percussive blow in the provocative position. The sensitivity of this and following "nerve root" tests has been compared to a final diagnosis of disc involvement. The sensitivity is extremely poor. With only clinical testing is may be as low as 40 percent. Adding the extra procedures of radiography and computed tomography (CT), the sensitivity reached about 60 percent.[10]

The distraction test can be used as an extension of a positive compression test or a separate procedure. If distraction relieves a positive compression response, the belief is that it is confirmatory for nerve root involvement. Increase in discomfort may be related to spasmed muscles or capsular adhesions.

Shoulder depression has been designed to first stretch the dural sleeve at the intervertebral foramina; however, the upper trapezius, scalenes, and supraspinatus are also included. If the examiner stretches the head and neck away from the side of shoulder depression after a negative first attempt in cervical neutral, the test will add in the brachial plexus if pain is produced on the side of shoulder depression (Fig. 17-5). If pain is produced on the opposite side, compression similar to the compression test is likely the cause and is indicative of similar processes.

Some authors suggest the brachial plexus stretch test[11] for evaluation (Fig. 17-6). The test is based on a sequence of maneuvers that first test local structural involvement and when not found or eliminated by position adds an additional positional element of stretch to the brachial plexus.

First the arm is abducted to a painful limit, then it is brought slightly below this level to eliminate the pain. The same procedure is used next with external rotation of the arm, then forearm supination without glenohumeral movement, followed by elbow flexion with forearm supination without glenohumeral movement. An increase in symptoms with the final maneuver is supposed to suggest brachial plexus involvement. Other maneuvers that may increase symptoms are wrist extension, contralateral arm abduction and external rotation, and cervical spine flexion. Finally, a Valsalva maneuver and Soto-Hall maneuver can help in exposing a space-occupying lesion (SOL).

Chiropractic Evaluation and Treatment

Coupled with the general orthopaedic findings, static and motion palpation of the cervical and thoracic spine will aid in determining a vertebrogenic cause of referred pain. Static palpation usually reveals local areas of tenderness and suggests areas of fixation. Occasionally transverse process pressure can cause a referral pain, but this is usually along the medial border of the scapula ("doorbell" sign). The intention of motioning a vertebral segment is to attempt a more functional appreciation of intersegmental motion. If blockages occur at the lower cervical area, it is more likely that referred pain from these areas is the cause due to the neurologic connection with the shoulder and arm. Radiographic evaluation can statically reveal degenera-

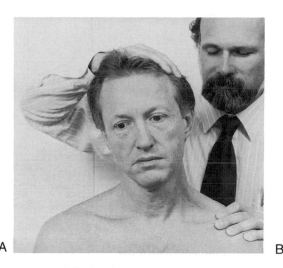 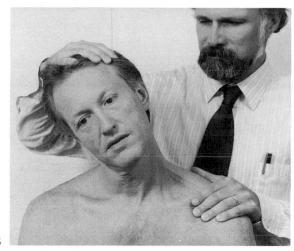

Fig. 17-5. (A) Shoulder depression without neck distraction. **(B)** Shoulder depression with coupled lateral cervical bending stretch.

tive changes in the lower cervical regions, again suggesting referral pain when frank objective neurologic signs are not present. Some authors recommend motion films to determine areas of hyper- and hypomobility. Oblique films will help determine if foraminal encroachment is a factor.

There are two explanations of why a patient may have foraminal encroachment visible on radiograph and although complaining of radiating pain have no objective neurologic signs. The first is that when a single nerve root is involved it is more likely that nondermatomal pain and paresthesias dominate the patient presentation without frank motor signs. This is probably because dermatomes overlap and most muscles are innervated by more than one nerve root. Therefore, objectifiable numbness and gross motor weakness are not evident. The second explanation is that the pain and paresthesias may be referred due to irritation of the facet joints and surrounding soft tissue. It is theorized by many chiropractors that this referred pain may be due to local intersegmental fixation of vertebrae corresponding to the neural level of involvement. It is also suggested that compensatory hypermobility may allow excessive movement, thereby causing irritation especially when complicated by bony degenerative changes.

Although treatment approaches vary in chiropractic, most have the intent of restoring normal movement by eliminating the areas of fixation. This may be accomplished through adjusting procedures or a variety of indirect approaches. Nansel et al.[12] have demonstrated increases in passive cervical end-range motion in asymptomatic individuals following cervical adjustments. In addition, many practitioners including this author suggest manipulation coupled with cervical traction in most cases of foraminal encroachment. If successful, home traction units are prescribed. Although the success rate seems empirically to be quite high, there is unfortunately little confirmation through research publication.

It has been theorized that disturbance of mechanical function in and about the cervical spine can neurologically affect reflexes that govern synchronization of muscle patterns for various body postures through processes of facilitation and inhibition. McCouch et al.[13] found that the upper cervical region contains receptors important to the neck righting reflexes (tonic neck reflex in infants). Stejskal[14] has demonstrated that facilitation of the deltoid and supraspinatus and inhibition of the pectoralis major occurred on the same side as head rotation. Cohen[15] produced imbalance and incoordination in animals who had the dorsal roots of C1, C2, and C3 anesthetized. These findings suggest, theoretically, that reflexes depend on accurate proprioceptive feedback and may demonstrate dysfunction with aberrant input that may arise from "fixated" vertebral segments. Therefore, balance of muscle tone and vertebral movement through soft tissue and manipulative approaches may affect these reflexes. It will probably be some time before the importance of these re-

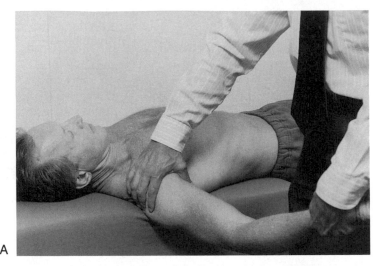

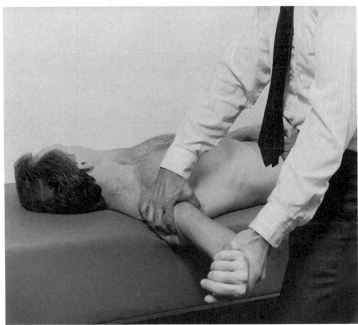

Fig. 17-6. (A) Beginning position. Each subsequent position is modified if pain is produced, ending in **(B)** brachial plexus stretch position.

flexes and the effect that manipulation has on them is determined.

THORACIC OUTLET SYNDROME

Thoracic outlet syndrome (TOS) consists of mainly neurologic and occasionally vascular signs and symptoms related to compression or entrapment of the bra-

chial plexus and/or subclavian-axillary vessels as they course downward to supply the arm. A suspicion of thoracic outlet involvement would be based on a presentation with somewhat diffuse upper extremity signs and symptoms. In 40 percent of cases there is a traumatic episode.[16] This means that in over half the cases no inciting trauma may be reported. Although any portion of the neurologic component can be affected, it is more common to see the lower brachial plexus presentation usually without a vascular component. The key historical clue is the relationship to positional induction and relief. Often when other extra-shoulder causes are involved, raising the arm or supporting the elbow with lift is the relieving position. The opposite is true for many cases of thoracic outlet involvement.

There are numerous theories regarding the etiology of TOS, including trauma as mentioned above. In addition, postural components, including either lack of muscular support or myofascial "contracture," have been suggested, alone or in combination, to result in a stooped posture (Fig. 17-7). Shortening of the pectoralis minor and scalenes is most commonly implicated. Entrapment by fibrous bands, anomalous slips of muscle, and muscle hypertrophy have also been postulated.

Sites of Entrapment

There are many potential sites of entrapment as the neurovascular bundle of the brachial plexus and subclavian-axillary vessels traverse down into the arm (Fig. 17-8). These sites are more easily differentiated ana-

tomically than clinically. There are essentially four vulnerable areas of compression:

1. Superior thoracic outlet—the more inferior aspects of the brachial plexus pass through this area.
2. Scalene groove or triangle—the roots of C5 to T1 and the subclavian artery pass through this area.
3. Costoclavicular interval—this is the space between the first rib and clavicle where the trunks or divisions of the brachial plexus and the subclavian-axillary vessels pass through.
4. Subcoracoid loop—this is the point at which the brachial plexus and axillary vessels pass under the coracoid process and pectoralis minor muscle.

Superior Thoracic Outlet

The superior thoracic outlet is an area bounded by the first rib, manubrium, and the first two thoracic vertebrae. It is more likely that brachial plexus compression at this site would be due to either an SOL or a cervical rib. Some potential SOLs would be tumors involving the thyroid gland, pleura, and lungs. An apical tumor

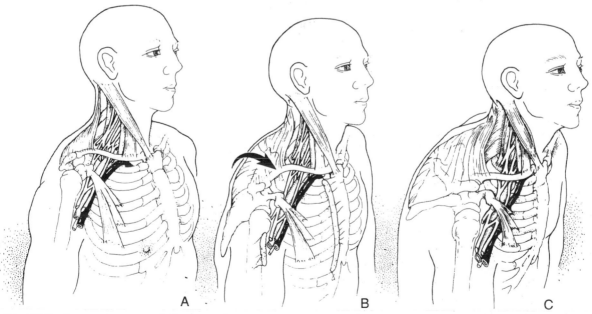

Fig. 17-7. Progressive postural distortion/decompensation with neurovascular compression. **(A)** Normal resting posture. **(B)** Shoulder protraction beginning; sternomastoid muscles are shortening, drawing head anteriorly and inferiorly. **(C)** Advanced deformity with adaptive shortening of scalene and smaller pectoral muscles. Note narrowed costoclavicular space as well (ribs 1 through 5 have been relatively elevated). Neurovascular compression is evident at all three sites. (From Sucher,[74] with permission.)

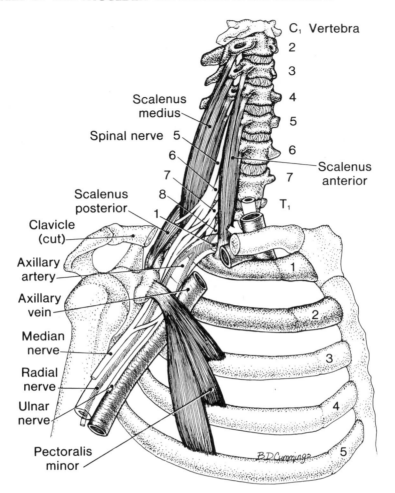

Fig. 17-8. Thoracic outlet entrapment by the scalene muscles. The neurovascular bundle is spread out to show the relations of its component parts. A portion of the clavicle has been removed. The brachial plexus and axillary artery emerge above the first rib and behind the clavicle between the scalenus anterior and scalenus medius muscles. The spinal nerves are numbered on the left, the vertebrae on the right. The T1 nerve lies dorsal to and beneath the subclavian artery. (From Travell and Simons,[8] with permission.)

such as a Pancoast should be considered if the history suggests and an associated Horner syndrome is evident. Although cervical ribs have often been associated with TOS, it is important to remember that fewer than 1 percent of the population have cervical ribs and that fewer than 10 percent of those individuals will ever have symptoms of TOS.[17,18] Beyond this observation is the finding that fewer than 10 percent of patients who required surgical decompression had cervical ribs.[19] If a short cervical rib or elongated C7 transverse process is present, compression may occur by a fibrous band that may connect this variation to the first rib.[20]

It should be noted that there is a strong correlation between cervical ribs and the development of a subclavian aneurysm.[21,22]

Scalene Triangle

The attachment of the scalenes is variable. There may be overlapping insertions of the anterior and middle scalenes onto the first rib or a conjoined tendon with an overlying fibrous band that may act as the offending structure.[23] The space between the anterior and middle scalene rib attachments are often no more than 2 cm leaving more of a groove than a space or triangle. Although arterial occlusion is theoretically possible, signs of involvement are rare. Venous occlusion is not possible due to the passage of the subclavian vein anterior to the anterior scalene.

Cervical spine movement into extension or rotation to the ipsilateral side can potentially diminish the anteroposterior dimensions (Fig. 17-9). Therefore, it is theoretically possible that shortening of the scalenes will augment this effect. Other components can include a cervical rib that decreases the vertical dimensions of the scalene triangle by elevating the base, and the position of abduction and external rotation, which may traction the brachial plexus.

Costoclavicular Interval

The costoclavicular interval is the space between the first rib and clavicle where the neurovascular bundle passes. The space can potentially be decreased by depression of the shoulder, poor posture, and fractures or exostosis of the clavicle or first rib (Fig. 17-10A). Depression of the shoulder can occur as a result of carrying heavy loads with the arms at the side or carrying a heavy backpack.

Given that the scapula migrates downward in development, the patient may be asymptomatic until such time as the alignment of structures causes tension or compression. It is important to note that TOS is uncommon in the younger age group before puberty. In addition, there is more scapular descent in females than males.[19]

Trauma can be the cause of muscular dysfunction either directly through local hemorrhage or pain leading to abnormal shoulder mechanics and indirectly through immobilization or protection. Acquired shoulder depression can occur in athletes. Commonly seen in tennis players, this "drooping" shoulder can be due to increased weight of the dominant arm or attenuation of the supporting muscles and capsule due to repetitive stretching and microtrauma.

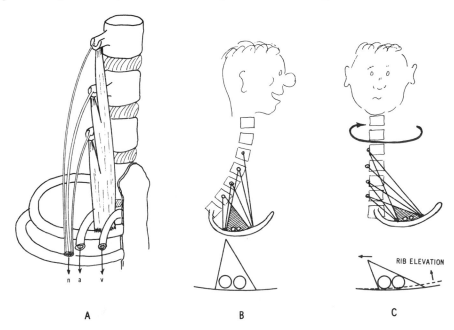

A   B   C

Fig. 17-9. Scalene anticus syndrome. **(A)** Relationship of the neurovascular bundle. The subclavian artery *(a)* passes behind the anterior scalene muscle, loops over the first rib, and is joined by the brachial plexus *(n)*. The artery is separated from the subclavian vein *(v)* by the anterior scalene muscle. The median scalene muscle (not shown) lies behind the nerve *(n)*. **(B)** The triangle formed by the scalenes and the first rib. **(C)** Distortion from turning the head toward the symptomatic side. Compression of the neurovascular bundle—the brachial plexus, the subclavian artery, and occasionally the subclavian vein—can be pictured from the test maneuver of the anticus scalene syndrome. (From Caillett,[75] with permission.)

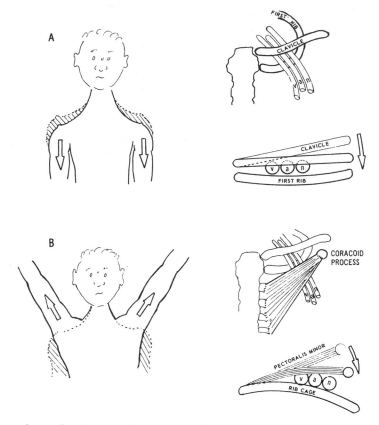

Fig. 17-10. Claviculocostal and pectoralis minor syndromes. **(A)** Claviculocostal syndrome. The neurovascular bundle is compressed between the clavicle and the first rib by retraction and depression of the shoulder girdles. **(B)** Pectoralis minor syndrome. The neurovascular bundle can be compressed between the pectoralis minor and the rib cage by elevating the arms in a position of abduction and moving the arms behind the head. (From Caillett,[75] with permission.)

The support of the scapula is essentially muscular, and therefore any fatigue or dysfunction of this muscular support may predispose to TOS. Furthermore, the addition of weight from a backpack, purse, child, or heavy breasts can accentuate the problem. Disuse or dysfunction of the serratus anterior or other stabilizing muscles may transiently predispose an individual to TOS. This "scapula suspensory insufficiency" should be evaluated in patients with vague upper extremity signs or symptoms.

Subcoracoid Loop

Another site of potential compression is as the brachial plexus loops under the coracoid and pectoralis minor insertion (Fig. 17-10B). Although not considered a very common cause of TOS, in the athlete the factor of re-

petitive hyperabduction should be considered. Hyperabduction is most commonly found with tennis serving, swimming, and some forms of throwing. The coracoid process and pectoralis minor act as a fulcrum over which the neurovascular structures are stretched. Hypertrophy of the pectoralis minor has also been implicated as a cause of TOS in swimmers.

TOS Testing

The standard sequence of testing is first to test the integrity of the distal arteries to determine if local occlusion may be responsible for any hand symptoms. The Allen's test is used for this purpose. The hand is elevated. The examiner occludes the ulnar and radial artery with the hands and asks the patient to pump his or her hand. This will eliminate blood supply through the venous system without arterial filling. Then one artery at a time is released to observe for a return of normal color within 10 seconds. Absence of this return of blood supply will be manifested by a blanched skin appearance that does not return or is markedly delayed.

A simple in-office test that attempts to reproduce the sense of weakness with overhead activity is the Roo's overhead grip test (Fig. 17-11). Simply by asking the patient to raise the hands overhead and repeatedly grip and release may reproduce weakness within 20 to 60 seconds. Some patients may experience a cramping of the forearms and occasionally the involved arm will develop pallor.

The other TOS tests address each of the possible geographic locations of compression with specific maneuvers. The following maneuvers are associated with a high incidence of false-positive and false-negative responses.[16] More definitive is the response of reproducing the patient's complaint rather than diminishing or obliterating the radial pulse (which may be found in 50 percent of normal individuals). The Adson's[24] and Halstead's tests are designed to test the anterior and middle scalenes, respectively. For the Adson's test, the patient's pulse is monitored while the patient turns the head toward the side of involvement (Fig. 17-12). Some authors indicated using a Valsalva maneuver to further magnify positive findings. Either a substantial decrease in the pulse or an increase in the patient's symptomatology is indicative of a positive response. Turning the head to the opposite side with some arm abduction

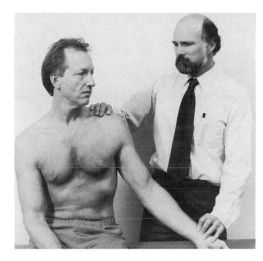

Fig. 17-12. Adson's test.

and extension tests for middle scalene compression (the Halstead's test, Fig. 17-13).

The Eden's test or costoclavicular test compresses the neurovascular bundles between the clavicle and first rib. The patient is instructed to draw the shoulders back with elevation (a military posture). The examiner palpates the pulses bilaterally. Again, an increase in symptoms or a significant decrease in pulse is indicative of a positive response.

Wright's (hyperabduction) test[25] is probably the most unreliable due to position (Fig. 17-14). The test is designed to determine if the neurovascular bundle is being compressed under the pectoralis minor mus-

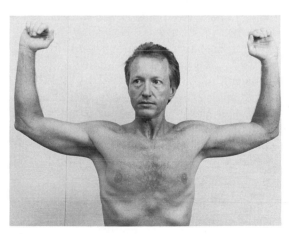

Fig. 17-11. Overhead grip test for TOS. Patient grips and releases repetitively in an effort to reproduce symptoms.

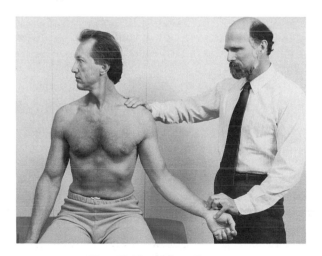

Fig. 17-13. Halstead's test.

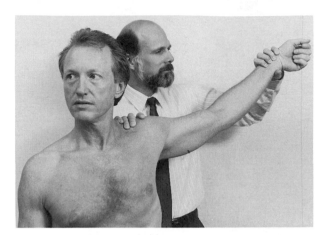

Fig. 17-14. Wright's (hyperabduction) test.

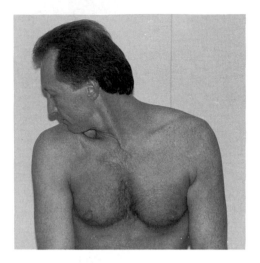

Fig. 17-15. Scalene cramp test.

cles. First, the examiner should raise the arm to 90 degrees and palpate the pulse with forward flexion. Then with varying degrees of abduction and external rotation, if positive, the pectoralis minor can be implicated. Many people will have a decrease with elevation alone, indicating a gravity response. However, the combination of a normal pulse with elevation with a significant decrease in abduction external rotation is suggestive of the pectoralis minor.

If, in addition to a diminution of pulse and reproduction of symptoms, a bruit is simultaneously heard over the subclavian, a confirmation of arterial compression is gained.

Travell and Simons[8] have devised the scalene cramp test and the scalene relief test (Figs. 17-15 and 17-16). The patient attempts to place the chin in the ipsilateral supraclavicular fossa. Relief of the symptoms should then occur with the relief test, which involves the patient returning to a neutral head position and then abducting the arm. By then bringing the arm across the front of the forehead, the clavicle is brought forward away from compression. Relief should occur within minutes.

Travell and Simons[8] also feel that general extensor digitorum involvement is associated with scalene trigger points. They advocate the finger flexion test. If all the fingers cannot be flexed enough to touch the palm, the test is positive indicating (indirectly) involvement of the scalenes. The suggestion is that fluid accumulation due to lymphatic blockage is the cause of the finger flexion restriction and the result of myofascial involvement of the scalenes. Mechanical and local possi-

bilities should be ruled out before making this assumption. The development of hand edema with a concomitant "frozen shoulder" is suggestive of reflex sympathetic dystrophy syndrome (see Ch. 16).

Other Diagnostic Testing

Radiographs of the cervical spine should be included to distinguish among the various cervicogenic mimickers of TOS. Entities to screen include disc degeneration and accompanying spondylosis. The apex of the lung should be well visualized to rule out pathologic processes in this area such as a Pancoast tumor. Causes of TOS that can be visualized or suspected from cervical films include adventitial ribs and elongated transverse processes. Again, the elongated transverse may have a fibrous band connecting it to the first rib. This is not radiographically demonstrable.

If available, it is occasionally helpful to include digital plethysmography or Doppler studies. They can be an important adjunct especially when there are positive plethysmography or Doppler findings on the symptomatic side and normal findings on the asymptomatic side.

Electromyography and Nerve Conduction Velocity Testing

Electromyography and nerve conduction velocity (NCV) testing are reserved for difficult cases where a

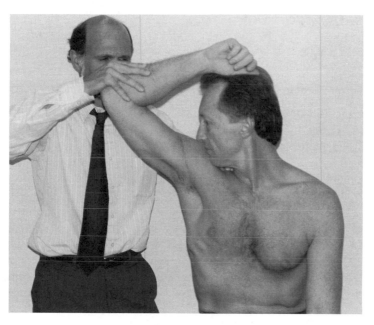

Fig. 17-16. Scalene relief test.

diagnosis is equivocal and needs further confirmation. Following is a brief description of each and how it may help in differentiating disorders of muscle, nerves, or the neuromuscular junction.

Electromyography is performed by inserting a concentric needle electrode into a specific muscle. Then specific patterns of electrical activity are monitored during several periods:

1. At insertion—electrical activity usually lasts only a few seconds. Prolongation is seen in patients with myopathy.
2. At rest—spontaneous activity such as fibrillations, potentials, fasciculations, and positive sharp waves usually indicates a neurogenic abnormality (usually indicating nerve degeneration).
3. During contraction—neurogenic disorders cause a reduction in the density pattern, interference pattern, and mean amplitude of motor unit potentials. Myopathies decrease the duration and amplitude of motor unit potentials but do not affect the interference pattern. Therefore, the main usefulness of electromyography is to differentiate between a myopathy and a neuropathy.

Limitations of electromyography include

1. Does not indicate specifically the etiology of the problem.
2. Due to persistence of neuropathic changes, timing of the onset of the problem is unreliable.
3. Testing is painful.
4. The test must be performed by a skilled examiner.

The velocity of both motor and sensory nerves can be evaluated through NCV measurement. This is done by stimulation at specific points and measurement of the latencies of each response. Sensory testing is usually more sensitive than motor in detecting metabolic disorders and nerve trauma. By dividing nerve problems into axonopathies; producing axon degeneration like diabetes and nutritional polyneuropathies, and myelinopathies; and producing myelin degeneration like nerve entrapment syndromes and Guillain-Barré syndrome one may differentiate based on the response to motor NCV. Axonopathies do not show abnormalities in the motor NCV until very late in the disorder, whereas myelinopathies show a decrease NCV due to the slowing of conduction with loss of myelin.

The use of electrodiagnostic studies should probably be reserved for cases of peripheral neuropathy or differentiation between these problems and cervical disc involvement. Although demonstrated by Urschel and Razzuk[26] as an accurate means of detecting TOS, most would agree that this means of testing should be reserved for difficult cases. There is a debate over the use of these studies based on the criticism that accurate measurement of nerve conduction velocity through the thoracic outlet is difficult. In fact, patients who were considered either mild or "nonspecific/disputed" neurogenic TOS had normal electrodiagnostic studies. When the patient had mainly a neurogenic TOS some of the consistent indicators were (1) low-amplitude median motor response with a normal sensory response, (2) low-amplitude ulnar sensory response, and (3) C8 to T1 neurogenic motor potentials.

F-waves have been suggested as a helpful indicator in diagnosing TOS.[27] F-wave or axillary F-wave latencies are very uncomfortable for the patient, which makes their inclusion questionable. They attempt to measure time for the impulse to loop through the brachial plexus.

Due to its noninvasiveness, it has been suggested that thermography is the ideal tool for evaluating TOS. Unfortunately, there is a problem in lack of specificity. Although able to detect changes in heat intensity, the ability to discern the location of the etiology is not possible. Also, autonomic changes may occur due to reflex activity that is unrelated to TOS. Venous stasis may increase the heat response; however, this is the opposite effect of arterial occlusion. Reflex sympathetic dystrophy can cause a diffuse finding on thermography. This entity has been associated by some authors with TOS while others considered it a separate diagnosis. The confusion with a neurogenic pattern on thermography in the C7 to C8 dermatome territory is that it does not differentiate between cervical radiculopathy and a common presentation of TOS.

Howell[28] has suggested the use of Semmes Weinstein monofilaments. These filaments are calibrated to bend when a specific amount of threshold pressure is reached. Ranging from 0.0045 to 447 g, these filaments can be used to map out the sensory aspects of the palms compared to a normal baseline. The entire extremity could be mapped with the other extremity acting as the normal comparison. Howell also suggested use of ninhydrin sweat testing for those with a strong sympathetic component.

Use of arteriography or venography should be reserved for cases where prior thoracic outlet surgery was unsuccessful and another attempt is planned or in patients with both long cervical ribs and a bruit. The latter is based on the correlation between aneurysm of the subclavian and long cervical ribs.

CONSERVATIVE TREATMENT

When the cause of TOS is soft tissue in nature there are two specific approaches that seem to be effective. The first is to correct postural imbalances through stretching and exercise. The second is to address trigger points that may exist in the primary muscles of compression. Some of the difficulties with this conservative approach is that many of the stretches and some of the exercises will temporarily exacerbate the patient's complaints. This is acceptable if the increase in symptoms is less than 2 hours following the exercise or stretch. It is important to stretch 5 to 10 times daily to effectively address contracture.

When shoulder pathology such as instability is present performance of the exercises or stretches may not be attainable. In this situation, correction of the underlying instability may be necessary first, either conservatively or surgically, before the TOS can be directly addressed. Interestingly, Leffert[16] observed that some patients who were rehabilitated following surgery for instability resolved their TOS symptoms without any direct attention.

In the 1940s there was recognition of the value in altering activities of occupation, daily living, and resting to help ameliorate the symptoms. By focusing on support of the arms during standing and sitting, symptoms can be reduced. The simple use of an arm rest while seated and support from a sling or the other hand if possible may help. For women with large breasts, extra support in the bra such as an underwire and padding of the shoulder straps to increase the surface area of contact can also be helpful. Arm slings and figure-eight type clavicular braces were used by Hansson[29] to relieve pressure from an unsupported arm. Interestingly, placing the arm behind the head in a rested position may relax the anterior scalene and provide relief, but this same position can aggravate the problem due to elevation and possible compression from the pectoralis minor.

Alteration of sleep patterns can help in the early phases of treatment. Often patients feel an aggravation with the arm above the head posture. This may relax the scalenes, as mentioned, previously, but provide entrapment around the coracoid.

Reichert[30] recommended an approach that would seem to mimic the offending posture. He had his patients sleep with three overlapping pillows with the intention of holding the cervical spine in flexion and the scapula abducted. He claimed success with 60 out of 74 patients.

In-office stretching should focus on the scalenes and pectoral muscles. The specifics are described in Chapter 18. Travell and Simons[8] recommend a supine or seated stretch of the scalenes for home care. The seated stretch involves grasping under a chair with the ipsilateral hand while stretching the head with the contralateral hand (Fig. 17-17). With the head turned slightly in the direction of pull the posterior scalene is addressed. With the head in neutral, the middle scalene is stretched. With the head turned toward the side of involvement, the anterior scalene is stretched. The supine stretch is performed with the patient's ipsilateral hand stabilized under the buttocks. The contralateral hand then stretches the relaxed neck in several ways to address each scalene.

Stretching of the pectorals can be performed by leaning through a doorway (Fig. 17-18) or into a corner with the arms elevated supporting body weight with the forearms or hands (Fig. 17-19). Different elevation levels stretch different aspects of the pectorals. Middle trapezius corner exercises can be performed by leaning back into a corner, taking a step away, and supporting body weight with the forearms; the shoulders are abducted and elbows flexed (Fig. 17-20). Contracting the muscles between the scapula in an attempt to bring the scapula together will result in the chest moving up and forward. No arm movement should occur. This is a difficult exercise due to the need to focus the contraction between the shoulder blades and not recruit the arm musculature. The contraction is held for 3 to 5 seconds and slowly released. Repetitions should start with 5 and over several weeks progress to 25 to 35 with three sets performed three times per day.

LEVATOR SCAPULA SYNDROME

The levator scapula muscles can be a source of painful shoulder movement due to their effect on shoulder and cervical spine movement. Referred to as levator scapulae syndrome by Estwanik,[31] superior scapula syndrome by Moseley,[32] and scapulocostal syndrome by Shull,[33] this syndrome may present with neck, shoulder, and arm pain. Reid[34] feels that this syndrome may be a variant of brachial neuritis (see below). Estwanik found that symptoms could be aggravated through sports such as wrestling, weightlifting, sailing, swimming, gymnastics, boxing, karate, and golf.

The levator scapula elevates the superior border of the scapula while lowering the glenoid. Working together, both levator scapula act as "checkreins" on cervical flexion. Postures involving chronic cervical flexion occupationally or with sports can cause a chronic irritative process. Attachment to the transverse process of the upper four cervical vertebrae may affect vertebral movement at these levels. Tightening of the levator scapula will cause lowering of the glenoid, which may affect the ability to use the shoulder in overhead activities.

Evaluation is recommended with the patient prone, supporting upper body weight onto the elbows. This elevates the superior border of the scapula away from the thorax allowing palpation. If injection is used in treatment this is also the ideal position (avoiding possible pneumothorax). It is important to compare both sides due to the common tenderness found in normal individuals. In other words, palpation should reveal a comparatively more tender point, and in classic cases reproduce the patient's complaint. Differential considerations should include cervical disc lesions, cervical osteoarthritis, cervical subluxation, and fibromyalgia. Visceral referred pain should be ruled out.

Treatment focuses on stretching the levator scapulae through the use of proprioceptive neuromuscular facilitation techniques and spray and stretch techniques described by Travell and Simons.[8] The patient is seated and using the hand grasps under the chair. The examiner stretches the neck forward and to the opposite side while applying fluoromethane spray or ice massage. Adjusting of upper cervical vertebra may be appropriate when restrictions are found.

Ischemic massage with a tennis ball and home stretching using the above position are prescribed. Avoidance of lifting heavy objects overhead or carrying heavy objects such as heavy briefcases should be followed for several weeks. Postural correction exercises coupled with ergonomic counseling regarding

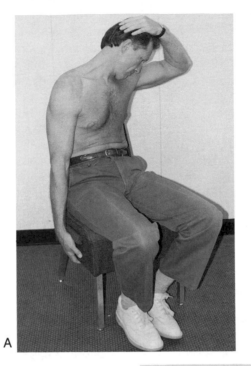

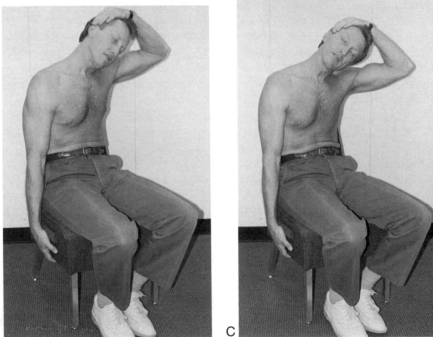

Fig. 17-17. (A) Stretch of posterior scalene and upper trapezius. **(B)** Middle scalene. **(C)** Anterior scalene.

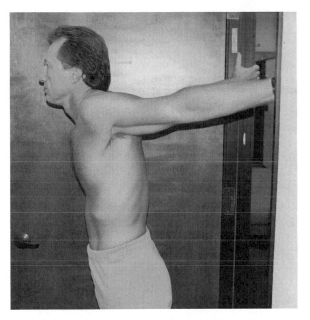

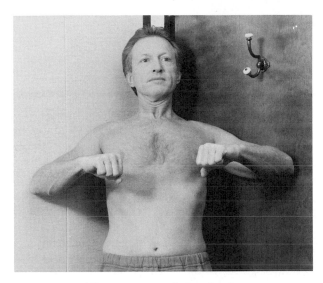

Fig. 17-20. Middle trapezius and rhomboid corner exercise.

Fig. 17-18. Pectoral stretching in the doorway.

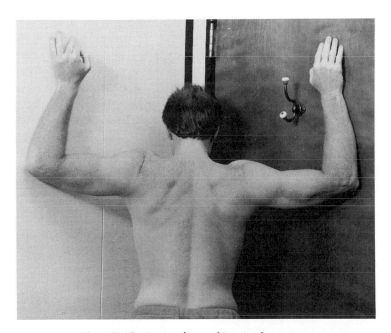

Fig. 17-19. Pectoral stretching in the corner.

stooped reading and work postures should be emphasized.

EFFORT THROMBOSIS

Effort thrombosis is considered a variant of TOS. Considered rare, it is still probably the most common vascular problem in athletes.[35] Although related mainly to trauma, it appears that compression of the subclavian or axillary veins by some of the same structures causing TOS may result in damage to the venous wall with subsequent thrombus formation. An interesting finding is that although complete obstruction is demonstrated by a venogram, evidence of a thrombus is not found at surgery.[33] The literature reports effort thrombosis occurring in swimmers[36] and hockey players,[37] also in baseball, gymnastics, volleyball, weightlifting, football, tennis, rowing, and basketball.[38]

The complications of thrombosis include (1) disability due to inability to use the arm because of swelling accompanied by a sense of heaviness or weakness, and (2) pulmonary embolism, which occurs in 12 percent of individuals with subclavian vein thrombosis.

The history and clinical presentation vary considerably from an immediate onset to a prolonged onset over a couple of weeks. The most common presenting complaint is a deep pain in the arm with associated swelling and rubor of the involved arm. Cyanosis with distension of the superficial veins may also be found. The swelling is usually relieved by elevation. The list of differentials with a patient complaining of upper extremity swelling, weakness, and/or pain is long including metastatic disease, infection, sarcoidosis, and multiple causes of poor circulation.

Further evaluation can be performed with a venogram. Although considered the standard, a venogram may cause extension of the thrombus.[38] CT and Doppler may also be helpful. Doppler seems particularly helpful in differentiating between compression and thrombosis.

Conservative treatment involves elevation of the arm. This will usually relieve the acute pain and swelling in 3 to 4 days; however, 60 to 85 percent of patients who receive no other treatment have persistent symptoms.[39] The athlete is usually placed on heparin for 10 days followed by warfarin. Intravenous streptokinase is used for clot dissolution if the clot is less than 2 weeks old. Sports activities are eliminated until the signs and symptoms resolve. Surgical treatment is of the thrombus (rare) and is only successful in local involvement. Other surgical treatment includes first rib resection and other forms of thoracic outlet decompression.

BRACHIAL PLEXUS AND PERIPHERAL NERVE INVOLVEMENT

The brachial plexus and peripheral nerves can become involved in shoulder dysfunction through several mechanisms:

1. Direct acute trauma to the nerve such as a blow
2. Direct acute trauma through surgery
3. Direct chronic trauma through stretching or compression (entrapment)
4. Indirect damage through injections (corticosteroids)
5. Idiopathic neuritis (brachial neuritis)

The severity of injury has been graded by various authors.[40,41] A synthesis of these classifications may be helpful with the caution that the distinction between these grades has been idealized. The delineation between a severe grade I and early grade II is not always so clear. The division into grades is based on the degree of damage, the longevity of signs and symptoms, and electromyographic documentation of denervation or lack thereof.

A grade I is considered a neuropraxia with only physiologic interruption of normal function. The symptoms usually include dysesthesias and weakness, which are transient, usually not lasting more than 10 to 12 hours in the most severe cases. Prognosis for full recovery is 100 percent. A grade II injury is considered an axonotmesis with some reaction of degeneration although with an intact neurilemma. This correlates to Sunderland's grade II and III injuries.[40] The less severe grade has motor and sensory loss lasting beyond 10 to 12 hours while the more severe grade has persistent loss beyond 2 weeks. The less severe has a prognosis of 100 percent full recovery while the latter carries with it a poorer prognosis of full recovery of between 60 and 80 percent. Finally, a grade III is considered a neurotmesis with reaction of degeneration in separated axons. If part of the neurilemma is still intact the prognosis is between 30 to 60 percent full recovery while total separation of the whole nerve is at best a 30 percent recovery potential.

Burner Syndrome

Damage to nerve roots or the upper brachial plexus can result from a stretch or compression injury in sports. Called "burner" or "stinger", this frequently occurring condition is common in sports, particularly football. A combination of shoulder depression with lateral flexion of the cervical region is the most common mechanism of injury. Injury can also occur as a direct blow to the supraclavicular region (Fig. 17-21). In football, protective padding prevents most of these injuries.

There is still some disagreement as to whether the lesion is with the cervical roots, the ventral rami, or the brachial plexus. Most authors feel that the true burner syndrome is due to a result of physiologic block, which is transitory. Using Seddon's[41] classification, this type

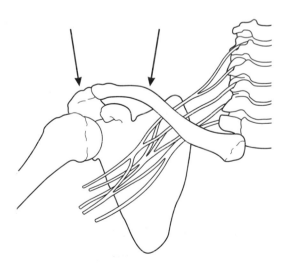

Fig. 17-21. The point of contact in burner injuries is over the clavicle, whereas in acromioclavicular injuries contact occurs at the acromion. In both situations the force applied drives the shoulder down, but different injuries occur. (Modified from Hershman,[76] with permission.)

of injury would be considered a neurapraxia. Axonotmesis can occur in severe injuries, but patients with residual symptoms do not usually have electromyographic evidence of this level of involvement.

The distinction between nerve root or plexus damage is often difficult. Lateral flexion will traction the contralateral nerve roots. The localization and degree of injury is based on the amount of lateral flexion and the amount of shoulder depression involved. The upper portion, particularly C5 to C6, is most often involved. It has been demonstrated that the upper trunk is affected to a greater degree with the combination of a neutral, arm-at-the-side position coupled with shoulder depression.

The athlete will experience a sharp pain, often described as burning, into the arm as far distal as the hand. Associated weakness will often occur immediately described as a heaviness or "dead arm" feeling. Weakness may also develop weeks after the initial injury. When present, the weakness is in the spinati, biceps, and deltoid muscles; therefore, abduction, external rotation, and elbow flexion may be comparatively weak.

Most symptoms last only a few minutes, but some injuries result in prolonged symptomatology from hours to months or longer. The incidence of prolonged recovery is probably on the order of 5 to 10 percent of the total injuries. A classification based on symptoms and duration has been presented by Clancy et al.[42]

It is important not to confuse a similar syndrome referred to as the burning hands syndrome. This is also due to trauma, particularly with the neck in flexion. The pertinent difference is that the burning hands syndrome represents a spinal cord injury, in most cases due to stenosis or fracture, and therefore carries a different protocol of management. Torg et al.[43] recommend an evaluation of a lateral cervical radiograph to determine possible stenosis. They have suggested a ratio between the width of the vertebral body and the spinal canal size. The canal size is estimated by measuring the distance between the posterior vertebral body and the spinolaminal junction. Torg and colleagues[43] suggest a ratio less than 0.8 is suggestive of stenosis (Fig. 17-22). Other factors to consider are stability of the cervical spine, which is usually based on lateral views of flexion and extension. More than 3.5 mm of

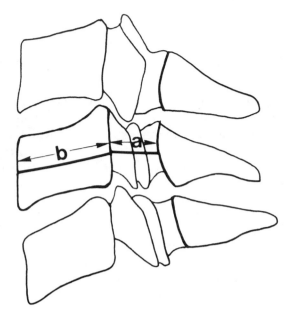

Fig. 17-22. The ratio of the spinal canal to the vertebral body is the distance from the midpoint of the posterior aspect of the vertebral body to the nearest point on the corresponding spinolaminar line *(a)* divided by the anteroposterior width of the vertebral body *(b)*. (From Torg et al,[43] with permission.)

movement between vertebrae or more than 11 degrees of angulation suggest instability.

Several studies have been performed to try to link electrodiagnostic and isokinetic testing to prediction of the amount of injury and to develop criteria for return to sports activity. The results indicated that although a large number of patients had abnormal findings up to 4½ years after the injury, the majority (63 percent) had returned to full strength compared to the opposite extremity.[43] Conversely, patients with weakness did not demonstrate abnormal electromyograms. This would indicate no significant axonal loss.

Based on the above findings, it has been recommended that the clinical evaluation of muscular function coupled with lack of symptoms is sufficient to determine re-entry into performance. It appears that certain individuals are prone to re-injury, but the criteria for determination is vague. It is recommended that proper shoulder padding be worn. Some authors indicate that a custom rubber neck roll can prevent some of the lateral flexion component of the injury and therefore serve as a prophylaxis.

Brachial Neuritis

An unusual disorder of unknown etiology that affects predominantly males in their 20s and 30s is referred to as brachial neuritis. Other names used in the literature include multiple neuritis, brachial plexus neuropathy, acute brachial radiculitis, paralytic brachial neuritis, and Parsonage-Turner syndrome.[44-48] Some cases have been reported as possible sequela to immunization, viral infections, other systemic infections, and serum sickness. There appears to be some relationship specifically with herpes zoster and radiation therapy. Although some patients report an episode following strenuous activity, there appears to be no connection with trauma. One study indicated that athletes in both contact and noncontact sports are affected.[49] Characteristic of this disorder is a rather acute onset of intense pain that may persist for hours to days. Reports of recovery taking months to 2 years have also been made.

Initially there are usually no neurologic signs and symptoms and the pain is irritated by neck and shoulder movement, which leads one to suspect a mechanical etiology. However, within days to weeks motor and sensory function are affected. The roots and spinal cord are usually spared with predominance in the long thoracic, axillary, suprascapular, and anterior interosseous nerves. Presentations are extremely variable including single muscle involvement sparing other muscles supplied by the same nerve trunk, and involvement of the motor component alone sparing the sensory component.

There is no documented successful treatment approach to this problem. In the acute stages, attention is placed on pain relief, which may require immobilization in a sling. As soon as possible movement and movement with resistance are introduced. Many athletes, although pain-free, will report residual weakness.

Nerve Entrapment Syndromes of the Shoulder

The Suprascapular Nerve

The suprascapular nerve (Fig. 17-23) originates off of the upper trunk of the brachial plexus at Erb's point. Formed from nerve roots C5 and C6, occasionally there is a contribution from C4. The nerve courses behind the upper trapezius. On reaching the superior border of the scapula, the nerve passes through the scapular

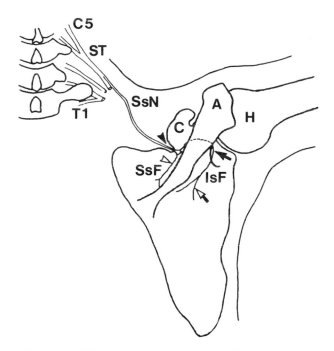

Fig. 17-23. The anatomic relationship of the suprascapular nerve (*SsN, outline arrowhead,* branch to supraspinatus muscle; *outline arrow,* branch to infraspinatus muscle) to the suprascapular *(black arrowhead)* and spinoglenoid *(black arrow)* notches of the scapula with the arm externally rotated in horizontal abduction. *C5,* cervical spinal root 5; *T1,* thoracic spinal root 1; *ST,* superior trunk of brachial plexus; *C,* coracoid process; *A,* acromion process; *H,* head of humerus; *SsF,* supraspinous fossa; *IsF,* infraspinous fossa. (From Ringel et al,[77] with permission.)

notch. The notch is covered by the transverse scapular ligament. In addition to motor supply to the supraspinatus, sensory branches supply the posterior capsule and acromioclavicular joint. Passing laterally, the nerve then passes around the base of the spine of the scapula to pass through the spinoglenoid notch. The infraspinatus is supplied after passage through this notch. About 50 percent of the normal population have a spinoglenoid ligament, an aponeurotic band that separates the supraspinatus and infraspinatus.[50,51] There are no cutaneous branches.

The literature reports varied etiologies of suprascapular nerve irritation in sports. Many are idiopathic,[52] but, some are due to traction injuries in throwing,[53] direct trauma from fracture or dislocation,[54] and possible transient problems due to compression or tractioning during supine weightlifting. Specific sports include throwing sports, backpacking, weightlifting, and volleyball.

The suprascapular nerve is susceptible to injury at three distinct locations: (1) at Erb's point, (2) at the scapular notch, and (3) the spinoglenoid notch. Each will present with slightly different clinical signs and symptoms. Injury at Erb's point is usually via stretch from a fall on a shoulder or other mechanism that distracts the shoulder from the neck. All elements of the nerve are affected leading to atrophy of both the supraspinatus and infraspinatus (Fig. 17-24). There may be associated posterior shoulder pain that is probably the result of irritation to the sensory component. Obvious weakness to abduction and external rotation would be evident.

There is a kinking effect of the suprascapular notch

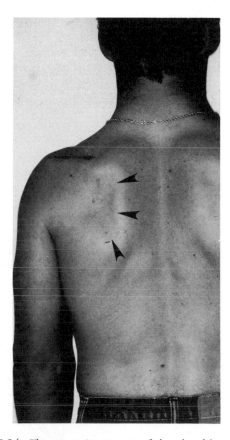

Fig. 17-24. The posterior aspect of the shoulder of a 27-year-old left-handed starting pitcher who experienced mild shoulder pain during the cocking and release phases of the pitching motion. Note the marked atrophy of the infraspinatus muscle *(arrowheads)* on the left side. (From Ringel et al,[77] with permission.)

due to the transverse ligament. As a result stretching due to cross-body adduction (horizontal) may irritate the nerve.[55] This can be found with throwing sports. It has also been reported that compression can occur due to healed fractures involving the scapular notch.[56] The presentation can be similar to the proximal compression with pain, atrophy, and weakness related to both the infraspinatus and supraspinatus. Radiographic evaluation can be helpful in demonstrating a narrowed scapular notch. This is an anteroposterior view with a 15 to 20 degree caudad orientation.[30]

Distinct from the above proximal compressions are lesions at the spinoglenoid notch. Often the lesion is distal to the sensory branches that innervate the acromioclavicular joint and posterior glenohumeral capsule. Therefore, patients may have mild or no complaint of shoulder pain. A relatively asymptomatic presentation with some mild discomfort and weakness may be found. This exact presentation was found by Ferretti et al.[50] with 12 top-level volleyball players competing in the 1985 European Championships. This was attributed to cocking and follow-through while serving.

Further evaluation can be performed with the use of electromyographic studies. Standard conduction latency times have been established by Kraft[57] for many of the nerves about the shoulder including the suprascapular nerve.

Conservative approaches include rest from any inciting activity, analgesics, and physical therapy. Injections may be the next avenue if the conservative approaches are unsuccessful. Surgery is reserved for cases that do not respond and may involve sectioning of a hypertrophied transverse scapular ligament, decompression of the suprascapular or spinoglenoid notches, or removal of a compressive ganglion.[58–61] Success is variable and if the strength of the infraspinatus is not fully restored there is a marked reduction in external rotation and stabilization of the humeral head.

Axillary Nerve

The axillary nerve (Fig. 17-25), formed from the 5th and 6th spinal nerve roots, arises from the posterior cord at the level of the coracoid process. Comparatively it has a very short route. Passing under the coracoid process and continuing anteriorly, it supplies the subscapularis. Near the inferior border of the subscap-

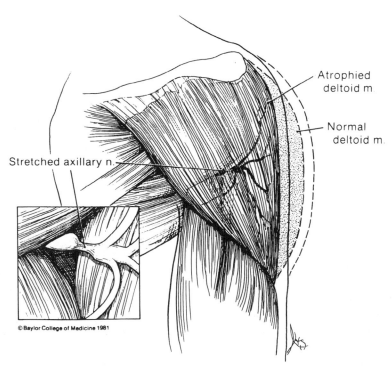

Atrophied deltoid m

Normal deltoid m.

Stretched axillary n.

© Baylor College of Medicine 1981

Fig. 17-25. Axillary nerve compression with shoulder. (From Tullos and Bennett,[73] with permission.)

ularis it joins the posterior humeral circumflex artery passing posterior through an open area referred to as the quadrilateral space. This space is bounded by the teres major and minor muscles, the long head of the triceps, and the shaft of the humerus. Branches to the inferior medial joint capsule occur during this route. Dividing into anterior and posterior branches, the teres minor, deltoids, and the skin overlying the deltoid are supplied.

Injury prior to entering the quadrilateral space is primarily due to stretch. The shorter the distance from the brachial plexus the more effect stretch has on the nerve. The three most common causes are dislocation,[62,63] fracture of the proximal humerus, and a direct blow to the shoulder.[64] Another possible cause is blunt trauma to the axilla resulting in hematoma and adhesions that compress the axillary nerve.[65] The most common sports in which axillary nerve injury occurs are football, wrestling, gymnastics, mountain climbing, and rugby.[66]

The typical presentation is weakness of the deltoid; however, weakness of the teres minor is more difficult to determine due to the predominance of the infraspinatus with external rotation. Interestingly, there may be no objectifiable numbness over the lateral arm in many cases of severe motor deficit.

Entrapment at the quadrilateral space is usually insidious. Fibrous bands or posterior glenoid osteophytes may be the source of irritation augmented by stretching of the arm into flexion or horizontal adduction such as occurs in throwing.[67]

The pain pattern and paresthesias associated with the quadrilateral space syndrome are not representative of clinical logic. The pain is often anterior. Tenderness may be found in several locations: anteriorly, laterally, and at the insertion of the teres minor. Paresthesias are nondermatomal and may extend down the arm into the hand. The apprehension position of abduction, and external rotation may exacerbate the symptoms.

Evaluation may include a subclavian arteriogram. It is interesting to note that almost 70 percent of patients with positive arteriograms demonstrating occlusion of the posterior humeral circumflex artery usually do not require surgery. The symptoms are tolerable by most individuals.

Electrophysiologic testing of the deltoid muscle is often normal although other neuropathies may be present in association with quadrilateral space entrapment.[68] Often there is no atrophy or weakness of the deltoid with this entrapment.

Conservative treatment may be helpful. Bateman[66] suggested using a splint with the arm in slight flexion coupled with exercise and electrical stimulation. Follow-up is monthly for a period of 2 to 4 months. Those cases that do not demonstrate improvement are referred for surgery as are cases of quadrilateral compression. Often the insertion of the teres minor is detached and reattached medially.

Long Thoracic Nerve

The long thoracic nerve (Fig. 17-26) is purely motor supplying the very important serratus anterior. It arises from the ventral rami of C5, C6, and C7 and is sometimes referred to as the external respiratory nerve of Bell. Due to its long, relatively superficial course, it is susceptible to injury either through direct trauma or stretch. Injury has been reported in almost all sports,

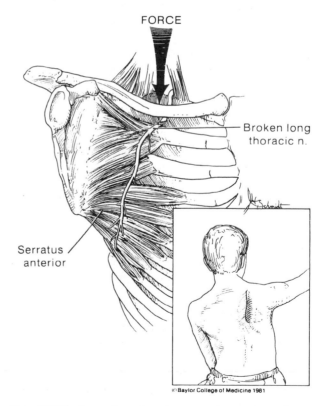

Fig. 17-26. Long thoracic nerve traction injury. (From Tullos and Bennett,[73] with permission.)

including weightlifting, archery, rowing, gymnastics, tennis, squash, soccer, shooting, discus throwing, football, ballet, bowling, basketball, and wrestling. With weightlifting, pull-overs may be the culprit due to the stretch effect with elevation of the arms combined with spinal extension. This is more likely to occur when performed standing as opposed to supine.[69]

Symptoms are often minimal. If symptomatic, a posterior shoulder or scapular burning type of pain may be reported. Often there is only asymptomatic winging of the scapula. However, even winging may not be evident until the trapezius stretches enough to reveal an injury several weeks prior. Testing of winging is performed with the patient facing a wall, flexing the shoulders to 90 degrees, internally rotating the shoulders, and performing a wall push-up. It is important to keep in mind the other causes of winging that may confuse the differential picture.

Musculocutaneous Nerve

Although rare, the musculocutaneous nerve can be affected through compression due to hypertrophy or entrapment between the biceps aponeurosis and brachialis fascia or it may be injured through stretch as occurs in dislocations and sometimes in surgery. The musculocutaneous nerve is motor to the coracobrachialis, biceps, and brachialis. It is sensory to the radial aspect of the forearm.

Origin of the musculocutaneous nerve is from the C5 to C6 levels with occasional contribution from C7. It arises from the lateral cord of the brachial plexus at about the level of the pectoralis minor muscle. Coursing through the coracobrachialis muscle (which it innervates) it enters the arm to supply the biceps and brachialis.

At about 2 to 5 cm above the cubital crease, the musculocutaneous nerve divides giving off a sensory branch that is divided into anterior and posterior fibers.

Injury can occur before entering the coracobrachialis due to dislocation or apparently due to stretch as has been reported in a throwing injury. Stretch is the proposed mechanism with the entity known as "backpack palsy."[70] Heavy backpacks (infantry type) used in camping/hiking and mountain climbing can cause damage to the upper trunk of the brachial plexus. Dysfunction can be severe and prolonged with similar injury as occurs with Erb's palsy from breech deliveries. The nondominant side is affected most, possibly due to relative weakness. The musculocutaneous and radial nerves are more commonly affected with minimal median nerve involvement. Early detection is important. The combination of time, avoidance of wearing a backpack, and strengthening of the shoulder muscles will probably be effective.

Distal to the coracobrachialis, the most common cause appears to be weightlifting. Either through compression due to hypertrophy or entrapment between the biceps and brachialis, the nerve may lead to a painless loss of muscles strength in flexion and supination of the forearm. Initial treatment should include avoidance of biceps curls or other biceps exercises. Over time, introduction of modified curls with lighter weight may be possible. Surgery is an option.

REFERENCES

1. Inman VT, Saunders JB de CM: Referred pain from skeletal structures. J Nerv Ment Dis 99:660, 1944
2. Feinstein R, Langton JNK, Jameson RM, Shiller F: Experiments of pain referred from deep somatic structures. J Bone Joint Surg 36A:981, 1954
3. Bogduk N, Marsland A: The cervical zygapophysial joints as a source of neck pain. Spine 13:610, 1988
4. Hildebrant J, Argyrakis A: Percutaneous nerve block of the cervical facet: a relatively new method in the treatment of chronic headache and neck pain. Pathological-anatomical studies and clinical practice. Man Med 2:48, 1986
5. Sluitjter ME, Koetsveld-Bart CC: Interruption of pain pathways in the treatment of the cervical syndrome. Anaesthesia 35:302, 1980
6. Peterson B: The Collected Papers of Irwin Korr. American Academy of Osteopathy, New York, 1979
7. Marks R: Distribution of pain provoked from lumbar facet joints and related structures during diagnostic spinal infiltration. Pain 39:37, 1989
8. Travell JG, Simons DG: Myofascial Pain and Dysfunction: The Trigger Point Manual. Williams & Wilkins, Baltimore, 1983
9. Grieve GP: Modern Manual Therapy of the Vertebral Column. Churchill Livingstone, Edinburgh, 1986
10. Vilkari-Juntura E, Porras M, Laasonen EM: Validity of clinical tests in the diagnosis of root compression in cervical disc disease. Spine 14:253, 1989
11. Elvey RL: Brachial plexus tension tests and the pathoana-

tomical origin of arm pain. p. 116. In Glasgow EF, Twomey LT, Scull ER et al (eds): Aspects of Manipulative Therapy. 2nd Ed. Churchill Livingstone, Edinburgh, 1985

12. Nansel D, Jansen R, Cremata E et al: Effects of cervical adjustments on lateral-flexion passive end-range asymmetry and on blood pressure, heart rate, and plasma catecholamine levels. J Manip Phys Ther 14:450, 1991

13. McGrouch GP, Deering ID, Ling TH: Location of receptors for tonic neck reflexes. J Neurophys 14:5, 1951

14. Stejskal L: Postural reflexes in man. Am J Phys Med 58: 1, 1979

15. Cohen LA: Role of eye and neck proprioceptive mechanism in body orientation and body coordination. J Neurophys 24:1, 1961

16. Leffert RD: Thoracic outlet syndrome: a correspondence newsletter to the American Society of Surgery of the Hand. December 12, 1988

17. Brown C: Compressive invasive referred pain to the shoulder. Clin Orthop 173:55, 1983

18. Brown SCW, Charlesworth D: Results of excision of a cervical rib in patients with thoracic outlet syndrome. Br J Surg 75:431, 1988

19. Roos DB: The place for scalenectomy and first rib resection in thoracic outlet syndrome. Surgery 92:1077, 1982

20. Minor NH: Anatomic structures of the thoracic outlet. Clin Orthop 207:17, 1986

21. Heyden B, Vollmer J: Thoracic outlet syndrome with vascular complications. J Cardiovasc Surg 20:531, 1979

22. Judy KL, Heymann RL: Vascular complication of the thoracic outlet syndrome. Am J Surg 123:521, 1972

23. Leffert RD: Thoracic outlet syndrome and the shoulder. Clin Sports Med 2:439, 1983

24. Adson AW: Surgical treatment for symptoms produced by cervical ribs and the scalenus anticus muscle. Clin Orthop 207:3, 1986

25. Leffert RD: Lesions of the brachial plexus including thoracic syndrome. Instructional Course Lectures 36:77, 1977

26. Urschel HC, Razzuk MA: Management of thoracic outlet syndrome. N Engl J Med 285:1140, 1972

27. Weber RJ, Piero DL: F wave evaluation of thoracic outlet syndrome. A multiple regression derived F wave latency producing technique. Arch Phys Med Rehabil 59:464, 1978

28. Howell JW: Evaluation and management of thoracic outlet syndrome. p. 151. In Donatelli RA (ed): Physical Therapy of the Shoulder. 2nd Ed. Churchill Livingstone, New York, 1991

29. Hansson KG: Scalene anticus syndrome. Surg Clin North Am 22:611, 1942

30. Reichert FL: Compression of the brachial plexus: the scalene anticus syndrome. JAMA 118:294, 1942

31. Estwanik JJ: Levator scapulae syndrome. Phys Sports Med 17:57, 1989

32. Moseley HF: Shoulder Lesions. p. 74. Charles C Thomas, Springfield, IL, 1945

33. Shull JR: Scapulocostal syndrome: clinical aspects. South Med J 62:956, 1969

34. Reid DC: Sports Injury Assessment and Rehabilitation. Churchill Livingstone, New York, 1992

35. Sotta RP: Vascular problems in the proximal upper extremity. Clin Sports Med 9:379, 1990

36. Vogel CM, Jensen JE: "Effort" thrombosis of the subclavian vein in a competitive swimmer. Am J Sports Med 13:269, 1985

37. Butsch JL: Subclavian thrombosis following hockey injuries. Am J Sports Med 11:448, 1983

38. Kleinsasser LJ: "Effort" thrombosis of the axillary and subclavian veins. Arch Surg 59:258, 1949

39. Pianka G, Hershman EB: Neurovascular injuries. In Nicholas JA, Hershman EB (eds): The Upper Extremity in Sports Medicine. CV Mosby, St. Louis, 1990

40. Sedden H: Surgical Disorders of the Peripheral Nerves. Churchill Livingstone, Edinburgh, 1972

41. Sunderland S: Nerve and Nerve Injuries. 2nd Ed. Churchill Livingstone, New York, 1978

42. Clancy WG, Brand RL, Bergfeld JA: Upper trunk brachial plexus injuries in contact sports. Am J Sports Med 5:209, 1977

43. Torg JS, Parlov H, Genuario SE et al: Neuropraxia of the cervical spinal cord with transient quadriplegia. J Bone Joint Surg 68A:1354, 1986

44. Hershman EB, Willbourn AJ, Berfled JA: Acute brachial neuropathy in athletes. Am J Sports Med 17:655, 1989

45. Burnard ED, Fox TG: Multiple neuritis of the shoulder girdle: report of 9 cases occurring in second New Zealand Expeditionary Force. NZ Med J 41:243, 1949

46. Parsonage MJ, Turner JWA: Neuralgic amyotrophy: shoulder girdle syndrome. Lancet 1:973, 1948

47. Tsairis P, Dyck PJ, Mudder DW: Natural history of brachial plexus neuropathy: report on 99 cases. Arch Neurol 27: 102, 1872

48. Bacevich BB: Paralytic brachial neuritis. J Bone Joint Surg 58A:262, 1976

49. Bergfeld JA, Hershman EB, Wilbourn AJ: Brachial injuries in athletes. Orthop Trans 12:743, 1988

50. Ferretti A, Cerullo G, Russo G: Suprascapular neuropathy in volleyball players. J Bone Joint Surg 69A:260, 1987

51. Mestdagh H, Drizenko A, Ghesten P: Anatomical basis of suprascapular nerve syndrome. Anat Clin 3:67, 1981

52. Drez D: Suprascapular neuropathy in the differential diagnosis of rotator cuff injuries. Am J Sports Med 4:43, 1976

53. Bryan WJ, Wild JJ: Isolated infraspinatus atrophy: a com-

mon cause of posterior shoulder pain and weakness in throwing athletes? Am J Sports Med 14:113, 1976

54. Zoltan JD: Injury to the suprascapular nerve associated with anterior dislocation of the shoulder: case report and review of the literature. J Trauma 19:203, 1979

55. Regachary SS, Neff JP, Singer PA et al: Suprascapular entrapment neuropathy: a clinical, anatomical, and comparative study. II. Anatomical study. Neurosurgery 5:447, 1979

56. Edeland HG, Zachrison BE: Fracture of the scapular notch associated with lesion of the suprascapular nerve. Acta Orthop Scand 46:758, 1975

57. Kraft GH: Axillary, musculocutaneous and suprascapular nerve latency studies. Arch Phys Med Rehabil 65:735, 1972

58. Ganzhorn RW, Hocker JT, Horowitz M, Switzer HE: Suprascapular nerve entrapment. J Bone Joint Surg 63:492, 1981

59. Rask MR: Suprascapular nerve entrapment: a report of two cases treated by suprascapular notch resection. Clin Ortho 134:266, 1978

60. Hirayama T, Takemitsu Y: Compression of the suprascapular nerve by ganglion at the suprascapular notch. Clin Orthop 155:95, 1981

61. Neviaser TJ et al: Suprascapular nerve denervation secondary to attenuation by a ganglionic cyst. J Bone Joint Surg 68A:627, 1986

62. Blom S, Dahlback LO: Nerve injuries in dislocations of the shoulder joint and fractures of the neck of the humerus. Acta Chir Scand 136:461, 1970

63. Pasila M, Jarona H, Kiviluto O et al: Early complications of primary shoulder dislocations. Acta Orthop Scand 40:260, 1978

64. Berry H, Bril V: Axillary nerve trauma following blunt trauma to the shoulder: a clinical and electrophysiological review. J Neurol Neurosurg Psychiatry 45:1027, 1982

65. Leffer RD, Seddon H: Infraclavicular brachial plexus injuries. J Bone Joint Surg 47B:9, 1965

66. Bateman JE: Nerve injuries about the shoulder in sports. J Bone Joint Surg 49A:785, 1967

67. Bennett GE: Shoulder and elbow lesions of the professional baseball pitcher. JAMA 117:510, 1941

68. Cahill BR, Palmar PE: Quadrilateal space syndrome. J Hand Surg 8:65, 1983

69. Stanish WD, Lamb J: Isolated paralysis of the serratus anterior muscle: a weight training injury. Case report. Am J Sports Med 6:385, 1978

70. Kulund DN: The Injured Athlete. JB Lippincott, Philadelphia, 1982

71. Foreman SM, Croft AC: Whiplash Injuries: The Cervical Acceleration/Deceleration Syndrome. Williams & Wilkins, Baltimore, 1988

72. Mannheimer JS, Lampre GN: Clinical Transcutaneous Electrical Nerve Stimulation. FA Davis, Philadelphia, 1984

73. Tullos HS, Bennett JB: The shoulder in sports. p. 110. In Scott WN, Nisonson B, Nicholas J (eds): Principles of Sports Medicine. Williams & Wilkins, Baltimore, 1984

74. Sucher BM: Thoracic outlet syndrome: a myofascial variant: Part 1: pathology and diagnosis. J Am Osteo Assoc 90:686, 1990

75. Caillett R: Shoulder Pain. 2nd Ed. FA Davis, Philadelphia, 1984

76. Hershman EB: Brachial plexus injuries. Clin Sports Med 9:311, 1990

77. Ringel SP, Theihaft M, Carry M et al: Suprascapular neuropathy in pitchers. Am J Sports Med, 18:80, 1992

18

General Treatment Approaches for Shoulder Disorders

THOMAS A. SOUZA

CRYOTHERAPY

Cold application can be administered through the use of various types of commercial or home modified cold packs, ice massage, immersion baths, and Freon sprays. The use of cold therapy is important for three major reasons:

1. Cold with compression is effective in reducing swelling. Through a combination of vasoconstriction and pressure, ice compression has been demonstrated to be appropriate for reducing the inflammatory response.[1]
2. Reduction of pain through a decrease in neural conduction. A sequence of changes occur with cold application beginning with a cold sensation, followed by a burning/aching sensation after 2 to 7 minutes, which is then followed by local numbness and a decrease in muscle spasm after 5 to 12 minutes. These effects are possibly directly related to a slowing of neural conduction.[2]
3. Reflex inhibition allowing stretching (spray and stretch). It is theorized that through a reflex inhibition, cold allows muscles to be stretched further with resetting of the muscle spindle.

Treatment time varies depending on the thickness of the tissue, type of cold application, and chronicity of the problem. With most cold pack application the time is usually between 10 and 20 minutes. In acute situations application may be as often as every waking hour.

Cryotherapy is important for the treatment of bursitis and tendinitis. For these conditions ice massage is a convenient approach. Freezing water in Dixie cups and applying for 5 to 10 minutes appears effective. Cryotherapy also may be used as an adjunct to other treatments such as mobilization and cross-friction massage. Contraindications include Raynaud's phenomenon, diabeties with vascular involvement, peripheral vascular disease, elderly patients with skin fragility, malignancies, cold hypersensitivity, and children and individuals unable to understand or communicate effectively. Ice massage of the carotids is also contraindicated.

HEAT MODALITIES

Hydrocollator

Hydrocollators (moist heat) packs are used generally for the purpose of reducing pain and inducing muscular relaxation through superficial heat penetration. The physiologic effects include vasodilation and an increase in metabolic activity. Heat decreases muscle spasm by inhibiting gamma nerve activity.[3] The packs are kept at a temperature between 150 and 170°F. Application is usually for 10 to 20 minutes with the pack wrapped in six to eight layers of toweling. Less toweling is often used, but caution is advised in leaving a patient unattended. One of the best uses of a hydrocollator is to place it on an abducted arm for up to 60 minutes in an attempt to increase range of motion (ROM). The weight of the hydrocollator plus gravity applies a mild load to the shoulder while the heat increases relaxation and decreases pain. Heat is contraindicated with acute inflammatory conditions.

Ultrasound

Joule, in 1847, was the first to discover that high-frequency sound energy could be produced from high-frequency electrical energy. Chilowsky and Langevin inadvertently found half a century later the destructive aspect of ultrasound when they directed an ultrasonic beam into water and found that fish who crossed the beam were killed instantly. It was not until 1937 that the first study reported the therapeutic aspects of ultrasound in the treatment of sciatica.

Ultrasound uses high-frequency acoustic energy in the range of 1 MHz to produce therapeutic effects of deep heat and vibration. The benefits can include pain relief, tissue healing, increased extensibility of connective tissue, reduction of muscle spasm and inflammation, and possibly assist in calcium resorption.[4] Penetration of ultrasound is reported to be as deep as 5 cm with a concentration occurring at the muscle-bone interface while superficial temperature is minimally elevated.[5] In general, continuous ultrasound is recommended in subacute or chronic stages of injury due to the thermal effects. Application is with either a linear or circular motion not to exceed 2 to 4 cm/s.[6] The treatment duration is determined by the following factors:

1. The size of the sound head determines the intensity; therefore, a smaller sound head may require twice the time application compared to a larger head. The intensity is determined by dividing the total wattage by the surface area of the crystal. The specific specifications of each machine will assist in the calculation.
2. The surface area to be treated is another factor in determining duration of treatment. A general recommendation is 5 to 6 minutes over an area of 5 to 6 square inches.[7] This is an average surface area when treating specific tendons about the shoulder.
3. The depth of and type of tissue being treated will affect the intensity and time of treatment.

For example, deep tissues such as the joint capsule will require a decrease in intensity with a concomitant increase in treatment time.[3] A property of ultrasound that must be considered is that the more homogeneous the tissue the more readily ultrasound penetrates. This is an important consideration when treating tendons in fatty areas because fat is fairly homogeneous. It is recommended that treatment of tendon injuries not exceed 1.5 W/cm^2 and not be longer than 5 to 7 minutes.[8] Ultrasound has been reported to penetrate deeper if the area has first been cooled.[9]

Continuous ultrasound at 1.0 W/cm^2 may help expose stress fractures.

Pulsed ultrasound is used when the thermal effects are not desired. The duty cycle is between 20 and 50 percent. The term micromassage effects is commonly used to describe these acoustic pressure changes. Nonthermal effects include cavitation and acoustic streaming. Cavitation is the effect of compression and expansion of gas bubbles. This results in vibration that may enhance cellular metabolism and at the same time mechanically break up scar tissue. Vibrating bubbles create movement in the cellular fluids around them with a result referred to as acoustic streaming. This may result in increased call metabolism and dissipation of fluid. Movement of fluid away from the acoustic energy source is the basis for phonophoresis, in which large complex molecules are driven through the tissue as deep as 10 cm in a 5 minute treatment.[10] Corticosteroids, salicylates, and local anesthetics are commonly used agents.

Caution must be used when applying over areas of joint effusion. An undesirable effect referred to as "unstable" or "transient" cavitation can occur with sudden collapse of large gas bubbles. Tissue damage can result. Ultrasound should never be used over ischemic areas because the heat generated cannot be properly dissipated by adequate blood flow.[11] Ultrasound over anesthetized areas is contraindicated due to the lack of patient feedback on perceived intensity or damage.

Dyson and Suckling[12] have noted an interesting effect on neural conduction. Conduction velocity decreases with intermediate intensities (between 0.5 and 1.5 W/cm^2), whereas conduction velocity increases with intensities below 0.5 and above 2 W/cm^2. Another interesting observation is that ultrasound in the range of 3 MHz of energy (not commonly used in the United States) may stimulate fibroblastic activity and enhance tissue healing.[9]

ELECTRICAL STIMULATION

Transcutaneous Electrical Nerve Stimulation

Although there are many models of transcutaneous electrical nerve stimulation (TENS) units manufactured with a multitude of reported effects, there are basically only two types: sensory stimulators used in the treatment of pain and neuromuscular stimulators that exercise muscle. There are two types of current. Direct current (DC) machines stimulate muscle and nerves, whereas alternating current (AC) machines stimulate nerves only. This neural stimulation can then cause muscle contraction.

Sensory Stimulators

Sensory stimulators include portable TENS units, high-volt stimulators, interferential units, Acuscope, and other microamperage units. Conventional TENS units use milliamperage stimulation of afferent nerves and modify pain through either the gate control mechanism or through stimulation of the production of neurohormonal substances such as enkephalins, endorphins, or serotonin. The gate control mechanism is based on a theory that stimulation of large fiber afferents has an inhibiting effect on small fiber nociceptors at the spinal cord level. Various parameters can be manipulated to emphasize one of the above pain inhibition mechanisms. These include frequency, pulse width and rate, and intensity. Table 18-1 lists common approaches with different combinations of these parameters. In general, a high-frequency/low-amplitude stimulation accesses the gate control approach, whereas low-frequency/high-amplitude stimulation results in a central/hormonal response.

Pulsed High-Volt Galvanic

Machines that deliver more than 100 V at a low average current (up to 1.5 mA) are called pulsed high-volt galvanic (PHVG) modalities. The pulse duration is very short at 1 microsecond.[13] High-volt galvanic gives primarily a TENS effect using a monophasic current with negligible polar effect (except for possible tissue healing). Due to a short pulse width, PHVG allows comfortable stimulation of both motor and sensory fibers. One unique feature is the ability to use the modality immersed in cold water to augment effects in acute injury. Table 18-2 lists the purported capabilities of PHVG with the associated modality setup to achieve the specific effect desired.

Interferential Stimulation

Interferential stimulation utilizes two medium frequency sinusoidal waves (4,000 to 5,000 Hz) to overcome skin impedance and allow stronger perception at a lower intensity. The reduced skin impedance is due to the higher-frequency carrier current that also

Table 18-1. Various Transcutaneous Electrical Nerve Stimulation (TENS) Approaches

Type	Pulse Width (pps)	Pulse Rate	Amplitude	Time of Treatment
High frequency	High: 75–150	Less than 200	Increase to discomfort	30 min–24 hr
Low frequency	Low: below 10	200–300	Increase to elicit strong rhythmic contractions	30–60 min
Brief and intense	TENS—150 Galvanic—1–5	150	Increase to tetanic contraction	15 min
Burst mode	50–100	75–100	Increase to strong but comfortable contraction	20–60 min

Table 18-2. Pulsed High-Volt Galvanic

Treatment Effect	Mode	Frequency (pps)	Type of Stimulation	Time (min)
Reduce edema	Continuous	High: 80–100	Sensory	20
Reduce muscle spasm	Continuous	High: 80–120	Sensory/motor	20–30
Autonomic response	Uninterrupted/pulsed	High: 80–100	Sensory	20–30
Neurohormonal	Uninterrupted/pulsed	Low: 2–5	Motor (twitch)	30–60
Muscle pump	Surged 1:3	Low: 30–50	Motor	20–30

shortens the pulse widths. The result is tolerance of stronger current with less discomfort. The stimulation is greater, signaling caution with the potential use of excessive average current. Where the two waves "interfere" with each other, a beat frequency ranging from 1 to 100 beats per second (bps) is created. This frequency can be changed by altering one of the carrier frequencies, which results in either a constant or rhythmic (sweep) mode. Various beat frequencies and their use clinically include 100 bps used for pain management, 50 to 60 bps used for tetanic contraction, and 1 to 50 bps used for muscle pumping effect (edema).

Concentration of the current is not always in the center of application. It is advisable to adjust the electrodes so that the patient perceives stimulation in the painful area.[14] Treatment time is usually between 20 and 30 minutes. Contraindications are the same for all forms of TENS, including cardiac pacemakers, pregnancy, thromboembolic disorders, and acute infections.[15]

Microamperage Stimulation

There are a number of devices that use microamperage stimulation in an attempt to effect healing on a cellular level. Sometimes referred to as "intelligent TENS," the basis for stimulation is reported by the manufacturer to be the ability to measure cellular electrical activity and compare it to a reference "normal" in the machine's circuitry. Purported effects have been acceleration of healing time through an increase in cell metabolism and dispersion of fluid.

Low-Volt Galvanic Stimulation

Low-volt galvanic is a unidirectional, waveless current referred to as "direct." The effects are chemical and vary depending on the polarity used. Essentially, the positive pole effects are "constrictive" and used in the treatment of acute conditions mainly through a reduction in congestion. The negative pole is used more in chronic settings through a "dilating" effect, increasing circulation to the area.

Neuromuscular Stimulators

Neuromuscular stimulators are used to stimulate muscles through an intact nervous system. There are numerous manufacturers and individual claims of superiority, but the approach and capabilities are essentially the same. The muscle is contracted either with stimulation alone or a voluntary co-contraction is incorporated.

CROSS FRICTION (TRANSVERSE) MASSAGE

Cross friction or transverse massage applies a graduated force 90 degrees to the long axis of a muscle, tendon, or ligament. This technique has been advocated by Cyriax,[16] Mennell,[17] Hammer,[18] and Hertling and Kessler.[19] Although controlled studies still are needed to compare its results with other therapeutic approaches, cross friction holds a strong place in the therapeutic armamentarium based on empirical success.

There is no single definitive theory as to why friction massage is effective, but there are several common suggestions. In the chronic phases of soft tissue disorders, there is the assumption that scar tissue may have formed in an irregular fashion and may represent a nociceptive focus. Cyriax believed that cross friction massage in the subacute phase could increase local circulation to the area (hyperemia). He assumed that friction at 90 degrees was less likely to harm healing or normal tissue; however, it may prevent disorganized scar tissue formation or in the chronic phase, break up abnormal adhesions. The idea of organizing scar tissue formation is based on two principles. First is the idea that new collagen formation follows along lines of stress similar to Wolff's law with regard to bone. This requires tension. The cross friction ingredient may involve another component described by Hertling and Kessler.[19] The analogy used is with pickup sticks. If pickup sticks are thrown down in disarray, one can organize them at a right angle to an applied force by rolling one's fingers back and forth over the pile. The suggestion is that this may also occur with cross friction massage; organization of scar tissue collagen is parallel to the fibers of a muscle, tendon, or ligament when rolled under the fingers at right angles. Therefore, increased blood flow to the involved area and/or organization of scar tissue with breaking down of old disorganized scar tissue are the main concepts regarding the effectiveness of cross friction massage.

An effect of cross friction is local anesthesia. This is

probably the result of gate control inhibition with large fiber proprioceptor stimulation inhibiting the small fiber nociceptors. The initial irritation probably also incorporates the counter-irritation response of central inhibition through endorphin release and dorsolateral funiculus stimulation.

The friction anesthesia may also be useful from a diagnostic perspective. If it was unclear whether a specific tissue was the cause of a particular restriction or site of pain and could not be differentiated by functional testing, friction anesthesia can allow subsequent testing to determine whether one of the original positives was now eliminated. For example, if impingement signs were positive yet testing of the supraspinatus and biceps produced equivocal findings, friction anesthesia could allow testing to determine which tendon is no longer producing positives. In the event of severely restricted abduction due to pain and weakness, friction anesthesia can allow retesting to determine if full abduction is possible, eliminating the possibility of a full tear of the supraspinatus.

Technique of Application

The decision of where to apply cross friction massage is based on a functional examination of the shoulder in an attempt to determine the involved tissues. These principles are outlined in Chapter 6. In essence, if pain were produced at a specific location by stretching of a tendon and not by contraction, combined with the finding of local tenderness at the insertion point, one would suspect the tendon. If contraction combined with stretch reproduced the complaint, the muscle would be implicated. If local tenderness and reproduction with stability testing only produced the pain, a ligament is more likely.

There are specific guidelines with respect to the application of cross friction massage. It is important to apply friction at right angles to the tissue being treated. No lotion is used on the skin. Application usually requires a reinforced contact with the thumb and fingers. A T-bar with a rubber tip can be used when finger or thumb pressure is not possible. It is important that the pressure be deep enough to move the tissue below the skin. Massage of the skin alone will not accomplish the desired effects.

With maximum pressure dictated by patient tolerance, a friction "anesthesia" can be accomplished within about 3 minutes of application allowing a much deeper pressure for subsequent treatment. Without a release in pressure, the friction massage is continued for at least 6 to 9 minutes as long as 20 minutes in rare cases. It is important throughout this process to monitor patient tolerance with questioning at least every 2 minutes before applying any substantial increase in pressure. Hammer[18] suggests the use of 5 minutes of ultrasound prior to cross friction massage. Others suggest the application of cold to accelerate the numbness potential.

Muscle bellies are usually treated in a relaxed position while tendons and ligaments are usually stretched to provide some tension with application.

Guidelines for management with cross friction have been suggested by Hammer.[18] If the patient's condition is aggravated by the procedure or does not develop the usual anesthesia within 3 to 5 minutes, continued care is not suggested. If there is no response in the patient's condition after three treatments, it is unlikely that further treatment will be effective.

For maximum effectiveness it is suggested that treatments occur three times per week. Pain or restriction is eliminated in several treatments over a period of 1 to 2 weeks in many cases. It is necessary in some cases to treat for as long as 2 months, particularly with chronic cases.

Contraindications for cross friction massage include direct massage over acute inflamed tissue, hematomas, calcifications, and peripheral nerves. Mennell[17] notes that friction massage over a trigger point (TP) can be exquisitely painful and that a distinction should be made before application. Usually the obvious difference is the typical "jump sign" found with a TP with possible referral pain into a related reference zone. One unpublished criticism of friction massage is that it may destroy the Golgi tendon apparatus with repeated usage.[20]

Although it has been suggested that bursitis is not an appropriate condition to treat with friction massage, Hammer[18] feels that due to the minimal inflammation of a chronic bursitis and the associated fibrosis, friction massage may be successful. He warns that there may be some irritation in the first three visits and that the normal anesthesia effect may be more difficult to attain.

Figure 18-1 through 18-8 illustrate the patient position and angle of application of cross friction for various muscles and ligaments about the shoulder.

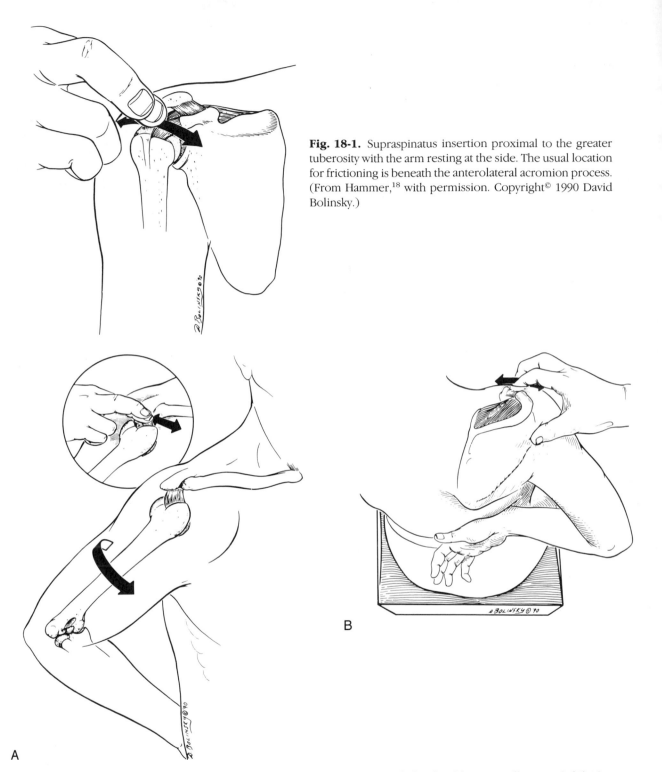

Fig. 18-1. Supraspinatus insertion proximal to the greater tuberosity with the arm resting at the side. The usual location for frictioning is beneath the anterolateral acromion process. (From Hammer,[18] with permission. Copyright© 1990 David Bolinsky.)

B

A

Fig. 18-2. Supraspinatus insertion proximal to the greater tuberosity with the shoulder internally rotated. **(A)** The tendon is brought into a more sagittal position just below the anterior acromion. **(B)** Superior view of the supraspinatus tendon beneath the anterior acromion with the shoulder internally rotated. The forefinger should be between the anterior acromion and the greater tuberosity. (From Hammer,[18] with permission. Copyright© 1990 David Bolinsky.)

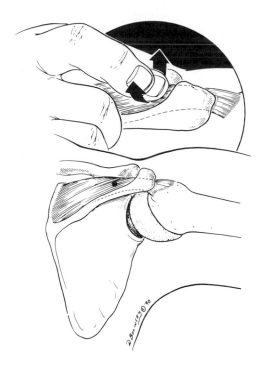

Fig. 18-3. Supraspinatus. To friction the musculotendinous portion of the supraspinatus, the shoulder should be in a rested position of 90 degrees abduction. This position allows the musculotendinous area to shift medially beneath the arch, where it can be treated. Deep pressure is required as the practitioner pronates and supinates the reinforced forefinger between the posterior clavicle and the anterior scapular spine. (From Hammer,[18] with permission. Copyright© 1990 David Bolinsky.)

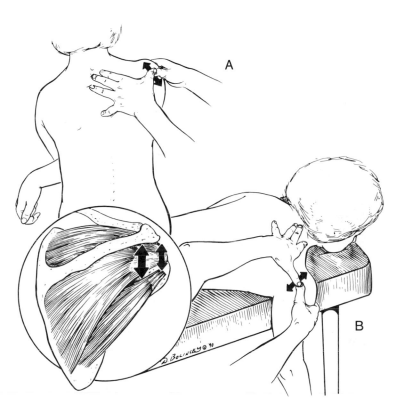

Fig. 18-4. Infraspinatus. The most tender area, either the tendon body or the insertion into the greater tuberosity, is frictioned. **(A)** This position creates a minimal stretch. **(B)** This position allows better penetration by relaxing the deltoid. (From Hammer,[18] with permission. Copyright© 1990 David Bolinsky.)

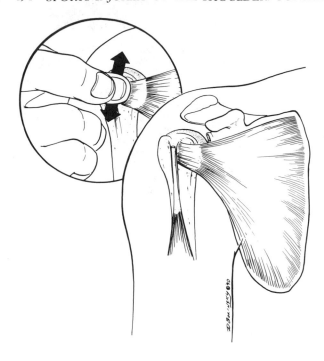

Fig. 18-5. Subscapularis. Friction is applied at the most tender level of the bony lesser tuberosity. The overlying deltoid may have to be moved laterally to achieve better bony contact. (From Hammer,[18] with permission. Copyright© 1990 David Bolinsky.)

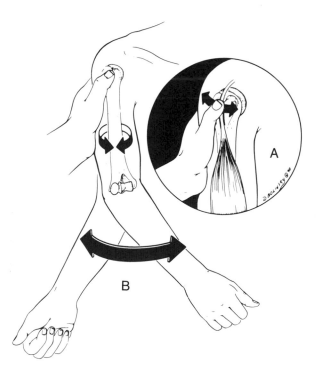

Fig. 18-6. Biceps tendon at the bicipital groove. The long head of the biceps tendon may be frictioned directly. The elbow should be flexed with the shoulder externally rotated **(A)** Another method is to maintain contact on the tendon while the patient moves the forearm medially and laterally **(B)** (From Hammer,[18] with permission. Copyright© 1990 David Bolinsky.)

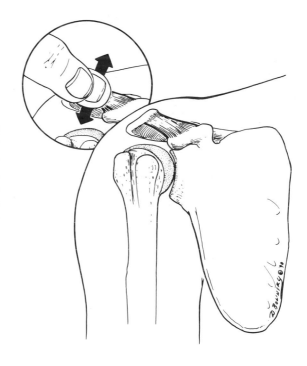

Fig. 18-7. Coracoacromial ligament. This ligament is not always palpable. Palpation should proceed from the superior lateral aspect of the coracoid tip. Frictioning should be considered when the ligament is tender to palpation or when the impingement test is positive with the shoulder flexed 90 degrees, the elbow flexed 90 degrees, and the forearm internally rotated. (From Hammer,[18] with permission. Copyright© 1990 David Bolinsky.)

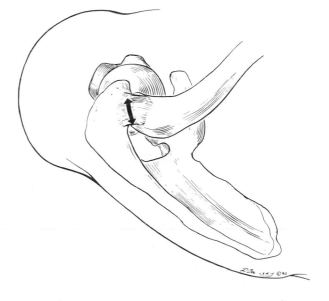

Fig. 18-8. Acromioclavicular ligament (superior view). Friction should be applied with the forefinger along the joint line. The angle of the acromioclavicular joint is variable. (From Hammer,[18] with permission. Copyright© 1990 David Bolinsky.)

Friction Massage with Motion

A variation of the application of cross friction massage is to introduce an active ROM with and without resistance. This approach has been utilized by the author with success only in conditions where acute inflammation is not present. Theoretically, the introduction of active movement may magnify the gate control inhibition of discomfort and allow deeper massage at a quicker rate.

Initially, cross friction is applied in the usual manner. After 1 to 2 minutes, the athlete is asked to attempt movement associated with the muscle or tendon being treated. The force is initially minimal by the patient. After 2 to 3 minutes of repeated contraction (20 seconds) with friction massage, the doctor then uses the other hand to provide a minimal resistance to the movement attempt. This involves an isotonic contraction and should not create substantial pain although mild discomfort is likely. This portion of the procedure is performed for approximately 2 to 3 minutes. The session is followed by icing and the prescription of mild isometric or isotonic exercises for the involved muscle at home. These exercises should be performed often throughout the day. Caution must be used when providing resistance to the patient's movement, and the patient should be reminded that the amount of force used in the home exercises is about a 25 percent contraction only.

Myofascial Release Technique

A different approach often referred to as a myofascial release technique (MRT) can be applied to the muscle.[21] Similar to the concept of motion with applied pressure, MRT utilizes a full ROM with pressure applied at an area of palpable adhesion or where a TP may be palpable. This "stripping" technique is best applied with skin lotion. Using a broad contact over the area of lesion, a firm pressure is applied as the patient actively moves through a full range. This procedure is repeated several times. Treatment is usually similar to cross friction (every other day). Improvement should occur within the first few treatments. MRT is applied along the axis of muscle fiber orientation, not perpendicular.

A variation of this technique is to perform a stripping massage while the muscle is under stretch with no active movement by the patient.

MYOFASCIAL TP THERAPY

The definition of a TP is more easily defined clinically than physiologically. TPs represent hyperirritable foci in muscle or fascia that are tender to palpation and may, upon compression, result in referred pain or tenderness in a characteristic "zone," which is distinct from a dermatome, myotome, sclerotome, or peripheral nerve area. Also associated with TPs are autonomic phenomena mediated through the sympathetic nervous system. Clinically, TPs are appreciated via palpation as taut bands of muscle or discrete nodules or adhesions. If the taut band is snapped it will usually result in a local "twitch" response.

It is apparent that TPs can mimic other musculoskeletal causes of pain and dysfunction. Referral zones can overlap other osseous or soft tissue structures or relay a sense of deep "joint" pain. Confusion can occur when radiographic degenerative changes accompany a complaint. Discrimination should be attempted consisting of:

1. Palpation. A search for characteristic TP location for a given muscle with an associated twitch sign, jump sign, and possible referral into a specific area (nondermatomal).
2. Stretch of the suspected muscle. Usually limitation will occur if a muscle is stretched to end range often accompanied by pain.
3. Active movement. Active movement into the pattern accomplished by a specific muscle may cause pain.

Travell and Simons[22] discuss the belief that TPs mimic specific named conditions. For example, they feel "frozen shoulder" is due to TPs found primarily in the subscapularis. TPs in the scalenes may be the cause of some cases of thoracic outlet syndrome. TPs in the levator scapulae are the cause of the levator scapulae syndrome. Although it would seem reasonable to consider TP involvement with these conditions, it would seem unwise to assume that all these conditions are TP-caused.

TPs have been classified by Travell and Simons[22] as follows:

1. Active TPs—symptomatic at rest with referral pain and tenderness. Associated weakness and contracture are often present.

2. Latent TPs—not painful unless compressed; they may manifest clinically as stiffness and/or weakness.
3. Further distinction is made between *primary TPs,* which are due to involvement of and found in a specific muscle, and *associated TPs,* which are found in a muscle that is located in the primary TP referral zone *(satellite TP)* or in a muscle that is functionally overloaded in compensation for a primary TP *(secondary TP).*

Travell and Simons[22] feel that activation of TPs may occur through direct stimuli such as acute overload, overwork/fatigue, chilling, and gross trauma or indirect stimuli such as other TPs, visceral disease, arthritic joints, or emotional stress. Maintenance of TPs is due to sensory hypersensitization. There are a plethora of ideas regarding how this occurs. Both chemonociceptors and mechanonociceptors are sensitized by various substances such as bradykinin, histamine, serotonin, potassium, prostaglandins, and probably substance P.[23,24] Interestingly, these nociceptors do not respond to phosphate or lactate (thought to be responsible for muscle pain after activity).[25] One study indicated that the source of some of these substances was degranulating mast cells (histamine) and platelet clusters (serotonin).[26] Although representing a local area of inflammatory reaction, therapeutic modalities used in the treatment of overt inflammation are not effective.

The above chemical theory of maintenance is only half of the story. Mechanical maintenance is due to continued actin/myosin interaction. Given that the taut bands associated with the TPs are electrically silent, it is likely that this "contraction" is not centrally mediated. Local events that may play a part are tearing of the sarcoplasmic reticulum (SR), which releases ionic calcium. This excess calcium maintains the actin/myosin interaction imposing increased metabolic demands. The local contraction impairs circulation preventing elimination of the affective metabolites.[27]

Treatment of TPs

Predicated on the assumption that TPs are local events and that maintenance of this local phenomenon is partly based on the availability of adenosine triphosphate (ATP) and the actin/myosin interaction, treatment is directed at eliminating this "physiologic" contraction via stretch and/or ischemic pressure.

The protocol suggested by Travell and Simons[22] is the "spray and stretch" approach. Theoretically, when the involved muscle is placed under tension and a vapocoolant spray such as fluoromethane is applied, cold receptors in the skin are stimulated that inhibit contraction and allow for a small window of time to further stretch the muscle, potentially eliminating the locally contracted TP. Precautions are based on avoidance of overcooling the skin and underlying muscle, which may exacerbate the condition. The procedure involves a passive stretch that is maintained and gradually increased as the coolant spray is applied. The position of stretch is often prescribed as a home stretch. Next, the area is warmed (usually with moist heat) and the muscle is placed through a full ROM several times to avoid residual soreness. Home instructions include avoidance of positions (especially occupational and sleep postures) that may allow a muscle to shorten or overstrain the muscle. Additionally, stretches are prescribed to augment the effects of the office treatment. Ice application may be substituted for the cold spray.

Another treatment approach includes the use of post–isometric techniques for stretching. Post–isometric relaxation (PIR) involves a minimal contraction of the muscle in a stretched position followed by relaxation and an attempt at accessing more ROM. The sequence involves first placing the muscle under stretch. Next the patient uses a 25 percent contraction to isometrically resist, followed by a stretch into a new position. This is a variation on the proprioceptive neuromuscular facilitation (PNF) technique referred to as hold-relax. Several attempts at increasing motion should be used followed by a full ROM and icing if post-treatment soreness occurs.

Myofascial release techniques combine stretching with various techniques of pressure application over the TP or muscle. While passively stretching the involved muscle, deep pressure or "stripping" massage is applied. The pressure is applied for up to 30 seconds in an attempt to get the muscle to "release." Caution must be exercised using this technique due to a tendency to overstretch or apply enough pressure that the patient has significant post-treatment soreness. Lotion is applied to the skin when using stripping massage.

Specific TPs

Referral patterns for various TPs can overlap, making distinction difficult. However, there are usually subtle clues related to restriction patterns or additional referral zones that can be helpful discriminators. Listed in Table 18-3 are potential myofascial causes of shoulder pain based on region.

Included with the description of each TP is a suggested position of stretch that can be used for any of the previously mentioned techniques. It is clear that often one position serves to stretch several muscles and also that the description for each specific muscle stretch varies with the author.

Infraspinatus

TPs in the infraspinatus (Fig. 18-9) are probably responsible for many posterior and deep shoulder complaints. The referral pattern is unique in that it is often perceived as "in the joint." In addition, referral down

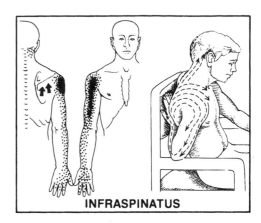

Fig. 18-9. TPs *(arrows)* for the infraspinatus. Pain pattern is indicated by dots. (From Basmajian and Kirby,[29] with permission.)

Table 18-3. Trigger Points of the Shoulder and Thoracic Regions

Upper thoracic back pain
  Scaleni
  Levator scapulae
  Trapezius
  Multifidi
Midthoracic back pain
  Scaleni
  Latissimus dorsi
  Infraspinatus
  Trapezius
  Serratus anterior
  Rhomboides
  Iliocostalis thoracis
  Multifidi
  Serratus posterior superior
Posterior shoulder pain
  Deltoid
  Levator scapulae
  Supraspinatus
  Subscapularis
  Teres minor
  Teres major
  Serratus posterior superior
  Triceps
  Trapezius
Anterior shoulder pain
  Infraspinatus
  Deltoid
  Scalene
  Supraspinatus
  Pectoralis major
  Pectoralis minor
  Biceps
  Coracobrachialis

(Adapted from Travell and Simons,[22] with permission.)

the anterior arm may simulate a biceps involvement. In more severe cases, this referral may extend to the wrist and hand laterally both on the anterior and posterior aspects. The main TP for the infraspinatus is in the belly of the muscle in the center of the scapula.

Restrictions can include difficulty and/or pain with attempts at reaching behind the back. Travell[22] describes a wraparound test to determine a shortening reaction. This is based on the observation that motion accomplished by a muscle is restricted by shortening when a TP is present. Other problems can include the inability to sleep on the affected side due to compression or on the uninvolved shoulder due to stretch. It is often helpful to have the patient sleep with a pillow between the involved arm and bed to prevent the relaxed position of internal rotation. This should eliminate the constant stretch that can occur during sleep.

Stretching the infraspinatus is usually via two positions. First, passively stretching the arm across the body in horizontal adduction places a stretch on the posterior structures. Secondly, passively stretching the arm up and behind the back can accomplish the same goal. In the latter position, having the patient press the elbow back against the examiner using the PIR technique may access more range.

Deltoid

TPs in the anterior and posterior deltoid refer locally. This may cause difficulty differentiating bicipital tendinitis from an anterior deltoid TP and infraspinatus ten-

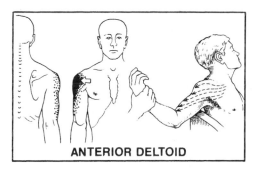

Fig. 18-10. TP *(arrow)* for the anterior deltoid. Pain pattern is indicated by dots. (From Basmajian and Kirby,[29] with permission.)

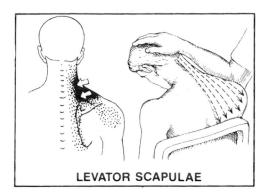

Fig. 18-12. TPs *(arrows)* for the levator scapulae. Pain pattern is indicated by dots. (From Basmajian and Kirby,[29] with permission.)

dinitis from a posterior deltoid TP. Referred pain and tenderness with anterior deltoid TPs may extend down the arm laterally to the elbow with associated restriction of external rotation and extension. Anterior deltoid TPs are often satellite TPs from the infraspinatus.

Stretching of the anterior deltoid is accomplished with the "cocking" position of abduction and external rotation (Fig. 18-10). The middle deltoid is stretched by horizontal adduction across the chest with the elbow at 90 degrees flexion. The elbow is used as the point of leverage. The posterior deltoid is stretched also with cross-body horizontal adduction, but the hand is brought over the opposite shoulder (Fig. 18-11).

Levator Scapula

The levator scapula TPs (Fig. 18-12) are probably a common source of the patient's complaint of shoulder pain. In other words, the patient includes the upper

trapezius area as representing the shoulder. Referral is primarily over the muscle and overlying upper trapezius.

Dysfunction is a potential indirect cause or effect of shoulder pain. Inability to couple with the other scapular muscles to properly position the scapula will affect the mechanics of the glenohumeral joint with impingement possible.

Travell and Simons[22] suggest a stretch with the patient seated. The patient grasps the bottom of the chair with the ipsilateral hand as the examiner stretches the neck to the contralateral side into a combined position of flexion and lateral flexion. This same position can be used by the patient as a home stretch using the opposite hand for stretching the neck.

Scalenes

As mentioned, Travell[28] suggests that signs and symptoms of thoracic outlet syndrome may be due to scalene TPs (Fig. 18-13). Referral occurs to the medial border of the scapula, anterior chest, and down the lateral arm to the wrist and hand. The pattern of arm and hand referral may need to be differentiated from a cervicogenic source of referral. It is interesting to note that the referral pattern differs from the typical thoracic outlet pattern, which is more manifest in the ulnar distribution. Perhaps compression/entrapment with thoracic outlet syndrome is distinct from TPs in the offending structures. Interestingly, one study indicated that 50 percent of an asymptomatic student group were found to have scalene TPs.[28]

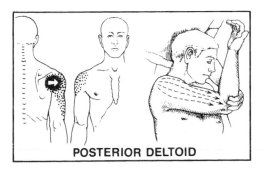

Fig. 18-11. TP *(arrow)* for the posterior deltoid. Pain pattern is indicated by dots. (From Basmajian and Kirby,[29] with permission.)

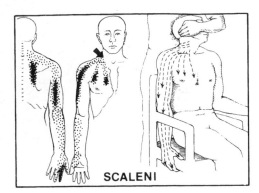

Fig. 18-13. TP *(arrow)* for the scalenes. Pain pattern is indicated by dots. (From Basmajian and Kirby,[29] with permission.)

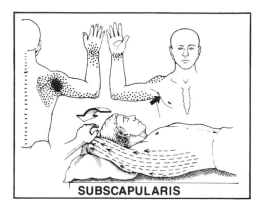

Fig. 18-14. TP *(arrow)* for the subscapularis. Pain pattern is indicated by dots. (From Basmajian and Kirby,[29] with permission.)

The stretch position for the scalenes is similar to that for the levator scapula. The patient grasps under a chair while the examiner stretches the neck to the opposite side. The variations for each division are (1) lateral flexion with the face rotated away from the involved side for the posterior scalene, (2) lateral flexion with the face facing forward for the middle scalene, and (3) lateral flexion with the face rotated to the same side for the anterior scalene.

These positions can be used as home stretches. If patients wish to perform them supine, they may place their hand under the ipsilateral buttocks for fixation. These stretches can be augmented at home with PIR techniques.

Subscapularis

The referral zone for the subscapularis TPs (Fig. 18-14) is the posterior aspect of the shoulder. This overlaps with the posterior deltoid, teres minor, and infraspinatus referral zones. An important differentiating feature when present is a straplike band of pain and/or tenderness around the wrist with the dorsal area most involved.

An important belief of Travell and Simons[22] is that TPs in the subscapularis may be the cause of pain and restriction simulating frozen shoulder or perhaps the cause of idiopathic frozen shoulder. Subsequent to development of TPs in the subscapularis, the pectoralis major, latissimus dorsi, and triceps are secondarily involved. The resulting restriction is mainly external rotation/abduction.

Stretching for the subscapularis is performed with the patient supine. The intent is to gradually increase abduction with some degree of external rotation to effectively stretch the muscle. PRI techniques may be helpful.

Supraspinatus

Although the supraspinatus is commonly involved with impingement and overuse, TPs in the supraspinatus are not considered common causes of shoulder pain (Fig. 18-15). Referral is local or into the deltoid area. Palpation for TP involvement is best performed with the patient lying prone. This position will relax the

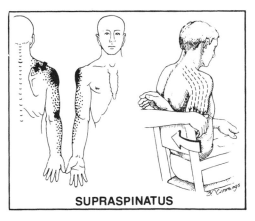

Fig. 18-15. TPs *(arrows)* for the supraspinatus. Pain pattern is indicated by dots. (From Basmajian and Kirby,[29] with permission.)

overlying trapezius making identification of the supraspinatus more assured.

Smolders[27] believes that dysfunction results in crepitus due to the unbalanced contraction of the deltoid. Travell[22] reported on resolution of early calcific deposits with TP treatment.

The supraspinatus is stretched by placing the patient's arm behind the back resting the hand on the back of the chair if possible.

Trapezius

Acromioclavicular pain and/or tenderness may be due to TPs in either the upper (Fig. 18-16A) or lower (Fig. 18-16B) trapezius. Distinction between local involvement and TP referral would be possible by finding referral zones, especially to the neck, and the lack of positive orthopaedic positives on acromioclavicular testing.

The upper trapezius is stretched with the hand grasping the chair and laterally flexing and rotating the head away from the involved side. Middle and lower fibers are stretched by having the seated patient cross the arms with elbows straight and lean forward.

Triceps

Two upper triceps TPs (Fig. 18-17) may refer pain to the posterior shoulder and/or elbow. Overlap would again occur with the teres minor, posterior deltoid, subscapularis, infraspinatus, and teres major referral zones.

Stretching of the triceps is accomplished with forward flexion of the shoulder. The elbow is flexed with the forearm supinated.

Biceps

Two TPs in the lower portion of the biceps (Fig. 18-18), just proximal to the cubital fossa, may refer pain or tenderness over the bicipital tendon area.

Biceps stretching occurs with 90 degrees abduction of the shoulder with some horizontal extension. The elbow is hyperextended with the forearm pronated.

Pectoralis Major

The clavicular portion of the pectoralis major may harbor TPs (Fig. 18-19) that refer over the anterior shoul-

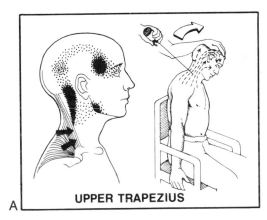

UPPER TRAPEZIUS

A

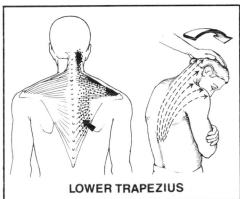

LOWER TRAPEZIUS

B

Fig. 18-16. TPs *(arrows)* for the **(A)** upper and **(B)** lower trapezius. Pain pattern is indicated by dots. (From Basmajian and Kirby,[29] with permission.)

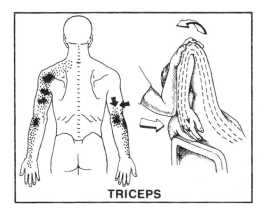

TRICEPS

Fig. 18-17. Tps *(arrows)* for the triceps. Pain pattern is indicated by dots. (From Basmajian and Kirby,[29] with permission.)

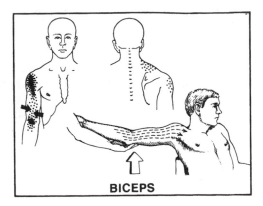

Fig. 18-18. TPs *(arrows)* for the biceps. Pain pattern is indicated by dots. (From Basmajian and Kirby,[29] with permission.)

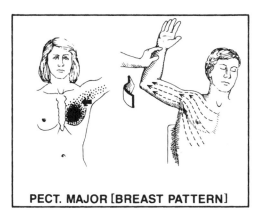

Fig. 18-19. TP *(arrow)* for the pectoralis major. Pain pattern is indicated by dots. (From Basmajian and Kirby,[29] with permission.)

der (deltoid area). The position of stretch for the clavicular section is with the shoulder abducted 90 degrees with external rotation. Stretching of the sternal section is performed supine with full flexion of the shoulder and external rotation. Doorway stretching with a PIR technique is quite effective. Caution must be used when performing the spray and stretch technique or home stretching due to the position of instability that must be acquired.

Pectoralis Minor

In addition to referral to the anterior shoulder by a pectoralis minor TP (Fig. 18-20), entrapment by a taut pectoralis minor may cause signs and symptoms of tho-

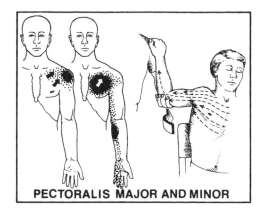

Fig. 18-20. TPs *(arrows)* for the pectoralis minor. Pain pattern is indicated by dots. (From Basmajian and Kirby,[29] with permission.)

racic outlet syndrome. These signs and symptoms would be increased by abduction of the arm.

Stretching of the pectoralis minor is similar to the position for the pectoralis major clavicular division. The arm is abducted slightly beyond 90 degrees with external rotation and some horizontal extension. It is not unusual for this position to temporarily reproduce the patient's referred pain. It is suggested that if this persists long after the treatment, that less aggressive yet persistent stretching be performed.

Latissimus Dorsi

The upper latissimus TP (Fig. 18-21) can refer pain down the posterior medial aspect of the arm to the fingers. The lower TP can cause a combination of lower

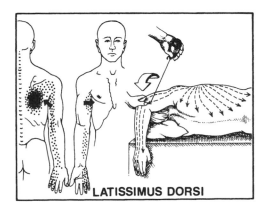

Fig. 18-21. TPs *(arrows)* for the latissimus dorsi. Pain pattern is indicated by dots. (From Basmajian and Kirby,[29] with permission.)

lateral back pain with an associated anterior shoulder pain.

Stretching is accomplished with the patient supine or side-lying with examiner assisted attempts at accessing full abduction.

ACUPUNCTURE/ACUPRESSURE

It is beyond the scope of this text to present a detailed description of the theories and practices of acupuncture. There are several texts that give a comprehensive

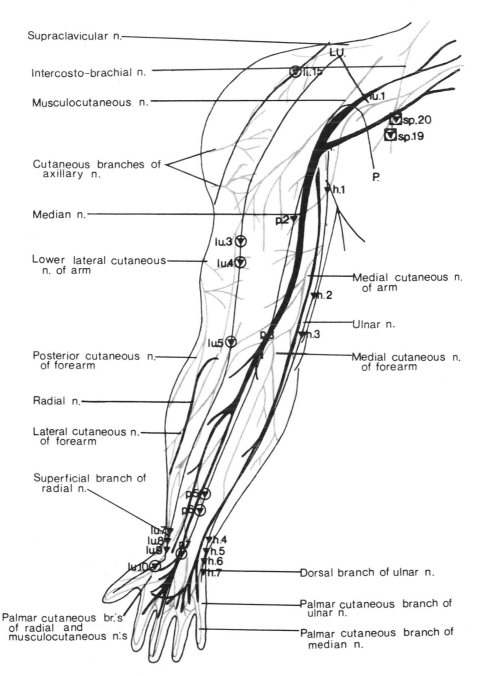

Fig. 18-22. Acupuncture points of the anterior upper extremity and their relationship to peripheral nerves. (From Mannheimer and Lampre,[30] with permission.)

presentation on the subject. In general terms, acupuncture can be divided into two schools of philosophy. The traditional school's diagnostic and treatment approaches are predicated on a system of "invisible" channels of energy called "chi" or "kl." There are 14 channels that are interdependent; energy is balanced among them. These channels start deep in the viscera (often named by the viscera of origin) and travel superficially where they may be accessed via needles and other apparatus. The diagnostic approach is to determine excesses or deficiencies of energy in each channel. Relationships among the channels exist temporally

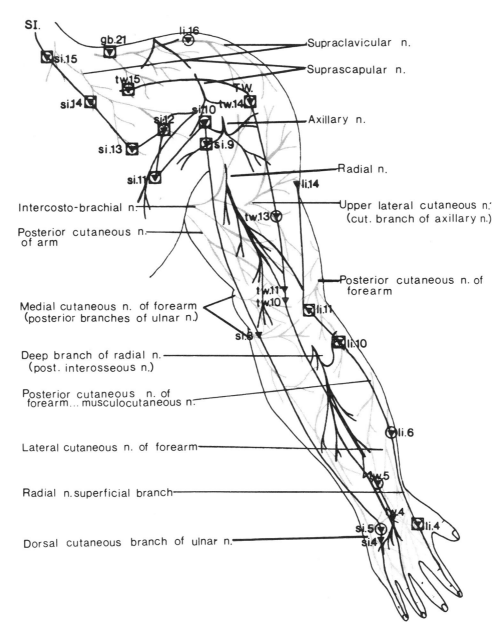

Fig. 18-23. Acupuncture points of the posterior upper extremity and their relationship to peripheral nerves. (From Mannheimer and Lampre,[30] with permission.)

Table 18-4. Optimal Stimulation Sites for Transcutaneous Electrical Nerve Stimulation (TENS) Electrodes. Anteromedial Shoulder and Volar Region of Upper Extremity.

Location	Superficial Nerve Branch	Acupuncture Point	Motor Point	Trigger Point	Segemental Level
Between first and second ribs, about 4″ lateral to sternum, medial to coracoid process	Musculocutaneous nerve	LU 1	Coracobrachialis is nearby (musculocutaneous) (C6)		C5–C7
Radial side of biceps brachii 2″ below anterior axillary fold. 3″ below anterior axillary fold	Musculocutaneous nerve and its lower lateral cutaneous branch	LU 3 LU 4	Biceps brachii (musculocutaneous) C5–C6		C5–C7
In antecubital fossa on crease at radial side of biceps tendon	Lateral cutaneous nerve of arm	LU 5	Brachialis (musculocutaneous) (C5–C6)		C5–C7
Just lateral to radial artery from first volar crease to just above radial styloid	Lateral cutaneous nerve of forearm communicating with superficial radial nerve	LU 7–9			C5–C7 C6–C8
Volar surface of hand at midpoint of first metacarpal	Superficial branch of radial nerve and palmar cutaneous of median	LU 10	Abductor pollicis brevis (median) (C8–T1)		C6–C8 C5–T1
Between heads of biceps brachii 2″ below anterior axillary fold	Musculocutaneous and intercostal brachial nerves, may communicate with medial cutaneous nerve of forearm	P 2			C5–C7 T2 C8–T1
Just medial to biceps tendon in antecubital fossa	Median nerve and anterior branch of medial cutaneous nerve of forearm	P 3	Pronator teres (median) (C6)		C5–T1 C8–T1
Between tendons of flexor carpi radialis and palmaris longus 2″ and 1½″ above volar crease, respectively	Median and anterior branch of medial cutaneous nerve of forearm	P 5 P 6 is 1″ below			C5–T1 C8–T1
Between tendons of flexor carpi radialis and palmaris longus at midpoint of transverse volar wrist crease	Median and anterior branch of medial cutaneous nerve of forearm and palmar cutaneous branch of median	P 7			C5–T1 C8–T1
Between ribs 2–3 and 3–4, midway between anterior axillary fold and sternum	Medial and intermedial supraclavicular nerves to second rib, lateral cutaneous nerves of thorax (2–4), the second nerve is the intercostal brachial nerve	SP 19–20	Pectoralis major (medial and lateral anterior thoracic nerves)	Pectoralis major	C3–C4 T2–C4
Medial to brachial artery in axilla	Ulnar nerve, intercostobrachial, medial cutaneous nerve of arm, and median nerve, which is just lateral to artery	H 1			C7–T1 T2 C9–T1 C5–T1
In groove medial to lower one-third of biceps brachii medial to brachial artery	Median and medial cutaneous nerve of arm	H 2			C5–T1 C8–T1

(continues)

Table 18-4. *(continued)*

Location	Superficial Nerve Branch	Acupuncture Point	Motor Point	Trigger Point	Segemental Level
Just superior to cubital tunnel by medial epicondyle	Medial cutaneous nerve of forearm	H 3			C8–T1
Ulnar aspect of wrist lateral to flexor carpi ulnaris tendon from 1½″ above first volar wrist crease to pisiform bone	Ulnar nerve and its palmar cutaneous branch	H 4–7			C7–T1
In depression anterior and inferior to acromion	Upper lateral cutaneous nerve branch of axillary	LI 15	Anterior deltoid (axillary) (C5–C6)		C5–C6

(From Mannheimer and Lampre,[30] with permission.)

Table 18-5. Optimal Stimulation Sites for Transcutaneous Electrical Nerve Stimulation (TENS) Electrodes. Posterolateral Shoulder and Dorsal Region of Upper Extremity.

Location	Superficial Nerve Branch	Acupuncture Point	Motor Point	Trigger Point	Segmental Level
1½″ lateral to spinous process of C7	Medial branch of supraclavicular	SI 15	Levator scapulae (spinal accessory and dorsal scapular (C3–C4)	Levator scapulae	Cranial C3–C4
1½″ above superior angle of scapula at the level of the spinous process of T1	Lateral (posterior) branch of supraclavicular	SI 14 TW 15 is just lateral	Middle trapezius (spinal accessory) (C3–C4)	Middle trapezius	Cranial C3–C4
Suprascapular fossa (medial end) 3″ lateral to spinous process of T2	Lateral (posterior) branch of supraclavicular and dorsal ramus of T2	SI 13	Middle trapezius (spinal accessory) (C3–C4)	Middle trapezius	Cranial C3–C4 T2
At midpoint of suprascapular fossa	Dorsal ramus of T2	SI 12	Supraspinatus (suprascapular) (C5–C6)	Supraspinatus	C5–C6 T2
At midpoint of infrascapular fossa	Dorsal ramus of T2	SI 11	Infraspinatus (suprascapular) (C5–C6)	Infraspinatus	C5–C6 T2
Directly above posterior axillary fold. Just below spine of scapula	Dorsal ramus of T2 and axillary (posterior branch), which continues as the upper lateral cutaneous nerve of the arm	SI 10	Posterior deltoid (axillary) (C5–C6)	Posterior deltoid	C5–C6 T2
Directly below SI 10. Just superior to posterior axillary fold	Axillary and dorsal ramus of T2	SI 9	Teres major (subscapular) (C5–C6)	Teres major	C5–C6 T2
In groove between olecranon and medial epicondyle of humerus	Ulnar nerve and its medial cutaneous branches	SI 8			C7–T1
In depression between pisiform bone and ulnar styloid	Dorsal and palmar cutaneous branches of ulnar nerve	SI 5			C7–T1
In depression between fifth metacarpal and triquetral	Dorsal and palmar cutaneous branches of ulnar nerve	SI 4	Palmaris brevis (median) (C8–T1)		C7–T1

(continues)

Table 18-5. *(continued)*

Location	Superficial Nerve Branch	Acupuncture Point	Motor Point	Trigger Point	Segmental Level
On cephalad surface of upper trapezius directly above superior angle of scapula	Supraclavicular	GB 21	Upper trapezius (spinal accessory)	Upper trapezius	Cranial C3–C4
In depression posterior and inferior to acromion and above greater tubercle of humerus with arm in anatomic position	Intercostal brachial, upper lateral cutaneous nerve—branch of axillary, and dorsal ramus of T2	TW 14	Posterior deltoid (axillary) (C5–C6)		C5–C6 T2
Just below deltoid insertion by lateral head of triceps	Upper lateral cutaneous nerve branch of axillary	TW 13	Lateral head of triceps (radial) (C7–C8)		C5–C6
In depression 1″ above olecranon with the elbow flexed to 90°	Posterior cutaneous of arm (radial), medial cutaneous of forearm (ulnar posterior branches), posterior cutaneous nerve of forearm	TW 10, TW11 is just above			C5–C8 C8–T1 C5–C8
Between radius and ulna on dorsal surface about 2″ proximal to transverse wrist crease	Posterior cutaneous nerve of forearm, branch of radial communicates with lateral cutaneous nerve of forearm, branch of musculocutaneous	TW 5	Extensor indicis proprius (radial) (C7)		C5–C8 C5–C6
In depression on dorsum of hand between tendons of extensor digitorum communis and extensor indicis proprius just distal to transverse crease of wrist	Posterior cutaneous nerve of forearm (radial, superficial radial and dorsal cutaneous branch of ulnar nerve)	TW 4			C5–C8 C6–C8 C8–T1
In depression between acromioclavicular joint and spine of scapula	Posterolateral branch of supraclavicular nerve	LI 16	Musculotendinous junction of supraspinatus		C3–C4
In depression anterior and inferior to acromion	Upper lateral cutaneous nerve branch of axillary	LI 15	Anterior deltoid (axillary) (C5–C6)		C5–C6
Lateral arm at deltoid insertion	Upper lateral cutaneous	LI 14			C5–C6
Lateral end of cubital crease in depression with elbow flexed	Posterior cutaneous nerve of forearm (medial), communicates with intercostal brachial nerve	LI 11	Brachioradialis (medial) (C5–C6)	Brachioradialis	C5–C8
Just below lateral epicondyle of humerus with forearm pronated	Superficial radial nerve superior to posterior interosseus nerve	LI 10	Extensor carpi radialis longus, supinator nearby (radial) (C6)	Extensor carpi radialis longus, supinator nearby	C6–C8
8–10 cm above radial styloid with arm in anatomic position	Superficial radial and lateral cutaneous nerve of forearm	LI 6	Extensor pollicis brevis (radial) (C7)		C6–C8 C5–C6
Midpoint of radial aspect of second metacarpal	Superficial radial in communication with distal branches of musculocutaneous	LI 4	First dorsal interosseus (ulnar nerve) (C8–T1)	First dorsal interosseus and adductor pollicis	C6–C8 C5–C7 C7–T1

(From Mannheimer and Lampre,[30] with permission.)

(a 2 hour peak of time for each channel) and in a "creative" or "destructive" manner. Both the radial pulses and various body points are used to determine need for treatment (taken together with a very elaborate system of historical review of the patient).

The Western view of acupuncture hinges on neural concepts. A relationship exists between acupuncture points and points where superficial nerves course close to the skin (Figs. 18-22 and 18-23). Specific locations of acupuncture points are listed in Tables 18-4 and 18-5. Treatment is therefore a form of neurostimulation inhibiting pain through a "counter-irritation" effect. Treatment may be with TENS, pulsed ultrasound, laser, or acupuncture/acupressure.

REFERENCES

1. Sloan JP, Giddings JP, Hain R: Effects of cold and compression on edema. Phys Sport Med 16:116, 1988
2. Waylonis GW: The physiological effects of ice massage. Arch Phys Med Rehabil 48:42, 1967
3. Lehmann JF, De Lateur BJ: Diathermy and superficial heat and cold therapy. In Kottke FJ, Stiwell GK, Lehmann JF (eds): Handbook of Physical Medicine and Rehabilitation. 3rd Ed. WB Saunders, Philadelphia, 1982
4. Ziskin MC, Michlovitz SL: Therapeutic ultrasound. p. 141. In Michlovitz SL (ed): Thermal Agents in Rehabilitation. FA Davis, Philadelphia, 1986
5. Gersten JW: Effect of ultrasound on tendon extensibility. Am J Phys Med 34:662, 1955
6. Kramer JF: Ultrasound: evaluation of its mechanical and thermal effects. Arch Phys Med Rehabil 65:223, 1984
7. Giek JH, Saliba ES: Application of modalities in overuse syndromes. Clin Sports Med 6:427, 1987
8. Rivenburgh DW: Physical modalities in the treatment of tendon injuries. Clin Sports Med 11:645, 1992
9. Lehmann JF, De Lateur BJ, Stonebridge JB, Warren CG: Therapeutic temperature distribution produced by ultrasound as modified by dosage and volume of tissue exposed. Arch Phys Med Rehabil 48:662, 1967
10. Griffin JE, Karselis TC: Physical Agents for Physical Therapists. 2nd Ed. Charles C Thomas, Springfield, IL, 1982
11. Lehmann JF, De Lateur BJ, Silverman DR: Selective heating effects of ultrasound on human beings. Arch Phys Med 47:331, 1966
12. Dyson M, Suckling J: Stimulation of tissue repair by ultrasound: a survey of mechanisms involved. Physiotherapy 64:105, 1978
13. Newton RA, Karselis TC: Skin pH following high voltage-pulsed galvanic stimulation. Phys Ther 63:1593, 1983
14. Alon G: High Voltage Stimulation. Chattanooga Corp, Chattanooga, TN, 1984
15. Nippel FJ: Interferential Current Therapy. An Advanced Method in the Management of Pain. Nemectron Medical, Temecuta, CA, 1979
16. Cyriax J: Textbook of Orthopaedic Medicine. Balliere-Tindall, London, 1982
17. Mennell J: The manipulatable lesion: joint play, joint dysfunction, and joint manipulation. p. 191. In Hammer WI (ed): Functional Soft Tissue Examination and Treatment by Manual Methods: The Extremities. Aspen, Rockville, MD, 1991
18. Hammer WI: Friction massage. p. 235. In Hammer WI (ed): Functional Soft Tissue Examination and Treatment by Manual Methods: The Extremities. Aspen, Rockville, MD, 1991
19. Hertling D, Kessler RM: Management of Common Musculoskeletal Disorders: Physical Therapy Principles and Methods. Harper & Row, New York, 1990
20. Carrick FR: Lecture Notes from NYCC Diplomate on Neurology Program, November 1987
21. Leahy PM, Mock LE: Altered biomechanics of the shoulder and the subscapularis. Chiro Sports Med 5:62, 1991
22. Travell J, Simons DG: Myofascial Dysfunction: The Trigger Point Manual. Williams & Wilkins, Baltimore, 1983
23. Perl ER: Sensitization of nociceptors and its relation to sensation. Adv Pain Res Ther 1:29, 1976
24. Mense S: Nervous outflow from skeletal muscle following chemical noxious stimulation. J Physiol 267:75, 1977
25. Kniffke KD, Mense S, Schmidt RF: Response of group IV afferent units from skeletal muscle to stretch, contraction, and chemical stimulation. Exp Brain Res 31:511, 1978
26. Awad EA: Interstitial myofibrositis: hypothesis of the mechanism. Arch Phys Med 54:449, 1979
27. Smolders JJ: Myofascial pain and dysfunction syndromes. p. 215. In Hammer WI (ed): Functional Soft Tissue Examination and Treatment by Manual Methods: The Extremities. Aspen, Rockville, MD, 1991
28. Travell JG: Scalene muscles: the entrappers. p. 344. In Travell JG, Simons DG (eds): Myofascial Pain and Dysfunction: The Trigger Point Manual. Williams & Wilkins, Baltimore, 1983
29. Basmajian JV, Kirby RL: Medical Rehabilitation. Williams & Wilkins, Baltimore, 1984
30. Mannheimer J, Lampre G: Clinical Transcutaneous Electrical Nerve Stimulation. FA Davis, Philadelphia, 1984

19
Mobilization and Adjustive Procedures

THOMAS A. SOUZA

A distinction must be made between the terms mobilization and adjustment. Although the intent of each technique is to restore joint range of motion and indirectly influence reflex pain, the application of the technique requires different evaluation and treatment application parameters.

Based on the original model by Sandoz,[1] approaches for increasing accessory movement at a joint are in fact points along a continuum that first begins with active movement. Range of motion at a joint may be actively acquired or passively acquired (Fig. 19-1). Active ranging is limited by the resistance of contracted antagonists and to some degree by the shortening effect of the agonists. Further, muscles work "across" the joint not at the joint. Passively, an elastic endpoint is reached that exceeds the range of actively acquired movement. This endpoint signals the limits of passive movement and therefore mobilization techniques. If this elastic barrier is exceeded, a small amount of movement is still available before the restrictions of the anatomic endpoint are reached. This range has been estimated as 0.125 inches in any given direction.[2] Past this point the structural integrity of the stabilizing structures is violated. To gain access to this "paraphysiologic" zone, a short amplitude impulse of force is added to the endpoint of the elastic barrier. The direct intent is to increase or free movement across a joint that is not controlled voluntarily (accessory movement). Although not under voluntary control, accessory movement does occur with active movements. Therefore, it is possible for soft tissue contracture to passively block or increase accessory movement. Additionally it has been observed that restriction of accessory motion

may in fact affect active movement capabilities. Adjunctive techniques such as mobilization to stretch noncontractile tissue or other techniques to relax the surrounding musculature may be helpful and necessary in aiding and holding an adjustment.

Another distinction between mobilization and adjustment is that the patient has some control over the degree of mobilization; however, the adjustment is performed quickly enough that the patient cannot control it. If the elastic endpoint is not reached, due either to the patient's attempt (consciously or unconsciously) at control or if sufficient muscle spasm is present, the adjustment may be prevented.

When the elastic barrier is passed a "click" or "pop" may be heard. This observation led some researchers to investigate the mechanical properties of the adjustment. Using the metacarpophalangeal joint gradual pressure was directed in long-axis traction. Up to about 8 kg of force, there was only slight opening of the articular space. When more tension was added there was a click heard with simultaneous increase in the articular space. The suggested explanation has been the release of gases from synovial fluid under negative pressure. A radiolucent area is sometimes visible in the joint space following an adjustment. This release of gas with increase in joint space is referred to as cavitation. It must be recognized that any attempts at a second cavitation response will be unsuccessful and potentially dangerous within the first few minutes of the first response. Apparently, a reverse phenomenon occurs when the negative pressure is restored and gases have been reabsorbed. It may take as long as 15 to 20 minutes for this to occur. Until recently, the

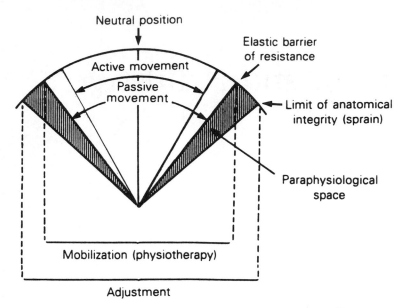

Fig. 19-1. Sandoz model of physiologic and paraphysiologic zones. (From Subotnick[12] as in Sandoz[1], with permission.)

negative pressure aspect of joint stability was largely ignored. However, especially in the shoulder, this aspect of joint stability is important. Therefore, subsequent attempts at adjusting a joint should be governed by the safety refractory period of 15 to 20 minutes. Also it is suggested that the joint not be exercised or otherwise stressed due to this relative instability for perhaps an hour after being adjusted. The extra added caution for most joints and, in particular, the shoulder, is that there may be relative inherent mobility of the joint. Individually, this mobility may be excessive due either to trauma or nontraumatic congenital/acquired laxity. These additional concerns must factor into the decision of whether an adjustment is given, and if given, the type of adjustment used.

MOBILIZATION

Mobilization techniques have been described by many authors.[3–6] An organized approach to classification of grading and application has been suggested by Corrigan and Maitland.[3] Mobilization is defined as a passive-movement approach that attempts to move the joint up to the paraphysiologic range. The majority of these movements are oscillatory and may be applied with either compression or distraction of the treated joint. The other variable is the position of the joint. Application can be within the available range or at end range.

Joint Positioning

Positioning of the joint is important in regards to the type of accessory movement that is being addressed. In general, rolling and gliding movements are the two movements recognized. Spin movement is similar to osteokinematic definitions. Rolling always follows bone movement and is independent of whether the joint is concave or convex. Using the humerus as an example, upward movement of the humerus is accompanied by upward rolling of the humerus.

Gliding, on the other hand, is relative to the type of joint surface that is moving. If the surface that is moving is convex, gliding occurs in a direction opposite to bone movement. For example, if the humerus is moving upward, downward gliding of the humerus must be added to assist this bone movement. The opposite rule applies to a moving concave surface on a convex surface: the gliding movement occurs in the same direction as bone movement. There are few opportunities for this application in the shoulder.

Gradations of Mobilization

Corrigan and Maitland[3] graded mobilization movements based on where in the range it was applied and the amplitude of application. It must be clear that these authors describe movements according to available range. Therefore, end-range mobilization refers to the individual patient's "pathologic" limitation not the limitations of the elastic barrier. Using this graded system, suggestions for application based on patient symptoms are given. Maitland divided mobilization into five grades:

Grade I movement is small amplitude and performed only at the beginning of the range.

Grade II movement is large amplitude performed within the available range not encroaching upon ranges that are resistive.

Grade III movement is also large amplitude performed up to the limited range.

Grade IV movement is small amplitude movement applied at the limit.

Grade V is equivalent to an adjustment where an impulse is added at the end of the paraphysiologic range.

Grade I through III movements are primarily applied in an attempt at pain relief. Grade IV movement is used primarily in the treatment of a hypomobile joint.

Determining a Treatment Approach

The application of a therapeutic approach to treatment is best determined by the selective tension approach of Cyriax[7] coupled with the joint play guidelines of Mennell,[2] and Schafer and Faye.[8] Cyriax[7] outlined an approach to define which process and structures were involved in any given joint complaint. By selectively differentiating first contractile from noncontractile tissues, one may determine the need for stretching of contractile tissues versus stretching of noncontractile structures. If hypermobile, avoidance of stretching techniques and emphasis on strengthening is recommended.

By combining the findings of active resistive movement coupled with passive movement, a sense of whether contractile or noncontractile involvement may be determined. Further differentiation may be added with the findings of "quality" of end range. It should be evident that contractile tissue may be painful due either to contraction or stretch. If both findings are present, it should be present in opposite directions (i.e., contraction into flexion hurts anteriorly as does passive extension). Unfortunately, this combination is not always evident. If inert or noncontractile tissue is involved, passive movement should be the major abnormality. Active movement should not affect noncontractile tissue unless compressed (i.e., bursa).

The quality of passive end range has been defined as normal and abnormal by Cyriax[7] and may help further define structure and process.

Normal

1. Soft tissue approximation. This is a soft end feel that occurs when muscle opposes muscle. (e.g., when the calf muscles hit the hamstrings or the forearm hits the biceps).
2. Muscular. This is an elastic feel that occurs when a muscle is stretched to its end range. This occurs with straight leg raising and the hamstrings.
3. Bone-on-bone or cartilaginous. This occurs when the joint anatomically stops as occurs with elbow extension.
4. Capsular. This occurs with a tight, slightly elastic feel such as with full hip rotation.

Abnormal

1. Spasm. When muscle spasm is present pain will prevent full range of motion.
2. Springy block or rebound. This occurs when there is a mechanical blockage such as a torn meniscus or labrum and the "end range" is before full range of motion is attained.
3. Empty. This occurs when there is an acute painful process such as bursitis. The patient prevents movement to end range.
4. Loose. This feeling is indicative of capsular or ligamentous damage and is in essence the "feel" that is sought on positive ligamentous testing.

Some authors will equate staging of injury with the timing of the pain on passive testing. For example, pain felt before end range is considered an acute process and would obviate the need for vigorous therapy. Pain felt at the same time as end range would indicate a subacute process and would be amenable to gentle stretching and mobilization. Pain felt after end range would indicate a chronic process that could respond to aggressive stretching and manipulation. If only patient presentation were so easily categorized, the life of the clinician would be much easier.

Although Cyriax[7] defined the springy abnormal end-feel of extremity movement, Mennell[2] and others feel that a springy end-feel at full end range of joint movement is a normal accessory finding that he refers to as joint play. The difference lies in the position of testing. Cyriax[7] defines an end-range position of a particular extremity movement (e.g., abduction/external rotation), whereas Mennell[2] and others speak of a more neutral assessment at the joint with one side of the articulation stabilized and the other motioned. When this springy end-feel is not present, joint dysfunction in the form of restriction is suggested. The appropriate treatment is to continue past this restriction with a thrust of high-velocity, short amplitude.

Harryman et al.[9] have demonstrated that, in cadavers, an obligate translation of the humerus occurs with specific movements when passively acquired. In addition, their findings coupled with the findings of Howell et al.[10] suggest the following:

1. Translation is a normal movement due in large part to the capsule tightening at end-range positions.
2. Lack of translation is evident in lax and pathologic glenohumeral joints.
3. Tightening of the capsule leads to an increase in translation sometimes occurring in planes not normal for that particular movement pattern, but often in a direction opposite of the restricted side (i.e., anterior translation with posterior tightening).
4. It is implied through research attempts that muscular contraction cannot eliminate the normal or abnormal translations.

Determination of abnormal accessory motion is distinctly different than the end-feel palpation findings outlined by Cyriax.[7] Cyriax is referring to the end range of an extremity movement such as abduction, flexion, and internal rotation. Accessory motion is palpated at the joint both with the joint in a neutral or open-packed position and with a coupled movement pattern taken to end range actively and passively. Therefore, the joint would not be restricted by the tension of the capsule or muscles with the first method. The latter techniques take advantage of the end-range position to determine whether the accompanying accessory motion is, in fact, occurring. There are specific guidelines for both assessment and application of treatment with accessory motion barriers.

It is of utmost importance that the patient is in a relaxed position. The examiner needs to stabilize one of the bones of the articulation while moving the other. This is analogous to the "load and shift" testing of shoulder stability, but the intent is the search for blockages as opposed to laxity.

Specific patterns of extremity movement are coupled with specific accessory motion so that restrictions in active movement may be indirectly an indicator of dysfunction of the accompanying accessory motion. It is interesting to note the disparity between observation and experimental evidence regarding which accessory movement is dysfunctional with a given active pattern. For example, Harryman et al.[9] have demonstrated anterior glide or translation of the humeral head with forward flexion, yet many authors suggest that posterior glide is necessary for forward flexion, and when not present restricts full movement. Other coupled patterns also seem antithetical to what has been previously suggested. Most glaring is the anterior movement assumed necessary for abduction coupled with external rotation. In fact, Harryman et al.[9] and Howell et al.[10] have demonstrated posterior movement of as much as 4 mm in the normal functioning joint. Perhaps this is merely a difference in semantics. The tenets of arthrokinetic movement state that rolling occurs in the same direction as bone movement and that gliding occurs in the opposite direction of bone movement when a convex surface is moving on a concave surface. This would explain most of the observations by Harryman et al.[9] and Howell et al.[10] The predicted gliding patterns would then fit the proposed accessory movement patterns proposed by Mennell[2] and others regarding specific movement patterns of rolling. Still, when objectifiably measured as actual translation it is apparent that the model proposed by Mennell and others may be in error.

The most important question to answer regarding the dilemma of which direction a thrust is needed is what causes the restriction. There are three proposed mechanisms that inherently will have some degree of overlap. First is the possibility of dysfunctional muscle firing. Unfortunately, it is unlikely that this is a cause but rather an effect of restricted accessory motion. Based on the unsuccessful attempts of Harryman et al.[9] and Howell et al.[10] to eliminate the obligatory end-range accessory movement using an external force or isometric contraction, it would appear that this movement is related mostly to capsular tightness and integrity opposite the direction of movement. Second is the possibility of trauma forcing the humeral head or other articulation into a subluxated position. This position would be less than the medical subluxated position, but would produce some symptomatology. For example, if a patient fell on an outstretched hand, the humerus might be forced posteriorly on the glenoid. If fixed a few millimeters posteriorly, restriction of movement may occur. Third is the possibility of adhesions. Interestingly, the observations of the above authors suggest that the opposite is true: capsular tightening causes an increase in obligatory movement and laxity decreases this effect. For example, tightening of the posterior capsule increases anterior translation with abduction/external rotation of the arm as would laxity anteriorly. However, the normal posterior translation would not occur with either. Using this third example it would seem possible that the restriction felt by the examiner on accessory movement testing is, in fact, tightening of the portion of the capsule being tested and that this tightening does not produce restriction of movement but creates excessive movement that is the cause of symptomatology. This would also correlate with the load and shift procedures that are intended to detect capsular integrity. For example, if while testing anterior glide a restriction (as opposed to laxity) was perceived, then posterior translation on extension or abduction/external rotation may be the source of dysfunction and/or pain.

Muscle Energy Technique

A muscle energy technique is applied as an indirect approach at increasing blocked accessory movement. Essentially a post–isometric relaxation technique, muscle energy techniques employ a mild to moderate contraction of the agonists followed by a stretch into a new position. Added to this may be pressure applied in the direction of desired movement for the joint while increasing the range. Greenman[11] and others have advocated this technique in the treatment of extremity disorders.

ADJUSTMENT OF THE SHOULDER

There are no clearly established criteria for determining the need or type of adjustment appropriate for a particular shoulder condition. Observation and hypothesis has led to a set of findings that may help direct the clinician. Tantamount to the understanding of need for adjustment is that no single evaluation finding is sufficient to warrant a specific maneuver. Taken as a group, there should be a consensus or near consensus of findings leading to the treatment decision. The following are a list of possible evaluation procedures that may assist in this decision:

1. The restricted pattern of active movement
2. Passive movement evaluation
3. Specific local or regional tenderness
4. Motion palpation
5. Tissues that are involved (i.e., muscle vs tendon vs capsule vs bursa)

For example, if a patient had signs of impingement with palpable tenderness over the supraspinatus or biceps tendons coupled with a painful arc, one might expect that (if gross instability was not present) an adjustment of the humerus inferiorly may be warranted. If another patient had restriction of posterior glide of the humerus coupled with findings of capsular tightness on horizontal adduction and anterior pain (due to excessive anterior movement), an adjustment of the humerus posteriorly may be appropriate.

Although radiograph analysis has been suggested by some chiropractors as a means of determining misalignment of an extremity joint, the difficulties with positioning and magnification render this tool unreliable. A very extensive approach as used by Howell et al.[10] would be required. Unfortunately, this would not be a practical, cost-effective approach.

There are contraindications to an adjustment maneuver, most involving common-sense discrimination. If the patient has an acute inflammatory condition of any type (e.g., acute phase of adhesive capsulitis, acute bursitis, infection, neoplasm, fracture), adjusting

Table 19-1. Area of Tightness Causing Excessive Accessory Movement

Shoulder Movement	Accessory Movement	Area of Tightness	Palpation Restriction/Direction of Correction
Forward flexion	Anterior	Posterior capsule	Posterior
Extension	Posterior	Anterior capsule	Anterior
Abduction	Superior	Posteroinferior capsule	Inferior
Horizontal adduction	Anterior	Posterior capsule	Posterior
Horizontal abduction	Posterior	Anterior capsule	Anterior

should be supplemented with an attention to pain control or medical alleviation of the underlying problem. It would seem obvious that adjusting into the direction of an observed instability pattern may be potentially detrimental.

Although there are numerous suggestions regarding the various accessory motions available for the shoulder girdle (Table 19-1), a combined approach will be used. With each restriction pattern a list of suggestive findings will be presented followed by several adjustive techniques for correction.

COMBINED TECHNIQUES FOR SPECIFIC JOINTS

Sternoclavicular Joint

Motion can be palpated statically in only one direction, anterior to posterior. All other motions of posterior to anterior and inferior to superior must use coupled movement patterns of the shoulder to detect restriction.

Motion may be palpated more easily with the sternoclavicular joint than the other articulations due to its relative superficiality as compared with acromioclavicular or glenohumeral joints. The obvious accessory movements that couple with active or passive movement are:

1. Depression of the shoulder complex—superior glide of the medial clavicle on the sternum
2. Elevation of the shoulder—inferior glide of the medial clavicle on the sternum
3. Horizontal adduction of the shoulder—posterior glide of the medial clavicle on the sternum
4. Horizontal abduction of the shoulder—anterior glide of the medial clavicle on the sternum

Restriction, in particular assymmetrical restriction, of one of these movement patterns may be due to re-

striction of the corresponding accessory motion. There are several procedures for restoring each.

The most simple yet effective approach to restoration of normal movement is the Mennell principle of palpating the movement of the joint while passively positioning the patient in a coupled movement pattern. If accessory motion is restricted at end range, the doctor simply imparts a high-velocity low-amplitude thrust into the direction of restriction while maintaining the coupled movement pattern. The following are some suggested approaches.

Superior Glide

Superior glide is performed by distracting the arm of the patient while standing and palpating the ipsilateral sternoclavicular joint. Passive mobilization through distraction with simultaneous upward pressure with the palm of the opposite hand may be effective. Adjusting is not usually necessary. This movement restriction is not as commonly found as others.

Inferior Glide

Inferior glide may be palpated via two movement patterns. First, the patient lies supine. The examiner palpates both sternoclavicular joints while the patient shrugs (Fig. 19-2). Absence of inferior glide is usually apparent with comparison to the assumed normal opposite. The other method is to have the patient actively elevate the arm while palpating the ipsilateral sternoclavicular joint. This may also be done by standing behind the patient and passively elevating the arm. The examiner should note that employing varying degrees of horizontal adduction with the elevation will often elicit consistent popping at the sternoclavicular joint.

Correction may be accomplished by a passive approach with the patient seated. The examiner stands behind the patient and elevates the involved arm with one hand while the other hand is placed over the sternoclavicular joint (Fig. 19-3). The sternoclavicular joint

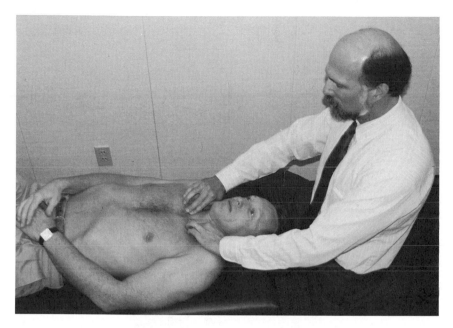

Fig. 19-2. Palpation of inferior glide of the sternoclavicular joint with passive elevation of the ipsilateral arm.

contact at the medial clavicle is with the thenar pad, which maintains an inferior directed force throughout the procedure. The examiner sweeps the arm up and out while maintaining the inferior pressure at the medial clavicle. This is repeated several times and the patient reassessed.

A muscle energy technique may be employed with the patient seated, examiner behind the patient. With the patient's arm controlled at the elbow and the opposite examiner's hand pressing inferiorward on the medial clavicle, the examiner lifts the arm until the motion barrier is met. At this point the patient is asked to attempt further abduction for 3 to 5 seconds against the resistance of the examiner. The additional slack is then passively taken up and the procedure is repeated several times.

A thrust may be used for correction with the examiner standing at the head of the supine patient (Fig. 19-4). Again the arm is elevated while the examiner uses the other hand to contact the sternoclavicular joint with the thenar pad and with fingers pointing inferiorward. With maximum elevation of the arm coupled with inferiorward pressure over the medial clavicle, a thrust is delivered inferiorward often accompanied by an audible release.

Posterior Glide

The patient lies supine and is asked to bring the palms of the straightened arms together in front of the face (Fig. 19-5). The examiner palpates the medial ends of the clavicle while the patient is instructed to push the arms forward (fingers toward the ceiling). Normally a posterior glide is easily palpated. Lack of movement requires an attempt at correction.

The passive approach involves applying pressure over the dysfunctional medial clavicle while bringing the horizontally abducted arm across the chest into horizontal adduction while maintaining a posterior compressive force at the medial clavicular end (Fig. 19-6). Traction may be applied to the arm by the examiner, further facilitating correction.

The muscle energy approach is to grasp the posterior aspect of the scapula and lift. The patient is asked to grasp behind the examiner's neck (Fig. 19-7). Using both hands may be easier to coordinate. With one-sided correction, the patient pulls down on the examiner's neck. The examiner extends back with the body weight while simultaneously pulling on the posterior shoulder girdle and compressing the medial clavicle. With a bilateral approach, the examiner uses compres-

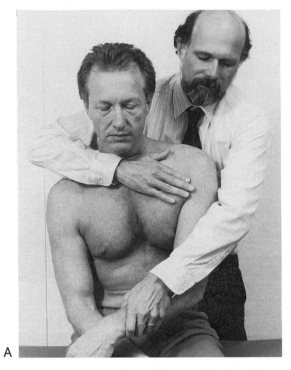

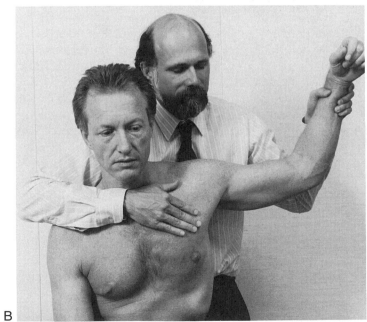

Fig. 19-3. (A & B) Correction of blocked inferior glide at the sternoclavicular joint.

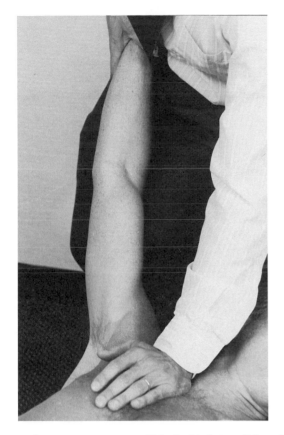

Fig. 19-4. Supine correction of blocked inferior glide at the sternoclavicular joint.

sion over the medial clavicles only. This procedure is repeated several times and then reassessed.

An adjustment may be accomplished with or without a drop-table apparatus. With the patient lying supine, the examiner distracts the humerus with one hand while applying posterior pressure with the palm of the opposite hand at the sternoclavicular joint (Fig. 19-8). A quick impulse with some distraction of the ipsilateral arm is used to adjust the sternoclavicular joint posteriorly.

Anterior Glide

To palpate anterior glide the seated or supine patient actively or passively horizontally abducts the arm. Forward protrusion of the medial clavicle is quite evident in the normal functioning sternoclavicular joint. Due to the restrictions of anatomy, it is impossible to em-

ploy an anteriorly directed force directly. The force then must come from the posterior movement of the lateral clavicle causing the coupled anterior movement of the medial end.

With the patient seated or supine, the examiner places the thenar pads over the crook of the middle third of the clavicle. Drawing the shoulders of the patient back with the forearms, the examiner imparts a thrust at end range flaring the medial clavicles forward (Fig. 19-9).

Acromioclavicular Joint

Movement at the acromioclavicular joint is less appreciable than at the sternoclavicular joint. First, the joint space becomes obscured often when the patient elevates the arm due to the contraction of the overlying deltoid. Second, movement is probably more discernible at the lateral end of the clavicle than at the joint itself. Movement is essentially fixed in that lateral clavicular and scapula movement occur more in concert than with one remaining fixed as the other moves upon it. The following is a suggestion of possible combined

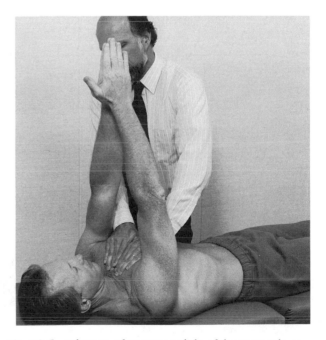

Fig. 19-5. Palpation of posterior glide of the sternoclavicular joint.

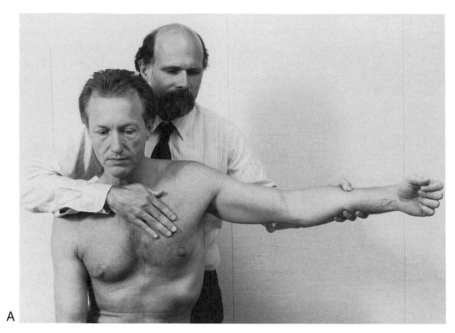

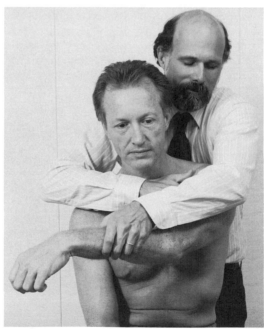

Fig. 19-6. (A & B) Passive correction of posterior glide restriction with horizontal adduction.

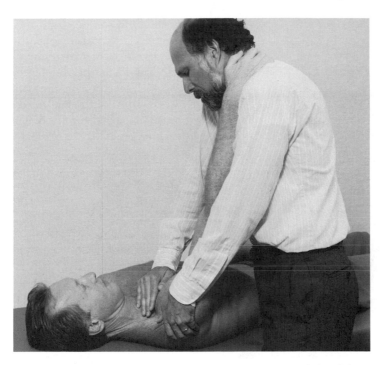

Fig. 19-7. Muscle energy technique for correction of restriction to posterior glide of the sternoclavicular joint.

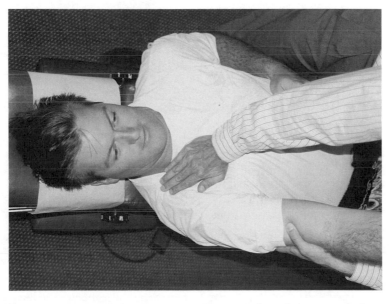

Fig. 19-8. Correction of posterior glide restriction at the sternoclavicular joint with drop-table technique.

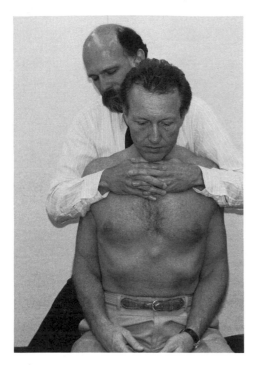

Fig. 19-9. Indirect correction of anterior glide at the sterno-clavicular joint with flaring of the shoulders.

movement patterns that correlate with specific accessory movements. Keep in mind that the acromial movement restriction could be due exclusively to a dysfunctional scapula mechanism. This may be entirely muscular in etiology. Correction is then targeted toward this end.

1. Superior glide—accompanies abduction
2. Inferior glide—accompanies adduction
3. Anterior glide—accompanies the coupled movement of flexion/abduction
4. Posterior glide—accompanies the coupled movement of extension/abduction
5. Combinations of the above movements occur with internal/external rotation. For example, internal rotation with the arm abducted allows palpation of anterior rotation with a component of superior accessory motion. These motions are more easily palpated at the lateral end of the clavicle.

Given that the most palpable movements are internal and external rotation, it is advisable to simply add a more static approach for the other movements. If the

patient lies supine, the overlying musculature is more relaxed. A distraction and compressive maneuver may be accomplished by pulling the clavicle and spine of the scapula in opposite directions in an attempt to discern a normal springy sensation. Compression may relieve pain in chronic instability (separation) of the acromioclavicular joint or irritate it with an acute separation or with osteoarthritis.

Due to the fact that the movements that accompany internal and external rotation are rotational, and given that adjustive thrusts are essentially uniplanar in corrective force, correction must be through indirect methods such as muscle energy techniques. With the patient seated, the examiner stands behind and controls the arm at the elbow. The arm is elevated to 90 degrees of abduction in the scapular plane (30 degrees horizontal adduction). Internal or external rotation is introduced while palpating the lateral clavicle. Resistance is offered to the internal or external rotation for a few seconds followed by further motion into the restricted range (Fig. 19-10). This effect is largely muscular and probably has little direct effect on the articu-

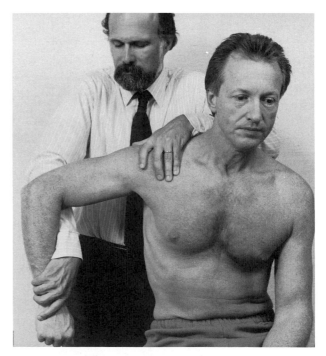

Fig. 19-10. Indirect correction of acromioclavicular joint movement through muscle energy technique applied to restrictions in internal and external rotation.

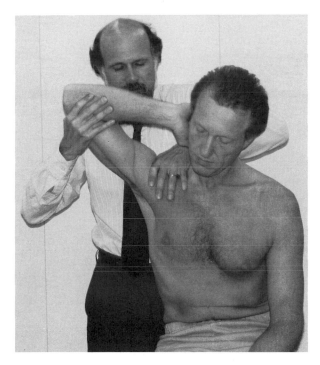

Fig. 19-11. Incorrect adjusting approach to correction of acromioclavicular joint dysfunction.

lation. It is important to remember that the rotational effect is due to the tension that develops with the costoclavicular ligaments in certain positions.

To release a restriction to the anterior-posterior capabilities of the joint, the patient is placed supine. A contact is made over the humerus bilaterally. A short quick impulse is given in an effort to leave the lateral clavicle behind. This is an attempt to free any adhesion development in the acromioclavicular joint itself.

Maneuvers that attempt to depress the lateral clavicle by placing the hand over the head as the examiner thrusts inferiorward are not recommended (Fig. 19-11). Although potentially useful in slowly resetting a second or third degree separation prior to stabilization, this maneuver offers little in terms of restoring any crucial accessory movement pattern.

Glenohumeral Joint

Most attempts at detecting accessory motion at the glenohumeral joint are performed with the arm in a relatively neutral position. Therefore, end-range move-

ment challenge is not being performed. Additionally, the concept of restoring *restricted* accessory motion by adjusting through restriction may be erroneous. From current data it seems much more likely that the restrictions are capsular and that dysfunction causing pain is due to *excessive* humeral translation as opposed to restricted translation. In general, the excessive accessory motion is opposite the side of capsular restriction. Based on these observations a different approach to listed restrictions combined with specific movement patterns is suggested:

1. Forward flexion—excessive accessory movement anteriorly occurs due to tightness or restriction palpated in the posterior capsule (posterior directed force).
2. Extension—excessive accessory movement posteriorly occurs due to tightness or restriction palpated in the anterior capsule (anterior directed force).
3. Abduction—excessive accessory movement superiorly occurs due to tightness or restriction palpated in the posterior capsule (posterior directed force).
4. Horizontal flexion—excessive accessory movement anteriorly occurs due to tightness or restriction palpated in the posterior capsule (posterior directed force).
5. Horizontal extension—excessive accessory movement occurs posteriorly due to tightness or restriction palpated in the anterior capsule (anterior directed force).

This new concept of restriction causing excessive movement does not change the palpatory findings of restriction and their correction. Correction, however, is probably more capsulo-adhesive. Although many subtle accessory movements patterns have been suggested for the glenohumeral joint, it seems likely that they represent palpation of distinct areas of capsular restriction. The primary movement restrictions to be addressed are (1) posterior, (2) anterior, (3) lateral, and (4) inferior. Combinations of these restriction patterns are possible.

Posterior Restriction

With the patient supine the examiner stabilizes the scapula with one hand placed on the posterior scapula and scapular spine while the other hand flexes the

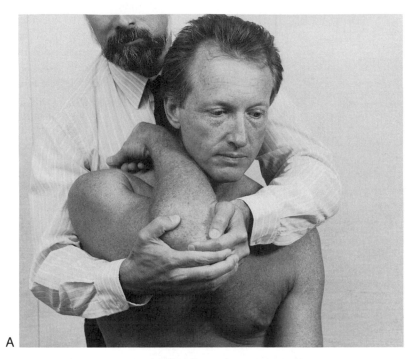

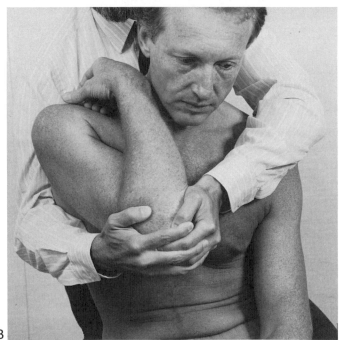

Fig. 19-12. Correction of posterior restriction at the glenohumeral joint **(A)** Direct posterior force; **(B)** slightly superior force. Care must be taken with the second approach due to the possibility of aggravating an underlying impingement.

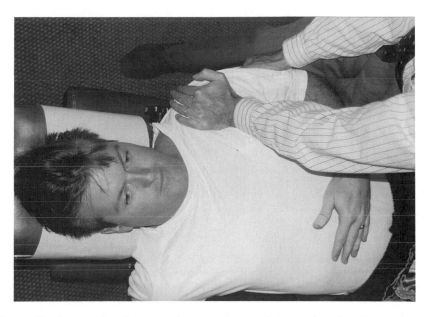

Fig. 19-13. Drop-table adjustment for posterior restriction at the glenohumeral joint.

arm at the shoulder to varying degrees. A posteriorly directed force is applied in an attempt to detect restriction. Note the similarity to the classic test for posterior instability. The difference is the detection of restriction and not laxity when addressing accessory motion. Correction may be performed supine or seated. Graded oscillations in a posterior direction can be applied for mobilization by the examiner. With a continuation into the restricted posterior direction with a short quick impulse an adjustment can be performed. In the seated position stabilization of the scapula is performed by "blocking" the scapula with the doctor's body (Fig. 19-12).

An alternative adjustment is possible on the drop-table apparatus (Fig. 19-13). With the patient lying supine, the examiner sets the thoracic section making sure that the shoulder is resting on the table. While supporting the back of the arm with one hand, the examiner directs a force posteriorly with the palm of the other hand in contact with the proximal humerus. The procedure may need to be repeated up to three times.

Home mobilization may be prescribed. The patient lies prone with body weight supported on the forearms (Fig. 19-14). By relaxing the shoulders and pushing the chest and abdomen downward, a stretch is applied to the posterior capsule. This is a passive stretch held for 30 to 60 seconds with no ballistic maneuvers allowed.

Anterior Restriction

The medial hand is brought high into the axilla with the thumb and index finger wedged superiorly and

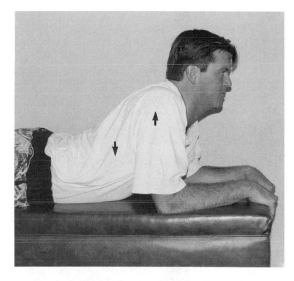

Fig. 19-14. Self-mobilization/stretch for posterior restriction.

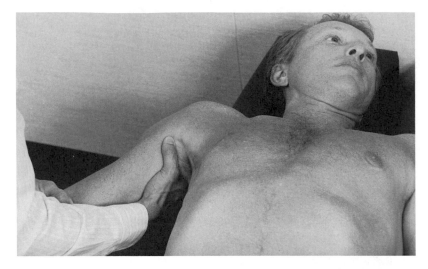

Fig. 19-15. Palpation and adjustment of anterior restriction at the glenohumeral joint.

the palm facing outward. The other examiner hand is at the flexed elbow of the patient. Downward pressure is applied at the elbow while the upper hand lifts the humerus anteriorly to take out slack (Fig. 19-15). End-range restriction is then tested with further pressure anteriorly. Restrictions are corrected by mobilization using graded oscillations. By applying a short quick impulse further anteriorly an adjustment is performed.

An alternative adjustment on the drop-table allows

positioning in a relatively neutral relaxed position (Fig. 19-16). The thoracic section is set with the patient's shoulder resting on the table. The patient lies prone while the examiner supports the arm. A thrust is directed anteriorly with the opposite hand. This maneuver may need to be repeated up to three times.

Restrictions anteriorly may also be accomplished with the arm in an abducted position using an anterior force or coupling with external rotation. A thorough

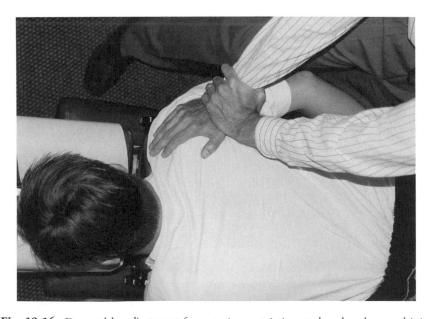

Fig. 19-16. Drop-table adjustment for anterior restriction at the glenohumeral joint.

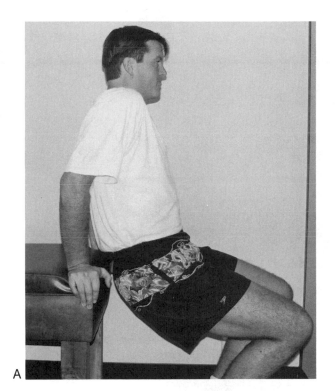

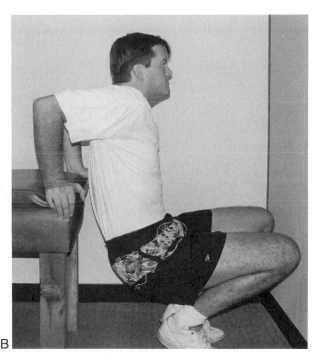

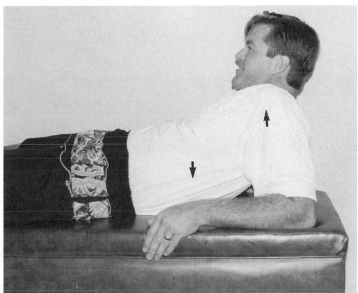

Fig. 19-17. Self-mobilization/stretch for anterior restriction. **(A & B)** Squatting method; **(C)** supine method.

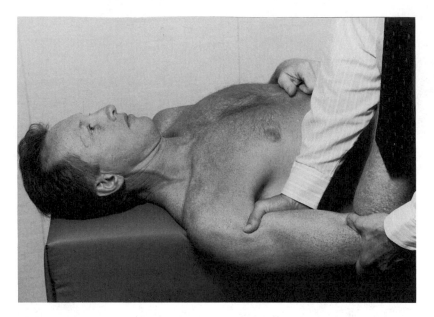

Fig. 19-18. Palpation and adjustment of lateral restriction at the glenohumeral joint.

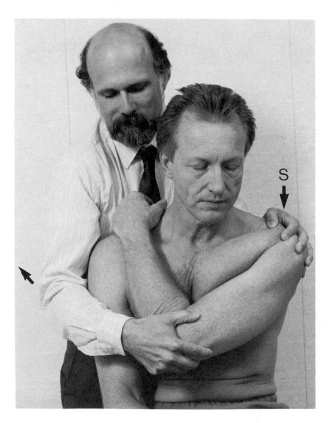

Fig. 19-19. Alternative adjustment of lateral restriction. *S*, stabilize.

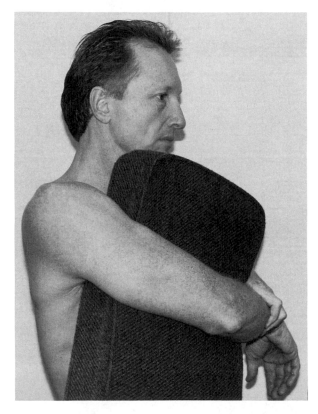

Fig. 19-20. Home stretch for lateral/posterior restriction using a pillow in the axilla with passive horizontal adduction.

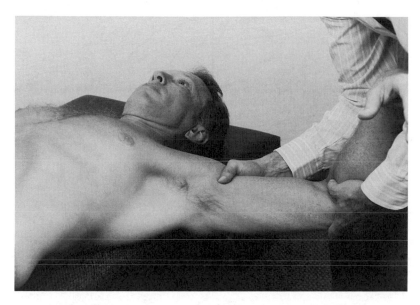

Fig. 19-21. Palpation and adjustment of inferior restriction.

examination for anterior instability and caution are needed when deciding to use these techniques. Adjusting into gross instability is contraindicated.

Home mobilization/stretching may be accomplished with several approaches. Two are demonstrated in Figure 19-17. The first method involves a squat while maintaining support on the hands. The second method involves support on the forearms in the supine position. In this latter method, the patient should relax the shoulders (as with all these maneuvers) and press the thorax down toward the table.

Lateral Restriction

The examiner places the medial hand high into the axilla cupping superiorly with the thumb and index fingers, palm facing outward. The other hand is placed over the lateral elbow. While pushing outward with the superior hand, the inferior hand offers a counterpressure toward the body (Fig. 19-18). Correction is accomplished with oscillations into the restriction or with a short impulse outward with the superior hand.

An alternative technique developed by the author is to stand behind the patient and use the patient's elbow to adduct the arm. While stabilizing the scapula with one hand and the other hand holding the patient's elbow, the doctor imparts a quick thrust into further adduction, often with an audible release (Fig. 19-19).

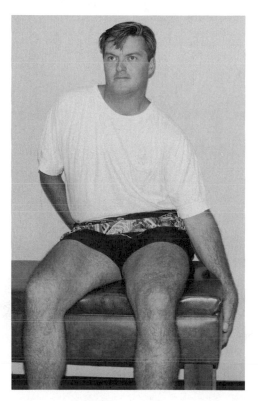

Fig. 19-22. Self-mobilization/stretch for inferior restriction performed by leaning away with the hand stabilizing the involved extremity.

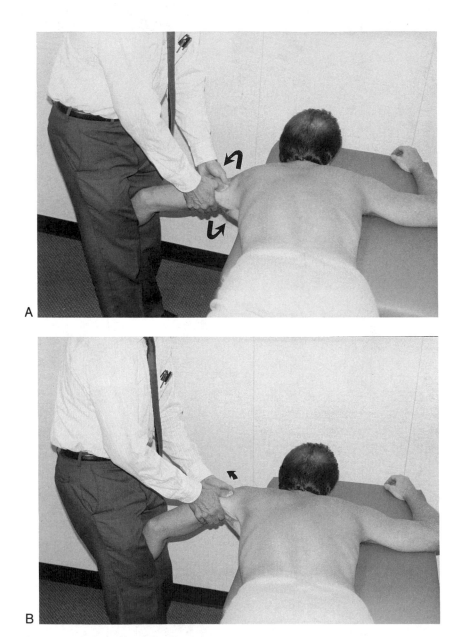

Fig. 19-23. **(A)** Circumduction of the shoulder in an attempt to locate subtle areas of restriction. **(B)** Correction is accomplished with a short quick impulse into the restriction.

A combination of lateral and posterior capsular stretching can be performed at home with a pillow placed in the axilla while the patient passively horizontally adducts the arm (Fig. 19-20).

Inferior Restriction

With the patient lying prone or supine, the examiner abducts the relaxed shoulder to about 90 degrees by lifting the bent elbow (Fig. 19-21). The other hand cups the proximal humerus between the web of the thumb and index finger and takes out the slack in an inferior direction. With a combination of abduction and inferior translation of the proximal humerus, the examiner finds the end-range restriction and either applies oscillations downward or thrusts with a short impulse inferiorly.

Self-mobilization may be accomplished by leaning away with the hand grasping under a chair or table (Fig. 19-22).

Global Approach

With the patient prone, the examiner may support the patient's elbow between the legs and use a firm grasp of the humeral head to impart a circumduction of the glenohumeral joint (Fig. 19-23). Areas of restriction can be addressed with short impulses in an attempt to break up local adhesions missed on the other testing and correcting procedures.

Scapulothoracic Joint

The various positions available to the scapula are best assessed in the prone position. While one hand pushes the shoulder posteriorly, the other examiner hand slides under the medial border of the scapula (Fig. 19-24). Restrictions due to shortened scapular musculature may be evident and can be treated in this position.

By using a circumduction maneuver, the scapula may be taken through a full range of movement possibilities in an attempt to detect restrictions. These restrictions may be treated with short impulse corrections.

A standing correction is possible by catching the inferior wing of the scapula between the web of the thumb and index finger of one hand and thrusting superiorly with a short quick impulse (Fig. 19-25).

In addition, it is important to always screen for cervical/thoracic spine and rib involvement. From either a purely mechanical perspective or perhaps a neurologic reflex perspective, these elements should always be evaluated and corrected when found.

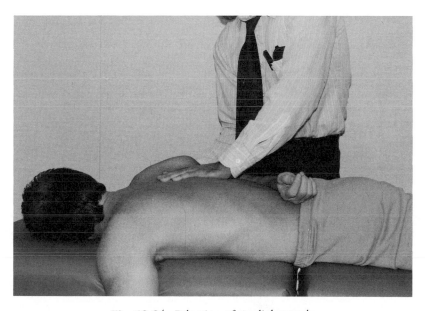

Fig. 19-24. Palpation of medial scapula.

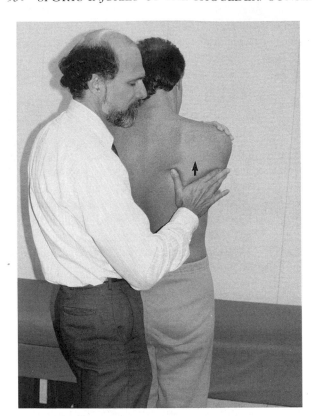

Fig. 19-25. Standing adjustment for scapula.

REFERENCES

1. Sandoz R: Some physical mechanisms and effects of spinal adjustments. Ann Swiss Chirop Assoc 6:91, 1976
2. Mennell JM: Joint Pain: Diagnosis and Treatment Using Manipulative Techniques. Little, Brown, Boston, 1964
3. Corrigan B, Maitland GD: Practical Orthopaedic Medicine. Butterworth-Heinemann, London, 1983
4. Kaltenborn FM: Mobilization of the Extremity Joints: Examination and Basic Treatment Techniques. Olaf Norlis Bokhandel, Oslo, 1980
5. Greenman PE: Principles of Manual Medicine. Williams & Wilkins, Baltimore, 1989
6. Paris SV: Extremity Dysfunction and Mobilization. Prepublication Manual, Atlanta, 1980
7. Cyriax J: Textbook of Orthopaedic Medicine. Balliere-Tindall, London, 1982
8. Schafer RC, Faye LJ: Motion Palpation and Chiropractic Technique: Principles of Dynamic Chiropractic. Motion Palpation Institute, 1989
9. Harryman DT, Sidles JA, Clark JM et al: Translation of the humeral head on the glenoid with passive glenohumeral motion. J Bone Joint Surg 72A:1334, 1990
10. Howell SM, Galinat BJ, Renzi AJ, Marone PJ: Normal and abnormal mechanics of the glenohumeral joint in the horizontal plane. J Bone Joint Surg 70A:227, 1988
11. Greenman PE: Principles of Manual Medicine. Williams & Wilkins, Philadelphia, 1990
12. Subotnick SI (ed): Sports Medicine of the Lower Extremity. Churchill Livingstone, New York, 1988

20

Rehabilitation and Prevention

THOMAS A. SOUZA

The design of a rehabilitation or prevention program has been largely based on empirical observation combined with current trends or tendencies in weight training. Unsupported by objective data, physicians, coaches, and trainers have had to devise a logical program that anecdotally met the needs of the specific sports activity the athlete was involved in. Recently, there has been a significant contribution of electromyographic data on specific exercises for specific muscles. Much of this data have been generated by the Biomechanics Laboratory at Inglewood, California, through the efforts of Townsend and colleagues.[1] Now it is possible to include some firm information to the database used for exercise prescription. What is noteworthy about these studies is that they contradict many of the accepted tenets of muscle activity. For example, it is assumed that if a muscle is at an optimal length and in a biomechanically advantageous position, its muscle activity will necessarily be more than other muscles that are less favorably positioned. This is not necessarily so because recruitment of muscular activity is not primarily a mechanical event. Also the possibility of eccentric activity of an antagonist exceeding the concentric activity of the agonist for a given movement was largely ignored or denied yet actions of many muscles (the subscapularis in particular) demonstrate the need for inclusion of this consideration.[2]

When devising a rehabilitative or preventative program for a given athlete it is essential to include the following information into the database before making decisions as to the appropriateness of a given exercise:

1. What are the requirements of the given sport or sports in which the athlete participates?
   a. What are the required (redundant) positions used to accomplish the sport?
   b. At what speed are these movements performed and for how long?
   c. What are the positions of risk that need to be supported?
   d. What cross body positions are needed? (coordination)
2. What is the level of participation and motivation of the athlete?
3. What is the biomechanical, physiologic, and psychological status of the athlete?

It is necessary to integrate current knowledge regarding training with the answers to these questions. The program should include the corresponding exercises that will challenge the specific muscles at a sufficient intensity and at the same time not risk irritation of an underlying disorder.

ELECTROMYOGRAPHIC DATA FOR SPECIFIC MUSCLES

A review of current understanding regarding exercise of the muscles of the shoulder complex is presented with an emphasis on those exercises that stimulate the greatest number of pertinent musculature. Emphasis is placed on safety considerations regarding risk to benefit ratio. In other words, although a particular position may be maximally stimulating for a particular muscle or group of muscles it may involve the danger of impingement or instability. Most of the studies used free weights or elastic tubing testing and isometric contractions. Therefore, transference of information to isokinetic or other mechanisms or approaches such as proprioceptive neuromuscular facilitation (PNF) may not be directly applied (although it is likely they are similar). Neither maximum weight nor speed of movement was included as a tested variable. The muscles are divided into groups and then discussed individually.

Rotator Cuff

Supraspinatus

Activity of the supraspinatus and other shoulder muscles was electromyographically evaluated by Townsend et al.[1] Activity of the supraspinatus was generally as expected. Peak activity was found to occur during the three positions of elevation: (1) abduction, (2) scaption (elevation in the scapular plane) especially with internal rotation, and (3) flexion. This activity was highest at the upper levels in the arc of 120 to 180 degrees (Table 20-1). The high activity with scaption/internal rotation agrees with the findings of Jobe and Moynes.[3] Interestingly peak activity was greatest with the military press in the beginning arc range of 0 to 30 degrees. The caution of performing scaption or abduction above 90 degrees in relationship to possible impingement can be avoided by the use of the first 30 degree arc of the military press. However, performing scaption or abduction below 90 degrees with a heavier weight can compensate for the difference and at the same time avoid the need to add the military press as one of the core exercises since flexion and scaption serve as maximal stimulators for many muscles.

A study by Blackburn et al.[4] suggests that supraspinatus activity can be activated by a prone exercise with horizontal abduction/external rotation. This position mimics the cocking phase of pitching and is used for stimulation of all rotator cuff musculature. Blackburn et al.[4] and a recent study by Worrell et al.[5] suggest that performing prone horizontal abduction with the arm positioned at 100 degrees abduction and externally rotated, elbow extended, is a maximum stimulator of the supraspinatus. The study by Worrell et al.[5] suggests that more electromyographic activity occurs in this position than with the standing scaption movement suggested by Jobe and Moynes.[3] The difference with the study by Worrell et al.[5] is that the subjects were asked to perform maximum isometric contractions.

Subscapularis

Although the subscapularis is primarily an internal rotator by design, it contracts maximally only when internal rotation is combined with abduction in the scapular plane (scaption) (Table 20-1). More importantly, the subscapularis demonstrates significant activity with external rotation eccentrically. Belle and Hawkins[2] found that the subscapularis fired both with external rotation/abduction and external rotation in neutral, significantly more than the infraspinatus. Another position of maximal stimulation was the push-up demonstrating significantly more activity than the serratus anterior.

Infraspinatus

The infraspinatus serves as the major external rotator of the shoulder. In addition, it serves a stabilizing role. This becomes evident with the substantial activity demonstrated on a number of exercises as listed in Table 20-1 including elevation in the frontal, sagittal, and scapular planes. Activity during these various phases of elevation suggests a coupling role with the deltoid.

The primary exercises exhibiting maximum activity were external rotation and external rotation/horizontal abduction. Similar results were obtained by Blackburn et al.[4] and Belle and Hawkins.[2] However, Blackburn et al.[4] found the most effective position to be prone demonstrating significantly more activity than in the standing position. All attempts at horizontal abduction demonstrated increased infraspinatus activity. Belle and Hawkins[2] found that a push-up with the arms away from the body (abducted) demonstrated significant infraspinatus activity. Finally, Pappas et al.[6] used a side-lying position with the bottom arm hanging off the table. The athlete then attempted external rotation from this position.

Teres Minor

In general, the teres minor acts in concert with the infraspinatus. Therefore, external rotation and external rotation/horizontal abduction were the top qualifiers (Table 20-1). However, Blackburn et al.[4] demonstrated isolation of the teres minor with the patient prone extending the externally rotated arm.

Deltoids

The deltoids, in particular the anterior and middle sections, are incorporated in most movements involving elevation in any plane. The leading exercises for the anterior deltoid were scaption with internal rotation,

Table 20-1. Qualifying Exercises for Each Muscle[a]

Muscle	Exercise	Peak (% MMT ± SD)	Duration (% Exercise)	Peak Arc Range (Degree)
Anterior deltoid	Scaption internal rotation	72 ± 23	50	90–150
	Scaption external rotation	71 ± 39	30	90–120
	Flexion	69 ± 24	31	90–120
	Military press	62 ± 26	50	60–90
	Abduction	62 ± 28	31	90–120
Middle deltoid	Scaption internal rotation	83 ± 13	70	90–120
	Horizontal abduction internal rotation	80 ± 23	38	90–120
	Horizontal abduction external rotation	79 ± 20	57	90–120
	Flexion	73 ± 16	31	90–120
	Scaption external rotation	72 ± 13	58	90–120
	Rowing	72 ± 20	43	90–120
	Military press	72 ± 24	38	90–120
	Abduction	64 ± 13	31	90–120
	Deceleration	58 ± 20	27	90–60
Posterior deltoid	Horizontal abduction internal rotation	93 ± 45	63	90–120
	Horizontal abduction external rotation	92 ± 49	57	90–120
	Rowing	88 ± 40	57	90–120
	Extension	71 ± 30	44	90–120
	External rotation	64 ± 62	43	60–90
	Deceleration	63 ± 28	27	60–90
Supraspinatus	Military press	80 ± 48	50	0–30
	Scaption internal rotation	74 ± 33	40	90–120
	Flexion	67 ± 14	31	90–120
	Scaption external rotation	64 ± 28	25	90–120
Subscapularis	Scaption internal rotation[b]	62 ± 33	22	120–150
	Military press[c]	56 ± 48	50	60–90
	Flexion[c]	52 ± 42	23	120–150
	Abduction[c]	50 ± 44	23	120–150
Infraspinatus	Horizontal abduction external rotation	88 ± 25	71	90–120
	External rotation	85 ± 26	43	60–90
	Horizontal abduction internal rotation	74 ± 32	38	90–120
	Abduction	74 ± 23	31	90–120
	Flexion	66 ± 15	23	90–120
	Scaption external rotation	60 ± 21	38	90–120
	Deceleration	57 ± 17	27	90–60
	Push-up (hands together)	54 ± 31	38	90–60
Teres minor	External rotation	80 ± 14	57	60–90
	Horizontal abduction external rotation	74 ± 28	57	60–90
	Horizontal abduction internal rotation	68 ± 36	43	90–120
Pectoralis major	Press-up	84 ± 42	75	½ peak–peak
	Push-up (hands apart)	64 ± 63	50	60–30
Latissimus dorsi	Press-up	55 ± 27	50	Peak—1 s

Abbreviation: MMT, manual muscle test.
[a] Ranked by intensity of peak arc.
[b] Criterion: two arcs greater than 50% MMT.
[c] Criterion: three arcs greater than 40% MMT.
(From Townsend et al,[1] with permission).

scaption with external rotation, and flexion. Most of the maximum activity occurred in the higher arcs of motion. Other exercises that qualified were the military press and abduction (Table 20-1).

The middle deltoid had similar findings with peak activity using scaption in internal rotation. Other top

exercises included horizontal abduction in internal and external rotation and the military press. Slightly lower in activity, yet still substantial, were scaption in external rotation, prone rowing, the military press, abduction, and deceleration.

The posterior deltoid showed significant activity

with horizontal abduction coupled with either internal or external rotation. Rowing was third followed by external rotation and deceleration.

Latissimus Dorsi

The press-up was the only exercise in the Townsend et al.[1] study that qualified for maximum stimulation. This would correlate with the generally accepted function of the latissimus dorsi with strenuous adduction of the arm.

Belle and Hawkins[2] noted an interesting recruitment of the latissimus dorsi on external rotation in the abducted position. Perhaps this again indicates the possibility of eccentric contraction at previously unrecognized levels.

Pectoralis Major

The two exercises that met contraction criteria for the pectoralis major were the press-up and the push-up with the hands apart. Horizontal adduction and the bench press did not meet the qualifying criteria. However, the press-up and push-up lift near full body weight whereas the latter exercises incorporated (at least in the testing environment) a small amount of weight.

Scapular Muscles

A similar study was performed by Moseley et al.[7] on the scapular musculature using the same exercises as in the previous study. Findings are described for each muscle (Tables 20-2 and 20-3).

Serratus Anterior

The middle and lower serratus anterior exhibited some possible subtle differences in function based on arc of contraction and specific movements incorporated. The middle serratus was active in a number of exercises. The top three were flexion, abduction, and scaption in that order. Most of the peak activity was in the higher elevations of 120 to 150 degrees. Other exercises with significant activity included the military press and both types of push-ups.

The lower serratus demonstrated similar incorporation with a different hierarchy. Although the top three exercises were the same, the sequence was different.

Scaption, abduction, and flexion was the order of ranking. Other qualifiers included both push-ups and the military press. It was interesting to note that peak activity for the push-up with a plus was as the chest rose away from the floor. The peak activity with the push-up/hands apart was during the isometric contraction with the chest close to the floor.

Rhomboids

The rhomboids were most active with several exercises: horizontal abduction in neutral, scaption, abduction, and prone rowing. All of these demonstrated peak activity in the extreme of the arc of motion.

Levator Scapulae

The levator scapulae is active with many exercises. Activity peaked during the isometric phase of each. There were six qualifiers including rowing, horizontal abduction in neutral, the shrug, horizontal abduction with external rotation, and extension. Scaption demonstrated some activity with a peak between 120 to 150 degrees of elevation.

Pectoralis Minor

The press-up was the only exercise that qualified for the pectoralis minor. With altered criteria, the two push-ups demonstrated enough activity to qualify.[7]

Trapezius

There were some interesting results with regard to prone rowing. It would seem likely that rowing would have more influence on the middle trapezius, but actually the upper trapezius seems more stimulated. An important point is that the rowing exercise used was performed prone and is more analogous to a bent-over row used primarily as a latissimus dorsi exercise. Also, all three sections of the trapezius were called into play for horizontal abduction maneuvers with some specific modification for each section.

Upper Trapezius

Individually, the upper trapezius was activated most with prone rowing, mainly with an isometric contraction held at the end range of the concentric contraction. The military press also was a maximal stimulator

Table 20-2. Qualifying Exercises for Each Muscle (Ranked by Intensity of Peak Arc)

Muscle	Exercise	Duration Qualified (% of Exercise)	Peak Arc (% MMT ± SD)	Peak Arc Range
Upper trapezius	Rowing	75	112 ± 84	Isometric[a]
	Military press	27	64 ± 26	150–peak
	Horizontal abduction with external rotation[b]	33	75 ± 27	Isometric[a]
	Horizontal abduction (neutral)[b]	33	62 ± 53	90–peak
	Scaption[b]	23	54 ± 16	120–150
	Abduction[b]	31	52 ± 30	90–120
Middle trapezius	Horizontal abduction (neutral)	78	108 ± 63	90–peak
	Horizontal abduction with external rotation	67	96 ± 73	Peak–90
	Extension (prone)	27	77 ± 49	Neutral–30
	Rowing	33	59 ± 51	90–120
Lower trapezius	Abduction	50	68 ± 53	90–150[c]
	Rowing	50	67 ± 50	120–150
	Horizontal abduction with external rotation	33	63 ± 41	90–peak
	Flexion	23	60 ± 18	120–150
	Horizontal abduction (neutral)	33	56 ± 24	90–peak
	Scaption[d]	23	60 ± 22	120–150
Levator scapulae	Rowing	78	114 ± 69	Isometric[a]
	Horizontal abduction (neutral)	67	96 ± 57	Isometric[a]
	Shrug	63	88 ± 32	Isometric[a]
	Horizontal abduction with external rotation	33	87 ± 66	Isometric[a]
	Extension (prone)	36	81 ± 76	Isometric[a]
	Scaption	46	69 ± 46	120–150
Rhomboids	Horizontal abduction (neutral)	33	66 ± 38	90–peak
	Scaption	25	65 ± 79	120–150[c]
	Abduction	31	64 ± 53	90–150
	Rowing	30	56 ± 46	Isometric[a]
Middle serratus anterior	Flexion[e]	69	96 ± 45	120–150
	Abduction[e]	54	96 ± 53	120–150
	Scaption	58	91 ± 52	120–150
	Military press	64	82 ± 36	150–peak
	Push-up with a plus	28	80 ± 38	Plus maneuver
	Push-up hands apart	21	57 ± 36	Last arc of push-up
Lower serratus anterior	Scaption	50	84 ± 20	120–150
	Abduction	54	74 ± 65	120–150
	Flexion[e]	31	72 ± 46	120–150
	Push-up with a plus[e]	67	72 ± 3	Chest moving away from floor
	Push-up hands apart	21	69 ± 31	Isometric as the chest was near the floor
	Military press	36	60 ± 42	120–150
Pectoralis minor	Press-up	75	89 ± 62	Isometric[a]
	Push-up with a plus	34	58 ± 45	Plus maneuver
	Push-up with hands apart	50	55 ± 34	Second to last arc of push-up

Abbreviation: MMT, manual muscle test.
[a] Isometric contractions were at the extreme of the range of motion.
[b] One or two of the consecutive arcs was between 40 and 50% MMT.
[c] Identical % MMT over two consecutive arcs for peak activity.
[d] One of the consecutive arcs was 49% MMT.
[e] Two exercises tied for the same ranking position.
(From Moseley et al,[7] with permission.)

Table 20-3. Muscle Function for the Qualifying Exercises

Muscle	Exercise	Function
Upper trapezius	Rowing	Retraction
	Military press	Upward rotation
	Horizontal abduction with external rotation	Retraction
	Horizontal abduction (neutral)	Retraction
	Scaption	Upward rotation
	Abduction	Upward rotation
Middle trapezius	Horizontal abduction (neutral)	
	Horizontal abduction with external rotation	Retraction
	Extension (prone)	
	Rowing	
Lower trapezius	Abduction	Upward rotation
	Rowing	Retraction
	Horizontal abduction with external rotation	Retraction
	Flexion	Upward rotation
	Horizontal abduction (neutral)	Retraction
	Scaption	Upward rotation
Levator scapulae	Rowing	Retraction
	Horizontal abduction (neutral)	Retraction
	Shrug	Elevation
	Horizontal abduction with external rotation	Retraction
	Extension (prone)	Elevation
	Scaption	Retraction
Rhomboids	Horizontal abduction (neutral)	
	Scaption	Retraction
	Abduction	
	Rowing	
Middle serratus anterior	Flexion	Upward rotation and protraction
	Abduction	
	Scaption	
	Military press	
	Push-up with a plus	
	Push-up with hands apart	
Lower serratus anterior	Scaption	Upward rotation and protraction
	Abduction	
	Flexion	
	Push-up with a plus	
	Push-up with hands apart	
	Military press	
Pectoralis minor	Press-up	Depression
	Push-up with a plus	Protraction
	Push-up with hands apart	Protraction

(From Moseley et al,[7] with permission.)

with peak activity with the last arc of concentric contraction. Finally, horizontal abduction in neutral and external rotation, scaption, and abduction were moderately stimulating for the upper trapezius.

Middle Trapezius

The middle trapezius was activated by horizontal abduction in neutral peaking in the last concentric arc and horizontal abduction with external rotation peaking in the first eccentric arc. Extension qualified with peak activity between neutral and 30 degrees of hyperextension. Finally, rowing qualified peaking between 90 and 120 degrees.

Lower Trapezius

The lower trapezius, as would be expected, is activated by positions with the arm elevated. Abduction, prone rowing, horizontal abduction with external rotation, flexion, and horizontal abduction in neutral were effective stimulators. The peak activity for abduction was above 90 degrees; for rowing and flexion peaking occurred at 120 degrees and above.

Summary

By integrating the current electromyographic evidence a general program including six exercises can be recommended. This rehabilitative or preventative program should maximally stimulate all of the glenohumeral and scapular musculature. For glenohumeral muscle strengthening the following exercises are suggested (Fig. 20-1):

1. Scaption
2. Flexion
3. Horizontal abduction with external rotation (prone)
4. Press-up

For scapular muscle strengthening there is an overlap of optimal exercises that include scaption and the press-up. In addition, two more exercises are included (Fig. 20-2):

5. Bent-over rowing
6. Push-ups with a plus

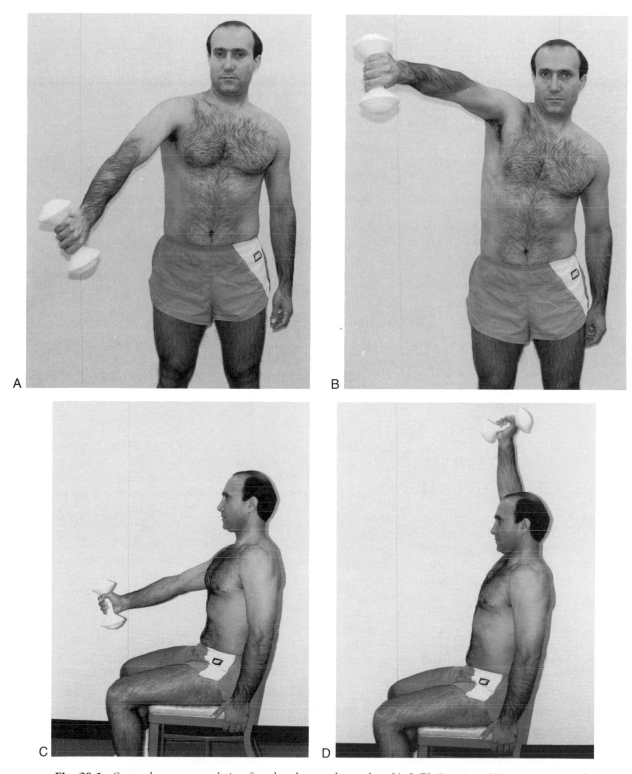

Fig. 20-1. General recommendation for glenohumeral muscles. **(A & B)** Scaption, (*Figure continues.*)

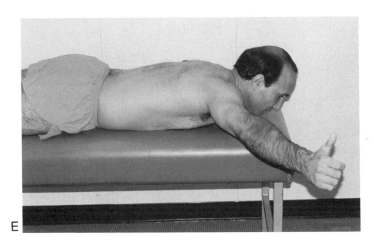
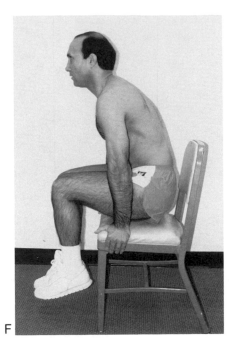

Fig. 20-1. (*Continued*). **(C & D)** flexion, **(E)** horizontal abduction with external rotation, **(F)** the press-up.

To prevent impingement, scaption should be performed shy of 90 degrees or substituted with flexion.

SPECIFIC REQUIREMENTS

Emphasis or modification of a generalized program is necessary based on the athlete's sport, the level of skill, age, and underlying pathology. Recent evidence regarding these aspects has been generated for a variety of specific sports. Distinctions between amateur and professionals,[8] normal and unstable shoulders,[9] and patients with impingement[10] have been studied in regard to altered muscle patterns of usage. This information can be applied with regard to an individual's needs. Following is a discussion of some individual sports.

Throwing

Although pitching is the specific activity most studied, some of the information is probably transferable to many of the throwing sports. Interesting conflicts have arisen between earlier findings by Inman et al,[11] in particular the description of the "force couple" between the deltoid and supraspinatus (and other rotator cuff muscles). In the nonthrower, the force couple may occur where a synergy exists between the two groups of muscles. Electromyographic evidence suggests more a sequence in the professional rather than equal synergy.[12] The deltoid positions the arm for early cocking whereas during late cocking the rotator cuff assumes dominance. This probably is the result of specific stabilization and positioning needs for the throwing act to follow.

Biceps activity in the normal shoulder probably functions more at the elbow. However, in the amateur pitcher both the biceps and rotator cuff are incorporated during the acceleration phase of pitching; this is a pattern not seen in the professional. Additionally, biceps activity increases in athletes with unstable shoulders. It appears to serve a function of stabilization compensating for the lack of capsular integrity.

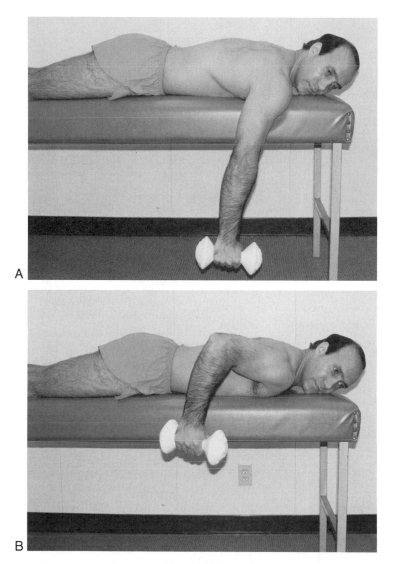

Fig. 20-2. General recommendation for scapular muscles include those in Fig. 20-1 plus: **(A & B)** bent-over row, (*Figure continues.*)

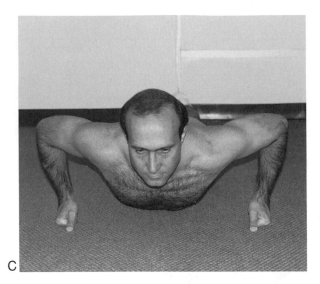
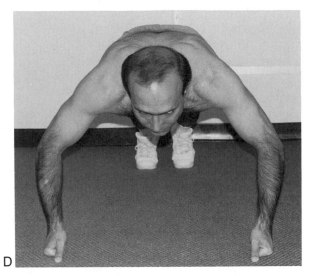

Fig. 20-2. (*Continued*). **(C & D)** push-up with a plus.

Rotator Cuff

The supraspinatus peaks in activity during late cocking. Therefore, it is not the essential initiator of abduction once believed. This peak activity in late cocking is decreased in the pitcher with impingement[10] and increased in the pitcher with instability.[9] Supraspinatus activity is increased in the amateur during the acceleration phase and decreased in the professional.[8] The professionals were apparently able to reduce the need for supraspinatus activity through timing and synchrony of the lower extremity contribution to the throwing act.

Generally the external rotators/abductors of the shoulder are weaker than the internal rotators/adductors. This is partially developmental. Neurologic inhibition can also occur due to contracture of the anterior musculature. In pitching and other throwing actions, it is requisite to have an almost abnormal degree of external rotation dependent on flexibility of the anterior structures and strength of the posterior musculature.

The teres minor and infraspinatus perform three functions dependent on the phase of pitching. First, they act to externally rotate the arm during the cocking phase. Second, they help stabilize the humerus in the late cocking phase. Third, they assist deceleration during the acceleration phase eccentrically. Generally, firing of the infraspinatus/teres minor was slightly later than the supraspinatus.

The subscapularis performs its peak activity eccentrically during late cocking, preventing excessive anterior shear forces on the humerus. Strong activity is also found concentrically during acceleration as the subscapularis functions as an internal rotator.

Interestingly, specific use of the rotator cuff is possible by the professional pitcher due to selective firing and contributions to force production through synchrony and timing of the lower body contribution. It has been demonstrated that over half of the force contribution is from the lower body in pitching.[13] Amateurs, on the other hand, seem to use the rotator cuff throughout the pitching act.[8]

Internal Rotators

The pectoralis major and latissimus dorsi act concentrically as strong internal rotators during the acceleration phase of pitching.[14] Also, they serve a protective role during late cocking by firing eccentrically with the subscapularis. This causes a prestretch prior to firing concentrically during acceleration. This plyometric action is essential for a powerful delivery.

Both impingement and instability apparently decrease activity of the pectoralis major and latissimus dorsi.[9,10] This could potentially allow anterior translation and superior migration during cocking leading to impingement. With instability, this could mean a further increase in shearing forces anteriorly increasing the laxity already present.

Scapular Rotators

Although the deltoid and supraspinatus were emphasized as the primary focus for arm elevation, it appears that the serratus anterior plays a significant role. Elevation up to 90 degrees caused about a 41 percent contraction.[7] Full elevation requires a 66 percent contraction. During pitching there is a short period when serratus activity exceeded 100 percent. Trapezius activity is lower than the serratus even though they are of equal size. The midtrapezius activity does increase during follow-through indicating a function of scapular protraction deceleration. The generalized decreased activity of the trapezius causes the serratus to perform at maximum levels.

Decreased activity is noted with both impingement and instability. The inability of the serratus to provide a stable platform for the humerus during the late cocking and acceleration phases will allow anterior and possibly superior migration of the humeral head, further stressing the anterior structures; shearing occurs during late cocking and acceleration, compression of subacromial structures during acceleration primarily.

The importance of serratus anterior specific exercise cannot be overemphasized. The apparent reflex inhibition found with instability and impingement may be intended as a protective mechanism; however, this only serves to further complicate the already existing pathology.

Integration of Electromyographic Information

The electromyographic data suggest several points of emphasis when dealing with a problem-free amateur or professional pitcher (and possibly for other throwing activities), or those compromised by instability or impingement (Table 20-4):

1. Given that most muscles contribute to the throwing act both concentrically and eccentrically, it would seem important to train for both functions accordingly for all participants. Training for the cocking

Table 20-4. Suggested General Approach to Training of Throwers

Eccentric training of posterior muscles for acceleration phase
Concentric training of posterior muscles for cocking phase
Eccentric training of anterior muscles for cocking phase
Concentric training of anterior muscles for acceleration phase
Eccentric training of biceps for cocking phase (in amateurs and those with instability) and for the deceleration of the elbow during the acceleration phase
Stretching of the posterior capsule
Concentric endurance/speed training of the serratus anterior for proper glenoid positioning
Focus on horizontal abduction/external rotation exercises (simulating the cocking position)

phase for the posterior musculature should be concentric focus; eccentric training would help support function during the acceleration phase. The opposite is true for the anterior musculature.

2. Given that the rotator cuff is used throughout most of the throwing phases, it would seem likely that early fatigue and consequent overuse would be the result. Due to the inability of amateurs to selectively activate the rotator cuff, they should train all the rotator cuff while continuing to develop synchrony between the lower and upper extremities with increasing focus on the subscapularis.

3. The biceps may be at risk, especially during acceleration, with the amateur and unstable pitcher. Emphasis should be placed on proper conditioning with emphasis on eccentric loading exercises due to its function during acceleration to decelerate the elbow.

4. Whether the decrease in activity of the pectoralis major and latissimus dorsi found with impingement is causative or reactionary, it would seem important to emphasize, in particular, the concentric function of these muscles. Tightness of the posterior capsule and musculature can neurologically inhibit the internal rotators even further. Stretching of the posterior capsule and muscles prior to strengthening can be helpful.

5. Serratus anterior function is paramount for proper positioning and the timing of the positioning of the humeral head during acceleration. Training concentrically is necessary to guarantee stamina for this controller of the movable scapular platform.

6. Due to the natural and sometimes acquired imbalance between the external rotators/abductors and

the internal rotators/adductors, it is necessary to emphasize horizontal abduction/external rotation exercises. This position simulates the cocking phase of pitching or throwing and is a primary ingredient in the successful contribution of the upper extremity to efficient throwing. This position has also been found to stimulate most of the rotator cuff musculature.[4]

Swimming

In addition to the exercise electromyographic data presented above, electromyographic analysis of swimmers with and without pain has been performed.[15,16] In the following discussion, emphasis is placed on the freestyle stroke, which if not used as the main competition stroke, is the most commonly used stroke during training. Added to this data are observations on flexibility and weight training to more effectively develop an approach to rehabilitative or preventative programs.

Deltoids

There are two peaks of activity for the deltoids. The first is at the end of pull-through where there is a sequential recruitment of each head. Starting with the posterior deltoid, the middle fires next, followed by the anterior head. The second peak is during hand entry. Peak activity is mainly in the anterior and middle heads with peak activity about 20 percent lower than at the end of pull-through. Activity through recovery drops dramatically.[15]

Electromyographic evaluation of the painful shoulder demonstrated marked reduction in activity of the anterior and middle deltoids during both periods of peak activity found in the nonpainful group.[16] Posterior deltoid activity did not differ significantly between the two groups. The decrease in the anterior and middle deltoid activity correlated well with the observation of a dropped elbow position. At hand entry the hand entered farther laterally and with a lower humerus. This is also commonly seen in fatigued swimmers. This positioning may be an attempt to avoid the classic impingement position of flexion with internal rotation.

Rotator Cuff

Each of the rotator cuff muscles appear to serve a specific role with the swimming act. Again, comparisons

between painful and nonpainful shoulders reveal some specific changes in pattern activity emphasizing that the rotator cuff does not act as a group. In other words, a decrease in one rotator cuff muscle is not necessarily accompanied by a reduction or increase in another.

The supraspinatus seems to aid the anterior and middle deltoids with similar peak activity during late pull-through and hand entry. Interestingly, the activity between the painful and nonpainful group was not significant.

The infraspinatus and teres minor, often grouped together as one functional unit, appear to have different roles. Peak activity of the teres minor was during middle pull-through, whereas peak activity of the infraspinatus was at midrecovery. Although the teres minor demonstrated no significant changes between groups, the infraspinatus demonstrated a significant increase in activity at the end of pull-through in the painful group. Apparently, this increase in activity was an attempt to avoid the impingement position of internal rotation found with the normal action at hand exit. The result of this increased activity of the infraspinatus visually is the dropped elbow recovery.

The subscapularis peaked during late pull-through and early recovery. However, it maintained a relatively consistent activity pattern throughout the stroke with a range between 26 and 71 percent maximum activity.[15] The most significant change in activity for the subscapularis with the painful shoulder was a decrease in activity during midrecovery. This decrease in activity may be yet another selective inhibition to decrease the tendency for impingement, which can occur with the internal rotation caused by subscapularis activity.

Internal Rotators/Extensors

Activity of the pectoralis major and latissimus dorsi are similar in both the painful and nonpainful shoulders. Peak activity occurs during pull-through with a sequential peak in firing of first the pectoralis and then the latissimus dorsi.

Scapular Rotators

The paired muscles for scapular rotation are the rhomboids and the upper trapezius, with both demonstrating peak activity during hand entry and then again at hand exit. Upper trapezius activity peaked slightly before the rhomboids at hand exit (early recovery). Activity was decreased in both muscles at hand entry in painful shoulders. There was an early peak of activity during mid pull-through in the painful group. There are two possible explanations. One is that the rhomboids are attempting to replace a concomitant decrease in serratus activity and prevent impingement. The second explanation is that in an attempt to avoid the impingement position, the rhomboids fire early to accomplish an early recovery (hand exit).

Serratus anterior activity is constant throughout the stroke cycle (somewhere between 20 and 40 percent).[15] Two peaks occurred, one during mid pull-through, the other at hand exit. Most significant was the generally lower activity of the serratus anterior in the painful shoulder.[16] In particular, during the propulsive phase of pull-through, the activity of the serratus anterior was greatly diminished with no real peak in activity. This may lead to a high risk position of impingement loss of the normal protraction of the scapula accomplished by the serratus anterior. Secondly, the power created by the reversal of origin and insertion of the serratus allowing the body to be pulled over the arms is substantially reduced. This same pattern of decreased activity is likely in the fatigued or untrained shoulder.

Integration of Electromyographic Information

The most striking features of the electromyographic analysis data are that the serratus anterior and subscapularis are prone to fatigue given their required attendance throughout the swimming stroke and that although deltoid activity decreases in the painful shoulder, supraspinatus activity remains relatively constant. The following are suggestions for exercise prescription based on all of the above findings (Table 20-5):

Table 20-5. Suggested General Approach to Training of Swimmers

High speed endurance training for the subscapularis and serratus anterior

Concentric focus on posterior musculature (prone horizontal abduction/external rotation)

Rotator cuff training

Simulated exercise with proprioceptive neuromuscular facilitation diagonal patterns or swim bench

1. Specific attention should be placed on training and endurance of the subscapularis and serratus anterior.
2. Emphasis on concentric training of the posterior musculature of the shoulder and scapula should be performed to guarantee a strong recovery.
3. Each rotator cuff muscle should be exercised (as best as possible) individually given their individual unique contribution to the swimming act.
4. Given the unique coupling patterns found in swimming, it is advisable to develop simulated exercise or training similar to the PNF concept of diagonal patterns of recruitment.

SOME SPECIFIC APPROACHES
Elastic Tubing Exercise

Elastic tubing can be used as an intermediate and occasionally advanced form of training. It offers the unique opportunity of being useful for isotonic (emphasis on either concentric or eccentric phases) or isometric exercise. Additionally, tubing can be modified to provide resistance in functional movement patterns.

The advantages of tubing are its portability and cost. Potential disadvantages are that the maximum amount of resistance is always at the end of the concentric phase and the tendency toward overuse. The beginning of the range of motion (ROM) places little tension on the tubing, thereby providing little resistance. As end-range concentric contraction is approached, resistance is increased. This type of variable resistance is not necessarily desirable, especially in patients with end-range discomfort. Patients who are used to heavy resistance exercise will often have a tendency to perform too many repetitions or sets with too much resistance, assuming that more is better. The result may be exacerbation of an existing complaint or creation of a new one.

Generally, two types of elastic resistance are available. The first is "surgical" types of tubing. The second is a Theraband type of elastic material that is more "sheet-like." Resistance can be varied several ways. First, the tubing can be shortened either by cutting, tying the attachment point closer to the exercised end, or stepping on or grasping the tubing closer to the exercised end. Secondly, different thicknesses (usually indicated by different colors) of tubing can be purchased.

There are several approaches to the use of elastic tubing in rehabilitation. The original approach involves a three- or four-stage progression. Each stage has a specific rehabilitative intent. Progression to the next phase requires successful completion of the preceding phase in an attempt to prevent injury from overenthusiastic and/or premature rehabilitation. The first phase involves a slow (if four phases) or fast (if three phases), mid-range, quick repetition for 60 seconds (pain or fatigue limited). This is the facilitation phase attempting to potentiate reflex pathways for future training. The second phase intent is strength. This phase involves contracting through a full ROM and holding at end range isometrically for up to 30 seconds. Release through the eccentric phase is slow and controlled. The third phase involves early endurance training. A full ROM is accomplished per second. The emphasis is on full range and speed and not on a specific range or phase of contraction. Figures 20-3 and 20-4 demonstrate various exercises performed standing and lying.

Another approach prefaced by a phase of lift freeweight exercise is a program accentuating the eccentric phase of contraction (Fig. 20-5). With this approach the opposite arm places the involved arm in an endrange position. Release of the opposite arm support allows focus on a slow negative or eccentric contraction. Caution must also be exercised with this approach. It is crucial that some form of conditioning be done prior to eccentric concentrated exercise.

A somewhat unique opportunity with elastic tubing involves the use of functional training. Functional training can be accomplished indirectly through the use of diagonal or spiral movements that mimic specific sports or phases of sports activities (Fig. 20-6). Directly, functional training can be accomplished through attachment of one end of the tubing to the apparatus specific to the sport (e.g., golf club, tennis racquet, baseball bat). In the case of swimming, resistance cords can be used to increase the force contribution of the upper extremity.

Finally, proprioceptive emphasis can be added through the use of balance or wobble boards accomplishing the same exercises while maintaining balance.

Eccentric Exercise

Recently, a surge of interest has occurred in relation to the possible need to specialize training through the selected emphasis of eccentric exercise. From a functional point of view, many sports activities require an eccentric component during deceleration phases of movement. In fact, an eccentric contraction is required in any situation where there is a sudden change in momentum. In sports and activities of daily living, the various aspects of eccentric function have been given synonyms. Negative work is a synonym best demonstrated by descending stairs or as one sits (quadriceps contraction). Another example is the term "negative," which simply implies the lowering of a weight or more specifically the tension maintained in a muscle as it is lengthening (the lowering phase of a biceps curl). Deceleration is probably the most common example in sports such as the decelerating phase of throwing and racquet sports or landing from a jump. The shock absorption aspect is synonymous, evident in landing from a jump or with a restraining activity like holding back a dog on a leash.

The interest in focused application of eccentrics centers around two important observations. First, eccentric loads seem to be a common culprit in the development of sprains and strains.[17] Secondly, isokinetic evidence indicates that patients with joint pain more often have eccentric deficits as compared to concentric testing.[18] Another suggested benefit is eccentric exercise's selective recruitment of type II fibers following immobilization.[19] This area of interest is still controversial and consensus as to the superiority of eccentric training does not exist. It would seem necessary, therefore, to include eccentric training emphasis as a component of total training. As will be discussed later, the concepts presented here are also in part used to explain the benefits of plyometric training given the important eccentric component of this approach. Some of the proposed benefits of eccentric exercise are based on several observations or theories. There suggested advantages center around a proposed superior efficiency of the eccentric contraction.

Apparently, an eccentric contraction is able to generate more force in a shorter period of time with less energy requirements than a concentric contraction. The Effman proposal[20] suggests a hierarchy with re-

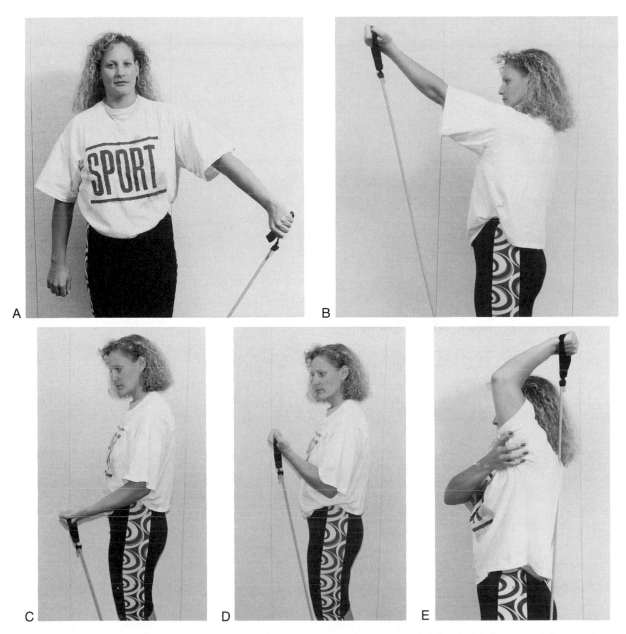

Fig. 20-3. Standing elastic tubing exercises. **(A)** Scaption-supraspinatus and deltoids (abduction 30 degrees forward), **(B)** forward flexion-deltoids/biceps, **(C & D)** forearm flexion/supination-biceps, **(E)** forearm extension-triceps, (*Figure continues.*)

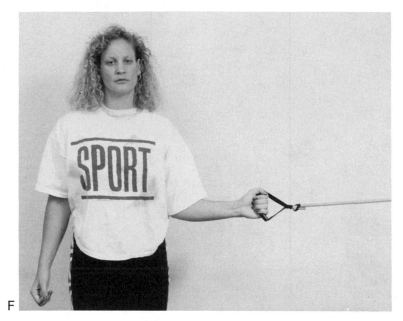

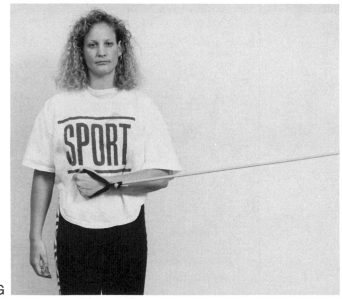

Fig. 20-3. (*Continued*). **(F & G)** internal rotation-subscapularis and other internal rotators, (*Figure continues.*)

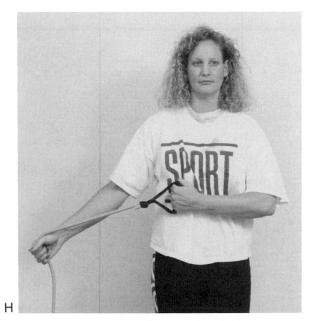

H

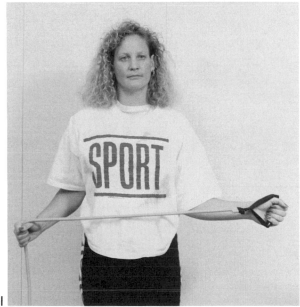

I

Fig. 20-3. (*Continued*). (**H & I**) external rotators-infraspinatus/teres minor, and (*Figure continues.*)

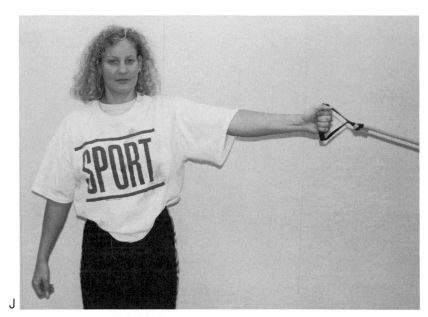

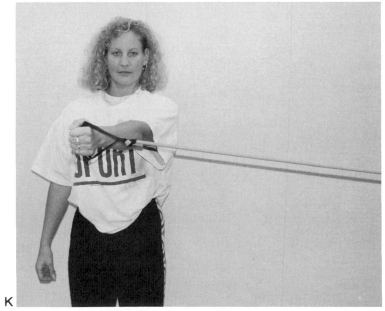

Fig. 20-3. (*Continued*). **(J & K)** horizontal adduction-pectorals.

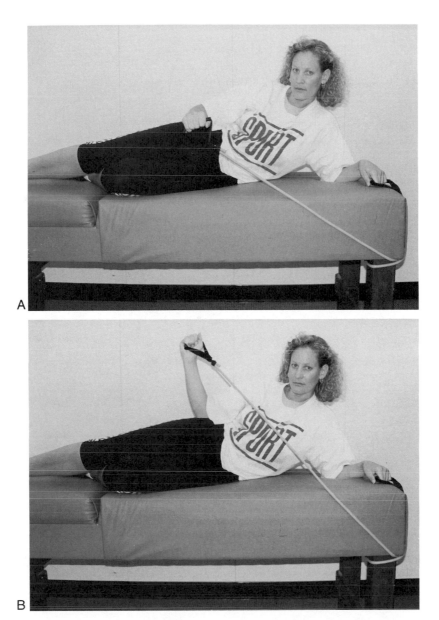

Fig. 20-4. Table elastic tubing exercises. **(A & B)** External rotation-infraspinatus/teres minor, (*Figure continues.*)

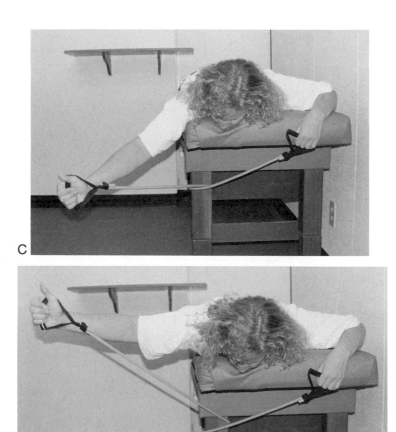

Fig. 20-4. (*Continued*). **(C & D)** horizontal extension with external rotation-midscapular muscles, posterior deltoid and supraspinatus, (*Figure continues.*)

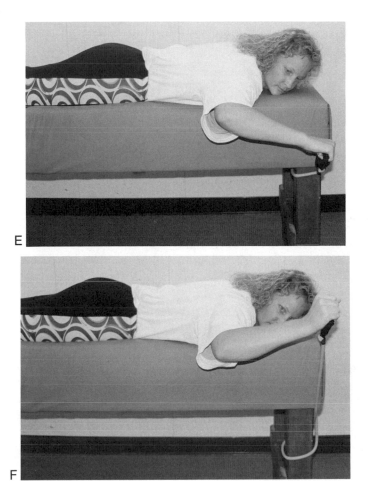

Fig. 20-4. (*Continued*). **(E & F)** prone external rotation-infraspinatus/teres minor, and (*Figure continues.*)

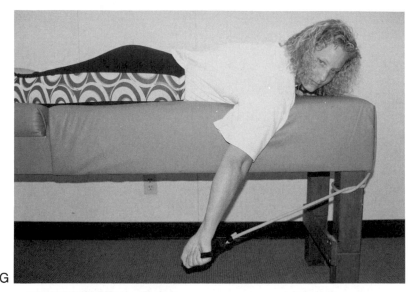

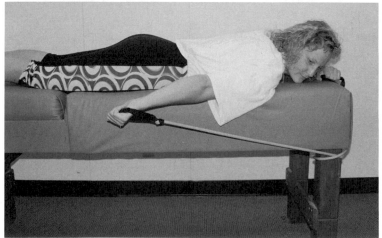

Fig. 20-4. (*Continued*). **(G & H)** prone extension-infraspinatus.

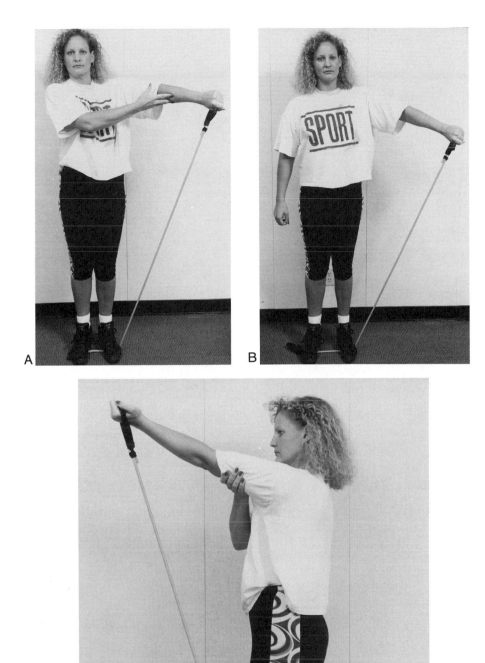

Fig. 20-5. Eccentric focus by lifting arm into starting position with other hand. The eccentric phase is unassisted. **(A & B)** Scaption, **(C)** forward flexion.

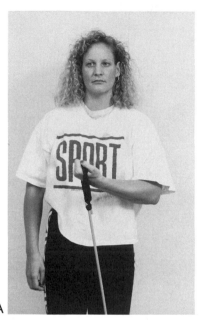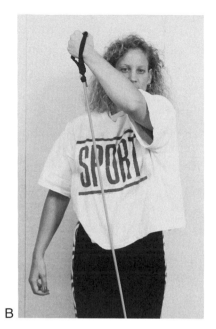

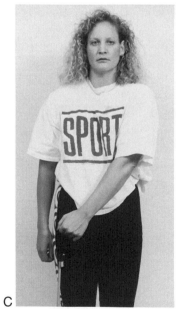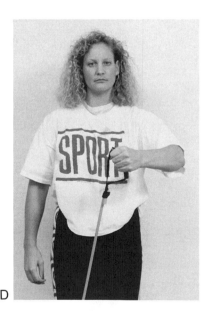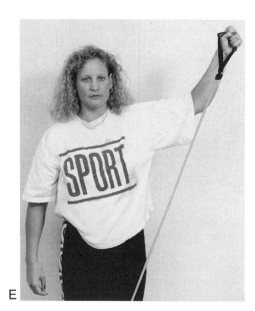

Fig. 20-6. Functional patterns with elastic tubing. **(A & B)** D_1 flexion pattern, **(C–E)** D_2 flexion pattern.

gard to force production. Eccentric contraction produces the most force, followed by isometric, followed by concentric. A general guideline suggested by Abbott et al.[21] is that an eccentric contraction of a given muscle is about 1.8 times that of an isometric contraction of the same muscle. This greater potential for eccentric contraction may, in part, be due to the different manner in which crossbridging of actin and myosin is produced and maintained.

Cavanagh and Komi[22] demonstrated a shorter response time with eccentric contraction. The principle of electromechanical delay is the amount of time between the biochemical response and the onset of subsequent muscle tension. The eccentric mode was found to be 4.4 milliseconds faster than the isometric contraction and 6 milliseconds faster than the concentric contraction.

The efficiency of oxygen utilization for eccentrics has been demonstrated by Knuttgen et al.[23] They found that 70 to 75 percent less oxygen was needed for eccentric as compared with concentric exercise. Davies and Barnes[24] also demonstrated that eccentric exercise required only 20 percent of the oxygen level of concentric contraction when examining downhill walking. Bigland-Richie and Woods[25] have shown that, in general, oxygen uptake per unit of muscle is three times greater for concentric contraction.

The training effect of eccentric exercise is not significant with regard to the cardiorespiratory systems but is apparently effective in decreasing the demands of oxygen uptake per unit of muscle activity. Development of tension with eccentric contraction does not require the normal splitting of adenosine triphosphate or creatinine phosphate as concentric contraction does.

An extremely important concept used in training, the stretch shorten cycle, focuses on the ability of the eccentric contraction to store and release energy. This is one of the main principles of plyometric exercise, which involves a prestretch to potentiate the following concentric contraction. In general, this is created by storage of energy in the series elastic component of the muscle and released as energy if a quick opposite movement is used or dissipated as heat if not. Therefore, to take advantage of this effect, there must be a quick stretch followed by a quick reversal from eccentric to concentric contraction usually within a relatively short ROM.

Guidelines for the prescription of eccentrics is still controversial yet includes some general agreement common to all exercise approaches, particularly the concept of a phased program with specific cautions and goals as progression signposts. It is generally agreed that eccentrics should begin during the subacute phase of healing. There is some disagreement as to when this phase begins. The distinction is based to some degree on the extent and severity of injury. However, somewhere between 3 and 7 days seems appropriate. Albert[19] has outlined a general program. The first phase begins at 7 days depending on the particular athlete's condition. Within this phase there is a progression from two-arm submaximal concentric and eccentric exercise. If performed pain-free the second phase places emphasis on preparation with two-arm concentrics followed by injured arm eccentrics. The first two phases are usually completed within 3 weeks. In the third phase initial functional eccentrics are started in preparation for plyometrics. This phase usually lasts 2 to 3 weeks. The fourth phase is not always applicable to all individuals, but if incorporated the emphasis is on plyometrics. This phase rarely is initiated before 3 weeks of training.

The initial phase should begin with concentrics combined with gravity (plus limb) resistance only. In some situations, the eccentrics may need to be doctor or patient assisted. The goal is to reach a stage where eccentrics against gravity are performed. In the second phase, eccentrics may progress to submaximal loading. Slow (less than 120 degrees/second), submaximal eccentrics are the initial type given in this second phase. The risk of injury using this type of eccentric is low. With regard to strength, Mannheimer[26] demonstrated a superiority of eccentrics over concentrics during the first 19 days postinjury yet not after. Loads can be increased to concentric-acceptable levels rather early. Johnson and Adamczyk[27] have demonstrated safety up to 20 percent above the one repetition maximum for a corresponding concentric contraction. Loads above 40 percent are contraindicated.

This phase of eccentrics can be accomplished with a variety of apparatus including elastic tubing, free weights, and a variety of weight machines. To access the starting position for the eccentric a well-limb concentric contraction is used. For example, if performing a biceps curl on a weight machine or similar apparatus, early phase eccentrics can be performed by lifting the weight with the uninvolved arm only and lowering it with the involved arm only. Another approach is to assist the involved arm into the beginning position. For example, elevate the right arm (involved side) with the left hand into a position to begin the negative. Release the involved arm to perform an unassisted negative.

Rest periods with eccentrics are not as necessary due to the low oxygen demand. Somewhere between 30 seconds to 1 minute is probably sufficient. The suggested application of sets and repetitions has been averaged to be somewhere between 3 and 20 repetitions with a three-set maximum. Curwin and Stanish[28] developed a program for tendonitis using eccentrics (see Ch. 14). This graduated program progresses from slower to faster speeds before increasing resistance. This approach adds a factor of safety by progressing from a four-count movement to finally a one-count movement. Frequency is influenced by tissue damage and delayed onset muscle soreness associated with eccentrics. Ideally, somewhere between two and three times per week is appropriate. More than three times a week result in minimal strength improvements.

Trudelle-Jackson et al.[29] reported that young females had a large disparity between concentric and eccentric strength and suggest a predisposition to knee disorders based on this difference. If this exists with the shoulder, as suggested by Ng and Kramer,[30] it is possible that eccentrics may play a preventative role with a higher potential for results in the female population. Ng and Kramer also demonstrated a significant advantage of internal rotational eccentric torque production over external rotation.

With regard to the elderly, eccentrics can be an optimal initiating approach. Due to the low oxygen demands, the ability to use more of a load than the concentric phase, and the observed difficulty with isometrics, eccentrics may be an optimal preparatory exercise before progressing with rehabilitation.

Criticism of eccentrics focuses on two aspects. First, it is easier to overload a muscle or tendon with eccentrics thereby increasing risk of damage.[28] Second, there is the observed effect of delayed onset muscle soreness (DOMS).[31] The first concern can be prevented with the use of an appropriately graded program. The second concern of DOMS is related to the initial concern with muscle overload. It has been dem-onstrated that eccentrics or eccentrics with concentrics will produce DOMS, but that concentrics alone will not.

The onset of DOMS is within a few hours, peaking around 48 hours. The symptoms include diffuse pain that is dull in nature and often aggravated by contraction of the involved muscle(s). Signs that are often evident include diffuse tenderness, muscle swelling, and loss of strength and active ROM, with a corresponding increase in electromyographic activity for a given load compared to normal.

Theories of causation are abundant and yet many are readily discounted. A theory of lactic acid accumulation[32] seems unlikely given the lack of circulation impairment with eccentric exercise.[33,34] The suggestion of tonic muscle contraction[35] as a cause is also unlikely given the finding that sore muscles do not demonstrate a consistent elevation in electromyographic activity.[36,37] It has been demonstrated that eccentric does damage muscle at the subcellular level.[38] The Z band appears to be the weakest mechanical component. Type IIb fibers, having the weakest Z bands, are most susceptible. With regard to connective tissue, eccentrics seem to damage the series elastic component of muscle (SEC). This tissue damage combined with the buildup of local fluid pressure and collagen/protein metabolites is probably the combined cause of DOMS.

Treatment of DOMS focuses on the above elements of fluid and metabolite accumulation coupled with tissue damage. Many approaches have been investigated. Nonsteroidal anti-inflammatory medications, exercise, and transcutaneous electrical nerve stimulation (TENS) have proved the most effective modalities. Rest, iontophoresis, and cryotherapy have not been effective approaches.[19]

Isokinetic Exercise

Isokinetics can play a valuable role in evaluation and rehabilitation of the athlete. In particular, as a form of advanced training, isokinetics can offer the advantage of variable speed, eccentric focus, and functional patterns (with modified apparatus). The disadvantages are the equipment cost for individual practitioners. As a result, few chiropractors have state-of-the-art isokinetic equipment. In the treatment of the professional athlete it is often necessary to refer to a facility with isokinetic equipment for rehabilitation and/or postsurgical evaluation. Chapter 8 addresses this issue in more detail.

Plyometrics

An extension of the eccentric concept is the plyometric approach. Plyometrics is an attempt at maximizing some of the physiologic characteristics of eccentric contraction and its effect on a subsequent concentric contraction. Through the ability of the elastic component of soft tissue to store energy and the muscle spindle response to quick stretch with an eccentric contraction, a quickly following concentric contraction can be augmented.[39]

The term plyometrics was first coined by track and field coach Fred Wilt.[40] The rationale for creation of the term is uncertain given that direct translation from the two Greek words of derivation *plyo* and *metric* means "more measure." The plyometric approach has existed for many years, but it was not until 1972 when this "new" system was incorporated into the training of Eastern bloc countries for the Olympics did it attain world recognition in the athletic community. The development of this training concept is attributed to Verhoshanski and Chormonson.[41]

The three general structures of muscle that affect tension are the contractile component, SEC, and parallel elastic component (PEC). The SEC is the main determinant of stored energy potential. The total force generated is the sum of the contractile component and SEC. The SEC stores the load of an eccentric contraction as energy and releases this energy if a concentric contraction follows closely.

Upper body plyometric programs have not been developed as much as lower body programs. Some common examples of plyometric exercises for the shoulder include bouncing wall push-ups (with and without resistance), rebound push-ups on a minitramp, and plyoball ball toss (Fig. 20-7). Progression to the advanced stage of plyometrics requires the ability of the athlete to perform regular push-ups prior to the bouncing type.

Proprioceptive Neuromuscular Facilitation

PNF techniques were first developed by Kabat[42] with the intent of rehabilitating the neuromuscular system as a whole. Drawing from several related areas, Kabat integrated the work of Sherrington[43] and Pavlov[44] on reflex and habitual actions, the theories of Gessell and Amatruda[45] and Coghill,[46] and Gellborne's[47] work on cortically controlled movement and proprioception. The techniques that were developed address both therapeutic and rehabilitative goals including decreasing of pain, increase in flexibility and ROM, and increase in strength and endurance. The general underlying principle is described as irradiation, where the incorporation of all muscles used to perform a functional movement is gradually stimulated.

PNF is a therapist/doctor directed series of movements that offer several unique advantages over conventional exercise, whether machine or therapist assisted.

Manual contacts offer the advantage of subtle control not available with a machine. The therapist/doctor adapts to the requirements suggested by the patient's response to a specific movement pattern. Generally, maximum resistance is suggested throughout the stronger ranges with diminishing resistance in the weaker ranges. Assistance through painful ranges is also encouraged. Manual contacts, if broad enough and not over tender areas, provides proprioceptive inhibition of pain through the large fiber afferents. Other forms of proprioceptive input can be incorporated, such as quick stretch (tapping over specific muscles or tendons) and vibration. Finally, approximation of joints can be included to simulate a weight-bearing posture and traction can be applied to decrease pain with some conditions.

Single movement patterns such as flexion/extension and internal/external rotation are commonly used with free weights or machines. An advantage of PNF is the use of spiral or diagonal patterns, which more realistically imitate functional patterns. Additionally, each link in the extremity being exercised may become a part of the functional pattern. In other words, in addition to exercising the shoulder, an upper extremity technique can also incorporate the elbow, wrist, and hand. To some degree, diagonal patterns can now be accomplished on some isokinetic equipment. However, this approach still lacks the fine control provided by a sentient assistant.

All forms of exercise can be accomplished within a single session incorporating isometric, concentric,

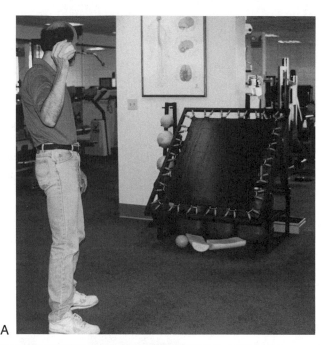

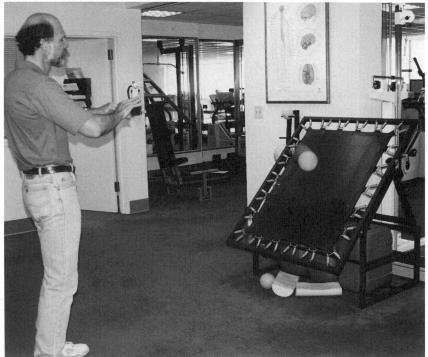

Fig. 20-7. (A & B) Throwing drills for the shoulder.

eccentric, reciprocal, and co-contractions. Each of these approaches can be combined to provide a specific therapeutic effect. A pattern of movement can include both isometric and isotonic components. The isometrics are often used at end range. Single isometrics of antagonists or agonists are used to assist stretch. Repeated contractions or reciprocal contractions as isometrics are used for both stretch and endurance.

Simulated sports activities can be performed using PNF techniques that involve both the functional pattern of the activity and the positional stabilization required whether weight-bearing and nonweight-bearing.

General PNF Principles

A thorough discussion of PNF techniques and principles can be found in the works of Knott and Voss[48] and Sullivan et al.[49] A more generalized description of approaches is presented here. The vocabulary of PNF can be a deterrent to learning the techniques. Unfortunately, many therapeutic approaches require acquisition of a new language in addition to the skill of performance. A selected list of terminology is given in an attempt to simplify understanding and encourage use of this valuable approach.

The diagonal movement pattern, used often in full ROM PNF, is comprised of three components. Either flexion or extension, internal or external rotation, and abduction or adduction are combined into a pattern for a particular joint. Other related joints may also have associated patterns that accompany a selected pattern. For example, shoulder flexion is coupled with external rotation and scapular elevation/upward rotation. External rotation of the shoulder is combined with forearm supination. Wrist and finger extension are combined with shoulder abduction. The reciprocal patterns combine respectively.

A designated abbreviation is given to each of these patterns for both the upper and lower extremity. For the upper extremity:

Diagonal 1 Flexion Upper Extremity (D$_1$F UE). This pattern is comprised of scapula elevation, and upward rotation. The shoulder is flexing, adducting, and externally rotating. The elbow may flex or extend or remain extended throughout the movement. The wrist and fingers flex and radially deviate while the thumb adducts (Fig. 20-8).

Diagonal 1 Extension Upper Extremity (D$_1$E UE). This pattern is comprised of scapular depression, adduction, and downward rotation. The shoulder is extending, abduction, and internally rotating. The elbow may flex, extend, or remain extend throughout the movement. The wrist and fingers extend and ulnar deviate while the thumb adducts (Fig. 20-9).

Diagonal 2 Flexion Upper Extremity (D$_2$F UE). This pattern involves scapular elevation, adduction, and upward rotation. The shoulder is flexing, abducting, and externally rotating. The elbow may flex, extend, or remain extended throughout the movement. The wrist and fingers extend and radially deviate while the thumb extends (Fig. 20-10).

Diagonal 2 Extension Upper Extremity (D$_2$E UE). The scapula depresses, abducts, and rotates downward. The shoulder extends, adducts, and internally rotates. The elbow may flex, extend, or remain extended throughout the movement. The wrist and fingers flex and ulnar deviate while the thumb opposes the fingers (Fig. 20-11).

It has been theorized and supported by one study that a specific muscle is optimally stimulated by a particular pattern (Table 20-6).[50] The anterior deltoid pattern is D$_1$F, the middle deltoid pattern is D$_2$F, and the posterior deltoid pattern is D$_1$E. The pectoralis major, sternal division is most active with a D$_2$E pattern. Flexion and extension of the elbow also affects optimizing the activity. The anterior and middle deltoid are more active with shoulder flexion patterns with the elbow also flexing, whereas the pectoralis major and poste-

Table 20-6. Optimal Pattern of Movement for a Specific Muscle

Muscle	Pattern
Anterior deltoid	Diagonal 1 flexion (D$_1$F
Pectoralis major (clavicular)	[elbow flexing])
Serratus anterior	
Coracobrachialis	
Middle deltoid	Diagonal 2 flexion (D$_2$F
Supraspinatus	[elbow flexing])
Infraspinatus/teres minor	
Trapezius	
Posterior deltoid	Diagonal 1 extension (D$_1$E
Teres major	[elbow extending])
Latissimus	
Rhomboids	
Levator scapulae	
Pectoralis major (sternal)	Diagonal 2 extension (D$_2$E
Subscapularis	[elbow extending])

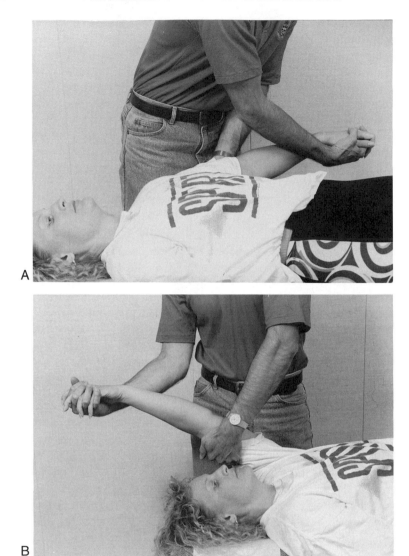

Fig. 20-8. D_1 flexion. **(A)** Patient initiates with flexion at the fingers. Movement pattern at shoulder is flexion, adduction, external rotation. **(B)** Final position.

rior deltoid are more active with the elbow extending.[50]

A recombination of proximal and distal D_1 and D_2 patterns results in a thrusting pattern and the reverse of a thrust (a withdrawal pattern). For example, a D_1 thrust (ulnar thrust) combines a D_1E for the forearm, wrist, and hand together with a shoulder D_1F pattern while the elbow extends (Fig. 20-12). The resulting pattern involves scapular protraction, shoulder flexion/adduction/external rotation, elbow extension, and forearm pronation as the hand opens. The reverse D_1 thrust or withdrawal pattern involves scapular retraction, shoulder extension/abduction/internal rotation with elbow, wrist, and hand flexion.

These patterns can be performed unilateral, bilateral, or with the assistance of the opposite upper extremity. They are usually performed supine initially to provide passive stability of the patient. Movements can then be performed in various other positions including prone. The prone position offers some advantages in the treatment of the swimming athlete in an attempt to simulate sport specific movements. In the supine

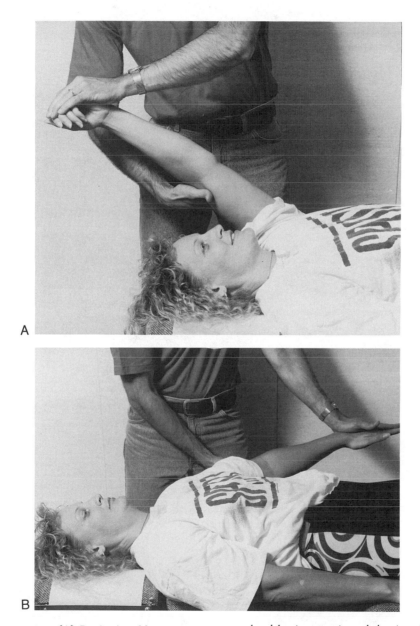

Fig. 20-9. D_1 extension. **(A)** Beginning. Movement pattern at shoulder is extension, abduction, internal rotation. **(B)** Final position.

position patterns are easily accomplished without the restrictions of the table. The flexor movements are resisted by gravity until midrange but assisted by gravity through the remaining concentric phase. Gravity will assist most extension movements. Unfortunately, similar to weightlifting, the supine position can limit scapular movement. In the prone position there is some restriction of full range due to the table; however, the

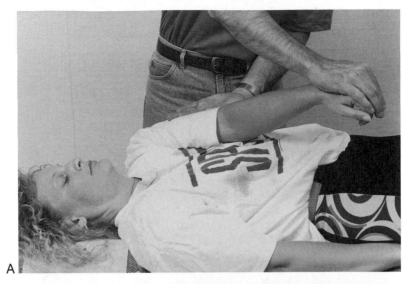

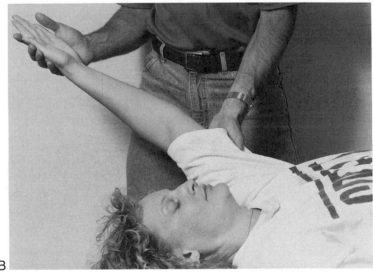

Fig. 20-10. D_2 flexion. **(A)** Beginning. Movement pattern at shoulder is flexion, abduction, external rotation. **(B)** Final position.

scapula is not fixed. Flexion and extension are both resisted by gravity (there is no mid-range switch as occurs in the supine position). The two patterns used are D_2F and D_1E (Fig. 20-13). $D_1 E$ closely resembles the swimming act.

There are four possible bilateral patterns including symmetrical, asymmetrical, reciprocal, and cross-diagonal. These patterns can be very helpful in simulating sports activities.

Bilateral symmetrical. Symmetrical patterns combine

the same pattern in the same direction (Fig. 20-14).

Bilateral asymmetrical. Asymmetrical patterns combine the two different patterns in the same direction. For example, D_1F for the right extremity is combined with D_2F of the left resulting in movement to the left (Fig. 20-15). Both symmetrical and asymmetrical patterns facilitate trunk flexion and extension, but the asymmetrical patterns add an element of trunk rotation.

Bilateral reciprocal. Reciprocal patterns involve the same pattern bilaterally moving in opposite directions. For example, D_2F of one extremity would be combined with D_2E of the opposite (Fig. 20-16). Again, rotation of the trunk is involved.

Cross-diagonal (reciprocal-asymmetrical). Cross-diagonal patterns incorporate the opposite pattern moving in opposite directions. For example, D_2E is performed by one extremity while the opposite performs D_1F (Fig. 20-17). The reciprocal patterns can be useful in simulating the backstroke pattern in swimming.

In addition to diagonal patterns, thrusting patterns can be performed bilaterally in either a symmetrical or reciprocal manner (Fig. 20-18).

Trunk Patterns

Trunk patterns involving the upper extremity (upper trunk patterns) combine the head and neck with upper trunk movements. Concomitantly, an asymmetrical upper extremity pattern is used with contact of the contralateral hand with the leading forearm. There are two patterns used, a chop and a lift.

A chop is an asymmetrical upper extremity exten-

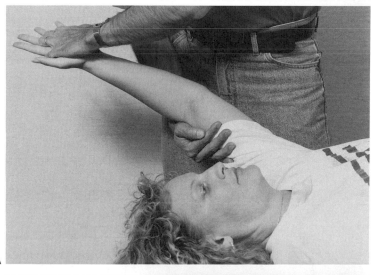

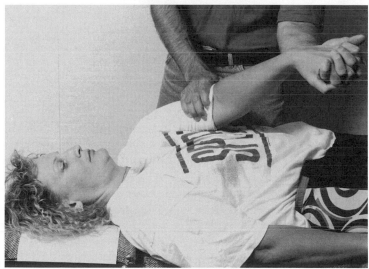

Fig. 20-11. D_2 extension. **(A)** Beginning. Movement pattern at shoulder is extension, adduction, internal rotation. **(B)** Final position.

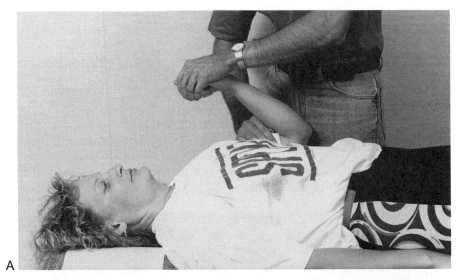

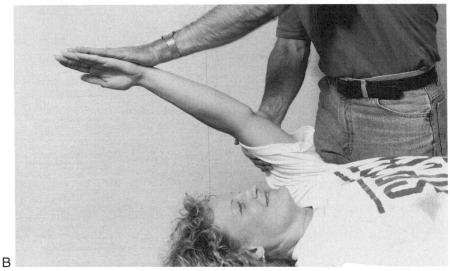

Fig. 20-12. (A & B) Thrust pattern.

sion movement. For example, right chopping involves a D_1 extension of the right upper extremity with a D_2 extension pattern for the left (Fig. 20-19 A & B). There is body contact with the opposite hand providing a closed kinematic chain. This may be easier than with the hands separate. A reverse chop can also be used.

The lift is the opposite of the chop involving an asymmetrical upper extremity flexion movement. Lifting to the right would involve D_2 flexion of the right upper extremity with D_1 flexion of the left (Fig. 20-19 C & D). This also involves a hand to hand contact.

Although there are many techniques possible with PNF the following techniques are commonly employed:

1. *Hold-relax*. This is an isometric contraction performed at end range to facilitate stretching.
2. *Rhythmic stabilization*. This is a pattern involving alternating isometric contractions of the agonist and antagonist in a stretch position followed by relaxation and further stretch.
3. *Contract-relax*. Either the athlete actively acquires

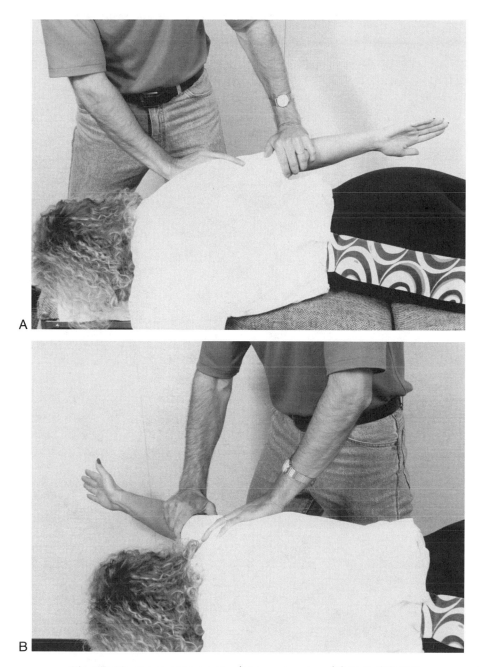

Fig. 20-13. Prone patterns simulating swimming. **(A)** D_1E, **(B)** D_2F.

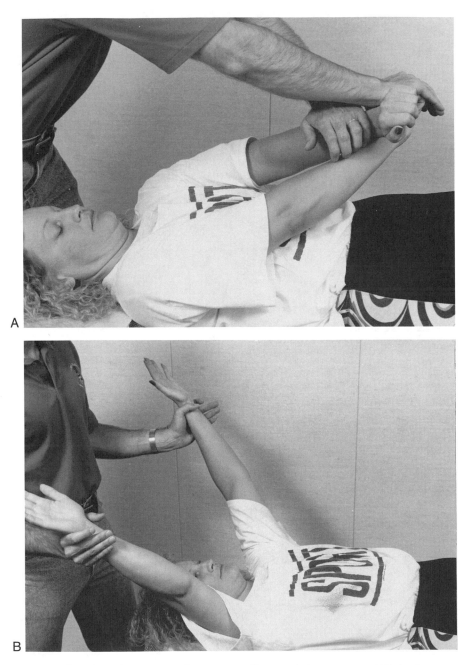

Fig. 20-14. Bilateral symmetrical pattern. D_2 flexion. **(A)** Beginning, **(B)** final position.

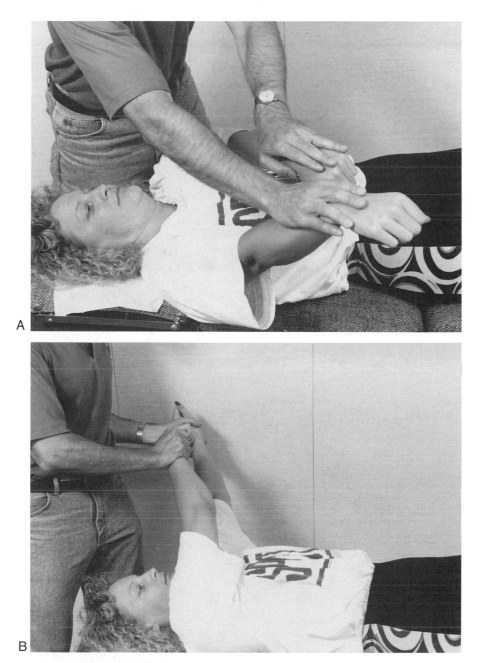

Fig. 20-15. Bilateral asymmetrical pattern. D_1F-right with D_2F-left. **(A)** Beginning, **(B)** final position.

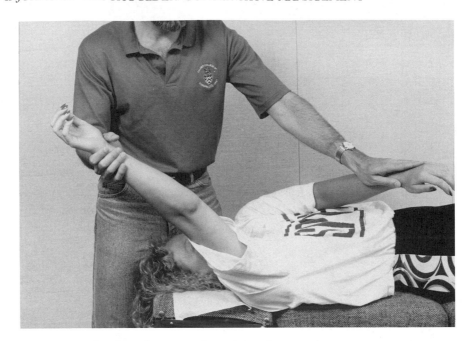

Fig. 20-16. Bilateral reciprocal. D₂F-left with D₂E-right. Beginning position.

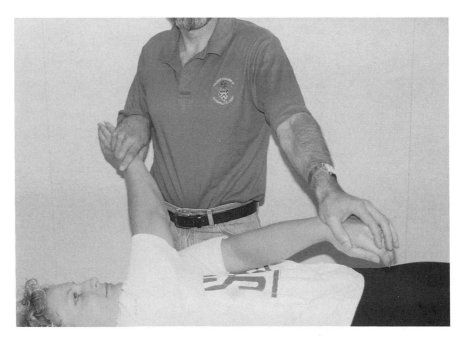

Fig. 20-17. Cross-diagonal pattern. D₂E-left with D₁F-right. Beginning.

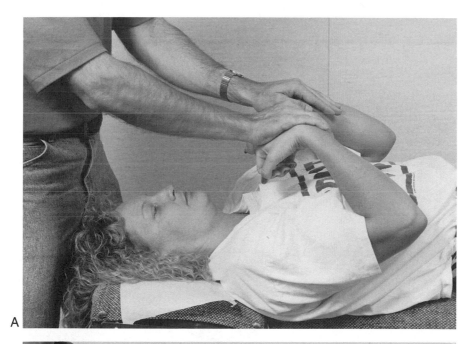

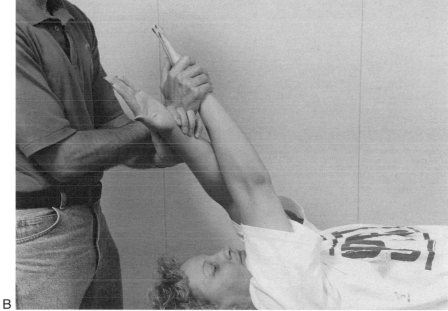

Fig. 20-18. **(A & B)** Symmetrical bilateral thrusting pattern. (*Figure continues.*)

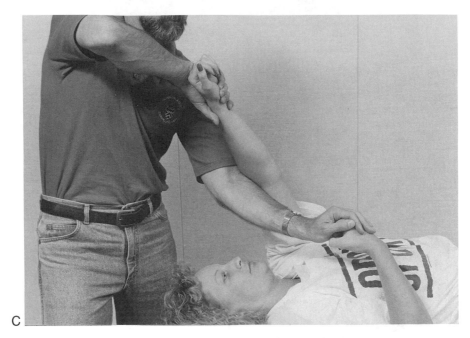

Fig. 20-18. (*Continued*). **(C)** Reciprocal bilateral thrusting pattern.

or the examiner passively acquires an end-range position. From this position, the athlete isotonically contracts through the antagonistic pattern against examiner resistance. The extremity is then brought back to the initial starting position. Similar to hold-relax, contract-relax is used as an alternative stretching technique.

4. *Repeated contractions*. This technique involves the use of a series of isotonic contractions through a full range either with diagonal patterns or unidirectional patterns in one direction only. The doctor can use an isometric hold pattern at a weak point in the movement pattern before progressing through the entire full range. Many trainers will accommodate decreases in strength with a decrease in resistance or assist through the weaker range.

5. *Slow reversal and slow-reversal-hold*. This involves the use of a full range isotonic contraction in one direction followed by the opposite pattern to end range. An isometric "hold" can be incorporated at the end of the agonist and antagonist pattern. This is then referred to as slow-reversal-hold.

Generalized Approach for the Shoulder

Probably the single most important diagonal pattern for the shoulder is the D$_2$F movement comprised of flexion, abduction, and external rotation. This pattern is requisite for the cocking phase of throwing, and for swimming and racquet sports. It also is often the most restricted pattern associated with shoulder pain or dysfunction. To access this pattern requires an approach that "sneaks up" on the restriction. Several suggestions include

Begin with isometrics with hold-relax and rhythmic stabilization to facilitate neural patterning, reduce pain, and reduce overuse of the scapula.

Use a D$_2$F pattern with the opposite extremity to facilitate a reciprocal spillover effect.

Before using the D$_2$F pattern with the involved extremity, begin with a D$_1$F pattern. This offers several advantages. While incorporating two of the patterns of restriction, flexion and external rotation, the D$_1$F pattern involves less movement into these ranges. Secondly, the more restricted and often painful movement of abduction is avoided. Finally, a D$_1$F pattern is less likely to cause impingement because it has such a restricted elevation pattern coupled with external rotation.

By combining these ideas with assisted bilateral movements, it is possible to initiate a program for the shoulder (Table 20-7). These initial movement patterns are performed supine. Next, it is necessary to incorpo-

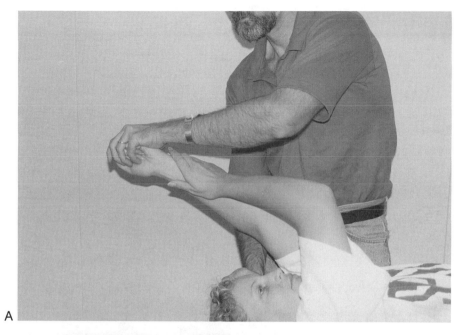

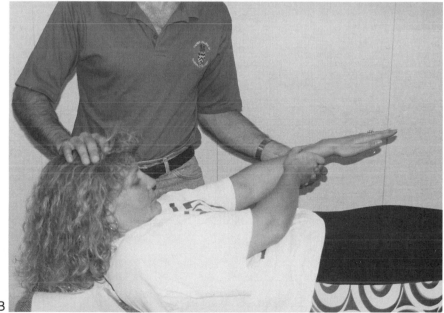

Fig. 20-19. Trunk patterns. **(A & B)** Chop. (*Figure continues.*)

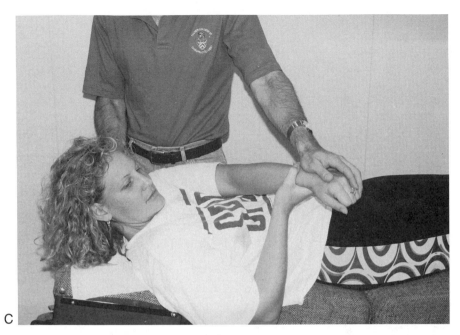

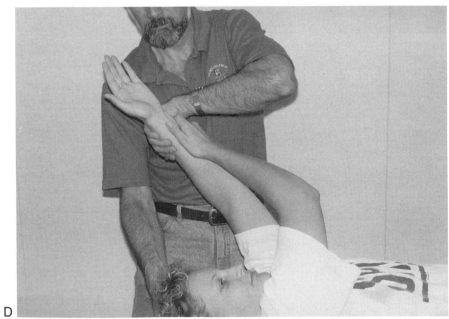

Fig. 20-19. (*Continued*). **(C & D)** lift.

rate various weight-bearing positions with the goals or stabilization and controlled mobility. These may begin with sitting (Fig. 20-20) and eventually involve a quadruped or standing position. Finally, the advanced stage incorporates bilateral symmetrical and reciprocal patterns.

Prevention

A preventive program has been developed by Janda and Loubert[51] for the throwing athlete. First, the athlete is tested for throwing speed and accuracy, and then isokinetically tested for various movement patterns.

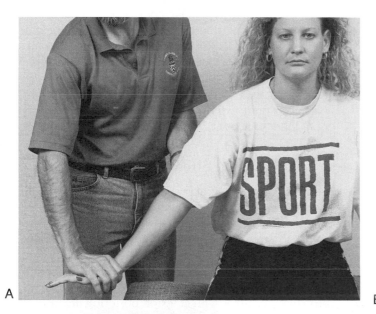

A

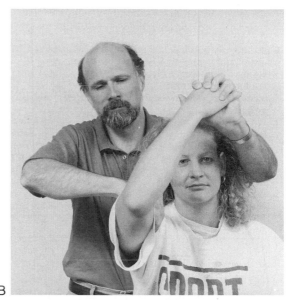

B

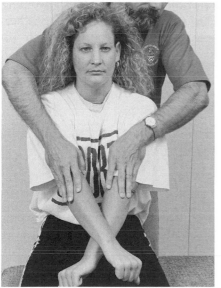

C

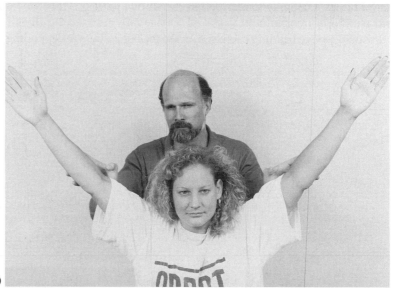

D

Fig. 20-20. Seated PNF patterns. **(A & B)** D₁F pattern, **(C & D)** bilateral pattern.

Table 20-7. General Proprioceptive Neuromuscular Facilitation Program for the Shoulder

Initial phase—decrease pain/increase ROM

1. Contralateral limb patterns
2. Isometrics of involved extremity with distal contact (to avoid painful shoulder area)
3. Rhythmic stabilization and hold-relax techniques for diminishing reflex scapular elevation
4. Mobility of the involved extremity be facilitated with a D_1F pattern (to avoid the more commonly restricted D_2F pattern initially). Techniques include
   a. Reverse chop
   b. A D_1 thrust with assistance from uninvolved limb
   c. If the above are not possible due to pain a reverse chop may be used

If the above is possible, D_2F patterns can be initiated with a lifting pattern first, followed by a unilateral D_2F pattern

5. Supine full patterns such as slow reversal and slow reversal hold are incorporated next

Intermediate stage—stability/controlled mobility with weight-bearing

1. Prone D_2F and D_1E patterns should be performed first
2. D_1F followed by D_2F patterns using alternating isometrics or rhythmic stabilization patterns followed by slow reversal hold beginning seated and progressing to standing procedures

Advanced stage—skilled movement/sports specific simulation

1. Bilateral patterns such as bilateral symmetrical/asymmetrical or cross-diagonal/reciprocal performed first supine or prone
2. Bilateral or unilateral patterns that simulate sport activity of athlete

Based on these results, specific patterns are emphasized. As with many PNF approaches, the shoulder is not exclusively trained. Both the neck, trunk, and associated upper extremity joints such as the elbow, wrist, and hand are incorporated.

Proprioceptive training can also be accomplished by challenging the shoulders in a weight-bearing posture requiring balance. By having the athlete perform push-ups on a medicine ball or "wobble or sliding boards," balance and strength are combined (Fig. 20-21). A new concept is to have the athlete lie on a table with only the lower body supported. The hands are used to support the upper body weight on a giant ball. These balls have been used in the rehabilitation of low back injuries using the concept of stabilization through proprioceptive training. A similar approach is appropriate for the shoulder. Athletes attempt ROM exercises and push-ups while supporting their weight onto the ball.

Full body proprioceptive training can be accomplished by having the athlete perform diagonal patterns with light free-weights or elastic tubing while balancing on a wobble board (personal communication; John Sousa, D.C. [Fig. 20-22]).

Stretching

Stretching is an integral part of a full rehabilitation and prevention program. Although there is some disagreement as to when to stretch, how often to stretch, how much to stretch, and how to stretch, it is generally agreed that flexibility is an important component for optimum performance. Of course, overstretching is a potential hazard as is stretching already lax or damaged structures. Athletes with anterior, posterior, and multidirectional instability must stretch cautiously avoiding the direction of laxity or avoid stretching altogether, depending on their age or sport requirements. Ironi-

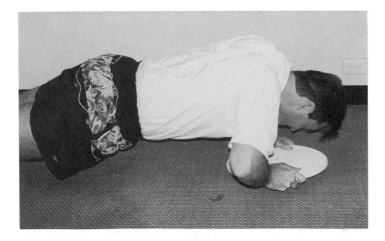

Fig. 20-21. Wobble board push-ups for proprioceptive training.

Fig. 20-22. (A–D) Wobble board Apley's exercises for proprioceptive training.

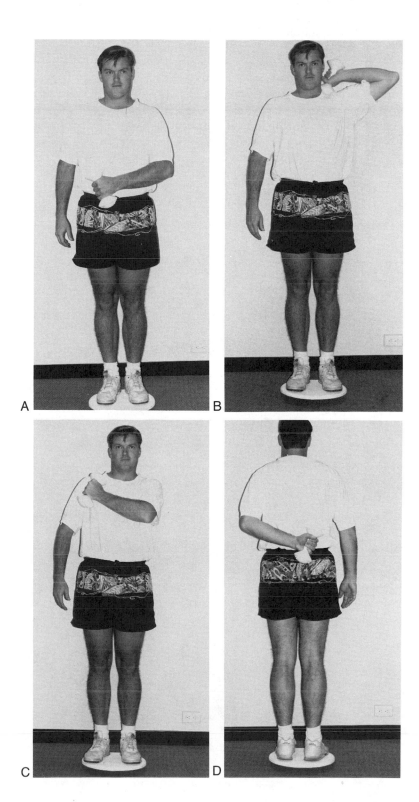

cally overstretching can result in a tightened muscle as a reflex reaction.

Although not thought of as a method of acquiring increased ROM, it appears that dynamic ROM exercises result in a greater degree of muscular relaxation than passive or ballistic maneuvers. As a result, dynamic exercise may be more effective at increasing ROM.[52,53]

It is important to distinguish between the terms *stretch* and *warm-up* or *cool-down*. The warm-up and cool-down should occur prior to any stretching. The intent of each is mainly cardiovascular and should not be analogous to stretching.

Stretching can focus primarily on muscles, the capsule and ligaments, or both. Methods of stretching are varied and include (1) static, (2) ballistic, (3) postcontraction (PNFs hold-relax, post–isometric relaxation,

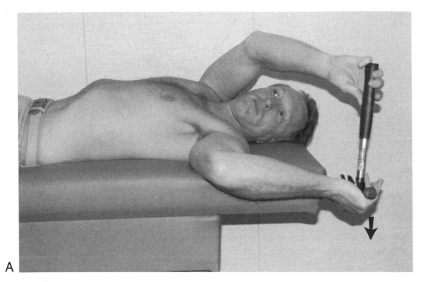

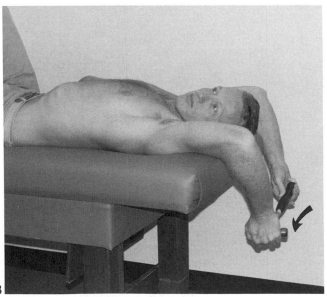

Fig. 20-23. T-bar (hammer) stretching. **(A)** External rotation stretch at 90 degrees. **(B)** External rotation stretch at full elevation. **(C & D)** Internal rotation stretch in two positions. (*Figure continues.*)

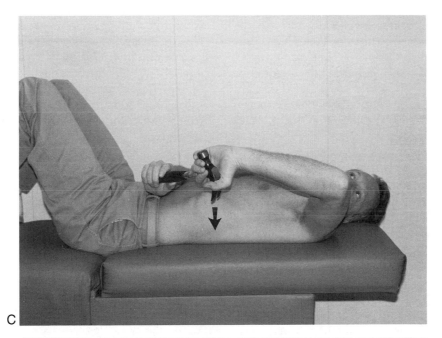

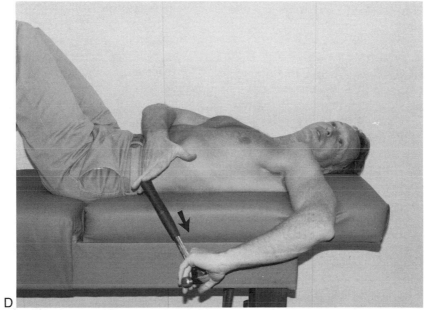

Fig. 20-23. (*Continued*).

muscle energy technique), and (4) cold-assisted (vapo-coolant spray or ice).

Most authors agree that the safest approach is a modified PNF technique that employs a minimum contraction in a stretched position for several seconds followed by a stretch into the new position.[54,55] Ballistic stretching is acceptable if prior warm-up has occurred and the ballistic maneuver is part of the plyometric pattern.

The pectoral muscles in particular are often in need of stretching. Posteriorly, the interscapular muscles may have a sense of tightness. Stretching of these muscles may be palliative at best unless accompanied by strengthening exercises.

Capsular stretching should in most cases focus on the posterior aspect. It has been noted that athletes with impingement have posterior capsular tightness. Additionally, it seems that this tightness can contribute to excessive anterior translation of the humeral head in patients with instability.

Some suggested stretch positions for specific structures are shown in Chapter 19. There are many other approaches available, yet the principles of self-stretching remain the same. From the stretch position a minimum resistance is applied in the direction opposite the stretch for 8 to 10 seconds followed by a cautious stretch into a new baseline position.

Another common approach is through the use of a T-bar to aid in rotational stretching. This can be modified through the use of a hammer, which obviates the need for special equipment. T-bar/hammer stretching for internal and external rotational stretching is demonstrated in Fig. 20-23. Pressure applied by the opposite hand induces the stretch.

REHABILITATION OF SPECIFIC DISORDERS

Rehabilitation of the shoulder complex is based on two major concepts: the condition (and specific structures involved) and the specific sport performed by the athlete. There are generally four major categories of conditions that require specific cautions and focus. These include (1) impingement, (2) instability and laxity (traumatic with associated damage or nontraumatic without damage); (3) tendinitis/tendinosis or bursitis (primary or secondary to the above), and (4) acromioclavicular separations.

Overlap of the first three conditions is common and requires a combined approach avoiding irritation or worsening of one condition while trying to correct another. After any acute processes are stabilized, it is of primary importance to focus on any underlying laxity or instability before progressing to any other concerns. A discussion of instability follows with a brief discussion of other conditions. Specific rehabilitation for the remaining conditions is outlined in the corresponding chapter.

Anterior Instability

Traumatic anterior instability is usually less responsive to conservative care due to the concomitant capsular, labral, humeral head, and rotator cuff damage. Therefore, when capsular damage is isolated, the remaining stability provided by the labrum and rotator cuff allows a more successful outcome. Similarly, atraumatic instability without labral damage or the shoulder with generalized laxity carries a much better prognosis.

With anterior instability recommendations include

1. Initial avoidance or modification of the stretching, strengthening, or sports activities that use or approximate the apprehension position
2. Avoidance of excessive stretching (in particular the extremes of flexion and horizontal adduction, which cause anterior translation of the humeral head due to posterior capsule tightening)
3. Initial emphasis on subscapularis and supraspinatus strengthening for lower abduction stability followed by strengthening of the posterior muscles including the infraspinatus and teres minor for higher abduction stability
4. Emphasis on the eccentric function of anterior musculature

A unique approach is to attempt to stabilize dynamically the humeral head by using rhythmic stabilization in the position(s) of instability. After assuring stability in positions shy of the patient's particular apprehension position, cautious application of submaximal isometrics is begun. The isometrics increase in intensity over several training sessions.

Through the use of a pulley-weight system Brostrom et al.[56] demonstrated a high success rate with anterior unstable shoulders. The emphasis was on shoulder flexion, internal rotation, and external rotation exercised three times a week for 8 weeks. The unsuccessful rehabilitation attempts were in 5 out of 29 cases. Most had decreased retroversion or a traumatic cause of their instability.

Posterior Instability

Selective cutting experiments seem to suggest that for significant posterior humeral head movement to occur, there must be laxity of the anterior capsule as well. The more common occurrence is recurrent posterior subluxation, both voluntary and nonvoluntary. Various conservative approaches have been recommended including proprioceptive feedback techniques and various PNF approaches. The concern is that successful surgical repair is difficult and that conservative care should be attempted first in all cases. The one exception is when there is an associated glenoid labrum or full-thickness rotator cuff tear. In these instances, response to conservative care is compromised. When small labrum tears or rotator cuff tears are undiagnosed, lack of response to conservative care can give a diagnostic clue to further evaluation.

The primary concerns with posterior instability are

1. If voluntary, it is crucial to have the patient discontinue this habitual practice (occasionally it may be necessary to have professional psychological counseling).
2. Avoidance of the bench press maneuver emphasizing alternative exercises such as cable crossovers. Other exercises that may need to be avoided are forward flexion as occurs with deltoid raises.
3. Avoidance of the dislocation position of forward flexion/internal rotation especially coupled with horizontal adduction.
4. Avoid excessive stretching, especially of the posterior capsule.

A basic approach to stabilization should follow a sequential approach: (1) stabilize the scapula, (2) strengthen the rotator cuff, (3) performance of functional movements with an emphasis on eccentric control.

TRAINING AND PREVENTION APPROACHES FOR SPECIFIC SPORTS

In addition to focusing on the specific muscular requirements of specific sports, a general year-round training approach should be used for peak performance and prevention of injury. Although it is beyond the scope of this text to cover all sports, some specific sports are addressed with the hope that transferral of principles is possible. Prefacing this discussion is a review of the principles of periodization.

Periodization

Developed in the Soviet Union in the 1950s, periodization focuses on increasing peak performance and maintaining a level of fitness and interest throughout the year by varying the type of exercise, intensity, volume, and load. This is accomplished by dividing the year into phases or training cycles (Fig. 20-24). This division may be in three or the original four phases of Matveyev.[57] The basic three division consists of (1) a preseason (preparatory) phase, (2) an in-season (competitive) phase, and (3) a postseason (transition) phase. Matveyev's divisions include (1) a preparation phase, (2) the first transition, (3) a competitive phase, and (4) a second transition or active rest phase.

The initial preseason or preparatory phase is intended to prepare the athlete through development of basic skills for the sport coupled with the high-volume, low-intensity workouts. Toward the end of the first phase (first transition) the athlete switches to more high-intensity training emphasizing power and strength when the sport is more anaerobic.

The in-season or competitive phase switches primarily to a power approach to training. Technique is emphasized coupled with high-intensity training using short workouts. It is important not to overtrain.

Finally, the focus in the postseason or transition phase is on active, rest, which includes participation in recreational sports and training that is mild to moderate with low-volume, low to moderate intensity.

Throwing Sports

Rehabilitation for throwing sports should include a gradual transition. Various approaches have been sug-

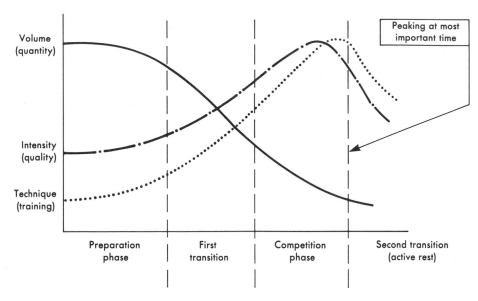

Fig. 20-24. Matveyev periodization model. (From Matveyev,[57] as adapted in Kirkendall,[70] with permission.)

gested, yet they all vary the aspects of long and short tosses, speed, and accuracy. The initial intent is to get the athlete to throw without an intent of accuracy or speed. Most programs such as the Fungo type emphasize proper warm-up with appropiate rest periods.[58] The intervals are usually 2 days throwing, one day rest. The day rest in between 2 consecutive days of pitching is an "active" rest day. This means that no throwing is allowed, yet all rehabilitation exercises are performed. Throwing practice is usually limited to 30 minutes. A long toss is used initially from center field. The ball should barely reach home plate. The second interval starts on the next interval (days 4 and 5) when the athlete throws between center field and second base. The ball should bounce several times before reaching home plate. In the next interval (days 7 and 8) they pitch from second base so that the ball clears by 1 to 2 feet. Normal pitches should be possible in the next interval (days 10 and 11), but individuality is the rule.

Several drills have been recommended that emphasize different elements of form. Some of these are described in Chapter 3. Others include the chair throw and the standing throw.[59] The chair throw is an attempt at trying to get the pitcher to pitch over the stride leg. By keeping the back foot on the edge of a chair the athlete is forced to pitch without as much lower body contribution focusing on position rather than speed

or accuracy. The standing throw is similar. The thrower must keep the weight on both feet while throwing until follow-through. This drill allows a focus on hip participation to the throwing act.

A recent study by Watkins et al.[60] on trunk participation in the throwing act used electromyographic analysis to determine the muscles most recruited in efficient pitching. Contralateral to the pitching arm side, the abdominal obliques, lumbar paraspinals, and rectus abdominis showed activity between 75 and 100 percent during the pitching act as did the ipsilateral gluteus maximus. Using this information, emphasis can be placed on testing and training these muscles to maximize performance and decrease stress to the pitching shoulder.

A periodization model for throwing sports is presented in Appendix 20-1. A preventative PNF approach is presented in Table 20-8.

Similar to the Fungo routine for pitchers, a modification can be applied to tennis. The training period is again 30 minutes with a program of 2 days serving, 1 day off. A single can of three balls is used. When they are all used the player must retrieve them before proceeding. This adds another element of imposed rest. A court with a high backstop is used. The player first hits at about eye level. In the next interval (days 4 and 5) the player hits down toward the junction of the fence

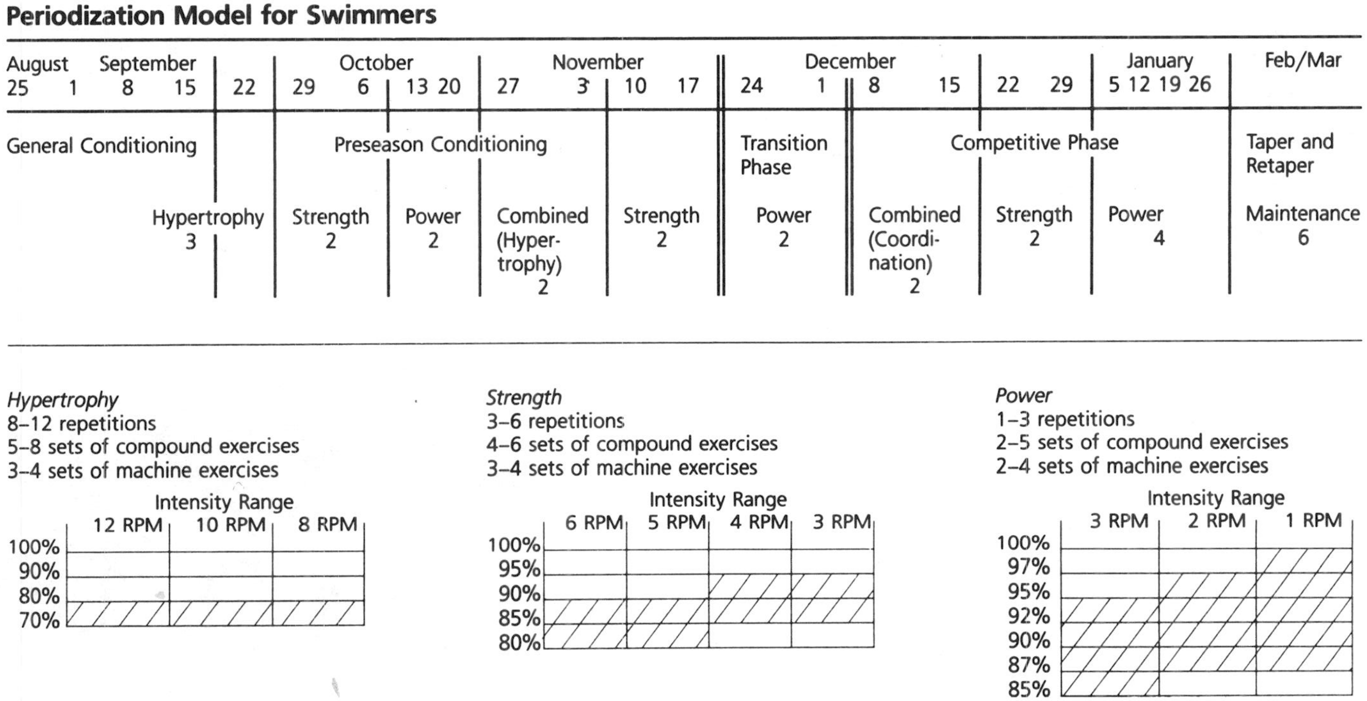

Periodization Model for Swimmers
August September
25 1 8 15
22
October
29 6 13 20
November
27 3 10 17
December
24 1 8 15
22 29
January
5 12 19 26
Feb/Mar
General Conditioning
Preseason Conditioning
Transition Phase
Competitive Phase
Taper and Retaper
Hypertrophy 3
Strength 2
Power 2
Combined (Hyper-trophy) 2
Strength 2
Power 2
Combined (Coordi-nation) 2
Strength 2
Power 4
Maintenance 6
Hypertrophy
8–12 repetitions
5–8 sets of compound exercises
3–4 sets of machine exercises
Intensity Range
12 RPM
10 RPM
8 RPM
100%
90%
80%
70%
Strength
3–6 repetitions
4–6 sets of compound exercises
3–4 sets of machine exercises
Intensity Range
6 RPM
5 RPM
4 RPM
3 RPM
100%
95%
90%
85%
80%
Power
1–3 repetitions
2–5 sets of compound exercises
2–4 sets of machine exercises
Intensity Range
3 RPM
2 RPM
1 RPM
100%
97%
95%
92%
90%
87%
85%

Fig. 20-25. Periodization model for swimmers. (From Uebel,[68] with permission.)

Table 20-8. Preventative Proprioceptive Neuromuscular Facilitation Program for the Pitcher

1. Neck diagonal patterns—full range resisted (athlete supine)
2. Rhythmic stabilization (RS) or hold relax (HR) for scapular protraction/retraction with shoulder flexed/elbow extended; punch and retract against resistance (athlete supine)
3. RS and HR for scapular protraction/retraction, arms next to side; resistance at shoulders (athlete prone)
4. RS and HR for horizontal extension/flexion with elbow bent, arm behind back; chicken movement (athlete prone)
5. RS and HR for extension/flexion with arms overhead; airplane exercise (athlete prone)
6. D_1 UE and D_2 UE
7. Throwing motion with elbow extended (athlete supine)
8. Throwing motion with elbow flexed (athlete supine)

and ground. The next interval (days 7 and 8) has the player serving to the backcourt boundary line. In the last interval (days 10 and 11) the player serves normally.

Swimming

Flexibility exercises should be stressed, but not overstressed (in particular with the young swimmer).[61] Ciullo[62] demonstrated in one study that the incidence of impingement symptoms dropped from 90 percent to approximately 14 percent with adolescent swimmers using a stretching program. Results in Master's swimmers were less dramatic. Griepp[61] demonstrated in his study a predictive relationship between reduced flexibility and the development of tendinitis. Ironically, Fowler and Webster[63] demonstrated a relationship to the development of tendinitis and posterior laxity. Therefore, a balance must exist between stretching for flexibility and strengthening for prevention of instability. The first recommendation is to not allow pairs stretching (assisted by a team member) under the age of 15. The rationale is that these athletes are less likely to understand the dangers of overstretching.[64] It is important, that paired stretching be taught and not assumed to be understood by the athlete. As mentioned previously gradual PNF types of stretching are preferred. With regard to posterior laxity, it may be theorized that due to the excessive translation posteriorly with anterior capsular tightness, capsular stretching should be emphasized for these swimmers. On the other hand, with athletes presenting with anterior laxity, anterior capsular stretching should be avoided; posterior capsular stretching may be beneficial.

Other suggestions are found in Chapter 4. A periodization protocol for swimming is presented in Fig. 20-25.

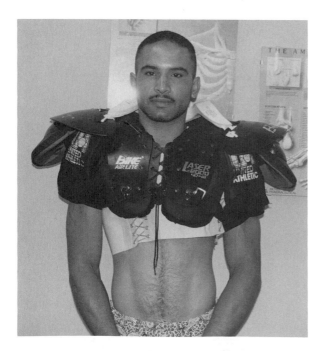

Fig. 20-26. Protective football equipment.

Fig. 20-27. Protective taping for acromi-oclavicular injury. **(A)** Three anchor strips with protective gauze over nipple. **(B & C)** Basket weave over anchors. **(D)** Shoulder spica (figure eight) taping with Elasticon.

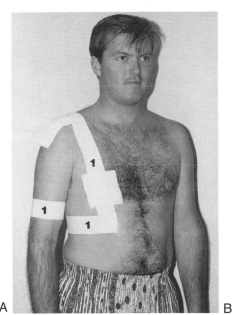

A

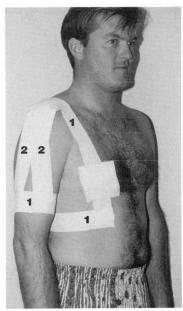

B

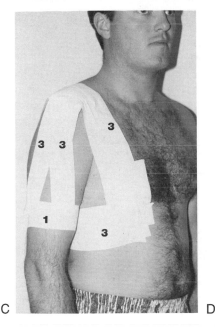

C

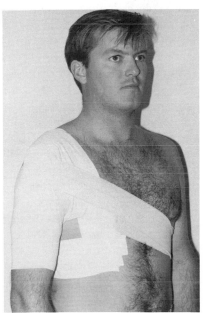

D

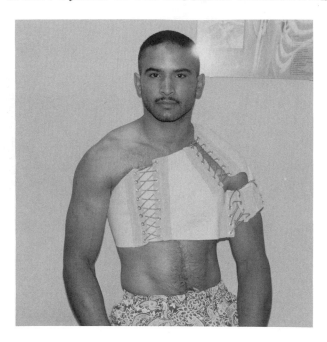

Fig. 20-28. Anterior instability brace/harness.

Football and Other Contact Sports

The most unique aspect of contact sports is the need for protection. Protection in the form of prevention is accomplished through the use of various sports equipment and padding as demonstrated in Fig. 20-26 for football. These devices protect the shoulder girdle and to some degree the cervical spine and brachial plexus. The other aspect of protection is for specific injuries that need taping or bracing to prevent further injury.

Acromioclavicular injuries are best protected with padding that is taped in place. Additional taping can add support to the acromioclavicular joint (Fig. 20-27). This taping usually consists of a basic basket weave approach stabilized and supported by a shoulder spica (figure eight Elasticon taping).

Anterior instability can be supported with taping or bracing. There are many forms of bracing with essentially the same feature of a restricting harness preventing excessive abduction external rotation (Fig. 20-28). Taping involves a figure eight approach either with the arm beginning in internal rotation behind the back or in a functional playing position (Fig. 20-29).

When handling on-the-field injuries it is often necessary to immobilize the shoulder until further evaluation or treatment is rendered. One common example is the Velpeau type of support (Fig. 20-30). Using an elastic ace bandage begin distally on the arm and proceed upward then circle around the shoulder and over the chest. Repeat the chest wrap twice followed by two sling supports under the forearm. Finish with two more wraps around the chest for stabilization.

Tennis

Tennis injuries can be minimized with proper racquet size, technique, and playing surface. Specific recommendations for prevention and rehabilitation of tennis injuries include a general shoulder exercise program as described previously plus the addition of elastic tubing resistance exercises. Figure 20-31 illustrates the use of elastic tubing resistance with each stroke. This functional training emphasizes mainly the concentric phase of activity.

Figure 20-32 demonstrates one example of bad form. A backhand is executed with a high shoulder and leading elbow. Both of these errors can contribute to both shoulder and elbow problems. Although with tennis the lower body contribution is significant to the production of force, other racquet sports such as racquetball utilize mainly arm and wrist activity due to the speed of the game.

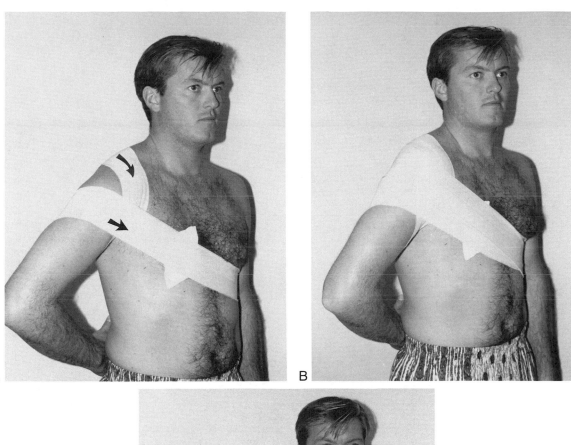

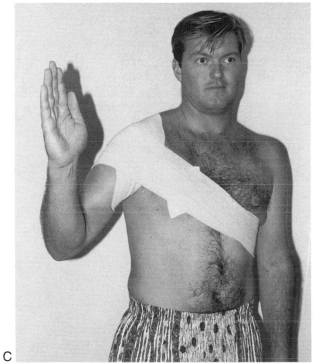

Fig. 20-29. Two approaches to restrictive taping for anterior instability. **(A)** Using 3 in Elasticon start at superior medial border of scapula. Wrap under shoulder and around chest. **(B)** Repeat 2 to 3 times. **(C)** Restriction of taping. (*Figure continues.*)

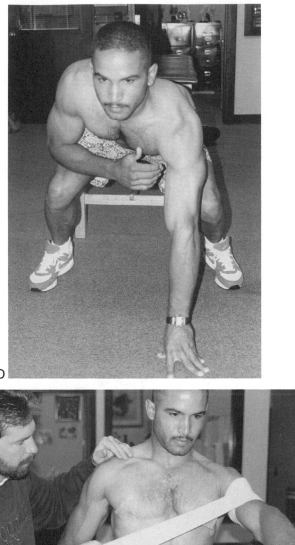

Fig. 20-29. (*Continued*). **(D)** Alternative method starts with athlete in functional position. **(E–H)** Same general approach. **(I)** Athlete supported in functional position. (*Figure continues.*)

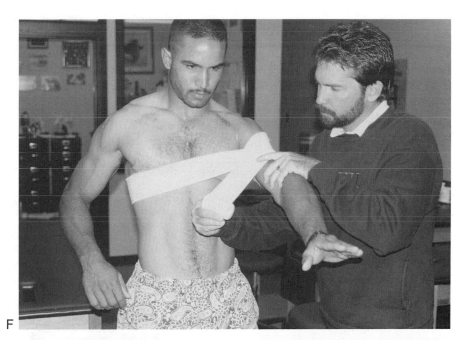

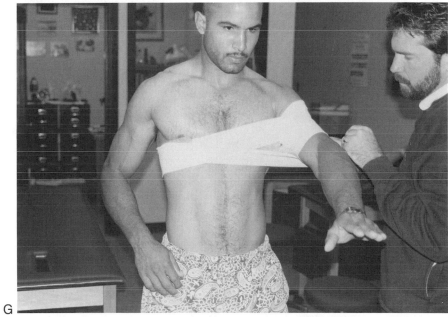

Fig. 20-29. (*Continues*).

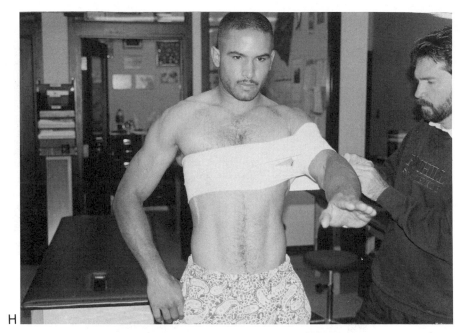

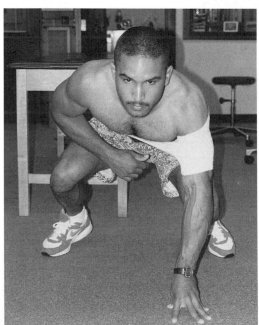

Fig. 20-29. (*Continued*).

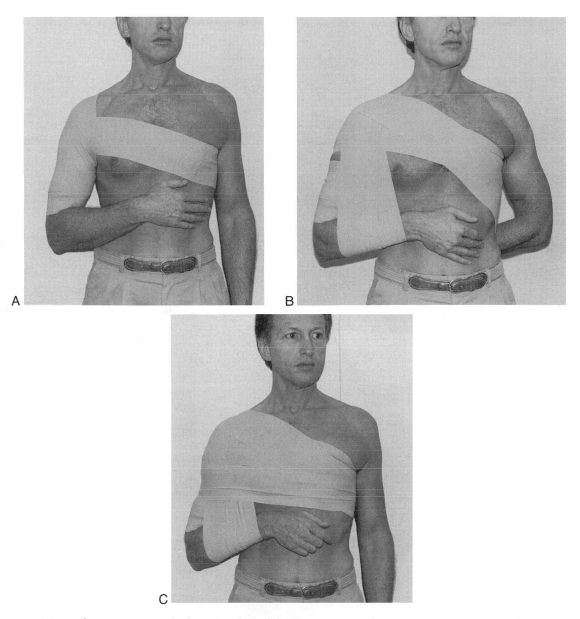

Fig. 20-30. Velpeau support with elastic bandage. **(A)** Wrap up arm and around chest. **(B)** Support forearm with two wraps. **(C)** Wrap around chest twice for stabilization.

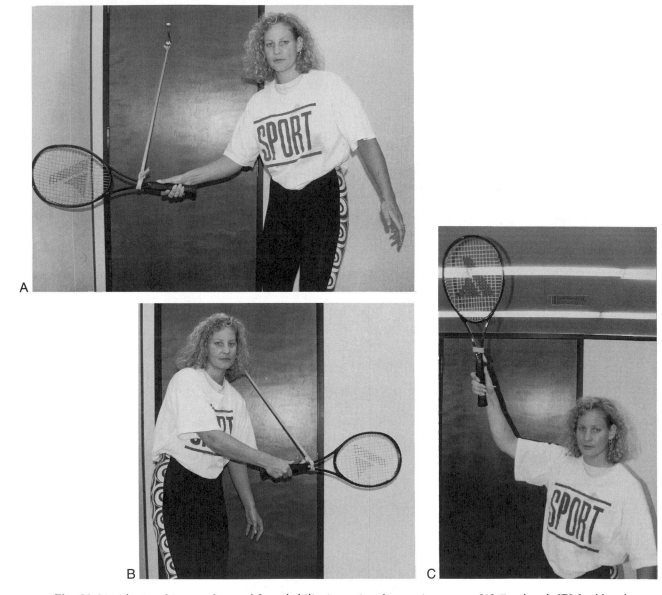

Fig. 20-31. Elastic tubing can be used for rehabilitation using the tennis racquet. **(A)** Forehand, **(B)** backhand, **(C)** the serve.

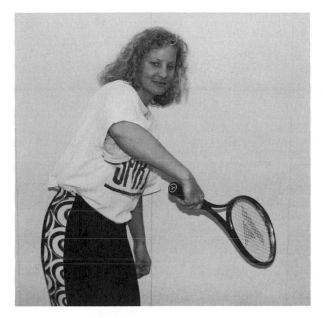

Fig. 20-32. Example of poor form leading with the elbow and elevating the shoulder.

SPECIAL CONCERNS FOLLOWING POSTSURGICAL REHABILITATION

There are a vast number of surgical procedures used for correction of a multitude of specific problems. However, by using some prototype examples of common surgical procedures, an outline of postsurgical rehabilitation is suggested.

Impingement and Rotator Cuff Tears

Following an unsuccessful attempt at conservative treatment for up to 24 weeks (depending on the specific lesion and activity requirement), surgery is often performed. Common procedures involve open and closed rotator cuff repair, and acromioplasty. Table 20-9 presents a general rehabilitation protocol for rotator cuff debridement, labral repair, or acromioplasty. Rehabilitation following a deltoid-on procedure for rotator cuff repair is given in Table 20-10.

Anterior Instability

Generally, surgical procedures for anterior instability are based on the requirements of the athlete following

Table 20-9. Protocol: Rotator Cuff Debridement, Labrum Tear, and Acromioplasty

I. Preoperative instructions
  A. Explain that the sling is used for the first day after surgery for comfort and that the athlete is then weaned out of it.
  B. Instruct in circumduction exercises, to be performed frequently.
  C. Explain about application of ice to shoulder at 20-minute intervals for pain and soreness.
II. Exercises[a]
  A. Initial phase: 2 to 7 days postoperatively
    1. Begin following exercises:
      a. Supine flexion
      b. Supine 90°–90° external rotation
      c. Supine 90°–90° internal rotation
      d. Supine abduction
      e. Horizontal adduction stretch
      f. Rope-and-pulley in abduction
      g. Rope-and-pulley in flexion
      h. Shoulder shrugs
    2. Goal: exercises above to be done 1 × 10, two times daily, progressing to 3 × 10. Expect soreness but do not discontinue. Reduce repetitions as needed.
    3. Use modalities as indicated for pain and inflammation.
  B. Intermediate phase: 7 to 10 days postoperatively
    1. Initiate the following active exercises after full active-assisted exercise is achieved:
      a. Shoulder flexion
      b. Shoulder abduction
      c. Supraspinatus
      d. Prone horizontal abduction
      e. Shoulder extension
      f. Prone external rotation
      g. Biceps curl
      h. Triceps or French curl
      i. Initiate PNF patterns for upper extremity, as tolerated
      j. Goal: begin with 3 × 10 as tolerated 2 or 3 times daily and progress to 5 × 10. When 5 × 10 is possible, begin adding weight 1 lb at a time, not to exceed 5 lb. Always work from 3 × 10, progressing to 5 × 10 before increasing weight.
    2. Continue stretching exercises that began day 2 postoperatively
  C. Advanced phase: week 3 postoperatively
    1. Continue exercise program with additional exercises:
      a. Sitting dip
      b. Progressive push-up
  D. Weeks 4 to 6 postoperatively
    1. Begin medium- to high-speed isokinetic work in all planes.
    2. Begin eccentric shoulder program, if indicated.
  E. Weeks 8 to 10 postoperatively
    1. Begin interval golf program, if indicated.
    2. Begin progressive resistance exercise (PRE) maintenance program.
  F. Weeks 12 to 16 postoperatively
    1. Begin interval tennis or throwing program, if indicated.
    2. Begin upper extremity plyometrics.

[a] Continually monitor daily for residual pain and effusion. If this occurs reduce program in frequency and intensity.
(From Harrelson,[69] with permission.)

Table 20-10. Rotator Cuff Repair: Deltoid-On Procedure

I. Immediate postoperative phase
  A. Postoperative day 1: Hospital discharge
    1. Patient immobilization (abduction pillow)
       Sling with arm placed at side of body or 45° to 60° of abduction with neutral rotation (position varies with severity of tear)
    2. ROM
       a. Passive ROM
       b. Rope and pulley
       c. T-bar exercises
       d. Pendulum exercises
       e. Gentle joint mobilization (grades I and II)
       f. Elbow, wrist, and hand ROM
       g. Cervical ROM exercises to deter neck stiffness
    3. Shoulder elevation, sagittal and scapular planes emphasized. Progress coronal elevation carefully.
       External rotation/internal rotation (begin 0° to 20° abduction).
    4. Strengthening
       a. Shoulder isometrics as tolerated
       b. Hand putty
    5. Decrease pain/inflammation
       a. Ice 15 to 20 minutes every hour
       b. Nonsteroidal antiinflammatory drugs
       c. Other modalities as needed
II. Early motion phase (postoperative day 4 to week 6)
  A. Hospital discharge to 3 weeks postsurgery
    1. Goals
       a. Increase ROM
       b. Decrease pain/inflammation
       c. Minimize muscular atrophy
    2. ROM
       a. Passive ROM (progress to active assisted ROM)
       b. Rope and pulley
       c. Shoulder flexion/extension to 90°
       d. Shoulder abduction to 90°
          • Shoulder flexion/extension
          • External rotation to tolerance with arm abducted to 35°
       f. Pendulum exercises
       g. Joint mobilization (grades I and II) to scapulothoracic, sternoclavicular, and acromioclavicular joints
       h. Continue elbow, wrist, and hand ROM
    3. Strengthening
       a. Isometrics (submaximal); may augment with electrical stimulation in flexion, abduction, external rotation, and internal rotation
       b. Hand putty
       c. Shoulder shrugs
    4. Decrease pain/inflammation
       a. Ice
       b. Other modalities as needed
  B. Weeks 3
    1. Goals
       a. Increase ROM
       b. Promote healing
       c. Regain and improve muscle strength
    2. ROM
       a. ROM exercises continued (progress external rotation/internal rotation ROM from 40° abduction to 90° abduction)
       b. Continue joint mobilization

    3. Strengthening
       a. Isometrics (submaximal to maximal)
       b. Continue shoulder shrugs
       c. Initiate elbow flexion/extension isotonics
       d. Initiate surgical tubing for external rotation/internal rotation at 30° abduction
    4. Promotion of healing
       a. Modalities as indicated
       b. Ice after treatment session
III. Intermediate phase (weeks 6 to 10)
    1. Goals
       a. Normalize ROM
       b. Normalize arthrokinematics
       c. Increase strength/endurance
    2. Criteria to progress to next phase
       a. Normal ROM
       b. Minimal pain/tenderness
       c. Manual muscle testing score of 4/5 in flexion, external rotation, internal rotation
  A. Week 6
    1. ROM
       a. Continue shoulder ROM exercises with T-bar
    2. Strength
       a. External/internal rotation with tubing
       b. Dumbbell isotonic exercises in shoulder flexion, abduction, extension, external rotation, and internal rotation
       c. Initiate upper body ergometer (UBE)
       d. Diagonal PNF patterns, manually
       e. Initiate neuromuscular control exercises
       f. Continue joint mobilization (advance grades)
    3. Decrease pain/inflammation
       a. Modalities as needed
  B. Weeks 8 and 9
       a. Continue ROM exercises
    1. Strength
       a. Continue isotonic/tubing exercises for rotator cuff/deltoid muscles
       b. Initiate empty can exercise
       c. Begin dumbbell program for scapular muscles
       d. Initiate wall push-ups for serratus anterior
       e. Continue PNF patterns
       f. Continue upper extremity endurance exercises
       g. Continue neuromuscular control exercises
    2. Decrease pain/inflammation
       a. Modalities as needed
       b. Ice after treatment session as needed
  C. Week 10 to month 4
       a. Advance all exercises to tolerance
IV. Advanced strengthening phase (months 4 to 6)
  A. Dynamic strengthening phase
    1. Goals
       a. Normalization of muscle strength/power/endurance
       b. Improve neuromuscular control
       c. Prepare patient/athlete to return to preinjury activity level
  B. Criteria to progress to phase IV
       a. Full, pain-free ROM
       b. No pain or tenderness
       c. Strength 70 to 80% vs contralateral side

(continues)

Table 20-10. *(continued).*

1. ROM
   a. Continue ROM exercises as needed to maintain full ROM
   b. Self capsular stretches
   c. T-bar (flexion, external rotation at 90°, internal rotation at 90°)
2. Strengthening
   a. Initiate tubing exercises
      (1) Diagonal patterns
      (2) Biceps
      (3) External/internal rotation
      (4) Scapulothoracic
   b. Initiate isokinetic exercises
   c. Continue isotonics
      (1) Deltoid
      (2) Supraspinatus
      (3) Triceps
   d. Continue PNF diagonals manually or with tubing
C. Month 5
   1. Strengthening
      a. Continue isokinetic exercises

b. Continue dumbbell program with emphasis on eccentrics and supraspinatus/deltoid muscles
c. Initiate plyometrics for rotator cuff (slow/fast sets, external rotation/internal rotation, 90/90)
d. Continue PNF diagonals with tubing or isokinetics
e. Medicine ball exercises (progress from below shoulder level to overhead)
f. Isokinetic testing (shoulder strength should be 80% before sport-specific activities are started)
2. Neuromuscular control
   a. Continue exercises for months 1 to 4
   b. Isokinetic examination fulfills criteria to throw
   c. Pass clinical examination
   d. No pain/tenderness
4. Initiate interval program
5. Upper extremity strengthening and stretching continued on a maintenance basis

(From Harrelson,[69] with permission.

surgery, the amount of damage, and the preference and expertise of the surgeon. There are two categories of procedures: (1) dynamic procedures, and (2) static procedures (Table 20-11). The dynamic procedures focus on stability through transfer of soft tissue and/or bone in an attempt to statically and dynamically reinforce the capsule. The static approaches attempt repair of capsular and labral damage and/or reattachment or tightening of the capsule. There is usually more residual restrictions in external rotation with the dynamic procedures. Therefore, it is sometimes suggested that the static procedures are more appropriate for the athlete. A protocol for rehabilitation of a dynamic (Bristow) procedure is presented in Table 20-12. Rehabilita-

tion following an anterior capsular shift is presented in Table 20-13.

Posterior Instability

The success of posterior repairs is not consistent. For this reason, most surgeons recommend a long-term conservative approach before considering surgery. The presence of a labrum tear will usually serve as a portent for surgery. The causes of recurrent posterior subluxation or dislocation vary. Based on the underlying pathology, various surgical approaches may be found to be more appropriate. Generally, there are three procedures used: (1) posterior capsulorrhaphy,

Table 20-11. Common Surgical Approaches to Anterior Instability

Dynamic Procedures

There are many variations of the following surgical techniques. The major disadvantage is the loss of external rotation ability, which averages between 10 and 20 degrees.

Bristow—The Bristow procedure involves transfer of the coracoid process to the glenoid. The entire coracoid with its tendon attachments is taken through the subscapularis muscle and attached with a screw to the glenoid in an attempt to provide a mechanical block to anterior movement.

Magnuson-Stack—The Magnuson-Stack procedure involves lateral transfer of the subscapularis tendon off of the lesser tubercle and across the bicipital groove onto the shaft of the humerus.

Putti-Platt—The Putti-Platt procedure involves various attempts to shorten the subscapularis tendon increasing the static and dynamic functions of this muscle/tendon to anterior stability.

Static Techniques

Static techniques are often preferred in treating athletes due to the loss of external rotation found with the dynamic techniques.

Bankart—The Bankart technique involves correction of a Bankart lesion with reattachment of the avulsed bone and capsule to the labrum.

Capsular Shift (capsulorrhaphy)—Various procedures have been developed to reattach or tighten the capsule.

Table 20-12. Protocol: Bristow Procedure

I. Preoperative instruction
  A. Explain that the sling is used for the first day after surgery for comfort, and then the athlete is weaned out of it.
  B. Instruct in circumduction and exercises (to be performed frequently).
  C. Explain about application of ice to shoulder at 20-minute intervals and as needed for pain and soreness.
  D. Explain rehabilitation progression.
II. Exercises
  A. Postoperative day 1
    1. Hand and elbow
      a. Putty
      b. Wrist ROM
      c. Elbow ROM
    2. Shoulder isometrics (with 0° shoulder adduction)
      a. Flexion
      b. Abduction
      c. Extension
      d. External rotation
      e. Internal rotation
    3. Shoulder ROM initiated as tolerated
      a. Circumduction ("saws, swings")
      b. Supine flexion
      c. Supine abduction
      d. Supine 0°–90° external rotation
      e. Supine 0°–90° internal rotation
      f. Supine horizontal adduction
      g. Rope-and-pulley in flexion and abduction
      h. Shoulder shrugs

    4. Gradually progress to 5 × 10, 2 or 3 times daily.
    5. Use ice pre- and postexercise for 20 minutes.
  B. Intermediate phase (weeks 2 to 8)
    1. Continue with above exercises twice daily.
    2. Add following exercises, as tolerated:
      a. External rotation stretch in 90–90° position, as tolerated
      b. Upper body ergometer (UBE)
      c. Shoulder flexion
      d. Shoulder abduction
      e. Supraspinatus
      f. Prone horizontal abduction
      g. Prone shoulder extension
      h. Prone external rotation
      i. Shoulder shrugs
      j. Biceps curl
      k. Triceps extension
      l. Rope-and-pulley in flexion and abduction, as tolerated.
    3. May progress PRE, as tolerated.
    4. Continue flexibility at 10 to 20 repetitions.
  C. Advanced phase (months 2 to 3)
    1. If progressing well, decrease program to maintenance 3 times weekly.
    2. Begin progressive return to functional weightlifting and activities.
    3. Begin eccentric shoulder program and isokinetics.
    4. Begin upper extremity plyometrics.
    5. Begin appropriate interval activity program, if appropriate.

(From Harrelson,[69] with permission.

Table 20-13. Protocol: Anterior Capsular Shift

I. Preoperative instructions
  A. Explain that athlete must wear immobilizer to sleep for 4 weeks, and then the athlete will be out of the immobilizer into a sling during the daytime as soon as possible. The sling should be used for 3 to 4 weeks.
  B. Stress no overhead activity for 6 weeks.
  C. Discuss rehabilitation program and progression.
II. Phase I (weeks 0 to 6)
  A. Weeks 0 to 2
    1. Use modalities (e.g., ice, electrical stimulation) for pain.
    2. Immediate postoperative hand and elbow exercises:
      a. Gripping with putty
      b. Wrist ROM
      c. Elbow ROM
      d. Goal: obtain full wrist and elbow ROM on first postoperative day.
    3. Initiate following exercises:
      a. Pendulum
      b. Rope-and-pulley, active assisted
        (1) Shoulder flexion to 90°
        (2) Shoulder abduction to 60°
      c. T-bar exercises
        (1) External rotation to 45° with arm abducted at 40°
        (2) Shoulder flexion and extension
        (3) Active ROM—cervical spine

        (4) Isometrics
          (a) Flexion
          (b) Extension
          (c) Abduction
          (d) External rotation
          (e) Internal rotation
      d. Goal: 90° flexion, 45° abduction, 45° external rotation, active assisted
  B. Weeks 2 to 4
    1. All exercises performed to tolerance—take to point of pain and/or resistance and hold.
    2. Exercises:
      a. External rotation to 60° with 90° of shoulder abduction with T-bar
      b. Internal rotation to 65° with 90° of shoulder abduction with T-bar
      c. Shoulder flexion and extension to tolerance with T-bar
      d. Shoulder abduction to tolerance with T-bar
      e. Shoulder horizontal abduction and adduction with T-bar
      f. Rope-and-pulley in flexion and abduction, as tolerated
      g. Continue isometrics
      h. External and internal rotation with tubing at 0° shoulder abduction

(continues)

Table 20-13. *(continued)*

3. Begin PRE with elbow program.
4. Begin joint mobilization techniques.
  C. Weeks 4 to 6
    1. Continue all exercises listed above to tolerance, except:
      a. External rotation to 75° at 90° of shoulder abduction with T-bar
      b. External rotation to 40° at 30° of shoulder abduction
      c. Internal rotation to 80° at 90° of shoulder abduction
III. Phase II (weeks 6 to 10)
  A. Weeks 6 to 8
    1. ROM exercises:
      a. Continue all T-bar exercises listed above.
      b. Gradually increase ROM to full ROM by week 8.
    2. Begin strengthening exercises (progress 0 to 5 lb):
      a. Shoulder flexion
      b. Shoulder abduction
      c. Supraspinatus
      d. Prone extension
      e. Prone horizontal abduction
      f. Prone horizontal abduction at 100°
      g. Side-lying external rotation
      h. Biceps curls
      i. Triceps curls
      j. Shoulder shrugs
      k. Progressive push-ups

  l. Continue tubing at 0° of abduction for external and internal rotation
    3. Begin neuromuscular control exercises for scapular stabilizers.
  B. Weeks 8 to 10
    1. Continue all ROM and strengthening exercises listed above.
    2. Initiate tubing exercises for rhomboids, latissimus dorsi, biceps, and triceps.
IV. Phase III (weeks 11 to 16)
  A. Weeks 11 to 13
    1. Continue PRE program.
    2. Continue tubing program.
    3. Begin shoulder eccentric program.
    4. Begin tubing in diagonal patterns.
    5. Begin isokinetic exercise, as tolerated.
    6. Initiate high-speed tubing exercise, as tolerated.
  B. Weeks 14 to 16
    1. Continue all exercises above.
    2. Emphasize gradual return to recreational activities.
Phase IV (weeks 18 to 26)
  A. Maintenance PRE, tubing, and ROM programs
  B. Isokinetic testing (18 to 20 weeks)
  C. Begin interval programs between weeks 20 and 24.

(From Harrelson,[69] with permission).

(2) posteroinferior capsular shift, and (3) posterior glenoid osteotomy. If the patient has a unidirectional instability with normal bony morphology, it is recommended that a posterior capsulorrhaphy be performed. If there is excessive glenoid retroversion the glenoid osteotomy is recommended.[65]

With recalcitrant multidirectional instability Bigliani[66] has developed the inferior capsular shift procedure. With this procedure and the above posterior instability procedures, caution should be used in attempting forward flexion too early.

REFERENCES

1. Townsend H, Jobe FW, Pink M, Perry J: Electromyographic analysis of the glenohumeral muscles during a baseball rehabilitation program. Am J Sports Med 19:264, 1991
2. Belle RM, Hawkins RJ: Dynamic electromyographic analysis of the shoulder muscles during rotational and scapular strengthening exercises. In Post M, Morrey BF, Hawkins RS (eds): Surgery of the Shoulder. CV Mosby, St. Louis, 1990
3. Jobe FW, Moynes DR: Delineation of diagnostic criteria and a rehabilitation program for rotator cuff injuries. Am J Sports Med 10:336, 1982
4. Blackburn TA, McLeod WD, White B, Wofford L: EMG analysis of posterior rotator cuff exercises. Athl Train 25:40, 1990
5. Worrell TW, Corey BJ, York SL, Santiestaban A: An analysis of supraspinatus EMG activity and shoulder isometric force development. Med Sci Sports Exerc 24:744, 1992
6. Pappas AM, Zawacki RM, McCarthy CF: Rehabilitation of the pitching shoulder. Am J Sports Med 13:223, 1985
7. Moseley JB Jr, Jobe FW, Pink M et al: EMG analysis of the scapular muscles during a shoulder rehabilitation program. Am J Sports Med 20:128, 1992
8. Gowan ID, Jobe FW, Tibone JE et al: A comparative electromyographic analysis of the shoulder during pitching: professional versus amateur pitchers. Am J Sports Med 15:586, 1987
9. Glousman R, Jobe FW, Tibone JE et al: Dynamic electromyographic analysis of the throwing shoulder with glenohumeral instability. J Bone Joint Surg 70A:220, 1988
10. Miller L, Jobe FW, Moynes DR et al: EMG analysis of shoulders in throwers with subacromial impingement.

Unpublished study. Biomechanics Laboratory, Centinela Hospital, Inglewood, CA, 1985

11. Inman VT, Saunders JR, Abbott LC: Observations on the function of the shoulder joint. J Bone Joint Surg 26:1, 1944

12. Jobe FW, Tibone JE, Perry J, Moynes D: An EMG analysis of the shoulder in throwing and pitching: a preliminary report. Am J Sports Med 11:3, 1983

13. Toyoshima S, Hoskikawa T, Miyashita M et al: Contribution of the body parts to throwing performance. p. 169. In Nelson RC, Morehouse CA (eds): Biomechanics IV. University Park Press, Baltimore, 1974

14. Jobe FW, Moynes DR, Tibone JE, Perry J: An EMG analysis of the shoulder in pitching: a second report. Am J Sports Med 12:218, 1984

15. Pink M, Perry J, Browne A et al.: The normal shoulder during freestyle swimming: an electromyographic and cinematographic anlaysis of twelve muscles. Am J Sports Med 19:569, 1991

16. Scovazzo ML, Browne A, Pink M et al: The painful during freestyle swimming: an electromyographic cinematographic analysis of twelve muscles. Am J Sports Med 19:577, 1991

17. Garrett WE: Basic science of musculotendinous injuries. p. 42. In Nicholas JA, Hershman EB (eds): The Lower Extremity and Spine in Sports Medicine. CV Mosby, St. Louis, 1986

18. Grace TG, Sweetsser ER, Nelson MA et al: Isokinetic muscle imbalance and knee joint injuries. J Bone Joint Surg 66A:734, 1984

19. Albert M: Eccentric Muscle Training in Sports and Orthopaedics. Churchill Livingstone, New York, 1991

20. Effman H: Biomechanics of muscle. J Bone Joint Surg 48:363, 1966

21. Abbott BC, Aubert XM, Hill AV: The absorption of work by a muscle stretched during a single twitch or a short tetanus. Proc R Soc B 139:86, 1951

22. Cavanagh PR, Komi PV: Electro-chemical delay in human skeletal muscle under concentric and eccentric contractions. Eur J Appl Physiol 42:159, 1979

23. Knuttgen HG, Patton JF, Vogel JA: An ergometer for concentric and eccentric muscular exercise. J Appl Physiol 53:784, 1982

24. Davies CTM, Barnes C: Negative (eccentric) work: physiological responses to walking uphill and downhill on a motordriven treadmill. Ergonomics 15:121, 1972

25. Bigland-Ritchie B, Woods JJ: Integrating electromyogram and oxygen uptake during positive and negative work. J Physiol 260:267, 1976

26. Mannheimer JS: A comparison of strength gain between concentric and eccentric contractions. Phys Ter 49:1207, 1969

27. Johnson BL, Adamczyk JW: A program of eccentric-concentric strength training. Am Correct Ther J 29:16, 1975

28. Curwin S, Stanish W: Tendonitis: Its Etiology and Treatment. DC Heath & Co, Lexington, KY, 1985

29. Trudelle-Jackson E, Meske N, Highgenboten HH, Jackson A: Eccentric/concentric torque deficits in the quadriceps muscle. J Orthop Sports Phys Ther 11:144, 1989

30. Ng LR, Kramer JS: Shoulder rotator torques in female tennis and nontennis players. J Orthop Sports Phys Ther 13:40, 1991

31. Frances KT: Delayed muscle soreness: a review. J Orthop Sports Phys Ther 5:10, 1983

32. Assumssen E: Observations on experimental muscle soreness. Acta Rheumatol Scand 1:109, 1956

33. Schwane J, Johnson S, Vandermakker C, Armstrong R: Blood markers of delayed-onset muscle soreness with downhill treadmill running. Med Sci Sports Exerc 13:80, 1981

34. Waltrous B, Armstrong R, Schwane J: The role of lactic acid in delayed onset muscular distress. Med Sci Sports Exerc 13:80, 1981

35. deVries HA: Prevention of muscular distress after exercise. Res Q 32:177, 1961

36. Abraham WM: Factors in delayed muscle soreness. Med Sci Sports Exerc 9:11, 1977

37. Abraham WM: Exercise induced muscle soreness. Phys Sports Med 7:57, 1959

38. Friden J, Sjostrom M, Ekblom B: A morphological study of delayed muscle soreness. Experientia 37:506, 1981

39. Chu D, Plummer L: The language of plyometrics. Natl Strength Cond Assoc J 6:30, 1984

40. Wilt F: Plyometrics-what it is and how it works. Athl J 55B:76, 1975

41. Verhoshanski Y, Chormonson G: Jump exercises in sprint training. Track Field Q 9:1909, 1967

42. Kabat H: Proprioceptive facilitation in therapeutic exercise. In Licht S (ed): Therapeutic Exercise. Williams & Wilkins, Baltimore 1965

43. Sherrington C: Integrator Activity of the Nervous System. Yale University Press, New Haven, CT, 1960

44. Pavlov T: Conditioned Reflexes. Oxford University Press, London, 1927

45. Gesell G, Amatruda C: The Embryology of Behavior. Harper and Brothers, New York, 1945

46. Coghill G: Anatomy of the Problem of Behavior. Macmillan, New York, 1942

47. Gellborne E: Proprioception and the motor cortex. Brain 12:35, 1949

48. Knott M, Voss DF: Proprioceptive Neuromuscular Facilitation: Patterns and Techniques. Paul B. Haeber, New York, 1956

49. Sullivan PE, Markos PD, Minor MAD: An Integrated Ap-

proach to Therapeutic Exercise: Theory & Clinical Application. Reston Publishing Co, Reston, VA, 1982

50. Sullivan PE, Portney LG: Electromyographic activity of shoulder muscles during unilateral upper extremity proprioceptive neuromuscular facilitation patterns. Phys Ther 60:283, 1980

51. Janda DH, Loubert P: A preventative program focusing on the glenohumeral joint. Clin Sports Med 10:955, 1991

52. Guissard N, Duchateau J, Hainaut K: Muscle stretching and motor neuron excitability. Eur J Appl Phys 58:47, 1988

53. Kametzke CA: The effects of dynamic range of motion exercises and static stretching on strength and range of motion of the hip joints. Master's Thesis. South Dakota State University, SD, 1983

54. Wallin D, Ekblom B, Grahn R, Nordenborg T: Improvement of muscle flexibility: a comparison of two techniques. Am J Sports Med 13:263, 1985

55. Osternig LR, Robertson RN, Troxel RK, Hansen P: Differential response to proprioceptive neuromuscular facilitation (PNF) stretch techniques. Med Sci Sports Exerc 22:106, 1990

56. Brostrom LA, Kromberg M, Nemeth G, Oxelback U: The effect of shoulder muscle training in patients with recurrent shoulder dislocations. Scand J Rehab Med 24:11, 1992

57. Matveyev L: Periodisierang des sportichen training. Berlin Berles & Wemitz.

58. Kerlan JK et al: Throwing injuries of the shoulder and elbow in adults. Curr Pract Orthop Surg 6:41, 1975

59. Greene CP: Spring training conditioning for the throwing shoulder. p. 261. In Zarin B, Andrews JR, Carson WG (eds): Injuries of the Throwing Arm. WB Saunders, Philadelphia, 1985

60. Watkins RG, Dennis S, Dillin WH et al: Dynamic EMG analysis of torque transfer in professional baseball pitchers. Spine 14:404, 1989

61. Greipp JF. Swimmer's shoulder: the influence of flexibility and weight training. Phys Sports Med 13:92, 1985

62. Ciullo JV, Guise ER: Adolescent swimmer's shoulder. Orthop Trans 7:171, 1983

63. Fowler PJ, Webster MS: Shoulder pain in highly competitive swimmers. Orthop Trans 7:170, 1983

64. Fowler PJ: Upper extremity swimming injuries. p. 893. In Nicholas JA, Hershman EB (eds): The Upper Extremity in Sports Medicine. CV Mosby, St. Louis, 1990

65. Bell RH, Noble JS: An appreciation of posterior instability of the shoulder. Clin Sports Med 10:887, 1991

66. Bigliani LU: Multidirectional instability. In: 1990 Advances on the Knee and Shoulder. Cincinnati, 1990

67. Auferoth F: Power training for the developing thrower. Nat Strength Cond Assoc J 8:740, 1986

68. Uebel R: Weight training for swimmers: a practical approach. Natl Strength Cond Assoc J 9:739, 1987

69. Harrelson GL: Shoulder rehabilitation. p. 402. In Andrews J, Harrelson GL (eds): Physical Rehabilitation of the Injured Athelete. WB Saunders, Philadelphia, 1992

70. Kirkendall DJ: Mobility: conditioning programs. p. 726. In Gould JA III, Davies GJ (eds): Orthopedic and Sports Physical Therapy. CV Mosby, St. Louis, 1990

Periodization Model for Track Throwers*

Variable Weight Throwing Program

SEP	OCT	NOV	DEC	JAN	FEB	MAR	APR	MAY	JUN	JUL	AUG

60% Heavy & 40-% Light

60% Light & 40% Heavy

40% Heavy & 60% Normal

100% Normal

Sample Workout for Basic-Strength Cycle

Monday
Warm-up with flexibility exercises: 10–15 min
Light throwing: 30–45 min
  use light and heavy implements
Weightlifting: 60–90 min
  emphasis on absolute strength
Warm-down: 10–15 min

Tuesday
Warm-up with flexibility exercises: 10–15 min
Medium to heavy throwing: 60–70 min
Plyometrics: 20–30 min
  low hurdle hopping: 3–8 hurdles
  double leg bounding: 20–30 meters
Warm-down 10–15 min

Wednesday
Warm-up with flexibility exercises: 10–15 min
Weightlifting: 45–60 min
Warm-down: 10–15 min

Thursday
Warm-up with flexibility exercises: 10–15 min
Easy technique drills: 15–30 min
Wind sprints, 75–85% intensity, full recovery: 30–40 min
  60 to 80 meters
Warm-down and restorative methods: 10–15 min

Friday
Warm-up with flexibility exercises: 10–15 min
Weightlifting: 60–90 min
Warm-down: 10–15 min

Saturday
Warm-up with flexibility exercises: 10–15 min
Medium to heavy throwing:45–60 min
  light and normal implements
Plyometrics: 20–30 min
  alternate leg bounding: 20 to 30 meters
Warm-down: 10–15 min

Sunday
Active rest

Totals for week
Warm-up and warm-down = 60–115 min
Throwing = 135–175 min
Technique drills = 15–30 min
Weightlifting = 165–240 min
Plyometrics = 40–60 min
Wind sprints = 30–40 min

Sample Workout for Strength-Power Cycle

Monday
Warm-up with flexibility exercises: 10–15 min
Light throwing: 30–45 min
  heavy and normal implements
Weightlifting: 60–90 min
  emphasis on absolute power
Warm-down: 10–15 min

Tuesday
Warm-up with flexibility exercises: 10–15 min
Medium throwing: 45–60 min
Plyometrics: 15–30 min
  double and single leg bounding: 30–40 meters
Warm-down: 10–15 min

Wednesday
Warm-up with flexibility exercises: 10–15 min
Technique drills: 45 min
Wind sprints, 80–90% intensity, full recovery: 25–35 min
  50 to 60 meters
Warm-down and restorative methods: 10–15 min

Thursday
Warm-up with flexibility exercises: 10–15 min
Weightlifting: 70–100 min
Warm-down: 10–15 min

Friday
Warm-up with flexibility exercises: 10–15 min
Medium throwing: 30–45 min
  normal implement
Plyometrics: 20–30 min
  alternate leg bounding: 30–40 meters
Warm-down: 10–15 min

Saturday
Warm-up with flexibility exercises: 10–15 min
Weightlifting: 45–60 min
Warm-down: 10–15 min

Sunday
Active rest

Totals for week
Warm-up and warm-down = 60–115 min
Throwing = 105–150 min
Technique drills = 45 min
Weightlifting = 175–250 min
Plyometrics = 35–60 min
Wind sprints = 25–35 min

*From Auferoth,[67] with permission.

Sample Workout for Competition Cycle	
Early Competitive	Late Competitive

Early Competitive

Monday
Warm-up with flexibility exercises: 10–15 min
Weightlifting: 60–90 min
  emphasis on explosive power
Technique drills: 30 min
Warm-down: 10–15 min

Tuesday
Warm-up with flexibility exercises: 10–15 min
Hard throwing: 45–60 min
  95% normal, 5% light implements
Hill sprinting: 20–30 min
  30 to 40 meters
Warm-down: 10–15 min

Wednesday
Warm-up with flexibility exercises: 10–15 min
Technique drills: 30–45 min
Warm-down: 10–15 min

Thursday
Warm-up with flexibility exercises: 10–15 min
Throwing: 15–30 min
  4 hard stands
  6 all out throws
Light explosive lifting: 30–45 min
Warm-down: 10–15 min

Friday
Warm-up with flexibility exercises: 10–15 min
Technique drills: 10–15 min
Wind sprints: 10–15 min
  10 to 15 meters
Warm-down: 10–15 min

Saturday
Competition

Sunday
Warm-up with flexibility exercises: 10–15 min
Throwing: 30–45 min
  normal implement
Wind sprints: 15–20 min
  20 to 30 meters
Warm-down: 10–15 min

Totals for week
Warm-up and warm-down = 60–115 min
Throwing = 95–135 min
Technique drills = 70–90 min
Weightlifting = 90–135 min
Plyometrics = 0
Wind sprints = 45–65 min

Late Competitive

Monday
Warm-up with flexibility exercises: 10–15 min
Medium to hard throwing: 30–45 min
Wind sprints: 20–30 min
  10 to 30 meters
Warm-down: 10–15 min

Tuesday
Warm-up with flexibility exercises: 10–15 min
Technique drills: 20–30 min
Warm-down: 10–15 min

Wednesday
Warm-up with flexibility exercises: 10–15 min
Weightlifting: 45–60 min
  very explosive lifting
Warm-down: 10–15 min

Thursday
Warm-up with flexibility exercises: 10–15 min
Easy throwing: 15–20 min
  emphasis on technique only
Wind sprints: 10–15 min
  10 to 15 meters
Warm-down: 10–15 min

Friday
Warm-up with flexibility exercises: 10–15 min
Throwing: competitive situation
  3 to 4 stands
  3 all out competitive throws: the athlete must be able to achieve
    a good mark in the first three in order to make the finals.
Warm-down: 10–15 min

Saturday
Competition

Sunday
Warm-up with flexibility exercises: 10–15 min
Light lifting, throwing, or both or active rest: 30–45 min
Warm-down: 10–15 min

Totals for week
Warm-up and warm-down = 60–115 min
Throwing = 65–90 min
Technique drills = 20–30 min
Weightlifting = will vary
Plyometrics = 0
Wind sprints = 30–45 min

Power Training Schedule/General Guidelines							
September (60–70%)		**December (80–85%)**		**March (60–85%)**	
Exercise	*sets × reps*	*Exercise*	*sets × reps*	*Exercise*	*sets × reps*
Back squat	3 × 10	Back squat	4 × 5	Power clean	10·7·5·5·7
Dead lift	3 × 10	Front squat	4 × 5	Push press	10·7·5·5·7
Bench press	3 × 10	Incline bench	4 × 5	Incline bench	10·7·5·5·7
Military press	3 × 10	Power clean	4 × 5	Back squat	10·7·5·5·7
Tricep extension	3 × 10	Bench press	4 × 5	Incline sit-ups	5 × 20
Power clean	3 × 10	Russian twists	5 × 15	**April (85–100%)**	
Arm curls	3 × 10	Good mornings	3 × 20	Reduce second workout	
Russian twists[a]	3 × 10	**January (70–75%)**		by 25 lb	
October (75–90%)		*Exercise*	*sets × reps*	*Exercise*	*sets × reps*
Exercise	*sets × reps*	Front squat	4 × 7	(Twice weekly)	
Back squat	6·5·4·3·2	Leg press	4 × 7	Power clean	5·4·3·2·1
Dead lift	6·5·4·3·2	Incline bench	4 × 7	Jerk from rack	5·4·3·2·1
Incline bench	6·5·4·3·2	Power clean and jerk	4 × 7	Bench press	5·4·3·2·1
Power clean	6·5·4·3·2	Tricep extension	4 × 7	Back squat	5·4·3·2·1
Russian twists	4 × 10	Twisting sit-ups	4 × 20	Russian twists	4 × 20 fast
November (70–75%)		Good mornings	3 × 10	**May (85–100%)**	
Exercise	*sets × reps*	**February (90–95%)**		Reduce second workout	
Back squat	4 × 8	*Exercise*	*sets × reps*	by 35 lb	
Leg press	4 × 8	Power clean	5 × 3	*Exercise*	*sets × reps*
Bench press	4 × 8	Back squat	5 × 3	(First week)	
Push press	4 × 8	Bench press	5 × 3	Power clean	5·3·2·1
Tricep extension	4 × 8	Jerk from rack	5 × 3	Incline bench	5·3·2·1
Power clean	4 × 8	Russian twists	4 × 20	Back squat	5·3·2·1
Incline sit-ups	4 × 20	Good mornings	3 × 20	Incline sit-ups	3 × 20
Good mornings[b]	3 × 15	(Second week)		(Third week)	
(Fourth week) 1st workout		Reduce second workout		Reduce second workout	
Power clean	2 × 2 (95%)	by 45 lb		by 60 lb	
Incline bench	2 × 2 (95%)	Power clean	5·3·2·1	Power clean	4·2·1
2nd workout		Bench press	5·3·2·1	Incline bench	4·2·1
Power clean	1 × 2 (95%)	Back squat	5·3·2·1	Back squat	4·2·1
Incline bench	1 × 2 (95%)	Russian twists	3 × 20	Russian twists	2 × 20

[a] Russian twists: see Sports Fitness May: 111–112, 1985.
[b] Good mornings: see Nat Strength Cond Assoc J, 7(5):79, 1985.

Appendix 1
International Classification of Diseases Codes for the Shoulder

353.0	Thoracic outlet syndrome
718.31	Chronic (recurrent) dislocation
723.3	Cervicobrachial syndrome
723.4	Brachial neuritis
723.4	Cervical radiculitis
726.0	Adhesive capsulitis
726.0	Tendinitis (specify)
726.11	Calcific tendinitis
726.12	Bicipital tenosynovitis
726.19	Subdeltoid bursitis
726.2	Impingement syndrome
727.61	Rotator cuff rupture
729.1	Myofascitis (trigger points)
831.01	Anterior dislocation
831.02	Posterior dislocation
831.04	Acromioclavicular separation (specify degree)
840.4	Rotator cuff tear

Appendix 2
Shoulder Examination

Observation			Palpation	
	R	L	*(Indicate on Diagram)*	(Draw diagram here)
Head Tilt	___	___	Tenderness ___	
Shoulder High	___	___	*(Describe)*	
Deformities	___	___	Trigger Points ___	
Carrying Angle	___	___	*(Describe)* ___	
Atrophy	___	___	___	
Scars	___	___	Swelling ___	
Dermal Lesions	___	___	___	

Reflexes			Measurements			Dermatomes/Peripheral Nerve		
	R	L		R	L		R	L
Biceps	___	___	Biceps	___	___	Level(s)	___	___
Brachioradialis	___	___	Elbow	___	___	Hypo	___	___
Triceps	___	___				Hyper	___	___

Range of Motion

Movement	R	Rest. A	Pn	Rest. P	Pn	Lax	L	Rest. A	Pn	Rest. P	Pn	Lax
Flexion	___	___	___	___	___	___		___	___	___	___	___
Extension	___	___	___	___	___	___		___	___	___	___	___
Ext. Rot. (side)	___	___	___	___	___	___		___	___	___	___	___
Ext. Rot. (abd)	___	___	___	___	___	___		___	___	___	___	___
Int. Rot. (side)	___	___	___	___	___	___		___	___	___	___	___
Int. Rot. (abd)	___	___	___	___	___	___		___	___	___	___	___
Abduction	___	___	___	___	___	___		___	___	___	___	___
Scaption	___	___	___	___	___	___		___	___	___	___	___
Horizontal Add.	___	___	___	___	___	___		___	___	___	___	___
Horizontal Abd.	___	___	___	___	___	___		___	___	___	___	___
Scapula Protrac.	___	___	___	___	___	___		___	___	___	___	___
Scapula Retrac.	___	___	___	___	___	___		___	___	___	___	___

Abduction Findings

Painful Arc (circle) R Active Passive ___ L Active Passive ___   Range ___   Range ___

	R	L		R	L
Hesitation Sign	___	___	Capsular Pattern	___	___
Scapulothoracic			Non-Capsular Pattern	___	___
Rhythm	___	___	Describe		
Antalgic Lift	___	___	Crepitus ___		

Notes ___
___
___
___
___
___

Accessory Motion

AC Joint	R	L
A-P		
Inf.-Sup.	___	___
SC Joint		
A-P		
Sup.-Inf.	___	___
Scapula		
GH Joint		
P-A		
Lat.	___	___
Lat.-Inf.	___	___
A-P	___	___
Circumduc.	___	

Legend: Pn = Pain   Lax = Laxity   Rest = Restricted   AC = Acromioclavicular   SC = Sternoclavicular   GH = Glenohumeral   R = Right   L = Left   A = Active   P = Passive

General Impingement Tests

	R	L
Painful Arc	_____	_____
Passive Forward Flexion (Neer's)	_____	_____
Int. Rotation at 90 Deg. Abd	_____	_____
Locking Maneuver	_____	_____

Specific Muscle Tests *(Indicate Grade and if Pain)*

	R	L
Supraspinatus		
Empty Can	_____	_____
Stretch	_____	_____
Infrapsinatus/Teres Minor		
Muscle Test	_____	_____
Stretch	_____	_____
Subscapularis		
Muscle Test	_____	_____
Stretch	_____	_____
Lift Test	_____	_____
Biceps		
Speed's	_____	_____
Stretch	_____	_____
Yergason's	_____	_____
Abbott-Saunders	_____	_____
Booth-Marvel	_____	_____
Gilcrest's	_____	_____
Ludington's	_____	_____
Lippman's	_____	_____
Deltoid		
Anterior	_____	_____
Middle	_____	_____
Posterior	_____	_____
Pectoralis Major	_____	_____
Pectoralis Minor	_____	_____
Latissimus Dorsi	_____	_____
Serratus Anterior	_____	_____
Teres Major	_____	_____
Trapezius	_____	_____
Rhomboids	_____	_____

Instability Tests

Load & Shift	R Ant	Post	Inf	L Ant	Post	Inf
Seated	_____			_____		
45 Deg Lean	_____			_____		
Sup	_____			_____		

	R	L
Apprehension	_____	_____
Anterior Drawer	_____	_____
Posterior	_____	_____
Relocation Test	_____	_____
Feagen	_____	_____
Voluntary Dislocation	_____	_____
Other	_____	

Glenoid Labrum Tests

	R	L
Clunk Test	_____	_____
Kocher Maneuver	_____	_____

AC Tests

	R	L
Sulcus Sign	_____	_____
Shultz	_____	_____
End-range		
Horiz. Add.	_____	_____
Abduction	_____	_____
Compress./Distract.	_____	_____

Thoracic Outlet Tests

	R	L
Adson's	_____	_____
Halstead's	_____	_____
Wright's	_____	_____
Roos	_____	_____

Bursal Tests

	R	L
Palpation with extension (Prone)	___	___
Dawbarn's	___	___

Cervical Screening

Range of Motion	RA	RP	Pn	LA	LP	Pn
Flexion	—	—	—	—	—	—
Extension	—	—	—	—	—	—
Lateral Bending	—	—	—	—	—	—
Rotation	—	—	—	—	—	—

Comments _____

Orthopedic Tests

	R	L
Compression	___	___
Distraction	___	___
Shoulder Depres.	___	___
Soto-Hall	___	___
Valsalva	___	___
George's	___	___

Accessory Motion

Segments	O-C1	C1-C2	C3-C4	C4-C5	C5-C6	C6-C7	C7-T1
R	___	___	___	___	___	___	___
L	___	___	___	___	___	___	___

Notes _____

Appendix 3
American Shoulder and Elbow Surgeons Shoulder Evaluation Form*

Name _____ Hosp. # _____ Date _____ Shoulder: R/L

I. <u>PAIN</u>: (5 = none, 4 = slight, 3 = after unusual activity, 2 = moderate, 1 = marked, 0 = complete disability, NA = not available) _____

II. <u>MOTION</u>:
  A. Patient Sitting
    1. Active total elevation of arm: _____ degrees*
    2. Passive internal rotation:
      (Circle segment of posterior anatomy reached by thumb)
      (Note if reach restricted by limited elbow flexion)

1 = less than trochanter	5 = L5	9 = L1	13 = T9	17 = T5
2 = Trochanter	6 = L4	10 = T12	14 = T8	18 = T4
3 = Gluteal	7 = L3	11 = T11	15 = T7	19 = T3
4 = Sacrum	8 = L2	12 = T10	16 = T6	20 = T2

    3. Active external rotation with arm at side: _____ degrees
    4. Active external rotation at 90° abduction: _____ degrees
      (Enter "NA" if cannot achieve 90° of abduction)

  B. Patient Supine:
    1. Passive total elevation of arm: _____ degrees*
    2. Passive external rotation with arm at side: _____ degrees

*Total elevation of arm measured by viewing patient from side and using goniometer to determine angle between <u>arm</u> and <u>thorax</u>.

III. <u>STRENGTH</u>: (5 = normal, 4 = good, 3 = fair, 2 = poor, 1 = trace, 0 = paralysis)

  A. Anterior deltoid _____   C. External rotation _____
  B. Middle deltoid _____   D. Internal rotation _____

IV. <u>STABILITY</u>: (5 = normal, 4 = apprehension, 3 = rare subluxation, 2 = recurrent subluxation, 1 = recurrent dislocation, 0 = fixed dislocation, NA = not available)

  A. Anterior _____   B. Posterior _____   C. Inferior _____

V. <u>FUNCTION</u>: (4 = normal, 3 = mild compromise, 2 = difficulty, 1 = with aid, 0 = unable, NA = not available)

  A. Use back pocket . . . . _____   I. Sleep on affected side . . . . _____
  B. Perineal care . . . . _____   J. Pulling . . . . _____
  C. Wash opposite axilla . . . . _____   K. Use hand overhead . . . . _____
  D. Eat with utensil . . . . _____   L. Throwing . . . . _____
  E. Comb hair . . . . _____   M. Lifting . . . . _____
  F. Use hand with arm at shoulder level . _____   N. Do usual work . . . . _____
  G. Carry 10–15 lb with arm at side . . . . _____   O. Do usual sport . . . . _____
  H. Dress . . . . _____

* From Rowe CR: Evaluation of the shoulder. p. 633. In Rowe CR (ed): The Shoulder. Churchill Livingstone, New York, 1987. Courtesy of the American Shoulder and Elbow Surgeons.

Appendix 4
Shoulder Evaluation

Procedure	*Comments*
Inspection	
Masses or swelling	Check around acromioclavicular joint for swelling; humerus if direct contact trauma
Discoloration	Unusual, however, hemorrhage may produce discoloration especially with trauma
Deformity	Check acromioclavicular joint; indicates osteoarthritis or separation; pectoralis and deltoid contour for dislocation
Scars	Past trauma or "open" surgery; need to ask about arthroscopic surgery
Atrophy	Pay particular attention to the posterior muscles about the scapula
Palpation	
Masses	Include axilla check for lymph nodes
Tenderness	Some areas are tender on everyone; compare bilaterally
Anterior joint	Anterior deltoid, biceps, bursa, capsule, supraspinatus (anterolateral)
Medial (axilla)	Latissimus, teres major, subscapularis, serratus anterior, lymph nodes
Lateral joint	Teres minor/infraspinatus, middle deltoid, supraspinatus (The deltoid insertion point is a common referral site of pain/tenderness)
Posterior joint	Posterior deltoid, teres minor/infraspinatus, posterior capsule
Coracoid	Attachment for pectoralis minor, short head of biceps, coracoacromial ligament and there is a bursa
Acromion	On joint—osteoarthritis or sprain; close to joint might be shoulder pointer if direct trauma
Trigger points	If there is reference pain on palpation cross-reference with Travell charts
Other	Check scapula and surrounding muscles; rhomboids, levator scapulae, trapezius, etc.

Active range of motion

Make sure you check for scapulohumeral ratio with abduction and flexion; note any snapping or crepitus and specifically where; place a hand on the joint being careful not to impede motion

Flexion	Check ROM; if end-range pain possible impingement or acromioclavicular joint involvement (Inability to flex with a supinated arm may indicate a posterior dislocation)

Procedure	*Comments*
Extension	Be sure patient does not lean forward; perform standing
Abduction	Check for ROM, painful arc impingement
Horizontal abduction	Make sure patient does not rotate body; stabilize trunk
Horizontal adduction	Cross body movement; end-range pain may indicate acromioclavicular compression
Interior rotation	Performed with arm behind back; measure as highest vertebral level reached by fingers
Exterior rotation	Performed arm at side and 90 degrees (May indicate adhesive capsulitis if abduction restriction is also present with external restriction)

Passive range of motion

Make sure patient is relaxed. Check quality of end range and whether pain is present before or after this point. In addition to ROM check specific areas of interest in comments column.

Flexion	End-range pain may indicate impingement (same as Neer's test)
Extension	End-range pain may indicate biceps
Abduction	Possible painful arc (if non-contractile); end-range pain may indicate acromioclavicular joint
Horizontal abduction	Avoid body rotation; common position with throwing; pain may indicate instability
Horizontal adduction	End-range pain may indicate acromioclavicular joint
Internal rotation	Performed on supine patient at 90 degrees, abduction, elbow bent 90 degrees
External rotation	Performed with arm at side and 90 degrees abduction, elbow bend 90 degrees

Orthopaedic/neurologic evaluation

Note location of pain if test is "positive" correlate with patient's chief complaint area. Note that restricted ROM may prevent the use of many of the following orthopaedic tests.

Apley scratch	3 positions; hand to opposite shoulder, behind back, behind head
Painful arc	Pain between 70 to 110 degrees of abduction may indicate impingement
Hawkin-Kennedy's	Passive internal rotation at 90 degrees forward flexion, pain indicates impingement sign
Neer's	Same as passive flexion; end-range pain indicates impingement
Capsular sign	Same position as a supine apprehension test, however, looking for restriction
Stability test	There are many tests; at least perform a "drawer" test for anterior posterior, posterior anterior, and inferior laxity (Note: "sulcus sign" or depression below the acromioclavicular on inferior, testing indicates general laxity)

Procedure	*Comments*
Apprehension	Perform every 45 degrees of abduction; pain/apprehension with posterior anterior force = instability
Relocation test	Perform as a supine apprehension test with a anterior posterior force; relief confirms instability
Clunk test	Supine apprehension test with circumduction; "clunk" indicates glenoid labrum tear
Speed's	Resisted forward flexion at 90 degrees; pain may indicate biceps involvement
Yergason's	Resisted supination/flexion of the forearm for biceps involvement
Empty can test	Resisted abduction with internal rotation; arm at 30 degrees horizontal adduction for supraspinatus

For the neurological exam check dermatomes and always check the cervical region for referral; include thoracic out let syndrome testing.

Muscle Strength

Pectoralis	Patient supine, resisted horizontal adduction with arm flexed 90 degrees, arm internally rotated
Anterior deltoid	Resisted abduction with arm abducted 90 degrees with external rotation
Middle deltoid	Resisted abduction with arm abducted 90 degrees in neutral rotation
Posterior deltoid	Resisted abduction with arm abducted 90 degrees with internal rotation
Rhomboid	Hand behind back, patient pushes elbow back against resistance of examiner
Upper trapezius	Resisted shoulder elevation; ear to shoulder
Middle trapezius	Patient prone, horizontally abducts arm against resistance while at 90 degrees abduction
Lower trapezius	Same as middle, however, arm position is 120 degrees abduction
Supraspinatus	"Empty can" position of internal rotation, 90 degrees abduction, 30 degrees horizontal adduction
Infraspinatus/Teres minor	Resisted external rotation, arm at side and 90 degrees abduction, elbow flexed 90 degrees
Subscapularis	Resisted internal rotation, arm by side, elbow flexed 90 degrees
Latissimus dorsi	Arm by side, elbow straight, resisted adduction
Serratus anterior	Resisted forward flexion at 90 degrees while monitoring scapular stability

Index

Page numbers followed by f represent figures; those followed by t represent tables.

P